# HEAD AND NECK CANCER

## *Treatment, Rehabilitation, and Outcomes*

# HEAD AND NECK CANCER

## Treatment, Rehabilitation, and Outcomes

**Edited by**

**Elizabeth C. Ward, PhD**
**Corina J. van As-Brooks, PhD**

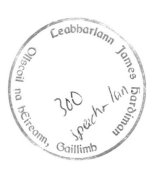

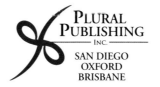

PLURAL
PUBLISHING
INC.

SAN DIEGO
OXFORD
BRISBANE

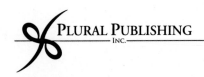

5521 Ruffin Road
San Diego, CA 92123

e-mail: info@pluralpublishing.com
Web site: http://www.pluralpublishing.com

49 Bath Street
Abingdon, Oxfordshire OX14 1EA
United Kingdom

Typeset in 10/13 Garamond Book by Flanagan's Publishing Services, Inc.
Printed in Hong Kong by Paramount Printing

ISBN-13: 978-1-59756-061-0
ISBN-10: 1-59756-061-8

**Library of Congress Cataloging-in-Publication Data:**

Ward, Elizabeth C., Dr.
  Head and neck cancer: treatment, rehabilitation, and outcomes / Elizabeth C. Ward, Corina J. van As-Brooks.
      p. ; cm.
  Includes bibliographical references and index.
  ISBN-13: 978-1-59756-061-0 (hardcover)
  ISBN-10: 1-59756-061-8 (hardcover)
  1.  Head—Cancer—Treatment. 2.  Neck—Cancer—Treatment. 3.  Deglutition disorders—Patients—Rehabilitation. 4.  Speech disorders—Patients—Rehabilitation.  I. As-Brooks, Corina J. Van.  II. Title.
  [DNLM: 1.  Head and Neck Neoplasms—therapy. 2.  Deglutition Disorders—rehabilitation. 3.  Larynx, Artificial. 4.  Speech Disorders—rehabilitation. 5.  Speech, Alaryngeal. 6.  Treatment Outcome.  WE 707 W257h 2006]
  RC280.H4H432 2006
  616.99'491—dc22
                                        2006023213

# CONTENTS

# PREFACE

In the past decade there have been numerous advancements in our understanding of head and neck cancer and its management. Recent years have seen an expansion of knowledge of cancer cell biology, new approaches and techniques introduced for cancer control, novel pharmaceutical products under investigation for minimizing the impact of treatment, an expansion of commercial products available to help meet the individual needs of patients, and increased importance placed on understanding the functional impact of various treatment approaches. The multidisciplinary team approach is now firmly recognized as optimal, and speech-language pathology practice has expanded, extending beyond the management of speech and swallowing to embrace the active rehabilitation of pulmonary function, olfaction, and taste. Throughout this textbook it is clear that the pursuit of optimal patient outcomes remains the firm goal of all multidisciplinary team members, and with the growing critical mass of researchers, medical staff, and clinicians dedicated to improving survival and post-treatment quality of life for patients with head and neck cancer, we are confident improvements will continue to be made into the next decade and beyond.

# ACKNOWLEDGMENTS

We would like to begin by acknowledging all of our contributing authors. Their extensive personal experience with patients, their families/caregivers, and other multidisciplinary team members has enabled them to provide the reader with research evidence and invaluable clinical insights into the current management techniques and support services for patients with head and cancer. We began this project with the intent to capture and represent international practices, and our contributing authors have embraced this in their chapters.

We are particularly indebted to those patients and their families who allowed videos and photographs of their personal experiences and believe the book is richer for these personal insights and demonstrations. We would like to thank them all for their openness and candor. To all the clinicians who assisted us in the filming and location of video footage, we also owe you our thanks.

We also wish to acknowledge the illustrations of Chris Edghill who brought many of the concepts here in the text to life with his illustrations. In addition, thanks are extended to those commercial companies and publishing houses who provided permission for their property to be reproduced within this text. We also wish to acknowledge the skills of James Kemp, who designed and created the CD that supports the current text. We hope the readers find that these audiovisual materials enhance their personal learning experience. Many of the images and video segments will be useful for patient education, and we hope that clinicians find these of assistance when counseling, educating, and preparing their patients for the challenges that lie ahead.

Finally, though most importantly, we would like to thank our husbands and families for their considerable support throughout this project. They have remained patient while family time has been sacrificed to allow us both to meet our author and editorial duties associated with this textbook. We thank them for their love, support, tolerance, and understanding.

# ABOUT THE EDITORS

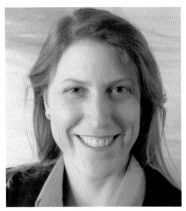

**Elizabeth C. Ward**

Dr. Ward, BSpThy, Grad Cert Ed, PhD, is a senior lecturer in the Division of Speech Pathology at the University of Queensland. Since receiving her PhD in 1995 from the University of Queensland, she has published numerous peer reviewed articles and book chapters in the areas of motor speech disorders, dysphagia assessment and rehabilitation, and the oncology population. Dr. Ward has a specific interest in the patient population with head and neck cancer and has a number of local, statewide, and national research projects running in collaboration with clinicians and laryngectomy support groups in Australia. The focus of her research in this area has been on improving speech and swallowing outcomes for patients following laryngectomy.

Dr. van As-Brooks, PhD, received her Bachelor's Degree in Speech Pathology from the College of Advanced Education in Rotterdam, the Netherlands and her Master's Degree in Phonetic Sciences from the University of Amsterdam, the Netherlands. In 2001 she obtained her PhD at the University of Amsterdam with a PhD thesis entitled "Tracheoesophageal Speech: A Multidimensional Assessment of Voice Quality."

She has been employed at the Netherlands Cancer Institute—Antoni van Leeuwenhoek Hospital since 1995 as a speech pathologist and researcher and has specialized in rehabilitation and research of voice and swallowing in head and neck cancer patients and rehabilitation of olfaction in laryngectomized patients. She has published widely in the area of laryngectomee rehabilitation and has lectured on this topic at numerous international meetings and workshops.

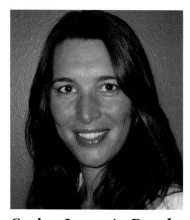

**Corina J. van As-Brooks**

Dr. van As-Brooks is currently employed as researcher and supervisor on various running research projects in the head and neck rehabilitation area at the Netherlands Cancer Institute—Antoni van Leeuwenhoek Hospital. She is a guest researcher at the Institute of Phonetic Sciences (Amsterdam Center for Language and Communication, the Netherlands) and since 2003 is also employed as clinical research manager of clinical trials on various new and existing products with Atos Medical AB (Hörby, Sweden).

# CONTRIBUTORS

**Annemieke H. Ackerstaff, PhD**
Research Psychologist
Department of Head and Neck Oncology and Surgery
Netherlands Cancer Institute—Antoni van
  Leeuwenhoek Hospital,
Amsterdam, the Netherlands

**Lynn M. Acton, MSc**
Speech-Language Pathologist
Yale-New Haven Hospital
New Haven, Connecticut, USA

**Alfons J. M. Balm, MD, PhD**
Otolaryngologist-Head and Neck Surgeon
Chairman of the Multidisciplinary Head and Neck
  Unit NKI/AVL-AMC
Department of Head and Neck Oncology and Surgery
Netherlands Cancer Institute—Antoni van
  Leeuwenhoek Hospital,
Amsterdam, The Netherlands
and Professor, Academic Medical Center
Amsterdam, The Netherlands

**Corina J. van As-Brooks, PhD**
Speech-Language Pathologist, Phonetic Scientist
Department of Head and Neck Surgical Oncology
Netherlands Cancer Institute—Antoni van
  Leeuwenhoek Hospital,
Amsterdam, The Netherlands
and Clinical Research Manager
Research and Development Department
Atos Medical AB, Hörby, Sweden

**Robyn A. Burnett, BAppSc (SpPath)**
Senior Speech Pathologist
Royal Adelaide Hospital,
Adelaide, Victoria, Australia

**William B. Coman, MBBS, FRCS (Edinburgh),
FRCS (England), FACS (United States),
FRACS (Australia) AM**
ENT Consultant,
Chair, Head and Neck Cancer Clinic,
Princess Alexandra Hospital,
Brisbane, Queensland, Australia

**Caterina A. Finizia, MD, PhD**
Otolaryngologist-Head and Neck Surgeon
Associate Professor,
Sahlgenska University Hospital,
Goteborg, Sweden

**Dennis P. Fuller, PhD**
Speech-Language Pathologist,
Associate Professor
Department of Communication Sciences and
  Disorders and Otolaryngology
St. Louis University,
St. Louis, USA

**Alexander D. Guminski, BSc (Med), MBBS,
FRACP, PhD**
Staff Specialist, Medical Oncology
Practitioner Fellow, Center for Immunology and
  Cancer Research
Princess Alexandra Hospital,
Brisbane, Queensland, Australia

**Kelli L. Hancock, BSpThy**
Senior Speech Pathologist
Princess Alexandra Hospital,
Brisbane, Queensland, Australia

**Frans J. M. Hilgers, MD PhD**
Otolaryngologist-Head and Neck Surgeon
Chairman of the Department of Head and Neck
  Oncology and Surgery
Netherlands Cancer Institute—Antoni van
  Leeuwenhoek Hospital,
Amsterdam, The Netherlands
and Professor, Institute of Phonetic Sciences
Amsterdam Center for Language and Communication
University of Amsterdam,
Amsterdam, The Netherlands
and Academic Medical Center
University of Amsterdam,
Amsterdam, the Netherlands

**Lyndell E. Kelly, MBBS, FRANZCR, PhD**
Radiation Oncologist
Oncology Department,
Dunedin Hospital,
Dunedin, New Zealand

**Sophie M. Kerle, BSpPath (Hons)**
Speech Pathologist
Division of Speech Pathology
The University of Queensland,
Brisbane, Australia

**Cathy L. Lazarus, PhD BRS-S**
Associate Professor, NYU Voice Center,
Department of Otolaryngology
NYU School of Medicine
New York, New York, USA
and Director of Hearing and Speech
Bellevue Hospital Center
New York, New York, USA

**C. René Leemans, MD PhD**
Head and Neck Surgeon
Professor and Chair
Department of Otolaryngology—Head and Neck
   Surgery
VU University Medical Center,
Amsterdam, The Netherlands

**Nadine R. Manison, BAppSc (SpPath)**
Senior Speech Pathologist
Royal Melbourne Hospital
Melbourne, Victoria, Australia

**Ann-Louise Morton, BSpPath (Hons)**
Senior Speech Pathologist
Royal Brisbane & Women's Hospital
Brisbane, Queensland, Australia

**Kylie A. Perkins, BSpThy**
Speech Pathologist—Private Practitioner,
Brisbane, Queensland, Australia

**I. Susan Reeves, MEd, CCC/SLP**
Senior Clinical Director
West Texas Rehabilitation Center
3001 S. Jackson
San Angelo, Texas, USA

**Rico N. P. M. Rinkel, MD**
Otolaryngologist/Speech Pathologist
Department of Otolaryngology—Head and Neck
   Surgery
VU University Medical Center,
Amsterdam, The Netherlands

**Nicholas A. Saunders, BSc (Hons) PhD**
Principal Research Fellow
Epithelial Pathobiology Group
Cancer Biology Programme
Center for Immunology and Cancer Research
The University of Queensland
Princess Alexandra Hospital,
Brisbane, Queensland, Australia

**Jeff P. Searl, PhD**
Associate Professor
The University of Kansas Medical Center
Hearing and Speech Department,
Kansas City, Kansas, USA
and Associate Professor
The University of Kansas Medical Center
Department of Otolaryngology: Head and Neck
   Surgery
Kansas City, Kansas, USA

**Ludwig E. Smeele, MD DMD PhD**
Head and Neck Surgeon
Department of Head and Neck Oncology and
   Surgery
Netherlands Cancer Institute—Antoni van
   Leeuwenhoek Hospital,
Amsterdam, The Netherlands

**Julie A. G. Stierwalt, PhD**
Assistant Professor
Department of Communication Disorders
Florida State University,
Tallahassee, Florida, USA

**Irma M. Verdonck-de Leeuw, PhD**
Psychologist, Speech Pathologist, Phonetic Scientist
Department of Otolaryngology—Head and Neck
   Surgery
VU University Medical Center,
Amsterdam, The Netherlands

**Elizabeth C. Ward, BSpThy (Hons), Grad.Cert.Ed, PhD**
Senior Lecturer, Division of Speech Pathology
School of Health and Rehabilitation Sciences
The University of Queensland
Brisbane, Queensland, Australia

**Kimberly R. Wilson, MS**
Doctoral Student
Department of Communication Disorders
Florida State University,
Tallahassee, Florida, USA

**Edwin M. Yiu, PhD**
Associate Dean, Faculty of Education
Division Head, Division of Speech and Hearing Sciences
University of Hong Kong,
Hong Kong, China

**J. Karel Zuur, MD**
Research Physician-ENT Resident
Department of Head and Neck Oncology and Surgery
Netherlands Cancer Institute—Antoni van
    Leeuwenhoek Hospital,
Amsterdam, The Netherlands

# Chapter 1

# CANCER OF THE HEAD AND NECK

Nicholas A. Saunders, William B. Coman, and
Alexander D. Guminski

## CHAPTER OUTLINE

# Introduction

Malignancy causes approximately one quarter of all deaths in Western countries. Although improvements in the treatment of many cancers have occurred, resulting in lower death rates or improved survival, the increasing proportion of older people in Western countries, along with adverse lifestyle changes such as increasing obesity, is likely to result in greater absolute numbers of cancer patients. Head and neck cancer is around the eighth most common cancer in Western countries and is more frequent in men. The most common form of such cancer is associated with smoking and alcohol consumption. In developing countries, head and neck cancers are more common than in the West. As developing countries become wealthier, mortality is reduced from other causes (especially infection), increasing the relative contribution from cancer. At the same time Western lifestyles are more commonly adopted and unfortunately are likely to contribute to rising cancer incidence. Head and neck cancer contributes significantly to the global cancer burden, currently ranked the sixth most common type overall, at approximately 640,000 cases per year (IARC-WHO GLOBOCAN Database, 2002).

Cancers of the head and neck are mostly squamous cell carcinomas (H&NSCC) arising from the mucosa, or lining, of the upper aerodigestive tract. Such tumors have frequent spread to local lymph nodes, but may be cured even at this stage by aggressive localized therapy. Some particular variants with specific features are recognized, such as nasopharyngeal carcinoma. A variety of other less common and rare tumors with diverse histology and origin (such as glandular, neurological, and structural elements) are seen, such as adenocarcinomas from salivary glands, carcinoids, sarcomas, and paragangliomas from the autonomic plexus of the carotid body. The sites of origin and main histological subtypes of head and neck tumors are shown in Table 1-1.

**Table 1-1.** Sites of Origin and Main Histological Sites of Head and Neck Cancer

| Site | Tumor Histology | Notable Features |
|---|---|---|
| Lip | SCC | |
| Tongue | SCC | |
| Oral cavity<br>Buccal mucosa<br>Alveolar ridges<br>Anterior tongue<br>Floor of mouth<br>Hard palate | SCC | |
| Oropharynx<br>Posterior/base of tongue<br>Vallecula<br>Tonsil<br>Soft palate | SCC | Most common forms of head and neck cancer overall |
| Hypopharynx<br>Piriform fossa<br>Postcricoid<br>Postpharyngeal wall | SCC | |
| Larynx<br>Supraglottic<br>Glottic<br>Subglottic<br>Transglottic | SCC | |

**Table 1–1.** *continued*

| Site | Tumor Histology | Notable Features |
|------|----------------|------------------|
| Parotid gland | Benign—pleomorphic adenoma, Warthin's tumor; malignant—mucoepidermoid carcinoma, adenoid cystic carcinoma, adenocarcinoma | Most common site of salivary gland tumor |
| Intraparotid lymph nodes | SCC | Often from previously excised skin primaries |
| Skin | SCC, basal cell carcinoma, melanoma | |
| Nasopharynx | SCC, varies from well differentiated to undifferentiated | Strongly associated with Epstein-Barr virus infection. Tumors spread early to lymph nodes, often bilaterally. |
| Thyroid | Papillary, Follicular, Medullary and Anaplastic | Papillary carcinomas have good prognosis and mostly occur in young adults, anaplastic carcinomas very poor prognosis. Medullary carcinomas may be part of a familial multiple endocrine neoplasia syndrome (MFN) |
| Nasal sinus | | Rare |
| Olfactory neurons | Esthiosoneuroblastoma | Rare |
| Carotid body | Paraganglioma | Two distinct tumors arising from cells of neural crest origin in the carotid body or from vagal nerve ganglia (glomus vagale; less common). Histologically resemble adrenal medulla phaechromocytomas but only rarely secrete catecholamines. May be familial |
| Minor salivary glands | Adenomas, adenocarcinomas | |
| Nerve sheaths | Neurofibroma, nerofibrosarcoma, schwannoma | Associated with familial neurofibromatosis |
| Any mesenchymal tissue | Sarcomas | Different subtypes—many best treated by surgery or radiotherapy and some (e.g., Ewing's sarcoma, rhabdomyosarcoma) benefit from chemotherapy. Includes vascular sarcomas such as angiosarcoma and Kaposi's sarcoma |
| Any | Neuroendocrine tumors | Spread early via the bloodstream, sensitive to chemotherapy but frequently recur |
| Any lymphatic tissue | Lymphoma | Usually treated with chemotherapy |
| Supraclavicular Lymph node (especially left side) | Metastatic carcinoma | Particularly from breast or stomach primaries |
| Bone | Benign tumors Malignant tumors | Similar to bone tumors arising at other sites |
| Dental tissue | Ameloblastoma | Most frequently arise in the molar region of the mandible, producing a locally aggressive and destructive lesion |

Note. SCC = Squamous cell carcinoma

Squamous cell carcinomas may arise from many different sites. The pattern and likelihood of spread, optimal treatment, and prognosis can differ according to the specific site from which the SCC has arisen. Management of head and neck cancers needs to accommodate the anatomical proximity and physiological requirements of structures vital to speech, swallowing, prevention of aspiration, sensory organs of smell, hearing, and vision, vascular supply to the brain, and critical neurological structures of the brainstem and facial nerves. The social and psychological impact of facial disfigurement and impaired communication can be invidious consequences of treatment. In this chapter we will discuss the biology underlying squamous cell carcinomas, the epidemiology of head and neck cancer both in developed and developing countries, and the approach to clinical management of the common forms of head and neck cancer.

## Introduction to Cancer Biology

Cancers occur when normal cells within the body accumulate a series of genetic and/or epigenetic lesions that disrupt key cell and tissue functions. The term genetic in this context refers to damage caused directly to the DNA sequence within chromosomes, and may be via mutations, translocations, deletions, or amplification, which ultimately lead to a corruption of the gene-based programming of cellular function. The term epigenetic refers to alterations to cells that may not directly affect the DNA sequence but may alter the regulation of gene expression, via DNA methylation or through the infection of the cell by transforming viruses such as the human papillomaviruses. Due to the nature of the genetic and epigenetic changes that occur in cancer cells, the progeny of the cancer cell inherits the defects in cell regulation. For this reason it is thought that the process of changing a normal cell into a cancer cell can only occur in dividing cells. In addition, it is apparent that the process of transforming a normal cell into a cancer cell requires more than one defect and in most instances requires a series of damaging events that accumulate within the replicating cell and ultimately lead to sufficient alterations in cellular regulation to manifest as neoplastic disease.

## The Biological Basis of Cancer Formation

Cancers are derived from normal cells that have received a number of sequential alterations to critical cellular functions. These alterations contribute to the defective behavior of the cells and ultimately lead to the development of tumors in situ. Since tumors arise from multiple lesional events, it is unlikely that all these defects occur simultaneously. Indeed, all the evidence suggests that tumors arise from an ordered progression, starting with normal cells passing through a precancerous phase in which cells display minimal levels of disrupted differentiation (i.e., dysplasia), through to cancers which display a transformed phenotype but may not show pathological signs of invasiveness or spread (see Figure 1–1). These benign cancers may then progress through to invasive cancers which have breached the normal tissue boundaries (such as the basement membrane in the case of epithelial tumors) and finally, these invasive tumors may progress through to metastatic disease, in which the cancer cells have spread to other tissues (e.g., lymph nodes) and organs in the body. It is now generally accepted that in order for a normal cell to become cancerous and exhibit metastatic behavior, a number of critical cellular functions must be disrupted, being namely (a) growth regulation, (b) apoptosis (programmed cell death), (c) differentiation, (d) replicative senescence, (e) angiogenesis, (f) DNA repair, (g) tissue remodeling and migration, and (h) immune evasion (Hanahan & Weinberg, 2000; Serewko et al., 2002).

### Growth Regulation

Growth regulation refers to the control of cell division. One of the hallmarks of cancer is that cancer cells are characterized by deregulated proliferation. This occurs in a number of ways. For instance, in normal cells certain cytokines (secreted proteins that activate cell surface receptors) and stimuli are able to stimulate cell division by activating signal transduction within the cells, leading to the initiation of a round of cell division or passage through the cell cycle. In contrast, many cancer cells exhibit semiautonomous growth in so far as they are being stimulated to replicate in the absence of normal stimuli. This constitutive activation of growth stimulatory pathways in cancer cells may come about

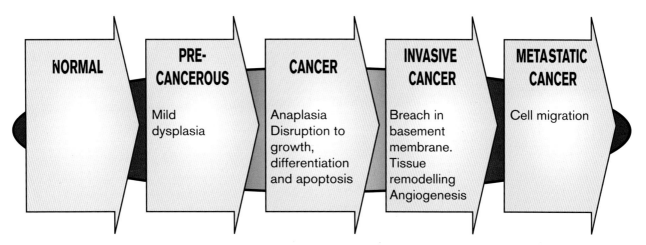

**Figure 1–1.** Simplified scheme of the progression from normal to metastatic disease.

through disruptions to the normal regulation of molecules involved in the regulation of proliferation. A prototypic example of this would be the mutation or amplification of the epidermal growth factor (EGF) receptor in a number of human cancers. EGF is a secreted cytokine that binds to receptors on the plasma membrane of cells and can activate a signal transduction pathway that results in the initiation of cell division. In many human cancers, such as head and neck cancers, the EGF receptor is either mutated or overexpressed (Ishitoya et al., 1989). Mutations in EGF receptor frequently result in changes that maintain the receptor in a constitutively active state. Alternatively, overexpression of the EGF receptor can lead to overactivity of this growth-promoting pathway, resulting in deregulated proliferative signaling in these cells.

Another mechanism by which growth can be deregulated in cancers is through the loss of growth inhibitory signaling pathways. A classic example of this would be the loss of TGFβ1 signaling in cancer cells (Dahler et al., 2001; Smith et al., 2004). Transforming growth factor-β1 (TGFβ1) is a secreted cytokine that can bind to receptors on the plasma membranes of most epithelial cells and activate a signal transduction pathway that can inhibit proliferation in cells. Many cancers, including head and neck cancers, have sustained defects in this pathway either through aberrant receptor expression or loss of the signaling proteins (SMADs) that mediate TGFβ1-mediated growth inhibition.

## Apoptosis

Apoptosis refers to a process of programmed cell death. Apoptosis is a normal process by which cells may be removed from the body. This removal is required to make way for younger maturing cells, as occurs on the external surface of the tongue. This process also occurs following DNA damage to the cells. For example, if cells were to be exposed to high concentrations of carcinogenic stimuli such as radiation or toxins, it can initiate apoptosis. This response is essential, since it protects the tissue from replicating DNA that is damaged. As with growth regulation, apoptosis is a complex process with many regulators some of which are pro-apoptotic (e.g., caspases) and some of which are anti-apoptotic (e.g., Bcl-2). Hence, the rate of apoptosis is dictated by the ratio of pro-apoptotic to anti-apoptotic signals. In normal circumstances, cancer cells that have a heavy burden of mutated and damaged DNA would be expected to be removed via apoptosis. However, evidence shows that a prerequisite for many cancers is that they have *disruptions* in the regulators of apoptosis, such that the ability of cells to undergo apoptosis has been deregulated (Hanahan & Weinberg, 2000). Thus, it is not uncommon to find that cancer cells overexpress anti-apoptotic genes such as Bcl-2 and/or are deficient in pro-apoptotic genes such as caspases.

## Differentiation

Differentiation refers to the process by which a cell changes to take on specific functions related to its stage of maturity. For instance, the stratified epithelial lining of the upper aerodigestive tract is comprised of cells that sit on a basement membrane. These cells have a basal cell phenotype and are capable of proliferation. Their primary function is to replace the older keratinocytes (epidermal cells that make keratin and which form the bulk of skin) as they are shed from the external surface of the epithelium (see Part A in Figure 1–2). When the basal cells have replicated they then pass into the next layer of the epithelium towards the external surface. As they do so they stop proliferating. This is an irreversible process. The cells then start to express genes that are important for the maintenance of the barrier function. This process is referred to as terminal differentiation since, once started, the process is irreversible and ultimately leads to apoptosis.

This process of terminal differentiation is a complex process since it involves both the loss of proliferative capacity and the gain of barrier functions. If a normal cell were to become transformed through exposure to carcinogens, yet retained the ability to terminally differentiate, then the transformed cell would simply eventually be shed from the epithelium without giving rise to cancer progeny. However, it is well documented that terminal differentiation is disrupted in head and neck cancer formation, and frequently there is an uncoupling between the regulation of growth and subsequent differentiation (Wong et al., 2003; 2005). Hence, it is common to have tumor cells that are proliferative and display aberrant control of differentiation. In this case, a normal cell transformed through exposure to carcinogens, and lacking the ability to terminally differentiate, then can give rise to cancer progeny. These disruptions to the appropriate control of proliferation and differentiation are complex and are only now being unraveled.

## Replicative Senescence

Replicative senescence is a term that refers to the irreversible loss of growth potential that all cells (except stem cells) undergo after a finite number of cell divisions (35–70 in tissue culture studies). Why cells senesce is currently debated. It may be a response to a growing accumulation of genetic damage over a large number of replication cycles that ultimately result in a cell's decision to not replicate any further. It may also be an inbuilt defense against cancer development, since it would stop cells with genetic damage from multiplying further. Whatever the reason for the evolution of senescence there is compelling evidence indicating that it is a genetically programmed event and that cells are "hardwired" to undergo a finite number of replications. This program is thought to involve a process by which cells sequentially lose a small portion of the ends of their chromosomes (telomeres) every time they divide. Once these telomeres get too short they then tell the cell that it can no longer divide or it will risk losing some of the genetic information at the end of the chromosomes. This process of telomere shortening does not appear to occur in cancers and stem cells due to the presence of an enzyme called telomerase, which adds the fragments back to the tips of the chromosomes thus maintaining a constant chromosome length. This allows for infinite replications to take place without eroding the genetic code on the ends of the chromosomes and hence allows for the immortalization of cancer cells (Hanahan & Weinberg, 2000).

## Angiogenesis

Angiogenesis refers to the process of vascularization. The process of vascularization is an essential step in allowing growth of new tissue. The best examples of this are in the developing embryo and in wound healing where there is a rapid growth of new tissue, which requires a blood supply to bring nutrients and remove metabolic byproducts. In normal tissues that are not subject to stresses or growth (such as most adult tissues) there is little requirement for the production of new vasculature and hence the genes and cytokines involved in this are kept in a state of stasis. This state of stasis is based on the sum of the actions of pro-angiogenic factors (e.g., vascular endothelial growth factors) and anti-angiogenic factors (e.g., thrombospondins). In the normal tissue, the ratio of pro-angiogenic to anti-angiogenic factors would favor the anti-angiogenic program. Evidence is now accumulating that during the process of carcinogenesis there is a selective disruption of this process such that pro-angiogenic signals predominate (Hanahan & Weinberg, 2000). This disruption is an essential part of solid tumor formation

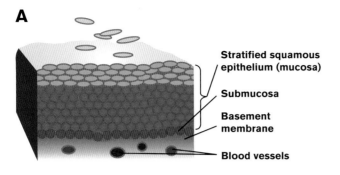

## NORMAL:
Schematic representation of the mucosal and submucosal layers of the upper aerodigestive tract

Stratified squamous epithelium (mucosa)

Submucosa

Basement membrane

Blood vessels

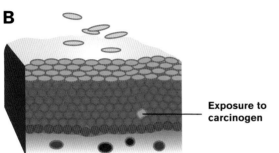

## INITIATION:
Schematic representation of how a carcinogen can induce a heritable alteration in a cell in the basal layer of the mucosal epithelium

Exposure to carcinogen

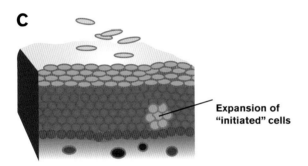

## PROMOTION:
The "initiated" cells (pale blue) can undergo expansion, either due to natural or deregulated proliferation or in response to specific mitogenic stimuli. This expanded pool of "initiated" precancerous cells increases the number of cells that could be further altered in response to another carcinogenic stimulus or via inherent genomic instability

Expansion of "initiated" cells

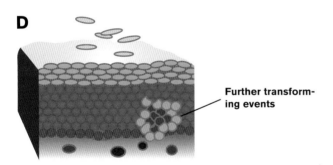

## PROGRESSION:
The expanded population of "initiated" precancerous cells (pale blue) is further transformed following exposure to another carcinogenic stimulus or due to genomic instability. This gives rise to a fully transformed cancer cell (dark blue)

Further transforming events

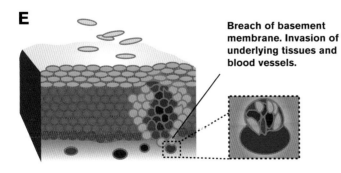

Breach of basement membrane. Invasion of underlying tissues and blood vessels.

## METASTASIS:
In the later stages of cancer development, the fully transformed cancer cells can breach the integrity of the underlying basement membrane and invade the underlying submucosal structures. Cancer cells will often enter the blood or lymphatic vessels and pass to other sites in the body to establish metastatic foci

**Figure 1–2.** Schematic representation of the stages from **B.** initiation to **E.** metastasis.

since in the absence of new vasculature within the developing tumor, the tumor mass would not be able to increase in size (see Figure 1–3). It is interesting to note that in recent years, inhibitors of tumor vascularization have been developed that have shown some promise as anticancer agents.

### DNA Repair

DNA repair is an important process by which a cell is able to monitor the integrity of its DNA or monitor the fidelity of DNA replication. This process is essential if cells are to avoid passing incorrect genetic information to their progeny. To achieve this cells have acquired complex regulatory mechanisms that allow them to monitor the DNA for damage and to repair any identified damage. Sensors of DNA damage include proteins such as the tumor suppressor gene, p53, or ATM gene. There are a large number of enzymes and factors involved in DNA repair. In general these enzymes/factors play a role in correcting errors introduced during replication. In addition, another series of enzymes/factors may be involved in the repair of DNA damage that occurs outside of replication.

Mutation of the p53 gene is one of the most important alterations that occur in cancer cells (Hanahan & Weinberg, 2000). It is estimated that approximately 50% of all human tissues have acquired defects in the activity of p53. The gene p53 is a transcriptional regulator that responds to DNA damage. In response to DNA damage (e.g., γ-irradiation or UV-irradiation), p53 can increase the expression of a factor called p21 which in turn prevents cells from undergoing cell division. This halt in cell division lasts until the DNA can be repaired and cell division is then resumed. Alternatively, if the damage to the DNA is perceived as too great, then p53 can initiate apoptosis of the cell. In this way, p53 ensures that the integrity of the DNA is maintained throughout cell division. For this reason, p53 is sometimes referred to as the "guardian of the genome." Given the central importance of p53 in normal cellular function, it is not surprising that in order for tumors to arise, defects in p53 control are frequently observed. Defects in p53 function are most frequently seen as a loss of function mutations. Such mutations are observed in head and neck cancers. Also noteworthy, is the observation that infection of the upper aerodigestive tract with oncogenic forms of the human papillomavirus (HPV) may also be associated with functional ablation of the p53 gene that is mediated via an interaction with the viral E6 protein. In particular, there is mounting evidence for HPV infection being involved in laryngeal carcinoma.

### Tissue Remodeling and Migration

In normal tissues, the borders of the tissue are bounded by strict anatomical boundaries, defined by structures such as the basement membrane. In order to metastasize, cancer cells must have the ability to disrupt their intercellular adhesions, digest or pass through the underlying basement membrane, traverse the underlying interstitium and gain access to either lymphatic vessels or blood vessels, and to then pass to other sites in the body and reestablish themselves as secondary cancers or metastatic foci (see Part E in Figure 1–2). The highly ordered structure that is char-

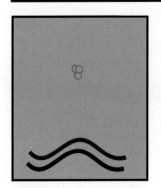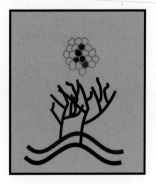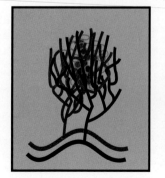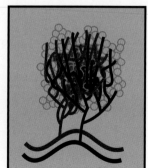

**Figure 1–3.** Schematic representation of the process of angiogenesis.

acteristic of all normal tissues is maintained via a process in which enzymes and factors involved in tissue remodeling or cell motility are inactive. Notable exceptions to this would be embryonic development, wound healing, and the cell motility characteristic of immunocytes. Thus, progression of cancer cells to invasive or metastatic disease requires that the cellular adhesion molecules such as integrins and cadherins are lost or suffer loss of function mutations, allowing cells to leave their original site. The digestion of extra cellular matrices and the basement membrane is normally associated with the activation of any one of a large family of proteases while the activation of motility is also associated with loss of cadherin function. It should be noted that the process of invasion and metastasis are complex and poorly understood processes that are under active study.

## Immune Evasion

The immune system plays an important role in monitoring tissues for evidence of cancer. The contribution of this surveillance differs between tissue sites. For example, there is a correlation between immune status and the occurrence of tumors in the skin and cervix. The most compelling evidence supporting this comes from the observation that patients who are immunosuppressed (e.g., renal transplant patients on immunosuppressive therapy) are predisposed to skin and cervical cancers (Westburg & Stone, 1973). The reason for this site selective role for the immune system in preventing tumors is complex and not well understood. Despite this, these observations indicate that in order for any mutation or transforming event to manifest as a tumor, they may also have to be able to evade the immune system in some way. Again, the basis for this evasion is still poorly understood.

## Causative Events in Head and Neck Cancer Formation

There are a number of known insults that can contribute to the development of cancers. For example, there is clear evidence that certain toxins can initiate cancers. The most widely known of these would be the toxins found in tobacco smoke or the exhaust from the older-style diesel engines. However, it is also estab-

lished that diet can contribute to a significant fraction of human malignancies although the specific causative agent(s) have not been identified yet. Other common causative agents are excessive UV or gamma irradiation and infection by tumor viruses (e.g., HPV or Epstein-Barr virus) or through agents or stresses that stimulate reactive oxygen species (e.g., so-called free radicals).

Of these factors the agents most relevant to head and neck cancer formation are tobacco smoke, alcohol consumption, Epstein-Barr virus (EBV), and HPV. Tobacco smoke is known to contain over 1000 different chemicals, many of which have been shown in in vitro tests to be carcinogens and mutagens. The link between alcohol consumption and head and neck cancer is less clear but is thought to be associated with the generation of aldehydes during alcohol metabolism. Aldehydes are relatively reactive molecules that can cause macromolecular damage. Viruses such as EBV are most frequently associated with the formation of nasopharyngeal carcinomas, while HPV is associated with laryngeal carcinoma and perhaps other types.

The types of damage done to the cells by these types of agents can be either epigenetic, genetic, or both. The genetic damage can be of several types and includes such things as translocations, mutations, deletions, and amplifications. Translocations occur when pieces of chromosomes can be moved to other chromosomal sites. This commonly occurs in Burkitt's lymphoma or acute promyelocytic leukemia. Mutations can occur as a result of irradiation or chemical mutagenesis and results in alterations in the coding sequence for genes. A common example of this is the mutations that occur in response to UV exposure. These mutations can alter the sequence and function of specific genes such as p53. Deletions may occur when pieces of genes are lost from the chromosomes. Such deletions occur to the tumor suppressor genes p16 in melanoma and pRB in retinoblastoma. Amplifications occur when the number of copies of a gene is increased in the genome. An example of this is cyclin D1 amplification in head and neck cancers.

The epigenetic damage can occur for a variety of reasons and serves to alter cellular function and may contribute to genomic instability and/or predispose the cell to subsequent genetic damage. An example of this phenomenon would be the infection of cells with the HPV. Postinfection, the viral DNA can exist episomally or be integrated into the host genome. The viral DNA then directs the expression of specific viral genes such as E6 and E7. The viral gene E6 binds p53 while E7 binds Rb. In both instances, this leads to a loss of function of p53 or Rb and can contribute to carcinogenesis.

The above examples show how endogenous and exogenous conditions/agents can lead to alterations in the genetic or epigenetic control of normal cellular function. If these alterations affect critical cellular regulators then they may contribute to the heritable alteration in normal cells that contributes to tumor formation.

# Epidemiology of Head and Neck Cancer

## Incidence Rates

The incidence of head and neck cancers shows considerable geographic, socioeconomic, and gender variation (see Tables 1–2, 1–3, and 1–4). Most tumor types show increasing incidence with age peaking in the 6th and 7th decade. The global incidence of head and neck cancer is approximately 640,000 cases per year, with mortality of over 300,000 (IACR-WHO, 2002).

In developed countries such as Australia, the incidence of head and neck SCC in men is falling from a peak in the 1980s, presumably due to a reduction in smoking rates. In women, the rates are lower but stable. Despite the fall in incidence rates, the absolute number of annual cases is projected to increase by almost 30% by 2011 due to anticipated changes in the age structure of the community. Squamous cell carcinomas are likely to remain the most common form of head and neck cancer. A representative distribution of the sites of origin of squamous cell carcinomas in a Western population (United Kingdom) is shown in Table 1–5. The global incidence of cancer overall is anticipated to rise substantially, from 10.9 million new cases per year to approximately 16 million new cases per year over the next 15 years, in the absence of specific interventions (World Health Organization, 2005).

**Table 1–2.** Highest, Lowest, and Selected Western Country Reported Incidences of Oral Cavity Cancer Worldwide

|  | Males | | Females | |
|---|---|---|---|---|
|  | **Country** | **ASR** | **Country** | **ASR** |
| Highest incidence | Papua New Guinea | 40.9 | Solomon Islands | 21.2 |
|  | Sri Lanka | 24.5 | Bangladesh | 16.8 |
|  | Botswana | 23.1 | Papua New Guinea | 16.3 |
|  | Puerto Rico | 20.6 | Pakistan | 14.7 |
|  | Hungary | 19.1 | Botswana | 9.5 |
| Western countries | France | 14.8 | Australia | 4.7 |
|  | Australia | 11.1 | United States | 3.4 |
|  | United States | 7.9 | New Zealand | 3.3 |
|  | Canada | 6.9 | Canada | 2.9 |
|  | New Zealand | 5.6 | United Kingdom | 2.7 |
|  | United Kingdom | 5.0 | France | 2.7 |
| Lowest incidence | El Salvador | 0.4 | Egypt | 0.2 |
|  | Egypt | 0.7 | El Salvador | 0.2 |
|  | Gambia | 1.0 | Nicaragua | 0.3 |
|  | Mali | 1.1 | Zambia | 0.4 |
|  | Congo Brazzaville | 1.7 | China | 0.7 |

Note. ASR = annual age standardized incidence rate per 100,000 population. (From Globocan 2002 database accessed at www.dep-iacr.fr.)

**Table 1-3.** Highest, Lowest, and Selected Western Country Reported Incidence of Nasopharyngeal Cancer Worldwide

|  | Males | | Females | |
|---|---|---|---|---|
|  | Country | ASR | Country | ASR |
| Highest five incidence | Brunei | 17.2 | Brunei | 7.3 |
|  | Singapore | 14.6 | Singapore | 5.1 |
|  | Malaysia | 11.4 | Malaysia | 4.2 |
|  | Guam | 7.1 | Vietnam | 2.7 |
|  | China | 3.9 | Guam | 2.5 |
| Western incidence | France | 1.2 | Canada | 0.3 |
|  | Canada | 0.9 | New Zealand | 0.3 |
|  | Australia | 0.8 | Australia | 0.3 |
|  | United States | 0.6 | United Kingdom | 0.2 |
|  | New Zealand | 0.6 | United States | 0.2 |
|  | United Kingdom | 0.4 | France | 0.2 |
| Lowest five incidence | Ecuador | 0.1 | Zambia | 0.1 |
|  | Chile | 0.1 | Liberia | 0.1 |
|  | Malawi | 0.1 | Argentina | 0.1 |
|  | Lesotho | 0.2 | Brazil | 0.1 |
|  | Swaziland | 0.2 | Haiti | 0.1 |

Note. ASR = annual age standardized incidence rate per 100,000 population. (From Globocan 2002 database accessed at www.dep-iacr.fr.)

**Table 1-4.** Highest, Lowest, and Selected Western Country Reported Incidence of Laryngeal Cancer Worldwide

|  | Males | | Females | |
|---|---|---|---|---|
|  | Country | ASR | Country | ASR |
| Highest five incidence | Lebanon | 15.7 | Iraq | 4.2 |
|  | Bangladesh | 15.4 | Bangladesh | 3.3 |
|  | Macedonia | 13.8 | Azerbaijan | 3.3 |
|  | Hungary | 13.5 | Myanmar | 2.3 |
|  | Poland | 13.2 | Colombia | 2.0 |
| Western incidence | France | 10.8 | United States | 1.3 |
|  | United States | 5.9 | Canada | 1.0 |
|  | Canada | 4.9 | United Kingdom | 0.8 |
|  | United Kingdom | 4.4 | France | 0.7 |
|  | Australia | 3.9 | Australia | 0.5 |
|  | New Zealand | 2.2 | New Zealand | 0.4 |
| Lowest five incidence | Samoa | 0.0 | Burkina Faso | 0.1 |
|  | Polynesia | 0.0 | Guinea | 0.1 |
|  | Gambia | 0.1 | Vanuatu | 0.0 |
|  | Guinea | 0.6 | Guam | 0.0 |
|  | Malawi | 0.7 | Samoa | 0.0 |

Note. ASR = annual age standardized incidence rate per 100,000 population. (From Globocan 2002 database accessed at www.dep-iacr.fr.)

**Table 1–5.** Approximate Distribution of Sites of Squamous Cell Carcinoma Arising in the Mucosa of the Head and Neck Region for the United Kingdom Population

| Site | Proportion of all Head and Neck Squamous Cell Carcinoma | Subsites | Proportion of Site |
|---|---|---|---|
| Tongue | 10% | – | – |
| Lip | 12% | – | – |
| Oral cavity | 18% | Floor of mouth | 33% |
| | | Anterior tongue | 33% |
| | | Alveolar ridge | 20% |
| | | Buccal mucosa | 10% |
| | | Hard palate | 4% |
| Oropharynx | 11% | Tonsillar fossa | 57% |
| | | Base of tongue | 33% |
| Hypopharynx | 10% | Piriform fossa | 60% |
| | | Postcricoid | 30% |
| Nasopharynx | <2% | – | – |
| Larynx | 36% | Supraglottis | 30% |
| | | Glottis | 66% |
| | | Subglottis | <4% |

## Identification of Risk Factors for Head and Neck Cancer

The upper aerodigestive tract is readily exposed to inhaled or ingested toxins, which may be occupational or cultural exposures, and identification of such factors has been a key aim in understanding the cause of head and neck cancers. Epidemiological studies seek to identify risk factors for the causation of disease, in this case head and neck cancer. Variations in incidence of H&NSCC within a community over time can usually be attributed to changes in exposure to risk factors, although changes in the provision of medical care (such as screening) can be a confounder.

### Evaluating and Applying the Results of Epidemiological Studies

There are different types of epidemiological studies and interpreting results requires an understanding of the methodology used and awareness of problems, such as confounding (discussed later in this section).

One type of methodology is a retrospective study. This type of research design is generally easier and quicker to perform, but the results may be affected by recall bias, particularly amongst participants who are trying to ascribe a cause for their disease. They are also less reliable, as participants must try to remember past exposures and lifestyle habits. In comparison, prospective studies generally give more reliable information, but can be diminished if many participants are lost to follow-up. Another methodology, such as a case control study, is useful for studying relatively infrequent events, such as head and neck cancers. In this study design a group of patients are matched for a variety of factors such as age, sex, place of habitation, etc., to a number of control individuals with similar matched factors who do not have the disease being studied. In addition to study design, consideration of both the factors considered in each type of study and the number of participants is also important. Studies that examine many potential factors are more likely to detect unsuspected associations. However they are also more likely to produce some spurious associations. Using a greater number of participants studied usually makes the results more reliable.

Interpretation of studies also needs to give consideration to the issue of confounding. Confounding is where an apparent association is not actually causal, but is itself associated with another exposure, which is the true cause of the head and neck cancer being studied. An example in head and neck cancer is the apparent occupational associations with laryngeal cancer, where the confounding factor is in fact the higher smoking rates in the occupations of participants compared with controls.

When interpreting research findings, the biological plausibility of the putative factor causing head and neck cancer needs to be considered. For example, one would expect that a risk factor would be one that damages the epithelial surfaces of the upper aerodigestive tract or affects cellular function in some way. An example is the identification of the human papillomavirus gene sequences incorporated into the DNA of oral squamous cell cancers, as this virus is known to cause malignant transformation in other epithelial surfaces, most notably the cervix. Repeated identification of the same factor across different studies further strengthens the association as causal. The practical significance of a risk factor depends on the strength of the association, the magnitude of the risk conferred (usually expressed as the relative risk compared with the unexposed population), and the ease with which it can be avoided or ameliorated. For example, increasing age is a risk factor for head and neck SCC but is not readily modifiable.

A study will normally report the confidence intervals associated with the absolute risk of the factor identified, which gives an estimate of the statistical likelihood of the value for the risk being true in the whole population from which a sample has been studied. For example a relative risk may be reported as 2 (i.e., individuals exposed to the factor have twice the risk of developing cancer compared with individuals not exposed to the factor). If the reported confidence intervals are 1 to 3, however, this indicates the real relative risk in the population has a 95% chance of being between 1 (i.e., no increased risk) and 3 (three times the incidence). Confidence limits are by convention set at the arbitrary level of 95%. The certainty of an association (or lack of association) between a risk factor and outcome is partly determined by the number of events observed in the study. Confirmation of the role of a risk

factor requires: (a) identification of a mechanism by which the risk factor causes head and neck cancer (often by laboratory studies), (b) demonstrating a relationship where increasing exposure increases the risk of head and neck cancer, and (c) evidence that reducing exposure reduces incidence of head and neck cancer.

## Current Known Risk Factors for Head and Neck Cancer

The most typical head and neck cancer patient seen in Western countries tends to be a male in his sixties usually with a long history of smoking and heavy alcohol use. A disproportionate number appear to be socially isolated and have limited financial resources; nutritional status is often compromised and coexisting medical conditions of emphysema, hypertension, and ischemic heart disease are often seen. They may also have a history of poor compliance with prescribed medical therapy or a delay in presentation despite significant symptoms or signs of their cancer. Another less common pattern is that of younger people, often in their thirties or forties, who have never smoked or have only a minimal smoking history. Human papillomavirus is suspected to contribute to these tumors. In developing countries, where oral cancer is more common, the typical patient usually comes from the demographic group where chewing of oral carcinogenic preparations, such as betel nut, is most commonly practiced. Aggressive cutaneous (skin) squamous cell cancers, often with early nodal involvement, are seen in patients who are immunosuppressed following organ transplants or from chronic lymphocytic leukemia.

**Tobacco and Alcohol Consumption.** Tobacco smoking is the risk factor most strongly associated with the most common form of H&NSCC in developed countries. Tobacco smoking has been recognized for over 40 years to be associated with an increased incidence of H&NSCC (Moore, 1965; Wynder, Bross, & Day, 1956). The association of tobacco smoking has been demonstrated consistently in several large studies and shows a dose-dependent relationship (see review in Sturgis et al., 2004). An increased risk of H&NSCC among those with increased alcohol consumption is also observed. Prolonged environmental exposure to smoking (passive smoking) has been recognized legally in Australia where a "never-smoked" bar worker was awarded compensation from her employer after developing incurable laryngeal cancer. Tobacco smoking and alcohol consumption are frequently associated, making the attributable risk of each alone and in combination more difficult to estimate. The interaction of the two risk factors appeared to be multiplicative among heavy users of both (Merletti et al., 1989). Heavy drinking has also been identified as a risk factor for delayed presentation of patients with head and neck cancer resulting in a higher proportion of more advanced tumors (Brouha, Tromp, Hordijk, Winnubst, & De Leeuw, 2005). An Italian case control study of oropharyngeal and oral cavity cancers estimated attributable risks for alcohol and tobacco of 23% and 72% respectively for men, and 34% and 54% for women (Merletti et al., 1989). Tobacco and alcohol were similarly identified as responsible for 95% of cases in a study in Puerto Rico (Almodovar et al., 1996). A German study (Ahrens et al., 1991) of risk factors for larynx cancer reported an odds ratio of 3.5 for smokers of more than 20 cigarettes/day for 30 years and 3.2 for daily consumers of alcohol. Ex-smokers showed a decrease in risk, although it took 15 years to return to that of "never" smokers.

The association of chewing tobacco with oropharyngeal cancer strengthens the association, as the same toxin delivered in a different manner is again carcinogenic, and may be more so due to the prolonged contact time of chewed tobacco with the buccal mucosa. Chewing tobacco, or snuff, is commonly used in parts of the United States and Scandinavia. In the developing world, where the incidence of oropharyngeal squamous cell cancer is high, exposure to chewing tobacco and other preparations, often using areca (betel) nut, appears causal. In Papua New Guinea, powdered slaked lime is added to chewed betel nut in the mouth, causing a rise in mean pH which has been found in vitro to result in release of reactive oxygen species from the chewed betel quid (Thomas & MacLennan, 1992). Concoctions of baked mixtures of betel nut, slaked lime, and tobacco, known as *Gutka* or *Paan Masalas*, are popular in India and Southeast Asia and are considered particularly risky as oropharyngeal carcinogens. Chewing preparations based on leaves of the *Catha edulis* shrub, a stimulant and mood enhancer, are commonly used in the Arabian Peninsula and East Africa, and are also considered to predispose to oropharyngeal cancer. The oral preparations described above have local names

and several English spellings, including *Paan, Khat, Kath, Q'at, Mate, Snus, Shamma,* and *Toombak.* These exposures are considered the likeliest cause of the high rates of oropharyngeal cancer in developing countries. They often have strong cultural associations and the use of different preparations in different societies frequently segregates according to gender or social status.

Socioeconomic status has a close association with H&NSCC of the oral cavity and larynx, although this association is probably due to the higher smoking rates and alcohol consumption with increasing social deprivation (Thorne, Etherington, & Birchall, 1997). Social deprivation is generally associated with delayed presentation and poorer access to specialist health care, compounding the disadvantage. Specific health interventions to target areas of deprivation are an important consideration in health service planning and provision seeking to lessen the impact of head and neck cancer.

The presence of powerful risk factors such as tobacco smoking and alcohol with H&NSCC can obscure the role of other environmental risks that are less potent or to which a much smaller proportion of the community may be exposed (e.g., some industrial toxins). Study of the exposures of individuals with head and neck cancer who do not have a history of tobacco or alcohol exposure, and of participants with head and neck cancer in whom tobacco and alcohol exposure is controlled for, has suggested causative roles for other factors (discussed in the subsequent section).

**Human Papillomavirus.** Infection with the human papillomavirus subtypes HPV16 and HPV18 is one of the strongest candidates, especially for cases of non-smokers and nondrinkers. A meta analysis of reported studies has suggested the strongest link being between HPV16 and oropharyngeal SCC (Kreimer, Clifford, Boyle, & Franceschi, 2005). A molecular mechanism for HPV oncogenesis is well established from other tumor types and expected changes in oncogenic pathways appear to be present in HPV16 oropharyngeal, especially tonsillar, tumors (reviewed in Hafkamp, Manni, & Steel, 2004). The overall HPV prevalence in H&NSCC tumor samples appears to be around 25%. Koch, Sewell, Zahurak, and Sidransky (1999) compared H&NSCC in 46 individuals who never smoked with 230 smokers and 29 ex-smokers with H&NSCC, and also performed some molecular studies. They found nonsmokers with H&NSCC included a disproportionate number of women, oral cavity tumors, patients at the extremes of age, and a lower incidence of both chromosomal losses, measured by loss of heterozygosity, and p53 mutation. The rate of HPV DNA incorporation into the tumor was only slightly higher in the nonsmokers.

**Gastroesophageal Reflux.** Gastroesophageal reflux has been postulated to account for some cases of laryngeal cancer, in particular among patients who are nonsmokers and nondrinkers (Wight, Palleri, & Arullendran, 2003), although this is a less certain association (Wilson, 2005).

**Particle Inhalation.** Some studies have observed exposure to asbestos (Gustavsson et al., 1998), industrial dust (Wunsch, 2004), oil fumes (Ahrens et al., 1991), cement dust (Dietz, Ramroth, Urban, Ahrens, & Becher, 2004), and atmospheric pollution (Wake, 1993) as causes of laryngeal cancer. However these associations are not yet confirmed. An association with occupational exposures to woodworking, metalworking, and the refining and textile industries has been associated with uncommon tumors of the sinonasal region (in particular sinonasal adenocarcinoma) (Mannetje et al., 1999).

**Marijuana.** Marijuana smoking has also been investigated (Hashibe et al., 2002) and has been associated with head and neck cancers with aggressive behavior in patients under 55 years of age. The active cannaboids in marijuana appear to cause DNA damage to cells in vitro which would support an association. The interaction between marijuana use and tobacco smoking has been reported to be synergistic (Zhang et al., 1999). A role for marijuana is relevant given the rise in incidence of marijuana smoking among young people in Western countries during the 1990s.

**Diet.** Dietary factors have received considerable attention but any association is complicated by the interaction between heavy tobacco and alcohol use and dietary deficiencies. Folate deficiency appears to interact with excessive alcohol ingestion multiplicatively increasing the risk of head and neck cancer, although at the same time this offers a potential opportunity for ameliorating the carcinogenic effects of alcohol. A toxic effect of high consumption of fried foods has been observed for oral pharyngeal cancer, which although statistically significant, conferred only a mod-

est increase in relative risk (Galeone et al., 2005). A comprehensive review of epidemiological studies has identified protective effects of fruit and vegetable intake, probably due to the combined effects of carotene, vitamin C, and vitamin E, but probably not vitamin A. Other micronutrients are likely to contribute a protective effect also as evidenced by the benefits of diet rather than specific nutrient supplementation (Chainani-Wu, 2002).

**Genetics.** Even for such a powerful risk factor as tobacco smoking, there is a postulated role for genetic responses, as clearly not all smokers develop H&NSCC. Considerable research effort has been expended attempting to identify individuals with polymorphisms in relevant genes such as detoxifying or DNA repair genes to elucidate the causal mechanism by which tobacco smoking provokes H&NSCC, and to better identify subgroups at the highest risk of developing H&NSCC, who may therefore benefit from interventions such as chemoprevention, screening, and intensive smoking cessation interventions. The study of Bongers et al. (1996) provides epidemiological evidence for genetic interaction, suggesting that even among smokers there are familial clusters of head and neck cancer.

Some types of head and neck cancer may show a significant difference in incidence between different communities, raising the possibility of genetic differences, or genetically determined responses to particular exposures, contributing to cancer causation. This is not observed for most commonly occurring H&NSCC, but is seen in nasopharyngeal carcinoma (NPC) where certain ethnic backgrounds (e.g., southern Chinese and some Pacific Islanders) have a higher incidence of NPC. The Epstein-Barr virus (EBV), which is endemic in most communities (with almost universal serological evidence of exposure), is believed to be implicated in NPC, illustrating the important interaction between environmental factors and genetic makeup. It appears that failure to clear the virus from primarily infected cells is the precursor to NPC. Expression of antiviral IgA antibodies has been identified as a risk for the subsequent development of NPC in a large cohort of Taiwanese men followed prospectively (Chien, et al., 2001). Quantitative measurement of EBV in blood has also been reported to correlate with the extent of the disease and prognosis (Lin et al., 2004).

## Risk Modification

The most important approach to head and neck cancer risk modification is tobacco control. Unfortunately even for only moderate smokers, an increased risk of H&NSCC compared to "never" smokers persists for up to 15 years following smoking cessation. For very heavy smokers, the risk probably never returns to normal. For those who continue to smoke, however, the risk increases with each year of cumulative smoking history. Reduction of alcohol consumption is also a modifiable risk factor. The benefits of dietary supplementation are still being studied but it seems there is no disadvantage from pursuing a diet high in vegetables and fruits and low in saturated fats, especially as this is likely to confer other health benefits. Chemoprevention, the use of biologically active supplements in people at risk of developing H&NSCC, has been studied in two main populations—individuals with premalignant oral lesions and patients who have had a previous H&NSCC and who thus have an approximate 4% annual incidence of developing a second upper aerodigestive tract primary. Agents tested in clinical trials so far include beta-carotene, alpha-tocopherol, ascorbic acid, and retinoids (Scheer, Kuebler, & Zoller, 2004). Retinoids appear to be the most promising of the compounds so far examined; however, their use is limited by toxic side effects and the development of resistance to their action by transformed cells. The formulation of new receptor selective synthetic retinoids and the combination of retinoids with nonretinoid agents are important areas of research currently (Smith & Saba, 2005).

## Clinical Assessment and Management

In the preceding sections we described some of the biological features of cancers in both general cancer and head and neck cancers in particular, as well as explored the risk factors for H&NSCC. In this final section of the chapter we will provide an introduction to the clinical aspects of staging and managing the head and neck cancer patient. More specific information regarding classification, staging, and multidisciplinary team management of specific types of head and neck cancers will follow in the subsequent chapters of this textbook.

## Anatomical and Functional Considerations in Treating Head and Neck Cancer

The head and neck region contains the most complex functional anatomy in the human body. It includes the central nervous system, vision, hearing and balance, olfaction, taste, deglutition, voice, endocrine and exocrine glands, and structures necessary for cosmetic appearance. As a result, the management of tumors of this area presents considerable functional and aesthetic problems. In some cases, a combination of radiotherapy with chemotherapy may offer an alternative to radical surgery with similar chance of cancer cure. In this situation, the patient's choice of treatment may be guided by the different side effects and treatment durations of the different modalities. In other situations the best survival outcome for a patient may be achieved with surgery followed by radiotherapy combined with chemotherapy, provided the patient is fit enough for these treatments. In all cases, management of acute side effects and rehabilitation of speech, swallowing, and appearance are integral to care. A multidisciplinary approach to the management of tumors is therefore mandatory, from primary assessment and planning of treatment, through definitive treatment, and during follow-up.

## Clinical Presentation

The typical presenting signs and symptoms of head and neck cancer are listed in Table 1–6. Patient symptoms may be due to local effects of the primary tumor mass, for example a laryngeal cancer causing hoarse voice and breathlessness. In other cases, the primary may be asymptomatic but the secondary tumor deposits in cervical lymph nodes cause neck swelling noted by the patient (Figure 1–4). Some asymptomatic oral lesions may be detected during dental examinations or by patients while brushing their teeth in front of a mirror.

A history should be taken from the patient and specific questions asked relevant to assessing the extent and spread of the tumor, as well the onset, duration, and progress of symptoms (this helps assess the rate of tumor growth). A careful history should be made inquiring about previous medical or surgical treat-

**Table 1-6.** Common Presenting Signs and Symptoms of Head and Neck Cancer.

| Sign or Symptom | Mechanism |
| --- | --- |
| Nonhealing ulcer | Primary cancer erodes mucosa |
| Neck lump | Lymph node replaced by metastatic cancer |
| Pain | Direct invasion of normal structures by cancer |
| Neuropathic pain | Invasion of sensory nerve by cancer cells, often at distance from where pain is felt; e.g., pain in part of face due to cancer infiltrating nerve ganglion near skull base |
| Difficulty swallowing (dysphagia) | Cancer obstructing the swallowing passage or affecting nerves or muscles required for swallowing |
| Pain on swallowing (odynophagia) | Act of swallowing causes distension of tissues invaded by cancer |
| Pain in the ear (otalgia) | May be referred pain due to oropharyngeal or hypopharyngeal tumors invading branches of the glossopharyngeal nerve |
| Reduced jaw opening (trismus) | Invasion of the muscles of jaw opening (e.g., the pterygoids) by cancer |
| Bad breath (halitosis) | Ulcerative lesion in the oral cavity with bacterial colonization |
| Ill-fitting denture | Tumor rubbing against denture |
| Reduced tongue movement | Invasion of primary tongue cancer into tongue base |
| Noise on breathing (stridor) | Obstruction of airway by tumor, especially laryngeal cancer |
| Breathlessness (dyspnea) | Tumor obstructing air entry into the upper airway |
| Hoarse voice (dysphonia) | Impaired mobility of the vocal folds due to direct tumor invasion or by invasion of the recurrent laryngeal nerve |
| Cough | Direct initiation of cough reflex by tumor |
| Coughing blood (hemoptysis) | Friable cancer surface causing bleeding into the upper airway or cancer invasion of blood vessel |
| Lung infection (pneumonia) | Aspiration due to impaired laryngeal function by tumor involvement |
| Fever | Infection in necrotic lymph node, in ulcerated tumor, or systemic effect of cancer due to cytokine release |
| Loss of appetite (anorexia) | Systemic effect of cancer |
| Weight loss | Systemic effect of cancer or physical inability to swallow preventing oral intake of food |

ments, concurrent health problems, past and current alcohol, tobacco, illicit drug, and medication use, and occupation and exposure to toxins relevant to head and neck cancer, as well as social and financial circumstances. These factors may influence the risks and complications of treatment and alter the management plan. Some issues may require urgent specific intervention, for example optimization of cardiac function or management of anticipated perioperative alcohol withdrawal.

The management of head and neck tumors requires a detailed evaluation of the disease extent using clinical examination and further investigations. Clinical examination aims to define the primary tumor and sites of spread by examining likely metastatic sites and by assessing the function of structures that may be

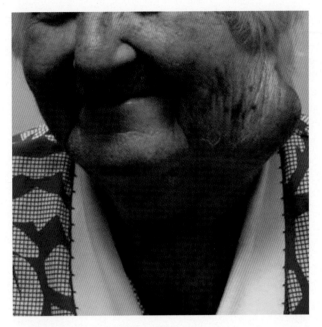

**Figure 1–4.** Example of grossly enlarged cervical lymph nodes secondary to metastatic squamous cell tonsillar carcinoma.

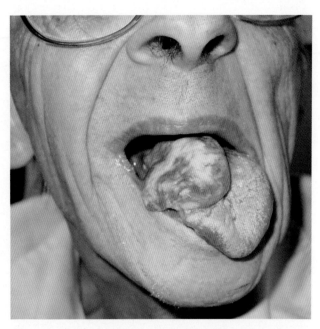

**Figure 1–5.** Large squamous cell carcinoma of the tongue.

involved (e.g., tongue mobility or fifth cranial nerve sensory function). Due to accessibility, the extent of the tongue or floor of mouth lesions can be gauged by direct palpation with the gloved finger (Figure 1-5). Careful manual examination of the lymph node groups is important. These nodal groups are shown in Figure 1-6 and explained in Table 1-7. Visual inspection of cancers in the nasopharynx and oropharynx in the awake patient can be achieved using flexible fiberoptic nasoendoscopy (Figure 1-7). Complete assessment frequently necessitates a panendoscopy in which the patient is anesthetized and a careful inspection made of the tumor and the whole region including the hypopharynx, larynx, upper esophagus, and trachea and main bronchi, as well as biopsies of suspicious areas. The findings of clinical examination are matched to the TNM staging system (detailed below) for the patient's tumor site of origin.

## Clinical Investigations

In addition to direct examination of the tumor, using manual or visual inspection, various imaging tech-

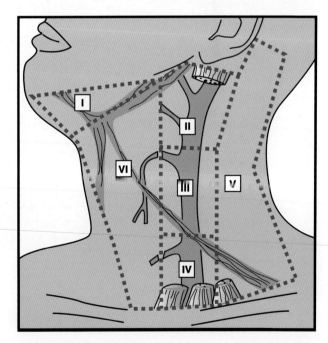

**Figure 1–6.** Lymph node groups of the neck.

niques are used to assess cancers in the head and neck region, including ultrasound in combination with fine

**Table 1–7.** Lymph Nodes Grouped in Levels

| Level | Lymph Nodes |
|-------|-------------|
| I | 1a Medial submental |
|   | 1b Lateral submental |
| II | Upper cervical |
| III | Midcervical |
| IV | Lower cervical |
| V | Posterior triangle of neck |
| VI | Supraclavicular |

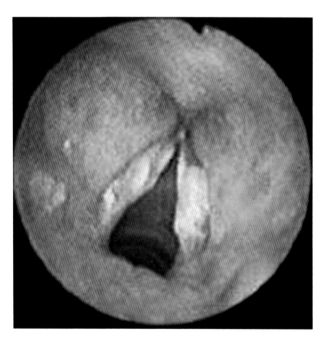

**Figure 1–7.** Early stage left vocal fold carcinoma (on the left of the picture) seen endoscopically.

needle aspiration cytology (USFNAC), computerized tomographic (CT) scan with contrast, magnetic resonance imaging (MRI) with contrast, positron emission tomography (PET) scan, and radionucleotide scanning (see Chapters 4 and 6 for detailed description of the application and benefits of each technique for different cancer sites). These scans supplement the visual tumor inspection and provide a good assessment of the bulk of the tumor and its spread into adjacent structures. Good communication between the clinician and radiologist prior to performing imaging, and alerting the radiologist to specific clinical questions, improves the efficiency and value of the studies. Most of the investigations used for initial evaluation of the tumor can be used in follow-up for the detection of recurrence.

## USFNAC

USFNAC is safe, rapid, and inexpensive and has become the standard tool for staging neck nodes. It avoids an open biopsy and its accuracy is over 90%. It gives information to the clinician on the presence or absence of malignant cells in a specific location.

## CT Scan

CT scanning is probably the most common investigation undertaken to stage head and neck cancers. The information obtained from CT is dependent on the quality of the scan and the specific scanning techniques performed, such as the distance between slices and the thickness of the reconstructed axial images, effective intravenous contrast, and, if appropriate, the use of scanning algorithms to image bone so that malignant invasion can be detected.

## MRI

MRI is not required in all situations but is particularly useful for assessing tongue, nasopharyngeal, and other base of skull tumors and for detecting tumor infiltration of cranial nerves (Figure 1–8). CT and MRI can also be useful to detect impalpable lymph nodes. Nodes that present with a maximum diameter of 1 cm or greater and a rounded appearance (due to the loss of the lymph node hilum) have increased probability of malignant involvement.

## PET Scan

PET scanning detects metabolic activity by measuring the uptake of radioactively labeled glucose ($^{18}$fluorine deoxyglucose or FDG), which is increased in cancers (and also in inflammatory lesions). PET can sensitively detect small secondary deposits of cancer or clarify lesions seen on CT, such as borderline enlarged lymph

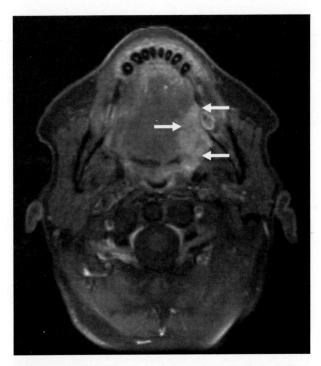

**Figure 1–8.** T2 weighted MRI image of left tongue squamous cell carcinoma. Area of tumor indicated by arrow.

nodes. PET scanning can be combined with CT (PET-CT fusion) to provide integrated anatomic and biochemical imaging. Currently, PET has a role in defining whether equivocal possible secondary tumor deposits seen on CT or MRI are more likely to be malignant or benign. PET can also be used to aid decision making when residual lymphadenopathy is seen after curative intent radiotherapy or chemoradiotherapy; a baseline (i.e., pretreatment) scan is performed to confirm FDG avidity of tumor deposits. The post-treatment scan is performed after at least 6 weeks, when radiation induced change has significantly resolved. If the slowly resolving lymph node masses are found to be PET negative then they can be safely observed, whereas if there is persistent PET positivity, a surgical resection can be offered. PET technology is a rapidly developing field. For example, it can be used to detect other biochemical properties such as hypoxia within tumor deposits (a possible marker of radiation and chemotherapy resistant tumors).

## Primary Tumors and Staging

In the TNM (tumor-node-metastasis) classification system (Sobin & Wittekind, 2002), *T* refers to the primary tumor. A higher T stage (e.g., T3 or T4) indicates a larger primary tumor. The T stage is determined either from the longest tumor diameter (expressed in centimeters) or from the structures invaded by the tumor. Examples of the T classification for the oral cavity and larynx are seen in Tables 1–8 and 1–9. In addition to the T1-T4 classifications, a primary tumor may be classified as Tx—primary tumor not assessable, or Tis—carcinoma in situ. The Tx classification is given when a patient may present with enlarged lymph nodes containing head and neck cancer cells proven on biopsy, but no primary tumor can be found despite careful examination of the mucosal surfaces of the head and neck area by endoscopic examination under anesthetic. Tx may also be used when an unsuspected primary may have been removed without proper assessment. Tis is used where malignant appearing cells are seen but have not invaded through the basement membrane of the epithelial surface from which the tumor has arisen. This lesion is not cancer by definition as the cells have not invaded beyond their normal location; however, it is known that there is a high risk of invasion developing so excision and careful follow-up are required.

*N* stands for local and regional nodal status. The nodal groups routinely examined in head and neck cancer have been presented previously in Figure 1–2. Lymph node involvement is the most important patient prognostic factor. Using the UICC TNM (Sobin & Wittekind, 2002) classification, an N0 node classification represents a neck in which there are no palpable nodes. An N1 node classification indicates a node less than 3 cm. An N2a indicates a node that is between 3 cm and 6 cm; an N2b node rating indicates there are two or more nodes in the neck less than 6 cm; while an N2c neck is one in which there are contralateral or bilateral nodes less than 6 cm. An N3 neck describes a neck in which the metastatic tumor volume in the neck is greater than 6 cm.

The *M* refers to the absence (M0) or presence (M1) of distant metastases, such as to the lung. Metastases usually, but not always, occur late in head and neck cancer. Secondary tumor, or metastasis, refers

**Table 1–8.** T (Tumor) Classification for Oral Cavity Tumors According to UICC TNM System

| T Classification | Explanation |
| --- | --- |
| Tx | Primary tumor cannot be assessed |
| T0 | No evidence of primary tumor |
| Tis | Carcinoma in situ |
| T1 | Tumor 2 cm or less in greatest dimension |
| T2 | Tumor more than 2 cm but less than 4 cm in greatest dimension |
| T3 | Tumor more than 4 cm in greatest dimension |
| T4a | Tumor invades through cortical bone into deep/extrinsic muscle of the tongue, maxillary sinus, or skin of the face |
| T4b | Tumor invades masticator space, pterygoid plates, or skull base, or encases internal carotid artery |

*Source:* Sobin & Whittekind, 2002

**Table 1–9.** T (Tumor) Classification for Larynx Cancers According to the UICC TNM System

| T Classification | Explanation |
| --- | --- |
| **Supraglottis** | |
| T1 | One subsite, normal vocal fold mobility |
| T2 | Mucosa of more than one adjacent subsite of supraglottis or glottis or adjacent region outside the supraglottis; without fixation |
| T3 | Fold fixation or invades postcricoid area, pre-epiglottic tissues, paraglottic space, thyroid cartilage erosion |
| T4a | Through thyroid cartilage, trachea, soft tissues of neck, deep/extrinsic muscle of tongue, strap muscles, thyroid, esophagus |
| T4b | Prevertebral space, mediastinal structures, carotid artery |
| **Glottis** | |
| T1 | Limited to vocal folds, normal mobility |
| T2 | Supraglottis, subglottis, impaired cord mobility |
| T3 | Fold fixation, paraglottic space, thyroid cartilage erosion |
| T4a | Through thyroid cartilage, trachea, soft tissues of neck, deep muscle of tongue, strap muscles, thyroid, esophagus |
| T4b | Prevertebral space, mediastinal structures, carotid artery |
| **Subglottis** | |
| T1 | Limited to subglottis |
| T2 | Extends to vocal folds with normal/impaired mobility |
| T3 | Fold fixation |
| T4a | Through cricoid or thyroid cartilage, trachea, deep/extrinsic muscle of the tongue, strap muscles, thyroid, esophagus |
| T4b | Prevertebral space, mediastinal structures, carotid artery |

*Source:* Sobin & Whittekind, 2002

to a deposit of cancer cells that have spread from the original site of the tumor, known as the primary tumor. Primary tumors of the head and neck can spread by direct invasion of surrounding tissues, by invasion of the lymphatic system, by invasion of the venous system, and via perineural spread. In head and neck cancer, metastasis is usually via the lymphatic system; that is, tumor cells from the primary enter local lymph channels and travel to draining lymph nodes where the tumor cells may lodge and begin to divide, establishing large masses. A feature of squamous cell cancers is that they may grow rapidly and outgrow their blood supply leading to necrosis in the central part of the tumor. This can often be detected radiologically, represented as an altered density in the middle of the malignant mass compared with the edges. Other mechanisms of spread of head and neck cancer cells include hematogenous (via the blood stream), which probably accounts for distant metastases, and perineural, whereby tumor cells invade small nerves close to the primary tumor and grow inside the sheath covering the nerve, typically growing back towards the origin of the nerve (in particular the fifth and seventh cranial nerves).

The TNM stage estimation is based on clinical examination, radiological or nuclear medicine imaging, and endoscopic examination at some sites. TNM staging can subsequently be confirmed by cytological examination (e.g., aspiration of enlarged lymph node suspicious for involvement by spread from the primary tumor) and from examination of tissue resected during an operation, which may lead to revision of the stage estimation (e.g., if examination of resected tissue reveals tumor deposits in lymph nodes not previously suspected as involved during earlier clinical or radiological examinations). This is referred to as pathological staging and is preceded by the letter $p$.

Staging of the cancer using the TNM system is essential to evaluate the extent of the tumor at presentation. It governs the ability of the management team to appropriately assign treatment modalities such as surgery, radiation, and/or chemotherapy for each patient. Formation of stage groups (Stages I, II, III, and IV) is made uniform by the use of the TNM classification, with individual TNM values grouped to identify patients with similar prognosis. For example, Table 1-10 shows the stage grouping for larynx cancers and it can be seen that T1N1, T2N1, T3N0, and T3N1 tumors are all

**Table 1-10.** Stage Grouping for Laryngeal Cancer Using the TNM System

|  | **Tis** | **T1** | **T2** | **T3** | **T4** |
|---|---|---|---|---|---|
| N0 | 0 | I | II | III | IV |
| N1 | N/A | III | III | III | IV |
| N2 | N/A | IV | IV | IV | IV |
| N3 | N/A | IV | IV | IV | IV |

Note. Tis, carcinoma in situ; I-IV, stage groups one to four

classified as Stage III. Having consistent classification and staging systems for cancers helps to standardize treatment between different centers and to test the value of treatments in trials by ensuring that patients with similar prognoses are being compared.

Although the TNM staging system provides the best way to standardize patients between different treating centers, it is not a perfect system. A significant deficiency is that the biological behavior of tumors is not considered. Similar T and N staged tumors can behave very differently in terms of their response to treatment. Predicting the biological behavior of tumors is an area of intense research interest. A further issue with TNM is that the one stage group may include patients with more advanced primary tumors and no nodal disease as well as patients with smaller primary tumors with nodal metastases. It is likely that the prognosis is in fact different between such patients, and the TNM classification of patients into different stages is a process that is regularly reviewed as more information is obtained. For example, in Table 1-10, Stage III includes T3N0 tumors as well as T1N1 tumors.

## Management of the Patient with Head and Neck Cancer

After staging, the patient is presented to a multidisciplinary clinic, whose therapeutic modalities include surgery, radiotherapy, and chemotherapy. The proven curative modalities are surgery and radiotherapy. Surgical management requires treatment of the primary and often separate dissection of the lymph nodes most likely to be the sites of spread. Examination of the surgically resected lymph nodes for microscopic tumor deposits not detected clinically is an important step in determining prognosis and the benefit of additional therapy.

Chemotherapy has a role in palliating advanced or recurrent disease. Although head and neck squamous cell cancers are quite sensitive to chemotherapy (i.e., they shrink in size), chemotherapy is not a curative treatment. It has been used before definitive surgery or radiotherapy, so-called induction chemotherapy, with the aim of reducing the size of the primary tumor and sterilizing micrometastases. Recent studies in patients at high risk of recurrence suggest combining radiotherapy with chemotherapy (chemoradiation) improves the patient outcome compared with radiotherapy alone.

Originally, radiotherapy had been used for patients not fit for surgery, or with only palliative intent for patients considered incurable. Subsequent improvements in technique and understanding of the doses of radiation required for effective treatment have led to radiotherapy becoming an effective alternative to surgery in some situations, for example early stage larynx cancer. Radiotherapy alone usually encompasses the primary tumor and an area of the neck containing the lymph node groups most likely to be involved by spread from the primary.

Advanced tumors such as some T2 tumors of the tongue and T3 and T4 regions of most areas of the head and neck require more than one modality of treatment. It is not uncommon for patients to have surgery followed by radiotherapy, or to have chemoradiation as an organ conserving rationale. In circumstances where a tumor is resected and extensive lymph node involvement is observed on histopathological examination of the specimen, the best patient outcome can be obtained by following surgery with radiotherapy, sometimes with concurrent chemotherapy. Using radiotherapy or chemoradiation has the potential advantage that if a tumor recurs locally (i.e., at the primary site or within the head and neck region) the patient can be salvaged by surgery. As a general principle increasing the number of modalities of treatment increases the side effects experienced by the patient. The timing of surgery following radiotherapy is influenced by the problem of tissue fibrosis which makes surgery more difficult. The optimal way to combine the different modalities of treatment is an area of active research and in practice often depends on local expertise, experience, and resources. Factors influencing the choice of treatment are shown in Table 1-11. A more detailed discussion of radiotherapy, chemotherapy, and chemoradiotherapy can be found in Chapter 3.

Newer novel treatments, such as immunotherapies targeting mutant p53 protein in tumor cells, antibodies to EGFR (epidermal growth factor receptor),

**Table 1-11.** Factors Influencing Recommended Treatment for an Individual Patient with Head and Neck Cancer

| Tumor Factors | Patient Factors | Physician Factors |
|---|---|---|
| Site | Medical condition and comorbidities | Expertise |
| Size | The impact of treatment on the quality of life of the patient | Availability of a comprehensive team—nursing, dental, speech therapy, dietitian, rehabilitation, and social support services |
| Depth of invasion | Performance status | Personal preference of members of the team |
| Degree of spread | Treatment cost | Preferences of the institution |
| Location and proximity to critical structures | Patient compliance | |
| Previous treatment | Previous treatment | |
| Need for reconstructive surgery | Patient preference | |

which is frequently overexpressed in head and neck squamous cell cancers, and antibodies to block the pro-angiogenic (blood vessel forming) substance VEGF (Vascular Endothelial Growth Factor), have been tested in patients with advanced disease and may become integrated into definitive treatment of primary tumors in the future.

## Multidisciplinary Care

Important members of the multidisciplinary management team include speech-language pathologists, who are able to assess and assist patients pre- and postoperatively with the assessment and management of swallowing and voice production; physical therapists, who are able to assist with patient coughing and clearance of the chest postoperatively; and social workers, who are able to assess the day-to-day needs of the patient and provide support to the patient during and following treatment. Experienced nursing care is also essential, both in the initial assessment of the patient and in providing care in the ward following surgery. Detailed discussion of the multidisciplinary team members and their roles will be outlined further in Chapter 14.

Most patients who have complex surgical procedures carried out spend some time in the intensive care unit, as these patients frequently suffer with comorbidities that may also be the result of their lifestyle (which in the majority of patients has induced the cancer of the head and neck). For instance, it is common for these patients to have cardiac, pulmonary, and liver diseases. These diseases increase the surgical risk of thromboembolism, bleeding, cardiac dysfunction, and postoperative chest infection.

## Outcomes

The outcome for most patients with head and neck cancer may be considered better than cancers arising from other areas. Compared to some other cancers, head and neck cancer has a greater tendency to spread or recur locally (i.e., around the primary site or in regional lymph nodes). Aggressive local therapy can, therefore, produce prolonged survival or cure. The 5-year survival rate for an advanced head and neck cancer with a lymphatic metastasis is around 50%. Certain tumor sites such as hypopharyngeal squamous cell carcinomas have a generally worse outcome. Attention to the functional outcomes and quality of life is essential in treating and assessing all patients with head and neck cancer.

## Conclusion

This chapter has discussed the molecular biology and epidemiology of head and neck cancers, in particular the most common form, squamous cell carcinoma. We have also attempted to illustrate some of the principles of clinical management of patients with head and neck cancer, in particular; the importance of careful and complete clinical and radiological staging and assessment of patients; the importance of review by a multidisciplinary team where the treatment modalities of surgery, radiotherapy, and chemotherapy can be individually selected or combined to give the patient the best chance of tumor cure or control for the most acceptable side effects; and the necessity of skilled intervention from nursing staff, speech pathologists, dietitians, physiotherapists, and social workers in managing these complex patients. Each of these key issues will be discussed further and expanded upon in the remaining chapters of this text. The collective term *head and neck squamous cell carcinomas* actually encompasses a large number of distinct clinical entities with differing natural histories, patterns of spread, manner of presentation, and response to treatment. The reader is recommended to pursue additional reading to fully appreciate the subtleties of underlying biological differences and hence differing management, as he or she gains experience in contributing to the care of head and neck cancer patients.

## References

Ahrens, W., Jockel, K. H., Patzak, W., & Elsner, G. (1991). Alcohol, smoking , and occupational factors in cancer of the larynx: A case-control study. *American Journal of Industrial Medicine, 20,* 477–493.

Almodovar, J., Perez., S. I., Arruza, M., Morrell, C. A., & Baez, A. (1996). Descriptive epidemiology of head and neck squamous cell carcinoma in Puerto Ricans. *Puerto Rican Health Sciences Journal, 15*(4), 251–255.

Bongers, V., Braakhuis, B. J., & Tobi, H. (1996). The relation between cancer incidence among relatives and the occurrence of multiple primary carcinomas following head and neck cancer. *Cancer Epidemiology, Biomarkers and Prevention, 5*, 595–598.

Brouha, X., Tromp, D., Hordijk, G. J., Winnubst, J., & De Leeuw, R. (2005). Role of alcohol and smoking in diagnostic delay of head and neck cancer patients. *Acta Otolaryngology, 125*, 552–556.

Chainani-Wu, N. (2002). Diet and oral, pharyngeal, and esophageal cancer. *Nutrition and Cancer, 44*, 104–126.

Chien, Y. C., Chen, J. Y., Liu, M. Y., Yang, H. I., Hsu, M. M., Chen, C. J., et al. (2001). Serologic markers of Epstein-Barr virus infection and nasopharyngeal carcinoma in Taiwanese men. *The New England Journal of Medicine, 345*, 1877–1882.

Dahler, A. L, Cavanagh, L. L., & Saunders, N. A. (2001). Suppression of keratinocyte growth and differentiation by transforming growth factor-$\beta$1 are mediated by different signaling pathways. *Journal of Investigative Dermatology, 116*(2), 266–274.

Dietz, A., Ramroth, H., Urban, T., Ahrens, W., & Becher, H. (2004). Exposure to cement dust, related occupational groups and laryngeal cancer risk: Results of a population based case-control study. *International Journal of Cancer, 108*, 907–911.

Galeone, C., Pelucchi, C., Talamini, R., Levi, F., Bosetti, C., Negri, E., et al. (2005). Role of fried foods and oral/pharyngeal and oesophageal cancers. *British Journal of Cancer, 92*, 2065–2069.

Gustavsson, P., Jakobsson, R., Johansson, H., Lewin, F., Norell, S., & Rutkvist, L. E. (1998). Occupational exposures and squamous cell carcinoma of the oral cavity, pharynx, larynx, and oesophagus: A case-control study in Sweden. *Occupational and Environmental Medicine, 55*(6), 393–400.

Hafkamp, H. C., Manni, J. J., & Speel, E. J. (2004). Role of human papillomavirus in the development of head and neck squamous cell carcinoma. *Acta Otolaryngology, 124*, 520–526.

Hanahan D., & Weinberg, R. A. (2000). The hallmarks of cancer. *Cell, 100*, 57–70.

Hashibe, M., Ford, D. E., & Zhang, A. F. (2002). Marijuana smoking and head and neck cancer. *Journal of Clinical Pharmacology, 42*, 103S–107S.

International Agency for Research on Cancer and World Health Organization. (2002). *Cancer incidence, mortality and prevalence worldwide, estimates for the year 2002.* Retrieved from IARC-WHO GLOBOCAN 2002 Database September, 2005, at: http://www-dep.iarc.fr/

Ishitoya, J., Toriyama, M., Oguchi, N., Kiatmura, K., Ohshima, M., Asano, K., et al. (1989). Gene amplification and overexpression of the EGF receptor in squamous cell carcinomas of the head and neck. *British Journal of Cancer, 59*, 559–562.

Koch, W. M., Lango, M., Sewell, D., Zahurak. M., & Sidransky, D. (1999). Head and neck cancer in nonsmokers: A distinct clinical and molecular entity. *Laryngoscope,109*, 1544–1551.

Kreimer, A. R., Clifford, G. M., Boyle, P., & Franceschi, S. (2005). Human papillomavirus types in head and neck squamous cell carcinomas worldwide: A systemic review. *Cancer Epidemiology, Biomarkers & Prevention, 14*, 467–475.

Lin, J. C., Wang, W.Y., Chen, K. Y., Wei, Y. H., Liang, W. M., Jan, J. S., et al. (2004). Quantification of plasma Epstein-Barr virus DNA in patients with advanced nasopharyngeal carcinoma. *New England Journal of Medicine, 350*, 2461–2470.

Mannetje, A., Kogevinas, M., Luce, D., Demirs, P. A., Begin, D., & Bolm-Audorff, U. (1999). Sinonasal cancer, occupation, and tobacco smoking in European women and men. *American Journal of Industrial Medicine, 36*, 101–107.

Merletti, F., Boffetta, P., Ciccone, G., Mashberg, A., & Terracini, B. (1989). Role of tobacco and alcoholic beverages in the etiology of cancer of the oral cavity/oropharynx in Torino, Italy. *Cancer Research, 49*, 4919–4924.

Moore, C. (1965). Smoking and cancer of the mouth, pharynx and larynx. *Journal of the American Medical Association, 191*, 283–286.

Scheer, M., Kuebler, A. C., & Zoller, J. E. (2004). Chemoprevention of oral squamous cell carcinoma. *Onkologie, 27*, 187–193.

Serewko, M. M., Popa, C., Dahler, A. L., Smith, L., Strutton, G. M., Coman, W., et al. (2002). Alterations in gene expression and activity during squamous cell carcinoma development. *Cancer Research, 62*, 3759–3765.

Smith, L., Dahler, A. L., Popa, C., Serewko-Auret, M. M. M., Wong, C. F., Barnes, L. M., et al. (2004). Modulation of proliferation-specific and differentiation-specific markers in human keratinocytes by SMAD7. *Experimental Cell Research, 294*, 356–365.

Smith, W., & Saba, N. (2005). Retinoids as chemoprevention for head and neck cancer: Where do we go from here? *Critical Reviews in Oncology/Hematology, 55*, 143–152.

Sobin, L. H., & Wittekind, C. (Eds.). (2002). *UICC TNM classification of malignant tumors* (6th ed.). Heidelberg, Germany: Springer Verlag.

Sturgis, E. M., Wei, Q., & Spitz, M. R. (2004). Descriptive epidemiology and risk factors for head and neck cancer. *Seminars in Oncology, 31*(6), 726-733.

Thomas, S. J., & MacLennan, R. (1992). Slaked lime and betel nut cancer in Papua New Guinea. *Lancet, 340*, 577-578.

Thorne, P., Etherington, D., & Birchall, M. A. (1997). Head and neck cancer in the South West of England—Influence of socio-economic status on incidence and second primary tumors. *European Journal of Surgical Oncology, 23*, 503-508.

Wake, M. (1993).The urban/rural divide in head and neck cancer—The effect of atmospheric pollution. *Otolaryngology, 18*, 298-302.

Westburg, S. P., & Stone, O. J. (1973). Multiple cutaneous squamous cell carcinomas during immunosuppressive therapy. *Archives of Dermatology, 107*, 893-895.

Wight, R., Paleri, V., & Arullendran, P. (2003). Current theories for the development of nonsmoking and nondrinking laryngeal carcinoma. *Current Opinion in Otolaryngology & Head and Neck Surgery, 11*, 73-77.

Wilson, J. A. (2005). What is the evidence that gastroesophageal reflux is involved in the etiology of laryngeal cancer? *Current Opinion in Otolaryngology & Head and Neck Surgery, 13*, 97-100.

Wong, C. F., Barnes, L. M, Dahler, A. L., Smith, L., Serewko-Auret, M. M., Popa, C., et al. (2003). A role for E2F in the modulation of keratinocyte squamous differentiation: Implications for the use of an E2F inhibitor in squamous cell carcinoma. *Journal of Biological Chemistry, 278*(31), 28516-28522.

Wong, C. F., Barnes, L. M., Dahler, A. L., Smith. L., Popa, C., Serewko-Auret, M. M., et al. (2005). Sp1 is a downstream effector of E2F-mediated suppression of squamous differentiation. *Oncogene, 24*, 3525-3534.

World Health Organization. (2005). *WHO Global Action against Cancer 2005*. Retrieved September, 2005, from http://www.who.int/cancer/media/GlobalActionCancerEnglfull

Wunsch, F. V. (2004). The epidemiology of laryngeal cancer in Brazil. *San Paulo Medical Journal, 122*(5), 188-194.

Wynder, E. L., Bross, I. J., & Day, E. (1956). A study of environmental factors in cancer of the larynx. *Cancer, 9*, 86-110.

Zhang, Z. F., Morgenstern, H., Spitz, M. R., Tashkin, D. P., Yu, G. P., Marshall, J. R., et al. (1999). Marijuana use and increased risk of squamous cell carcinoma of the head and neck. *Cancer Epidemiology, Biomarkers & Prevention, 8*, 1071-1078.

# Chapter 2

# EVALUATING THE IMPACT OF CANCER OF THE HEAD AND NECK

Irma M. Verdonck-de Leeuw, Rico N. P. M. Rinkel, and C. René Leemans

## CHAPTER OUTLINE

## Introduction

Worldwide, approximately 500,000 patients are diagnosed with primary head and neck cancer every year (Parkin, Bray, Ferlay, & Pisani, 2005). Next to the traditional outcome measures of overall survival, tumor control, and complications, health related quality of life and functional health status measures have grown to become standard outcome parameters in clinical studies. With the incorporation of such tools, research has demonstrated that head and neck cancer and its treatment have a distinct impact on daily life compared to other cancer types. In addition to general complaints such as pain and fatigue, head and neck cancer patients are often confronted with changes in facial appearance, voice, speech, and swallowing problems, and related social withdrawal and emotional distress (Bjordal et al., 1999; Bjordal et al., 2001; Borggreven et al., 2005; De Graeff et al., 2000; Fung & Terrell, 2004; Hammerlid et al., 1999; Hammerlid & Taft, 2001; Kugaya et al., 2000; List & Pinar Bilir, 2004; Morton, 2003; Pauloski et al., 1998; Pauloski et al., 2002; Perry, Shaw, & Cotton, 2003; Schliephake & Jamil, 2002).

The past years have shown an improvement in the technical, surgical, and medical possibilities available to optimize the functional outcomes of patients with head and neck cancer. For instance, laser surgery has become a preferred treatment modality in selected cases of early glottic cancer, surgical voice restoration has become available for laryngectomees, and reconstruction of ablated tissues in advanced oral cavity and oropharynx cancer using free flaps have been found to improve functional characteristics of dynamic structures such as the tongue and pharynx. Further progress is ongoing, and in many clinical trials, such as those which examine organ-preservation treatment modalities (e.g., chemoradiation), functional status and health related quality of life assessment are key components of outcome measurement. However, despite the medical/technical improvements, many head and neck cancer patients still have voice, speech, or swallowing problems after treatment and require ongoing management by speech-language pathologists. For this reason, measures of the functional status of voice, speech, and swallowing pre- and posttreatment are necessary to fully document patient outcome. Such data is also needed to document the efficacy of voice, speech, and swallowing intervention with this population. In order to compile this necessary data, a working knowledge of the generic and specific outcome measures available for use with the head and neck population is essential.

The purpose of the current chapter is to provide an overview of the main types of outcome measures and assessment tools used in the evaluation of health related quality of life, and functional voice, speech, and swallowing outcomes. Specifically, the reader will become familiar with many of the main questionnaires, rating scales, and instruments currently used to evaluate, monitor progress, and record outcomes for patients with head and neck cancer. This overview is not meant to be conclusive: in clinical practice, many assessment outcome measures have been developed worldwide. Rather this review will focus on validated outcome measures that are widely used throughout the world and published in peer-reviewed literature. For each type of outcome measure and assessment approach, an example of a recently published study using the tool/measure/technique has been provided to provide context for patients with head and neck cancer.

## Health Related Quality of Life

The World Health Organization (www.who.int) has declared health to be a "state of complete physical, mental and social well-being, and not merely the absence of disease." In recent years much interest has been focused on integrating quality of life as an endpoint for cancer clinical trials. The general purpose of health related quality of life (QOL) assessment in clinical trials is to evaluate the well-being of individuals or groups of patients. It is known that self-reported health predicts mortality and morbidity and that it can be used to screen for high-risk groups (Fayers & Sprangers, 2002). QOL evaluation can also be used to improve clinical management of patients by obtaining real-time feedback from individuals on quality of life issues. In addition, data from individual patients' QOL assessments can facilitate improved communication between patients and their clinicians.

A large number of instruments have been developed for health related quality of life assessment and can be divided into (a) generic, (b) disease specific, and (c) symptom specific questionnaires. In the following section, examples will be given of several instruments within each of these categories that are in current use throughout the world. Because in most cases user registration and licensing is required, only short descriptions will be provided here with key references supplied to assist the reader in further reading.

## Health Related Quality of Life Instruments: Generic

Generic instruments focus on broad aspects of quality of life and health status, and are intended for use in general populations irrespective of the disease or condition of the patient. Most instruments address the following issues: total well-being, physical functioning, physical symptoms, emotional functioning, cognitive functioning, role functioning, social well-being, sexual functioning, and spiritual issues. Widely used generic instruments are the COOP/WONCA charts, the Medical Outcomes Study 36-item Short Form (SF-36), the EuroQol (EQ-5D), and the SEIQoL, which will be detailed below.

### The COOP/WONCA Charts

The COOP/WONCA charts (Van Weel, 1993) are often used in primary health care to determine the functional health status of groups of patients with chronic diseases. The COOP/WONCA charts represent six dimensions: physical fitness, mental well-being, daily activities, social activities, change in health, and overall health. Each chart consists of a question referring to the status over the past 2 weeks and five response levels, supported by simple drawings. Lower scores refer to better functioning, except for the chart "change in health," where a middle score represents no change in health and a higher score represents better and a lower score worse health. The COOP/WONCA charts are validated for many languages. More information can be found on http://www.globalfamilydoct or.com/publications/coop-woncacharts/Coopwo ncacharts.htm.

> ■ Example: Peeters et al. (2004) used the COOP/WONCA charts in a study on patients treated for early glottic cancer. They reported moderate correlations between voice problems and the COOP/WONCA social

activities chart, indicating a negative effect of voice problems on daily social activities.

### The Medical Outcomes Study 36-Item Short Form (SF-36)

The SF-36 (Aaronson et al., 1992) is a health survey with 36 items comprising eight scales: Physical Functioning, Role Limitations Due to Physical Health, Bodily Pain, General Health, Vitality, Social Functioning, Role Limitations Due to Emotional Problems, and Mental Health. The SF-36 has proven useful in surveys of general and specific populations, in comparing the relative burden of diseases, and in differentiating the health benefits produced by a wide range of different treatments. The SF-36 has been translated in more than 50 countries as part of the International Quality of Life Assessment (IQOLA) Project. More information can be found on http://www.sf-36.org.

> ■ Example: In a study of 570 patients with upper aerodigestive tract cancers, Terrell et al. (2004) reported that the presence of a feeding tube had the most negative impact on QOL, with deterioration on six of the eight SF-36 scales. In descending order of severity, medical comorbid conditions, presence of a tracheostomy tube, chemotherapy, and neck dissection were also associated with significant decrements in QOL domains. Patients who took the survey more than 1 year after diagnosis had improved QOL.

### The EuroQoL (EQ-5D)

The EQ-5D (The EuroQoL Group, 1990) consists of five dimensions (mobility, self-care, usual activities, pain/discomfort, anxiety/depression), each of which can take one of three responses (in total 15 items). The EQ-5D is being widely used by clinicians and researchers including the pharmaceutical industry. More information can be found on http://www.euroqol.org.

> ■ Example: Homs, Essink-Bot, Borsboom, Steyerberg, and Siersema (2004) used the EQ-5D in a study of metal stent placement and single dose brachytherapy for the palliation of inoperable esophageal carcinoma. Dysphagia improved more

rapidly after stent placement than after brachytherapy, but long-term relief of dysphagia was better after brachytherapy. Generic HRQOL deteriorated over time on all functional scales of the EQ-5D.

### Schedule for the Evaluation of Individual Quality of Life (SEIQoL)

The SEIQoL was developed to assess quality of life from the individual's perspective (McGee, O'Boyle, Hickey, O'Malley, & Joyce, 1991). This semistructured interview allows individuals to nominate the domains they consider most important to their quality of life, and to use their own value system when describing the functional status and relative importance of those domains. The procedure is as follows: first, the patient is asked to nominate the five most important aspects of their quality of life. Then, the patient is asked to score each nominated aspect according to its severity. Finally, relative weights for the importance of each item are given, which is called judgment analysis. As judgment analysis is impractical for individuals with cognitive impairment and in many clinical situations, a shorter, direct weighting procedure has been developed: the SEIQoL-DW. More information can be found on http://www.isoqol.org/.

■ Example: Sharpe, Butow, Smith, McConnell, and Clarke (2005) used the SEIQoL-DW to investigate response shift. Patients diagnosed with metastatic cancer were interviewed. Surviving patients were then re-interviewed 3 and 6 months later. The majority of patients showed restricted priorities close to the diagnosis of metastatic cancer. Half the sample shifted their priorities from one area to another over time. Response shift was found to be helpful for those who nominated domains that were poorly rated, but unhelpful for those who shifted from a highly rated life domain.

### Health Related Quality of Life Instruments: Cancer Specific

Cancer specific instruments have been developed to detect more subtle disease and treatment-related effects on QOL. They are expected to have better sensitivity to the health states of the patients involved. A cancer specific instrument can be used in clinical trials and may also provide detailed information of clinical relevance to the management of patients. Next to total well-being, physical functioning, physical symptoms, emotional functioning, cognitive functioning, role functioning, social well-being, sexual functioning, and spiritual issues which are part of generic questionnaires, most cancer specific questionnaires address issues of fatigue, pain, nausea, vomiting, and dyspnea. Two examples of widely used cancer specific questionnaires include the Quality of Life questionnaire (QLQ-C30) from the European Organization for Research and Treatment of Cancer (EORTC) and the Functional Assessment of Cancer Therapy—General (FACT-G).

### The EORTC QLQ-C30 Questionnaire

The EORTC QLQ-C30 Questionnaire (Aaronson et al., 1993) consists of 30 items and was designed to be multidimensional, and brief and easy to complete. The QLQ-C30 includes a global health related QOL scale (2 items) and five functional scales: physical functioning (5 items), role functioning (2 items), emotional functioning (4 items), cognitive functioning (2 items), and social functioning (2 items). There are three symptom scales: fatigue (3 items), nausea and vomiting (2 items), and pain (2 items), and 6 single items relating to dyspnea, insomnia, loss of appetite, constipation, diarrhea, and financial difficulties. The QLQ-C30 is available in a range of languages and has been widely used in multinational cancer clinical trials. The QLQ-C30 is a core questionnaire with several cancer site specific modules such as the head and neck QLQ-H&N35 Module (described later in chapter). The 15-item EORTC QLQ-C15-PAL is a shortened version of the QLQ-C30 and is a "core questionnaire" for palliative care. More information can be found on http://www.eortc.be/home/qol/.

■ Example: Fang et al. (2005) studied changes in quality of life for patients with advanced stage head and neck cancer following primary radiotherapy or concomitant chemoradiotherapy. Sixty-eight (46%) patients dropped out during the study period. Thirty-nine (57%) died of cancer.

Those who were older, had stage IV disease, were treated by radiotherapy alone, or had worse pretreatment EORTC QOL scales were significantly more likely to drop out. Those with cancer of the hypopharynx/larynx had a 3.3-fold higher probability to report an improvement in global QOL than those with cancer of the oral cavity/oropharynx.

## The Functional Assessment of Cancer Therapy—General (FACT-G)

The FACT-G (Cella et al., 1993) has a modular approach with a core questionnaire (the FACT-G) and several modules such as the FACT-H&N for head and neck cancer patients (described in later in chapter). The FACT-G contains 27 items with four subscales: physical well-being (7 items), social/family well-being (7 items), emotional well-being (6 items), and functional well-being (7 items). The FACT-G is available in a range of languages and has been widely used in multinational cancer clinical trials. The FACIT-PAL is a questionnaire focusing on patients in the palliative phase. More information can be found on http://www.facit.org.

■ Example: Sehlen et al. (2002) used the FACT-G in a cohort of 124 head-and-neck cancer patients who were treated by radiotherapy. They found that QOL did not change during treatment. Four socio-demographic variables (children, currently employed, ethanol abuse, level of secondary education) accounted for 26% of variance in QOL at six weeks after radiotherapy. They concluded that by routinely obtaining clinical information from the patient's history, patients at risk of low QOL after radiotherapy can be identified.

## Health Related Quality of Life Instruments: Head and Neck Cancer Specific

Several validated instruments are available specifically for use with patients with head and neck cancer. Most dedicated head and neck cancer questionnaires address issues on (oral) pain, speech, swallowing, oral dysfunction (as xerostomia, dry mouth, trismus), and social interaction. Next to the already mentioned EORTC QLQ-H&N35 and the FACT-H&N, the UW-QOL-R (University of Washington Quality of Life Head and Neck Questionnaire), the HNCI (Head and Neck Cancer Inventory), and the HNQOL (University of Michigan Head and Neck Quality of Life survey) are validated and widely used instruments to assess quality of life for patients with head and neck cancer. Next to these self-rated instruments, expert-rated instruments such as the TOM (Therapy Outcome Measures) and the HNPSS (Head and Neck Performance Status Scale) are used to obtain insight into specific head and neck cancer symptoms.

## The EORTC QLQ-H&N35 Module

The EORTC QLQ-H&N35 Module (Bjordal et al., 1999) is a site-specific module of the EORTC QLQ-C30 questionnaire (discussed previously), which covers specific issues relating to head and neck cancer. The 35-item questionnaire comprises seven subscales: pain (4 items), swallowing (5 items), senses (2 items), speech (3 items), social eating (4 items), social contact (5 items), and sexuality (2 items). There are 10 single items covering problems with teeth, dry mouth, sticky saliva, cough, opening the mouth wide, weight loss, weight gain, use of nutritional supplements, feeding tubes, and painkillers. More information can be found on http://www.eortc.be/home/qol/.

■ Example: Petruson, Silander, and Hammerlid (2005) evaluated whether weight loss can be predicted with QOL questionnaires. At diagnosis, those patients who had greater than 10% weight loss after treatment scored significantly worse on 15 of 28 QOL variables than did patients who lost less than 10%. The largest differences were found for: role functioning, fatigue, loss of appetite, global quality of life, sticky saliva, and swallowing. The fatigue scale was the only significant predictor of weight loss at diagnosis. It was concluded that patients with head and neck cancer who are at risk of severe weight loss developing during treatment may be detected with the aid of QOL questionnaires at diagnosis.

### The Functional Assessment of Cancer Therapy—Head and Neck (FACT-H&N)

The FACT-H&N (List et al., 1996) is a 12-item extension of the FACT-G (discussed previously). Items address additional concerns or symptoms as dry mouth (1 item), oral pain (1 item), breathing (1 item), speech (2 items), swallowing (4 items), facial appearance (1 item), and smoking/drinking habits (2 items). The FACT-H&N is available in a range of languages and has been widely used in multinational cancer clinical trials. The FHNSI is a shortened version of the FACT-H&N. More information can be found at http://www.facit.org.

■ Example: Ringash, Bezjak, O'Sullivan, and Redelmeier (2004) stated that QOL scores can be difficult to interpret. Their study goal was to estimate the magnitude of difference in QOL that is noticeable to patients. Laryngeal cancer patients rated their own QOL as compared to each other. The FACT-H&N score had to differ by 6.22 for patients to rate themselves as "a little bit better" relative to other patients and by 12.4 for patients to rate themselves as "a little bit worse" relative to others.

### University of Washington Quality of Life Head and Neck Questionnaire Revised (UW-QOL-R, Version 3)

The UW-QOL-R (version 3) (Weymuller, Alsarraf, Yueh, Deleyiannis, & Coltrera, 2001) consists of 10 head and neck specific items on pain, appearance, activity, recreation, swallowing, chewing, speech, shoulder, taste, and saliva and 3 items on general quality of life. The UW-QOL also asks the patients to prioritize these 10 items in order of importance and invites the patients to write comments in the form of free text. More information can be found on http://depts.washington.edu/soar/projects/dxcat/hnca/ qol_uw.htm.

■ Example: Zuydam, Lowe, Brown, Vaughan, and Rogers (2005) used the UW-QOL to investigate the association between speech and swallowing status and selected clinical parameters in 278 consecutive patients undergoing primary surgery, presurgery and

postsurgery at 6 months, 1 year, and later. Multiple logistic regression showed that no radiotherapy and primary surgical closure/laser surgery were the main predictors of good swallowing, and primary surgical closure/laser surgery was the main predictor of good speech at 1 year.

### Head and Neck Cancer Inventory (HNCI)

The HNCI is a 30-item questionnaire covering four domains: speech (10 items), eating (10 items), aesthetics (2 items), and social disruption (7 items). The questionnaire and the administration and scoring procedures are described in Funk, Karnell, Christensen, Moran, and Ricks (2003).

■ Example: El-Deiry et al. (2005) compared 27 patients who underwent surgery and postoperative radiation therapy with a group of 27 patients after concurrent chemotherapy and radiation therapy, more than 12 months after treatment. The domain scores on eating, speech, aesthetics, and social disruption were similar. They concluded that as nonsurgical means of treating head and neck cancer have become more aggressive and surgical techniques have become more focused on function preservation and rehabilitation, the overall health related quality of life resulting from these different approaches is similar.

### University of Michigan Head and Neck Quality of Life Survey (HNQOL)

The HNQOL is a 20-item survey composed of four domains: pain, emotion, communication, and eating and a single item on overall disturbance of bother. The questionnaire is described in Terrell et al. (1997).

■ Example: Eadie and Doyle (2005) determined QOL in 30 laryngectomees who used tracheoesophageal (TE) speech as their primary method of postlaryngectomy communication. Results revealed a high level of self-perceived QOL in the domains of communication, eating, pain, and emotion. They speculated that possible reasons for this good self-reported QOL include use of TE speech for postlaryngectomy communication, a higher level of education, and membership in a support group.

### Therapy Outcome Measures (TOM)

The TOM is an expert rated instrument and comprises 10 scales relating to a range of communication and swallowing disorders, and was developed to assess the efficacy of speech and language therapy (Enderby & John, 1999). Within each of the 10 scales, there are four five-point rating scales used to rate impairment, disability handicap, and distress/well-being. An Australian version (AusTOMs) with extension of the scales to occupational therapy and physiotherapy was developed in 2004 (Perry et al., 2004). The AusTOMs incorporates four five-point rating scales including: impairment, activity limitation, participation restriction, and distress/well-being.

■ Example: Mady, Sader, Hoole, Zimmermann, and Horch (2003) compared TOM ratings of speech and swallowing with an intelligibility test and the EORTC H&N35 module. There was a high intercorrelation between the results of subjective TOM speech evaluation and the intelligibility test, but no correlation with any of these methods could be shown for the self-evaluation by the participants. Dsyphagia was a more severe problem than speech impairment.

### Head and Neck Performance Status Scale (HNPS)

The HNPS is an expert rated instrument and consists of three subscales: eating in public, understandability of speech, and normalcy of diet. The HNPS is developed and described by List, Ritter-Sterr, and Lansky (1990).

■ Example: Campbell et al. (2004) determined associations between objective assessments (swallowing function and weight change) and subjective quality of life measures in a

group of patients with head and neck cancer. Aspiration was associated with decreased QOL scores in chewing, swallowing, and normalcy of diet.

## Health Related Quality of Life Instruments: Symptom Specific

Several symptom specific instruments that relate to voice, speech, and swallowing are available, and these will be the primary focus of the following sections. Once again, it is beyond the scope of the present chapter to go into detail on all voice, speech, and swallowing scales available. Rather, in the following sections a number of the key scales in current use will be outlined and references will be provided to assist readers seeking further information. A research publication that has used one of each type of symptom specific scale (voice, speech, and swallowing) is also provided for the reader as an example of their application to the head and neck cancer population.

### Voice

Quality of life questionnaires that specifically relate to voice production include: the 30-item Voice Handicap Index (VHI) (Jacobson et al., 1997), the 10-item Voice Related Quality of Life questionnaire (VRQOL) (Hogikan & Sethuraman, 1999), the 28-item Voice Activity and Participation Profile (VAPP) (Ma & Yiu, 2001), a 5-item list for screening purposes (Van Gogh et al., 2005), and the S-Secel (Finizia, Palme, & Bergman, 2002). Of these, the VHI is the most widely used questionnaire in laryngeal cancer studies. The VHI consists of 30 statements on voice-related aspects in daily life (with five response levels). Summarizing the scores on the 30 statements leads to a total VHI score, ranging from 0 to 120. A higher score corresponds to a worse voice-related functional status. Furthermore, the VHI includes an overall question on the quality of the voice with four response levels including 0 (good), 1 (reasonable), 2 (moderate), and 3 (poor).

■ Example: Schindler et al. (2005) used the VHI in addition to voice quality analyses in 20 male subjects who underwent a supracricoid laryngectomy (SCL). Subjective and objective data showed a severely dysphonic voice after SCL; self-assessment data revealed only moderate functional and emotional consequences. They concluded that self-assessment explores a different dimension of the patient's voice and that even if a severe dysphonia is present the consequences on everyday oral communication may be only moderate.

### Speech

Regarding speech related quality of life, no specific questionnaires are available. Recently, Rinkel, Verdonck-de Leeuw, and Leemans (2005) developed the Speech Handicap Index (SHI) for patients with cancer of the oral cavity or pharynx. Similar to the VHI, the SHI consists of 30 items on speech problems in daily life (maximum SHI 120) and an extra question on overall speech quality.

■ Example: Rinkel et al. (2005) investigated psychometric characteristics of the SHI in a cohort of 92 patients after treatment of cancer of the oral cavity or pharynx and a cohort of 110 randomly chosen subjects from the normal population. SHI reliability appeared to be high with high internal consistency and test-retest stability. The SHI differentiated patients from controls. Tumor stage and location appeared to influence SHI scores.

### Swallowing

The two main swallowing specific quality of life questionnaires in current use include the SWAL-QOL and SWAL-CARE (McHorney et al., 2002), and the M. D. Anderson Dysphagia Inventory (MDADI) (Chen et al., 2001). The SWAL-QOL is a 44-item tool that assesses dysphagia related quality of life scales: general health, general burden, food selection, eating duration, eating desire, fear of eating, sleep, fatigue, communication, mental health, and social functioning. Furthermore, symptom items such as coughing, choking, saliva, gagging, drooling, chewing, and throat problems are evaluated. The SWAL-CARE is a 15-item tool that assesses quality of care and patient satisfaction. The scales differentiate normal swallowers from patients with oropharyngeal dysphagia and are sensitive to differences in the severity of dysphagia as clinically defined. The 20-item MDADI includes a global total score and an emotional, functional, and physical subscale.

■ Example: Lovell, Wong, Loh, Ngo, and Wilson (2005) used the SWAL-QOL in addition to the UW-QOL to determine the impact of dysphagia on QOL in 51 patients treated for nasopharyngeal carcinoma (NPC). Self-reported swallowing difficulty appeared to predict a lower HR-QOL score. It was recommended that future QOL studies relating to swallowing function associated with nasopharyngeal cancer use a swallowing specific questionnaire such as the SWAL-QOL, in addition to head and neck specific questionnaires.

## Assessing Functional Outcomes: Voice and Speech

In the following sections, the ways of measuring voice and speech will be discussed. These include perceptual ratings, acoustical analyses of the speech and voice signal, imaging techniques, and aerodynamic analyses of voice and speech production. Of these, it is acknowledged that clinicians often place primary reliance on their highly trained ears when conducting voice and speech outcome evaluations. Behrman (2005) reported that in common diagnostic practice of voice therapists, voice quality, observation of body posture and movement, and probing the patient's ability to alter voice production are each significantly more likely to be performed than the more objective stroboscopic, acoustic, aerodynamic, and EGG assessments. It is, however, recognized that a voice analysis protocol should be multidimensional, including more than just perceptual ratings, incorporating acoustic analyses, aerodynamics, and imaging techniques for comprehensive evaluation (Dejonckere et al., 2001).

Selection of voice and speech analyses is not easy and depends on a number of considerations including: the cancer site and treatment modality (e.g., evaluating voice outcome in laryngectomees requires different assessment tools and protocols than the measurement of voice outcome following radiation for early glottic cancer); the type of voice or speech disorder (e.g., assessing nasality requires a different acoustic analysis technique than assessing pitch); the skills of the investigator/clinician (e.g., performing perceptual ratings needs extensive training); the invasiveness of a technique for a patient (e.g., providing a "sustained /a/" for acoustical analyses is less invasive than endoscopic evaluation); and financial resources (e.g., costs associated with instrumentation versus perceptual assessment). The following sections provide an overview of various imaging, perceptual, acoustic, and physiological outcome measures for voice and speech that are in use throughout the world. Within each main section, an example of a recent study on head and neck cancer will be provided to exemplify the nature of the information provided by each type of assessment approach.

## Imaging Techniques

Visual inspection of the head and neck structures including the neck, ears, nose, oral cavity, and nasopharynx is standard procedure for patients with head and neck cancer. In addition to visual inspection of the easily accessible structures of the head and neck, various other techniques including laryngoscopy, nasopharyngoscopy, and ultrasonic imaging techniques are available to assist the clinician to conduct more detailed examination of internal structures.

Laryngoscopy is used to assess the supraglottic laryngeal structures as well as examine vocal fold movement and vibration. This procedure can be performed by means of a laryngeal mirror or a rigid laryngoscope introduced via the oral cavity. Using this type of assessment, laryngeal and vocal fold function can only be observed during sustained vowels. In comparison, the use of a flexible endoscope introduced via the nose, passed into the oropharynx and positioned above the level of the larynx, enables the clinician to view the larynx and vocal fold motion during connected speech.

To enable more detailed assessment of vocal fold vibration, assessment techniques such as laryngoscopy under stroboscopic illumination (laryngostroboscopy), videokymography, and high speed imaging can be utilized. Laryngostroboscopy combines a strobe light source with laryngoscopic assessment. Depending on the frequency of the stroboscopic light, portions of the vibratory cycle of the vocal folds are illuminated such that vocal fold motion appears either stopped or slowed by the optical illusion of stroboscopic light. This allows close examination of the vocal folds at a particular stage of the glottic cycle or slow motion representation of the full glottic cycle (see Figure 2-1). As the technique is based on the assumption of a regular glottic cycle, difficulties are encountered when examining patients with irregular vocal fold vibration.

In contrast, videokymography (VKG) and digital high speed imaging are new methods to investigate vocal fold behavior, including irregular vocal fold vibration. VKG involves the use of a modified video camera, coupled to a standard rigid endoscope and constant light source. VKG is capable of capturing high-speed vocal fold motion using high speed imaging of one preselected line (up to 8000 lines/second) which is recorded to a standard videocassette recorder for review and analysis. When the film is then viewed, the motion of the vocal folds is slowed, allowing close examination of vocal fold movement, including open and closed phases of the glottal cycle, opening and closing movements, displacements of the upper and lower vocal fold margins, and propagation of mucosal waves. The high image capture rate allows direct observation of vocal fold movement even if it is aperiodic. Figure 2-2 shows a VKG recording of regular (top) and irregular (bottom) vibrating vocal folds. Digital high speed imaging cameras have a lower recording rate of 2000 images per second with lower spatial resolution, but they do record the complete image of the larynx. If an image similar to a VKG is desired, one can choose a line on the high speed recording and a VKG can be produced.

Direct visualization of velopharyngeal function is conducted using endoscopic or nasoendoscopic procedures. Nasoendoscopy involves passing a flexible endoscope through the nasal passage until it is positioned above the velopharyngeal port. By having the patient produce a number of non-nasal and nasal sounds, words, and passages, as well as reflexive behaviors such as swallowing, the clinician can obtain information on velopharyngeal closure patterns and velopharyngeal competence during speech.

Ultrasound imaging is a harmless and non-invasive method of obtaining direct visualization of internal structures. It involves sending high-frequency sound

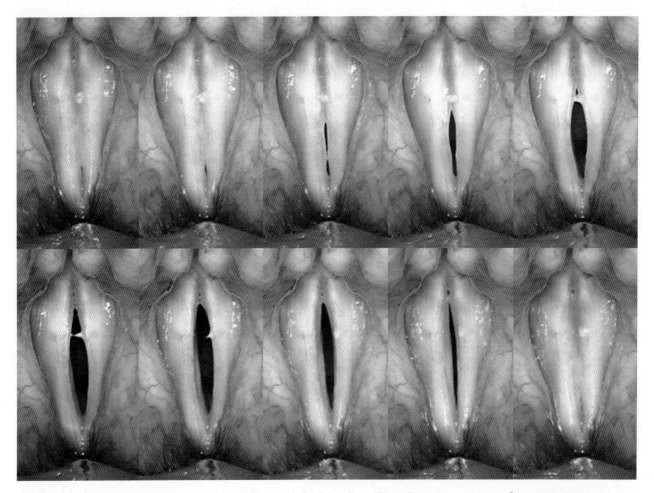

**Figure 2–1.** Stroboscopic images of a normal glottal cycle. (Photo courtesy of KayPENTAX)

waves into the body that are reflected, refracted, or absorbed, and the returning echoes carry information about the size, distance, and uniformity of the structure under investigation. A handheld transducer, generating ultrasound and detecting and transmitting the returning echoes, is placed on the area being examined and moved around. The ultrasound images can be displayed on a screen or recorded for further analyses. Ultrasound can be used to examine lingual function during speech. Some experience viewing ultrasound images is required to optimize the use of this technique.

■ Example: Bressmann, Uy, and Irish (2005) studied tongue movement using ultrasound imaging. The results revealed a protrusion and retraction component that is represented by the measurement points on the posterior

tongue, a tongue tip control component that is represented by the measurement points on the tongue blade, and a dorsal height and position control component that is represented by the measurement points on the tongue dorsum.

## Perceptual Ratings

To standardize perceptual ratings of voice and speech quality, several rating protocols have been developed which can be divided in global and detailed protocols. Detailed protocols are further subdivided into voice and speech rating protocols. Speech material required for completion of perceptual scales usually comprises standardized text or sentences. Adapted texts are used

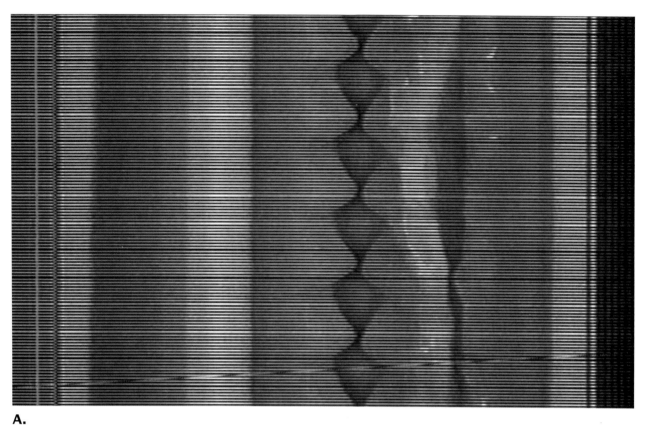

**A.**

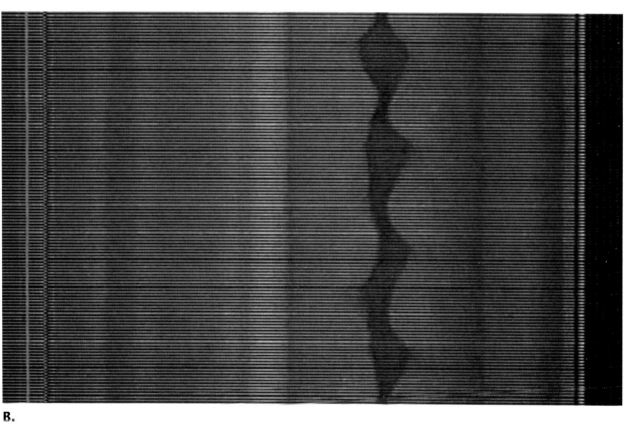

**B.**

**Figure 2–2.** Examples of videokymographic recordings of regular **A.** and irregular **B.** vibrating vocal folds. Each line captures the vocal folds at a preselected position.

for specific purposes; for example, to evaluate nasality, standardized text with and without nasals can be used.

Global ratings include ratings on overall voice or speech quality, intelligibility, acceptability, or communicative suitability. Ratings are usually based on a 3-item (for instance, good-moderate-poor), 4-item (for instance, good-reasonable-moderate-poor), 5-item (for instance, good-good/moderate-moderatemoderate/poor-poor), 10-item, or a visual analogue scale (ranging from good to poor). Global evaluations can be made by experts or naïve listeners.

The most widely used voice rating protocol is the GRBAS protocol as proposed by the Japanese Society of Logopedics and Phoniatrics (Hirano, 1981). The GRBAS protocol is used by clinicians to categorize the voice using five descriptive perceptual parameters: overall grade or severity (G), roughness of the voice (R), breathiness (B), asthenia (A), and strain (S). For head and neck cancer purposes, adapted voice rating protocols have been developed for patients after treatment for early glottic cancer (Verdonck-de Leeuw et al., 1999) and for laryngectomized patients (Van As, Koopmans-van Beinum, Pols, & Hilgers, 2003; Moerman et al., 2006).

Speech rating protocols include ratings on supralaryngeal, pharyngeal, or oral aspects. Laver's Vocal Profile Analysis Protocol (VPAP) is a phonetically based system consisting of four sections: vocal quality (supralaryngeal, pharyngeal, laryngeal features), prosody (pitch, consistency, and loudness), temporal organization (continuity, rate), and comments (breath support, rhythmicality, diplophonia) (Laver, 1991). VPAP as such is not widely used, but many institution-developed versions have been developed worldwide.

Other analytic speech transcription protocols feature analyses using the International Phonetic Alphabet (IPA). Feature analyses include consonant ratings regarding manner of articulation (plosive, fricative, liquidae, nasal, semivowel), place of articulation (bilabial, labiodental, dental, alveolar, retroflex, palato-alveolar, palatal, velar, and uvular), and voicing (voiced or not; voice onset time). Vowel ratings include grade of opening of the mouth, lip-rounding, and tongue position (front-back). For pathological speech, an extension of the IPA, the extIPA system, was developed (Duckworth, Hardcastle, & Ball, 1990). See also: http://www.arts.gla.ac.uk/ipa/ipa.html.

◼ Example: Borggreven et al. (2005) used tests on communicative suitability, intelligibility, articulation, nasality, and consonant errors with a control group and patients with advanced oral or oropharyngeal cancer before treatment, and 6 and 12 months after treatment. Speech tests were significantly worse for patients before and after treatment compared with the controls. Speech did not improve between 6 and 12 months. After treatment, patients with T3-4 tumors showed a significantly worse speech quality than patients with T2 tumors.

## Acoustic Analyses

Although perceptual ratings of voice and speech quality are a standard component of most assessment protocols, they are subjective and require extensive training procedures to increase reliability between different raters. Therefore, in clinical trials, perceptual ratings are often not feasible and sufficiently uniform. Acoustical voice analysis on the other hand can be performed quickly and objectively. There are several software packages available such as the Computerized Speech Lab (CSL) with VisiPitch and the Multidimensional Voice Program (www.kayelemetrics.com), dr Speech (www.drspeech.com), or PRAAT (www.praat.org). Speech material used for analyses of pitch, loudness, and speech rate usually consists of recordings of spontaneous speech or reading. Speech material for voice analyses usually consists of sustained vowels, while consonant-vowel utterances or short sentences are used for speech analyses. The most common forms of acoustic analysis examine the waveform of the speech sound (oscillogram), the spectrum, and the spectrogram.

### Oscillogram

In an *oscillogram*, the horizontal axis displays the time axis and the curve shows how the loudness increases and decreases in the speech signal. Figure 2–3 shows an example of the oscillogram of the whole word "cancer".

## Spectrum

A *spectrum* represents a distribution of frequency (horizontal axis) and amplitude (vertical axis) of the speech sound at one moment in time. Voiced speech sounds are the result of a combination of the glottal sound source (energy produced by the vibrating vocal folds) and the vocal tract filter (the resonator characteristics as produced by the tongue, lips, jaws, velum, oral cavity, nasal cavity, etc,). The vibration frequency of the sound source is determined by the mass, elasticity, and tension of the vocal folds (or neoglottis in case of laryngectomees). The vibration of the vocal folds creates a periodical waveform that can be described as the sum of a number of single harmonic sine waves, each with a particular amplitude, frequency, and phase. Figure 2-4 shows the periodical waveform of some

periods of the vowel /a/ in the word "cancer". Each pitch period is the result of one single vocal fold vibration. The number of pitch periods per second defines the fundamental frequency (F0, pitch) of the voice.

The harmonic with the lowest frequency is called the fundamental frequency (F0), and all other harmonics are ideally integer multiples of F0. Most energy is concentrated in the lower frequencies and the amplitude level decreases approximately 6 dB per octave. The glottal sound source is then modified by various configurations of the vocal tract with resonances on specific frequencies (called formants) which are numbered from the bottom up as F1, F2, F3, etc. Additional sound sources for consonants include frication noise (fricatives), turbulence noise (glides, liquids), aspiration noise (the /h/), and release bursts (plosives). The spectrum is created by means of Fourier analysis which

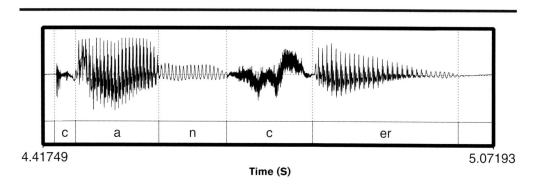

4.41749                                                                     5.07193

**Time (S)**

**Figure 2–3.** Oscillogram of the word "cancer".

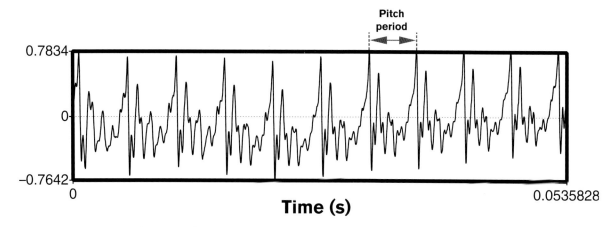

**Figure 2–4.** Periodic waveform from the middle of the /a/ sound in the word "cancer".

decomposes the complex speech wave into its constituent sine waves. Figure 2–5 shows the spectrum of the waveform of the /a/ sound displayed in Figure 2–4.

## Spectrogram

The *spectrogram* is a three-dimensional representation of the spectrum with the time axis on the horizontal axis and the frequency on the vertical axis. The amplitude is represented by shades of darkness. Narrow-band spectrograms have better frequency resolution showing individual harmonics of voiced sounds and are more often used in voice analyses; wide-band spectrograms have better temporal resolution showing rapid articulatory changes and are more often used in speech analyses. Figure 2–6 shows a wide-band spec-

trogram of the word "cancer", and Figure 2–7 a narrow-band spectrogram of the same word. Voiced sounds (like the vowels) are quasi-periodic with horizontal spectral bands representing the formants. The positions of the formants are different for different sounds. In plosive consonants (like the /k/ in cancer), there is a long period of silence followed by the burst with strong energy. In nasal sounds (like the /n/ in cancer), a clear energy drop can be seen. In the unvoiced fricative sounds (like the /s/ in cancer), the energy is noise-like and concentrated high up in the frequency band.

## Pitch and Loudness Measurements

Pitch is the perceptual correlate of frequency and is usually measured by the average fundamental frequency

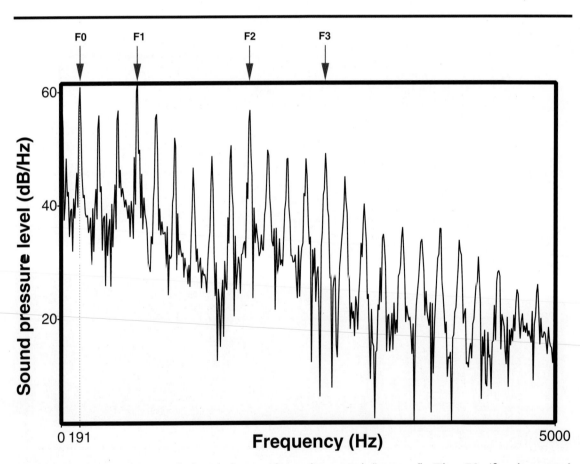

**Figure 2–5.** Spectrum of the /a/ sound in the word "cancer". The F0 (fundamental frequency, pitch) is 191 Hz. F1, F2, and F3 are the resonance peaks at the formant frequencies that determine the sound of the vowel.

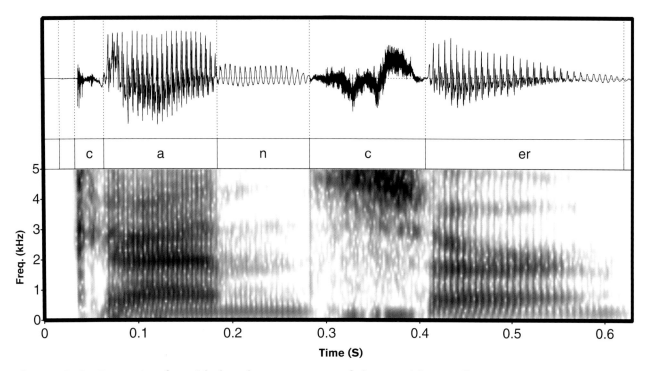

**Figure 2–6.** Example of a wide-band spectrogram of the word "cancer".

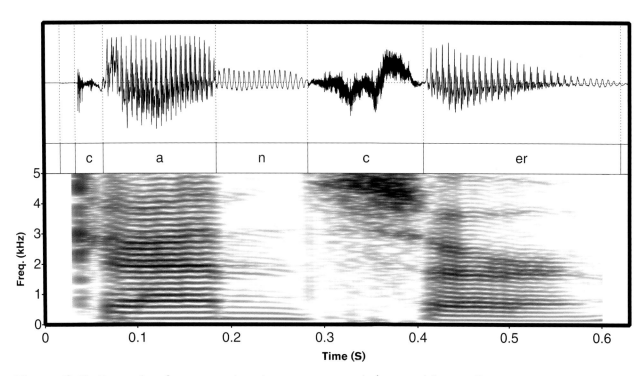

**Figure 2–7.** Example of a narrow-band spectrogram of the word "cancer".

(F0) during running speech (in Hz). Loudness is the perceptual correlate of intensity but is also related to pitch and spectral characteristics. Intensity is usually measured by the average sound pressure level (SPL) during running speech (in dB). Patients are typically asked to produce speech as soft and as loud as they can to obtain insight into minimal and maximal SPL levels. Also, patients can be asked to produce SPL levels at their conversational speech level. For all acoustic measures, though particularly for repeated measurements of intensity, the mouth-microphone distance should be kept constant, usually at 30 centimeters. Using a headset microphone can facilitate a constant mouth to microphone distance.

A Voice Range Profile (VRP), also called phonetogram, can also be used to give insight into the range of pitch and intensity of a speaker's voice. The basic instrumentation required to create a VRP consists of a tone generator and a sound pressure level (SPL) measuring device. The speaker is asked to produce a sustained /a/ as loud and as soft as possible at various frequencies (pitch) (Verdonck-de Leeuw et al., 1999). There are also programs available, such as the Voice Range Profile (www.kayelemetrics.com) or the Voice Profiler (www.alphatron.com), that help generate VRPs.

### Speech Rate, Speech Quality, and Temporal Measurements

Voice and speech quality analyses can be performed in the time domain (oscillogram) or the frequency domain (spectrum/spectrogram). Speech rate is usually measured by calculating the average number of words or syllables per minute during reading out loud a standardized text: the average speech rate. Other temporal characteristics such as the duration of single sounds can be measured either in the time or frequency domain. Speech quality analyses such as formant measures of vowels are performed in the spectral domain.

### Voice Quality Measurements

Spectral voice quality parameters include the harmonics-to-noise ratio (HNR), the signal-to-noise ratio (SNR) (Yumoto, Sasaki, & Okamuro, 1984), the difference between the amplitudes of the first and second harmonics, and the spectral slope. The spectral slope represents the ratio between the energy in the lower harmonics (below 1 kHz) and the higher harmonics (1–5 kHz) and higher (>5 kHz) and can be measured on a single vowel or from running speech. Temporal voice quality parameters include perturbation measurements: distortions in the period frequency (jitter) or period amplitude (shimmer).

Nasality can be measured by means of the nasalance score, which is defined as the ratio between the nasal sound pressure level and the nasal plus oral sound pressure level. To measure the nasalance score, specific instruments are available, such as the Nasometer (KayPENTAX, www.kayelemetrics.com).

Although the previous section has discussed a number of different acoustic measures that can be used to document changes in voice and speech, the major limitation of acoustic analysis for patients with pathological voice change is the high variability among voices and often weak signal periodicity, due to vocal fold irregularities. As many acoustical analysis programs calculate periodicity aspects in the time domain of the acoustical voice signal, this can lead to unreliable results for poor (nonperiodic) voices on time domain parameters such as pitch and perturbation measurements (Carding et al., 2004; Moerman, Pieters, Martens, Van der Borgt, & Dejonckere, 2004; Titze, 1994; Van As, Hilgers, Verdonck-de Leeuw, & Koopmans-van Beinum, 1998; Van Rossum, de Krom, Nooteboom, & Quene, 2002). Acoustical voice analysis using the spectral domain has proven to provide more robust acoustical parameters for pathological voices, as for instance tracheoesophageal (TE) voices of laryngectomized patients (Van Gogh et al., 2005).

Obviously, reliable acoustical parameters cannot be obtained in patients with chaotic, nonperiodic noisy voices, such as tracheoesophageal speakers. In that case, acoustic signal typing is recommended. Titze (1994) first introduced acoustic signal typing, which involved visual inspection of the speech signal and spectrogram and classifying each person's data using three categories of sound signals: (1) signals are nearly periodic, (2) signals contain intermittency, strong subharmonics, or modulations, and (3) chaotic or random signals. Reliable acoustical parameters as pitch and perturbation can be obtained for voice signals categorized as type 1, but not for type 2 or 3 signals. In a later study, Lawson, Jamart, and Remacle (2001) used the concept of acoustical signal typing with their patients who had undergone Tucker's reconstructive (partial) laryngectomy. They assigned spectrograms into five categories: 0—no phonation, I—noise present and no harmonics or fundamental frequency, II—noise and a fundamental frequency present but no or rudimentary harmonics, III—rudimentary fundamental frequency and harmonics, and IV—no noise and present fundamental frequency and harmonics. Van As-Brooks, Koopmans-van Beinum, Pols, and Hilgers (2006) defined four categories for laryngectomized voices, based on visual inspection of spectrograms: (1) stable and harmonic, (2) stable and at least one harmonic, (3) unstable or partly harmonic, and (4) barely harmonic. Van Gogh et al. (2005) used robust acoustical parameters to categorize tracheoesophageal voice into three categories. This simplification into three categories is helpful in clinical practice, because objective acoustical categorization can substitute the subjective categorization of patients as good, moderate, or poor based on perceptual ratings of TE voice quality.

■ Example: Van Gogh et al. (2005) demonstrated the efficacy of voice therapy for patients with voice problems after treatment for early glottic cancer. Multidimensional voice analyses (the Voice Handicap Index, acoustic and perceptual voice quality analysis, videolaryngostroboscopy, and the Voice Range Profile) showed significant voice improvement after voice therapy on the total VHI score, percent jitter, and noise-to-harmonics ratio in the voice signal and on the perceptual rating of vocal fry.

## Physiological Measures

Although acoustic analyses are used in clinical trials and to monitor efficacy of therapy or treatment, no direct link can be made between the acoustic data and physiological functioning. Therefore, for comprehensive assessment, physiological analyses are needed (Thompson-Ward & Murdoch, 1998). To obtain insight in voice and speech physiology, several physiological tests are available including electromyography, electroglottography, electropalatography, electromagnetic articulography, and aerodynamic performance. A brief overview will be given of the various techniques. More information can be found in Thompson-Ward and Mur-

doch (1998), Baken and Orlikoff (2000), and Maassen, Kent, Peters, Van Lieshout, and Hulstijn (2004).

Electromyography (EMG) is used to evaluate the motor system during voice, speech, swallowing status, or shoulder function after neck dissection. During EMG, the patient is laid down on an exam table and tiny needles are inserted into various muscles of interest to measure electrical activity. The patient is asked to perform certain vocal or swallowing tasks for each muscle tested. EMG examination takes less than 5 minutes and most patients tolerate the test well, although brief pain or discomfort during insertion of the needles can be experienced. Usually the resulting EMG signal is visually inspected on an oscilloscope, but quantitative measurements are also possible.

Electroglottography (EGG) is a non-invasive method to investigate vocal fold adduction by measuring the degree of conductance for a small high-frequency electrical current flowing between electrodes placed on opposite sides of the neck at the level of the larynx. The opening and closing of the vocal folds causes variation in the electrical resistance of the current. These changes in resistance are then displayed on a screen. The EGG signal of the fast vocal fold movements may be confounded by other movements such as laryngeal elevation or heartbeat. Visual inspection of the EGG signal gives insight into the opening and closing phase and maximum contact of the vocal folds.

Electropalatography (EPG) records the timing and location of tongue contact with the hard palate during continuous speech using a custom made acrylic palate fitted with electrodes (see Figure 2–8). When the tongue comes into contact with the plate, the electrode signals are conducted to a processing unit and displayed on a computer screen providing the viewer with a display of lingual-palatal contact from first initial contact, through to the point of maximum palatal contact, and until full release. From this information, articulatory closure patterns and temporal articulatory measures can be determined. While the majority of EPG research to date has focused on articulatory disorders in children and in experimental phonetics research, there is a growing body of research employing EPG in acquired motor speech disorders in adults. For further information, see McAuliffe and Ward (in press).

Electromagnetic articulography (EMA) utilizes alternating electromagnetic fields to track articulator movements over time during speech production.

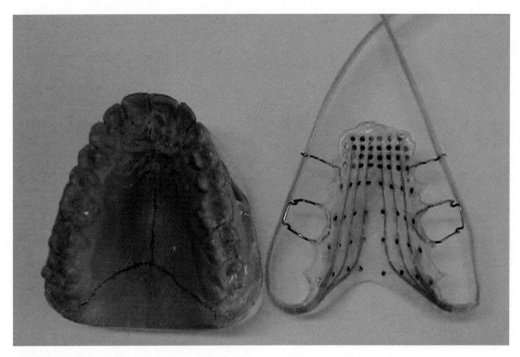

**Figure 2–8.** Example of an EPG palate (right) and plaster mold (left) used to create the individual patient palate.

Three transmitter coils are mounted equidistant from one another on a rigid helmet so that they generate a radially symmetric alternating electromagnetic field at different frequencies (see Figure 2-9). A number of receiver coils (sensors) are placed on the patient's articulators (tongue, jaw, lips, and teeth) along the mid-sagittal plane. The induced voltages on these receiver coils are sampled and stored in a computer. Software packages are available to analyze the data in the two- and three-dimensional domain, giving insight into parameters such as the displacement, velocity, and acceleration and deceleration of lingual function during the approach, closure, and release phases of target consonant productions.

Aerodynamic performance can be evaluated by measuring airflow, air pressure, and phonatory ability. Usually, a spirometer or pneumotachograph is used. Air volume is measured by the use of a mask fitted tightly over the face into a mouthpiece with nose clips to avoid nasal escape. The mean flow rate is calculated by dividing the total volume of air used during phonation by the duration of phonation. Maximum phona-

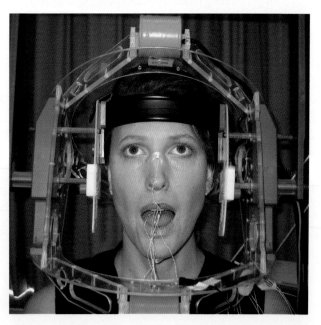

**Figure 2–9.** Example of an EMA system for assessment of articulatory function. Note receiver coils attached to lips and tongue and a reference coil on bridge of nose.

tion can be measured using a stopwatch. The patient is instructed to sustain the vowel /a/ for as long as possible following deep inspiration, vocalizing at comfortable pitch and loudness levels. The phonation quotient is defined as the vital capacity (the amount of air that can be forcefully expelled from fully inflated lungs) divided by the maximum phonation time. Pressure measurements require the use of a probe attached to a pressure transducer, which can be positioned either in the trachea or oral cavity. Tracheal and subglottic pressure requires an invasive procedure such as tracheal puncture or transglottal catheter. Determining intraoral pressure is less invasive, as the transducer can be simply positioned in the oral cavity during speech. Measuring intraoral pressure can be useful in obtaining insight in the relation between oral pressure and the production of speech sounds.

■ Example: Wakumoto et al. (1996) reported speech evaluation by means of electropalatography (EPG), acoustical analysis, and speech intelligibility for patients after two different glossectomy procedures: directly sutured (n = 5) or reconstructed with forearm flap (n = 5). Speech intelligibility and acoustical analysis were investigated presurgery, and 1, 6, and 12 months postoperation. EPG data were collected 6 months postsurgery. Acoustical analyses were carried out by consonant frequency characteristics and formant variance from consonant to vowel transitions. Results revealed that participants reconstructed with a forearm flap showed better speech function than those who were directly sutured. Articulatory characteristics determined from the acoustical analysis were more in agreement with the results of EPG assessment than with the results of the speech intelligibility test.

## Assessing Functional Outcomes: Swallowing

The swallowing sequence is divided into the oral, pharyngeal, and esophageal stages. Studies of swallowing function in patients with head and neck cancer reveal that dysphagia is common, especially in patients with advanced oral or oropharyngeal cancer. Any of the swallowing phases can be compromised, dependent on tumor size and site. In general, patients treated for larger, extended tumors have more swallowing problems; patients with resection of the anterior tongue and floor of the mouth experience problems in the oral phase while patients after resection of the tongue including the tongue base encounter swallowing dysfunction in the pharyngeal stage as well (see Chapters 5 and 7). Additional effects of radiotherapy such as fibrosis and xerostomia can have negative consequences on swallowing (see Chapter 3). Severe swallowing dysfunction can lead to aspiration pneumonia and/or the need for long-term alternative feeding to meet nutritional needs.

Various methods can be used to evaluate swallowing function in the head and neck cancer population including: clinical swallowing examination (medical history, oral/oropharyngeal examination, and observing symptomatic dysphagia), objective evaluation techniques (videofluoroscopy, fiberoptic evaluation [FEES], scintigraphy, manometry), and rating scales of dysphagia severity and disability levels. Each of these will be discussed briefly in the following sections. Additional references for further reading and an example of a recent study involving the head and neck cancer population have been provided for each form of assessment.

## Clinical Examination

Specific details regarding the clinical examination of swallowing can be found elsewhere (for example, see Logemann, 1998; Miller, 1997); however, in brief, the clinical swallowing examination includes a medical history, oral/oropharyngeal examination, and swallow trials. The medical history is compiled from the patient's medical record and consultation with the physician and nursing staff, the family, and the patient. Key indicators of swallowing problems include a history of swallowing complaints, incidents of coughing/choking or regurgitation, difficulty or avoidance of some food consistencies, poor nutrition, presence of a feeding tube, any prior oral/oropharyngeal resection or radiation (with or without chemotherapy), history of pneumonia or respiratory compromise/disease, and any prior neurological injury/insult.

Following a thorough medical history, the oral/oropharyngeal examination involves inspection of the oral cavity and oral health including dental status (prostheses) and saliva management (xerostomia, drooling), as well as direct evaluation of the strength, motion, and symmetry of the tongue, lips, jaws, and soft palate. Furthermore, sensation of the lips, cheeks, palate, tongue, and pharynx is evaluated. Observing symptomatic dysphagia in selected patients includes a swallowing trial, which incorporates trials of various food and fluid consistencies. Bolus size and characteristics (taste, temperature) can be modified to examine any change. Multiple swallows may be observed to explore fatigue effects throughout a meal.

Level of swallowing disability as determined from the clinical bedside assessment can be quantified using scales such as the Royal Brisbane Hospital Outcome Measure for Swallowing (RBHOMS, Ward & Conroy, 1999). The RBHOMS is a swallowing disability rating scale, designed to monitor difficulties in everyday swallowing function based on clinical indicators of swallowing, not specific diet/fluid consistencies. Psychometric analysis reveals it to be a valid clinical tool for documenting change in swallowing disability over time and across patients with different etiologies (Ward & Conroy, 1999). The RBHOMS contains 10 levels of function (Level 1: patient aspirates secretions, to Level 10: swallowing function better than premorbid/preadmission level) spread across four main functional stages (Stage 1: nil by mouth, Stage 2: commencing oral intake, Stage 3: establishing oral intake, and Stage 4: maintaining oral intake). Level of disability is recorded at each clinical assessment to chart progress and patterns of change during the course of dysphagia management.

■ Example: Su, Chen, and Sheng (2002) examined outcomes following two methods of tongue reconstruction, radial forearm free flap transfer (n = 19) and pectoralis major flap transfer (n = 6). Swallowing and speech function were evaluated 6 months to 5 years after the reconstruction. Speech intelligibility and an articulation test were used. Clinical evaluation of deglutition included a questionnaire on dietary habits and a swallowing rating of 1 to 7. Patients with free flap reconstruction had more intelligible speech. Assessment of data obtained by clinical questionnaire showed no significant difference between the two groups in swallowing function.

## Objective Assessment

Videofluoroscopic swallowing study (VFSS) and modified barium swallow (MBS) visualize movements in oral preparation, oral, pharyngeal swallowing stages. During VFSS, patients either stand upright or are seated in a special swallowing chair, in the videofluoroscopic suite. Assessment typically involves trials of thin liquids, thick liquids, semisolids, and solids (such as a cookie or a marshmallow) coated with barium paste. Anterior/posterior and lateral views of the oral cavity, pharynx, and upper part of the esophagus are then observed as the patients swallow. A carefully defined protocol incorporates administration of various bolus sizes and types and is described in detail in Logemann (1993, 1998). An example of a swallowing sequence as observed on MBS in a patient without swallowing problems is given in Figure 2–10.

MBS analysis typically involves discussion of oral, pharyngeal, and laryngeal anatomy as well as an evaluation of swallow physiology. Visual observations of aspiration and penetration can be observed (see Figure 2–11) and then quantified using scales such as the penetration-aspiration scale (Rosenbek, Robbins, Roecker, Coyle, & Wood, 1996), an eight-point, equal-appearing interval scale to describe penetration and aspiration events. Additional temporal measurements can be made from the MBS recording, including oral transit time (time it takes the bolus to move through the oral cavity) and pharyngeal transit time (time it takes the bolus to move through the pharynx). Estimates of oral residue (approximate percent oral residue after the first swallow) and pharyngeal residue (approximate percent pharyngeal residue after the first swallow) can also be documented. This information can be used to calculate oropharyngeal swallow efficiency (OPSE; Logemann & Kahrilas, 1990), which is determined by measuring the percentage of bolus swallowed into the esophagus divided by the total (oral and pharyngeal) transit time.

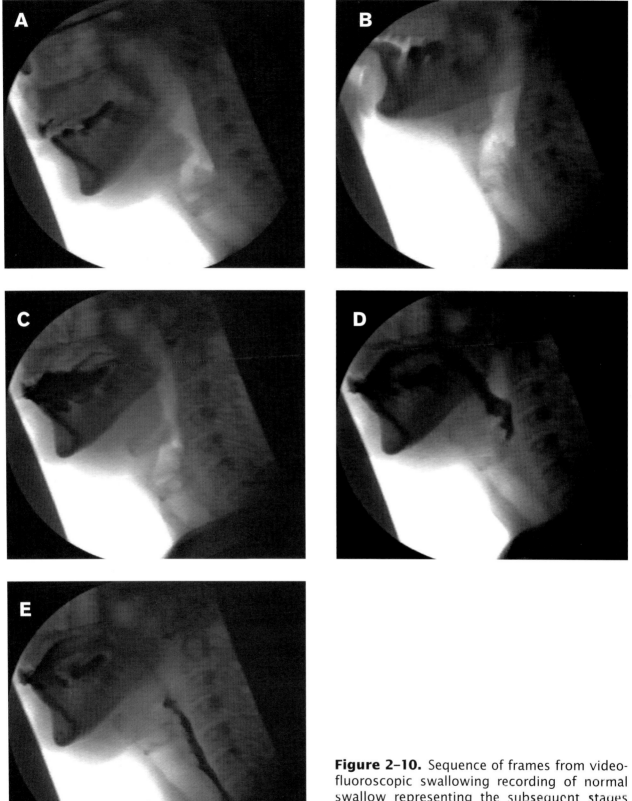

**Figure 2–10.** Sequence of frames from video-fluoroscopic swallowing recording of normal swallow representing the subsequent stages of the swallow: preparatory phase **A.**, **B.**, oral phase **C.**, pharyngeal phase **D.**, and esophageal phase **E.**

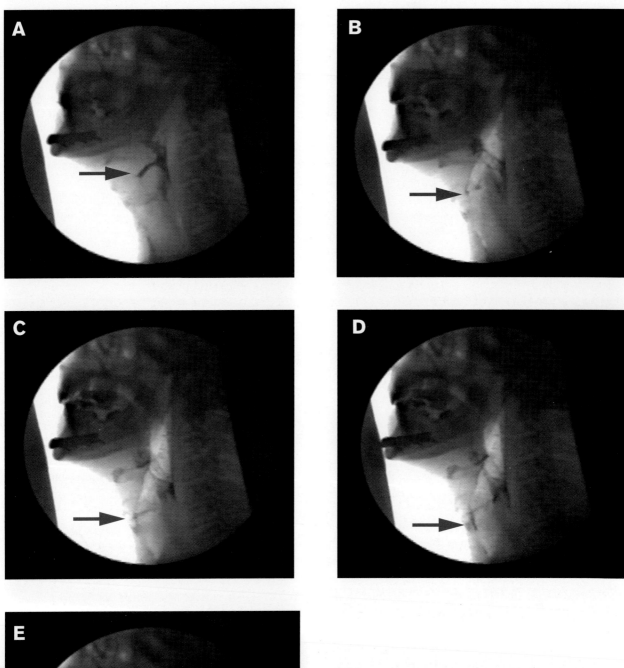

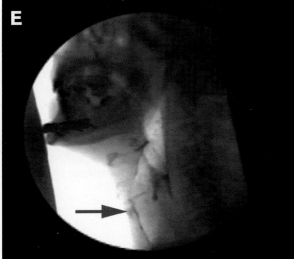

**Figure 2–11.** Sequence of frames from videofluoroscopic swallowing recording of aspiration. Arrows on frames **A.** through **E.** indicate the passing of the liquid into the larynx and being aspirated.

For a complete overview of the MBS assessment procedure and analysis the reader is directed to Logemann (1993, 1998).

Based on the MBS findings, classification of dysphagia severity and functional level for eating can be achieved using the Dysphagia Outcome and Severity Scale (DOSS; O'Neil, Purdy, Falk, & Gallo, 1999). The DOSS is a seven-point scale ranging from Level 1: severe dysphagia to Level 7: normal in all situations. As the DOSS is only relevant for patients who still have their laryngeal structures intact, Ward and colleagues at the Royal Brisbane and Women's Hospital, Australia (Ward, personal communication, June 2006) have developed a modified version of the DOSS for classifying dysphagia severity for total laryngectomy and pharyngolaryngectomy patients. The modified scale has descriptors for each of the severity levels which relate to the specific characteristics of the swallow in the laryngectomy population. The scale is currently undergoing psychometric analysis, and preliminary data suggests the scale has good validity and high reliability.

Fiberoptic endoscopic examination of swallowing (FEES) allows direct visualization of the oropharynx and larynx during swallowing. FEES assessment is conducted using a flexible endoscope (preferably connected to video camera and recorder to allow playback and detailed analysis) and a light source; software packages are available for digital recordings, monitoring, and measurements. During FEES assessment, the fiberoptic scope is inserted into the nose and passed over the velum into a position to view the pharynx and larynx from above. It allows the clinician to examine the structure and function of the soft palate, base of tongue, oropharynx, hypopharynx, larynx, and subglottis. Pooling, residue, and penetration/aspiration can be observed. Secretions and secretion management can be directly observed (see Figure 2-12). FEES provides an additional view of the pharynx and larynx to that provided by videofluoroscopy and is complementary to it. The advantage of FEES is that it does not involve exposure to radiation and can be conducted at the patient's bedside. It is, however, limited by an inability to examine both the oral and the esophageal stage of the swallow, and events during the actual swallow (during the whiteout) cannot be observed. For further details on FEES procedure the reader is directed to Langmore, Schatz, and Olsen (1988) and Bastian (1991).

Fiberoptic endoscopic evaluation of swallowing with sensory testing (FEESST) (Aviv et al., 1998) encompasses FEES assessment with additional evaluation of laryngopharyngeal sensation and airway protection as determined by delivering air-pulse stimuli to the mucosa. It is the only instrumental assessment of swallowing related sensation. Further research regarding FEESST testing is needed to fully determine normative data for sensory thresholds, the clinical application of the data, and the impact of potential confounding variables (e.g., distance from mucosa, impact of secretions, etc.).

Unlike MBS and FEES assessments, manometry is not an imaging study; rather, it is used to quantify pressure changes in the mouth, pharynx, and esophagus during swallowing. The technique involves the insertion of the manometric catheter (which may contain one or more pressure transducers) via the nasal passages and into the region being investigated (e.g., pharynx, esophagus) (see Figure 2-13). Manometry provides important but limited information on swallow physiology and is best paired with videofluoroscopy (referred to as manofluorography) such that the etiology of the observed pressure changes can be identified. Particularly in patients following total laryngectomy, where the surgical reconstruction causes disruption to the normal pressures facilitating bolus flow (see further discussion in Chapter 10), information from a manofluorographic assessment may be useful.

Scintigraphy assesses bolus movement by tracking a radionuclide within a bolus during and after ingestion, via special equipment including a gamma camera and computer. Using a gamma camera, the number of radiation particles in the bolus can be quantified as it passes through the digestive tract. The main advantage of scintigraphy is its ability to accurately quantify both the amount of radioactive material in any structure (e.g., aspirated in lungs, pooled in pharynx) and the transit time of the bolus (Sonies, 1991). The disadvantages of this procedure include the inability to view patient anatomy during the swallow, the fact that only one swallow of one consistency can be observed, and need for a physician trained in nuclear medicine.

■ Example: Eisbruch et al. (2004) used videofluoroscopy, direct endoscopy, and CT scans in 26 patients to identify

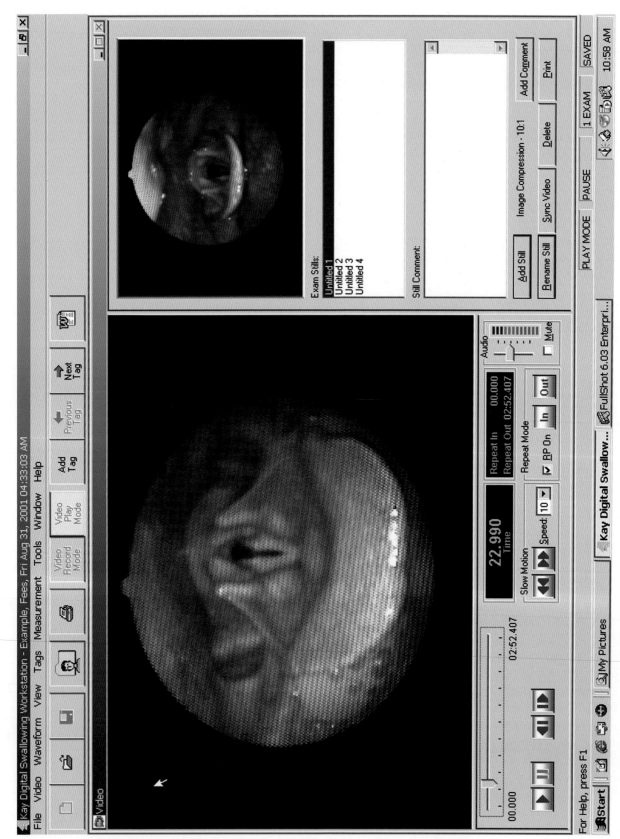

**Figure 2–12.** Example of a FEES view. Note green colored food in valleculae. (Photo courtesy of KayPENTAX)

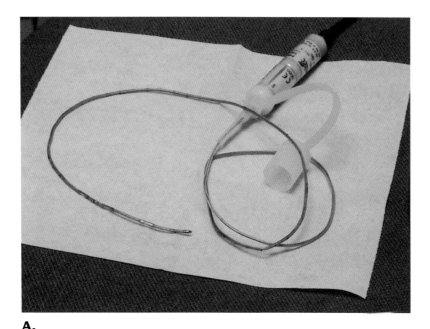

**A.**

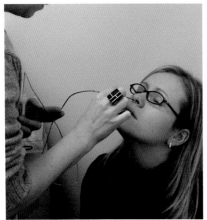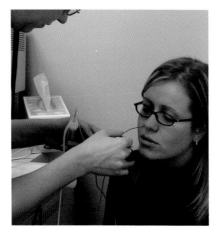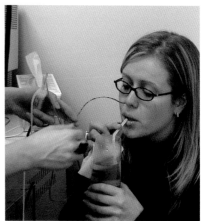

**B.**

**Figure 2–13.** Examples of **A.** a manometric catheter and **B.** its insertion for assessment.

the anatomic structures whose damage or malfunction causes late dysphagia and aspiration after intensive chemotherapy and radiotherapy for head and neck cancer, and to explore whether they can be spared by intensity-modulated radiotherapy (IMRT). The posttherapy abnormalities included weakness of the posterior motion of the base of tongue, prolonged pharyngeal transit time, lack of coordination between the swallowing phases, reduced elevation of the larynx, and reduced laryngeal closure and epiglottic inversion, contributing to a high rate of aspiration. The structures whose damage may cause dysphagia and aspiration after intensive chemotherapy and RT are the pharyngeal constrictors and the glottic and supraglottic larynx.

## Conclusion

The purpose of this chapter was to provide an overview of the main types of assessment tools and outcome measures used in the evaluation of health related quality of life, and functional outcomes of voice, speech, and swallowing. Selecting an outcome measure or outcome assessment protocol requires many considerations. These considerations include the purpose of the study, the content and length of the outcome assessment protocol, and psychometric characteristics of the various outcome measures, including reliability, validity, and availability of normative values. No consensus has been reached regarding the optimal choice of evaluation outcome measures. Further research is needed to obtain insight into the psychometric properties of many of the tools currently in clinical use, together with (international) consensus meetings if standard outcome protocols are to be developed in the near future for use with patients with head and neck cancer. In the meantime, it has been the intent of the current chapter to make the reader familiar with a range of outcome variables currently in use for evaluating the impact of cancer of the head and neck.

## References

Aaronson, N. K., Acquadro, C., Alonso, J., Apolone, G., Bucquet, D., Bullinger, M., et al. (1992). International Quality of Life Assessment (IQOLA) Project. *Quality of Life Research, 1*(5), 349–351.

Aaronson, N. K., Ahmedzai, S., Bergman, B., Bullinger, M., Cull, A., Duez, et al. (1993). The European Organization for Research and Treatment of Cancer QLQ-C30: A quality-of-life instrument for use in international clinical trials in oncology. *Journal of the National Cancer Institute, 85*(5), 365–376.

Aviv, J. E., Kim, T., Thompson, J. E. Sunshine, S., Kaplan, S., & Close, L. G. (1998). Fiberoptic endoscopic evaluation of swallowing with sensory testing (FEESST) in health controls, *Dysphagia, 13*(2), 87–92.

Baken, R. J., & Orlikoff, R. F. (2000). *Clinical measurement of speech and voice*, San Diego, CA: Singular.

Bastian, R. W. (1991). Videoendoscopic evaluation of patients with dysphagia: An adjunct to the modified barium swallow. *Otolaryngology Head and Neck Surgery, 104*(3), 339–350.

Behrman, A. (2005). Common practices of voice therapists in the evaluation of patients. *Journal of Voice, 19*(3), 454–469.

Bjordal, K., Ahlner-Elmqvist, M., Hammerlid, E., Boysen, M., Evensen, J. F., Biörklund, A., et al. (2001). A prospective study of quality of life in head and neck cancer patients. Part II: Longitudinal data. *Laryngoscope, 111,* 1440–1452.

Bjordal, K., Hammerlid, E., Ahlner-Elmqvist, M., deGraeff, A., Boysen, M., Evensen, J. F., et al. (1999). Quality of life in head and neck cancer patients: Validation of the European Organization for Research and Treatment of Cancer Quality of Life Questionnaire-H&N35. *Journal of Clinical Oncology, 17*(3), 1008–1019.

Borggreven, P. A., Verdonck-de Leeuw, I. M., Langendijk, J. A, Doornaert, P., Koster, M. N., de Bree, R., et al. (2005). Speech outcome after surgical treatment for oral and oropharyngeal cancer: A longitudinal assessment of patients reconstructed with a microvascular flap. *Head & Neck, 27*(9), 785–793.

Bressmann, T., Uy, C., & Irish, J. C. (2005) Analysing normal and partial glossectomee tongues using ultrasound. *Clinical Linguistics Phonetics, 19*(1), 35–52.

Campbell, B. H., Spinelli, K., Marbella, A. M., Myers, K. B., Kuhn, J. C., & Layde, P. M. (2004). Aspiration, weight loss, and quality of life in head and neck cancer survivors. *Archives of Otolaryngology-Head & Neck Surgery, 30*(9), 1100–1103.

Carding, P. N., Steen, I. N., Webb, A., Mackenzie, K., Deary, I. J., & Wilson, J. A. (2004). The reliability and sensitivity to change of acoustic measures of voice quality. *Clinical Otolaryngology, 29,* 538–544.

Cella, D. F., Tulsky, D. S., Gray, G., Sarafian, B., Lloyd, S., Linn, E., et al. (1993). The Functional Assessment of Cancer Therapy (FACT) scale: Development and validation of the general measure. *Journal of Clinical Oncology, 11*(3), 570–579.

Chen, A. Y., Frankowski, R., Bishop-Leone, J., Hebert, T., Leyk, S., Lewin, J., et al. (2001). The development and validation of a dysphagia-specific quality-of-life questionnaire for patients with head and neck cancer: The M. D. Anderson dysphagia inventory. *Archives of Otolaryngology-Head & Neck Surgery, 127*(7), 870–876.

De Graeff, A., de Leeuw, R. J., Ros, W. J. G., Hordijk, G., Blijham, G. H., & Winnubst, J. A. M. (2000). Long-term quality of life of patients with head and neck cancer. *Laryngoscope, 110,* 98–106.

Dejonckere, P. H., Bradley, P., Clemente, P., Cornut, G., Crevier-Buchman, L., Friedrich, G., et al.: Committee on Phoniatrics of the European Laryngological Society (ELS). (2001). A basic protocol for functional assessment of voice pathology, especially for investigating the efficacy of (phonosurgical) treatments and evaluating new assessment techniques. Guideline elaborated by the Committee on Phoniatrics of the European Laryngological Society (ELS). *European Archives of Otorhinolaryngology, 258*(2), 77–82.

Duckworth, M. A. G., Hardcastle, W., & Ball, M. J. (1990). Extensions to the International Phonetic Alphabet for the transcription of atypical speech. *Clinical Linguistics and Phonetics, 4,* 273–280.

Eadie, T. L., & Doyle, P. C. (2005). Quality of life in male tracheoesophageal (TE) speakers. *Journal of Rehabilitation Research and Development, 42*(1), 115–124.

Eisbruch, A., Schwartz, M., Rasch, C., Vineberg, K., Damen, E., Van As, C. J, et al. (2004). Dysphagia and aspiration after chemoradiotherapy for head-and-neck cancer: Which anatomic structures are affected and can they be spared by IMRT? *International Journal of Radiation Oncology * Biology * Physics, 1*(60), 5, 1425–1439.

El-Deiry, M., Funk, G. F., Nalwa, S., Karnell, L. H., Smith, R. B., Buatti, J. M., et al. (2005). Long-term quality of life for surgical and nonsurgical treatment of head and neck cancer. *Archives of Otolaryngology—Head & Neck Surgery, 131*(10), 879–885.

Enderby, P. M., & John, A. (1999). Therapy outcome measures in speech and language therapy: Comparing performance between different providers. *International Journal of Language and Communication Disorders, 34*(4), 417–429.

Fang, F. M., Tsai, W. L., Chien, C. Y., Chiu, H. C., Wang, C. J., Chen, H. C., et al. (2005). Changing quality of life in patients with advanced head and neck cancer after primary radiotherapy or chemoradiation. *Oncology, 68*(4-6), 405–413.

Fayers, P. M., & Sprangers, M. A. G. (2002). Understanding self-rated health. *Lancet, 359,* 187–188.

Finizia, C., Palme, C., & Bergman, B. (2002). A longitudinal study of the Swedish Self-Evaluation of communication experiences after laryngeal cancer questionnaire in patients treated for laryngeal cancer. *Acta Oncologica, 41*(3), 262–268.

Fung, K., & Terrell, J. E. (2004). Outcomes research in head and neck cancer. *Journal of Otorhinolaryngology and its Related Specialties, 66*(4), 207–213.

Funk, G. F., Karnell, L. H., Christensen, A. J., Moran, P. J., Ricks, J. (2003). Comprehensive head and neck oncology health status assessment. *Head & Neck, 25*(7), 561–575.

Hammerlid, E., Ahlner-Elmqvist, M., Bjordal, K., Biörklund, A., Evensen, J., Boysen, M., et al. (1999). A prospective multicentre study in Sweden and Norway of mental distress and psychiatric morbidity in head and neck cancer patients. *British Journal of Cancer. 80,* 766–774.

Hammerlid, E., & Taft, C. (2001). Health-related quality of life in long-term head and neck cancer survivors: A comparison with general population norms. *British Journal of Cancer, 84*(2), 149–156.

Hirano, M. (1981). *Clinical examination of voice. Disorders of human communication 5.* New York: Springer Verlag.

Hogikan, N. D., & Sethuraman, G. (1999). Validation of an instrument to measure voice-related quality of life (V-RQOL). *Journal of Voice, 13,* 557–569.

Homs, M. Y., Essink-Bot, M. L., Borsboom, G. J., Steyerberg, E. W., & Siersema, P. D. (2004). Quality of life after palliative treatment for oesophageal carcinoma—A prospective comparison between stent placement and single dose brachytherapy. *European Journal of Cancer, 40*(12), 1862–1871

Jacobson, G., Johnson, A., Grywalski, C., Sibergleit, A., Jacobson, G., Benninger, M. S., et al. (1997). The Voice Handicap Index (VHI): Development and validation. *American Journal of Speech and Language Pathology, 6,* 66–70.

Kugaya, A., Akechi, T., Okuyama, T., Nakano, T., Mikami, I., Okamura, H., et al. (2000). Prevalence, predictive factors, and screening for psychologic distress in patients with newly diagnosed head and neck cancer. *Cancer, 12,* 2817–2823.

Langmore, S. E., Schatz, K., & Olsen, N. (1988). Fiberoptic endoscopic examination of swallowing safety: A new procedure. *Dysphagia, 2*(4), 216–219.

Laver, J. (1991). *The gift of speech. Papers in the Analysis of Speech and Voice.* Edinburgh: Edinburgh University Press.

Lawson, G., Jamart, J., & Remacle, M. (2001). Improving the functional outcome of Tucker's reconstructive laryngectomy. *Head & Neck, 23*(10), 871–878.

List, M. A., D'Antonio, L. L., Cella, D. F., Siston, A., Mumby, P., Haraf, D., et al. (1996). The Performance Status Scale for head and neck cancer patients and the Functional Assessment of Cancer Therapy—Head and Neck (FACT-H&N) scale: A study of utility and validity. *Cancer, 77,* 2294–2301.

List, M. A., & Pinar Bilir, S. (2004). Functional outcomes in head and neck cancer. *Seminars in Radiation Oncology, 14*(2), 178–189.

List, M. A., Ritter-Sterr, C., & Lansky, S. B. (1990). A performance status scale for head and neck cancer patients. *Cancer, 66,* 564–569.

Logemann, J. A. (1993). *Manual for the videofluoroscopic study of swallowing* (2nd ed.). Austin, TX: Pro-Ed.

Logemann, J. A. (1998). *Evaluation and treatment of swallowing disorders* (2nd ed.). Austin, TX: Pro-Ed.

Logemann, J. A., & Kahrilas, P. J. (1990). Relearning to swallow after stroke: Application of maneuvers and indirect feedback: A case study. *Neurology, 40,* 1136–1138.

Lovell, S. J., Wong, H. B., Loh, K. S., Ngo, R. Y., & Wilson, J. A. (2005). Impact of dysphagia on quality-of-life in nasopharyngeal carcinoma. *Head & Neck, 27*(10), 864–872.

Ma, E., & Yiu, E. (2001). Voice activity and participation profile: Assessing the impact of voice disorders on daily activities. *Journal of Speech, Language and Hearing Research, 44,* 511–524.

Maassen, B., Kent, R., Peters, H. F. M., Van Lieshout, P., & Hulstijn, W. (Eds.). (2004). *Speech motor control in normal and disordered speech.* Oxford: Oxford University Press.

Mady, K., Sader, R., Hoole, P. H., Zimmermann, A., & Horch, H. H. (2003). Speech evaluation and swallowing ability after intra-oral cancer. *Clinical Linguistics and Phoniatrics, 7*(4–5), 411–420.

McAuliffe, M. J., & Ward, E. C. (In press). The use of electropalatography in the assessment and treatment of acquired motor speech disorders in adults: Current knowledge and future directions. *NeuroRehabilitation, 21*(2).

McGee, H. M., O'Boyle, C. A., Hickey, A., O'Malley, K., & Joyce, C. R. (1991). Assessing the quality of life of the individual: The SEIQOL with a healthy and a gastroenterology unit population. *Psychological Medicine, 21*(3), 749–759.

McHorney, C. A., Robbins, J., Lomax, K., Rosenbek, J. C., Chignell, K., Kramer, A. E., et al. (2002). The SWAL-QOL and SWAL-CARE outcomes tool for oropharyngeal dysphagia in adults: III. Documentation of reliability and validity. *Dysphagia, 17*(2), 97–114.

Miller, R. M. (1997). Clinical examination for dysphagia. In M. E. Groher (Ed.) *Dysphagia: Diagnosis and Management* (3rd ed.). Butterworth-Heinemann, Edinburgh, United Kingdom.

Moerman, M. B., Martens, J. P., Van der Borgt, M. J., Peleman, M., Gillis, M., & Dejonckere, P. H. (2006). Perceptual evaluation of substitution voices: Development and evaluation of the (I)INFVo rating scale.

European Archives of Otorhinolaryngology, 263(2), 183–187.

Moerman, M., Pieters, G., Martens, J. P., Van der Borgt, M. J., & Dejönckere, P. (2004). Objective evaluation of the quality of substitution voices. *European Archives of Otorhinolaryngology, 261*(10), 541–547.

Morton, R. P. (2003). Studies in the quality of life of head and neck cancer patients: Results of a two-year longitudinal study and a comparative cross-sectional cross-cultural survey. *Laryngoscope, 113,* 1091–1103.

O'Neil, K. H., Purdy, M., Falk, J., and Gallo, L. (1999). The Dysphagia Outcome and Severity Scale. *Dysphagia, 14,* 139–145.

Parkin, D. M., Bray, F., Ferlay, J., & Pisani, P. (2005). Global cancer statistics, 2002. *CA A Cancer Journal for Clinicians, 55,* 74–108.

Pauloski, B. R., Logemann, J. A., Colangelo, L., Rademaker, A. W., McConnel, F. M. S, Heiser, M. A., et al. (1998). Surgical variables affecting speech in treated patients with oral and oropharyngeal cancer. *Laryngoscope, 108*(6), 908–916.

Pauloski, B. R., Rademaker, A. W., Logemann, J. A., Lazarus, C. L., Newman, L., Hamner, A., et al. (2002). Swallow function and perception of dysphagia in patients with head and neck cancer. *Head & Neck, 24*(6), 555–565.

Peeters, A. J., van Gogh, C. D., Goor, K. M., Verdonck-de Leeuw, I. M., Langendijk, J. A., & Mahieu, H. F. (2004). Health status and voice outcome after treatment for T1a glottic carcinoma. *European Archives of Otorhinolaryngology, 261*(10), 534–540.

Perry, A. R., Shaw, M. A., & Cotton, S. (2003). An evaluation of functional outcomes (speech, swallowing) in patients attending speech pathology after head and neck cancer treatment(s): Results and analysis at 12 months postintervention. *Journal of Laryngology & Otology, 117,* 368–381.

Perry, A., Morris, M., Unsworth, C., Duckett, S., Skeat, J., Dodd, K., et al. (2004). Therapy outcome measures for allied health practitioners in Australia: The AusTOMs. *International Journal of Quality of Health Care, 16*(4), 285–291.

Petruson, K. M., Silander, E. M., & Hammerlid, E. B. (2005). Quality of life as predictor of weight loss in patients with head and neck cancer. *Head & Neck, 27*(4), 302–310.

Ringash, J., Bezjak, A., O'Sullivan, B., & Redelmeier, D. A. (2004). Interpreting differences in quality of life: The FACT-H&N in laryngeal cancer patients. *Quality of Life Research, 13*(4), 725–733.

Rinkel, R. N. P. M., Verdonck-de Leeuw. I. M., & Leemans, C. R. (2005). The speech handicap index: Better understanding of patients' complaints. *Abstract Bi-annual Symposium Netherlands Society for Otorhinolaryngology Head & Neck Surgery.*

Rosenbek, J. C., Robbins, J. A., Roecker, E. B., Coyle, J. L., & Wood, J. L. (1996). A penetration-aspiration scale. *Dysphagia, 11*(2), 93-98.

Sehlen, S., Hollenhorst, H., Lenk, M., Schymura, B., Herschbach, P., Aydemir, U., et al. (2002). Only sociodemographic variables predict quality of life after radiography in patients with head-and-neck cancer. *International Journal of Radiation Oncology, Biology, Physics, 52*(3), 779-783.

Schindler, A., Favero, E., Nudo, S., Spadola-Bisetti, M., Ottaviani, F., & Schindler, O. (2005). Voice after supracricoid laryngectomy: Subjective, objective and self-assessment data. *Logopedica Phoniatrica Vocology, 30*(3-4), 114-119.

Schliephake, H., & Jamil, M. U. (2002). Prospective evaluation of quality of life after oncologic surgery for oral cancer. *International Journal of Oral and Maxillofacial Surgery, 31*, 427-433.

Sharpe, L., Butow, P., Smith, C., McConnell, D., & Clarke, S. (2005). Changes in quality of life in patients with advanced cancer: Evidence of response shift and response restriction. *Journal of Psychosomatic Research, 58*(6), 497-504.

Sonies, B. C. (1991). Instrumental procedures for dysphagia diagnosis. *Seminars in Speech and Language, 12*(3), 185-197.

Su, W. F., Chen, S. G., & Sheng, H. (2002). Speech and swallowing function after reconstruction with a radial forearm free flap or a pectoralis major flap for tongue cancer. *Journal of Formos Medical Association, 101*(7), 472-477.

Terrell, J. E., Nanavati, K. A., Esclamado, R. M., Bishop, J. K., Bradford, C. R., & Wolf, G. T. (1997). Head and neck cancer-specific quality of life: Instrument validation. *Archives of Otolaryngology—Head & Neck Surgery, 123*(10), 1125-1132.

Terrell, J. E., Ronis, D. L., Fowler, K. E., Bradford, C. R., Chepeha, D. B., Prince, M. E., et al. (2004). Clinical predictors of quality of life in patients with head and neck cancer. *Archives of Otolaryngology—Head & Neck Surgery, 130*(4), 401-408.

The EuroQoL Group. (1990). EuroQol—A new facility for the measurement of health-related quality of life. *Health Policy, 16*(3),199-208.

Thompson-Ward, E. C., & Murdoch, B. E. (1998). Instrumental assessment of the speech mechanism. In B. E. Murdoch (Ed.), *Dysarthria: A physiological approach to assessment and treatment.* Cheltenham, England: Stanley Thornes.

Titze, I. R. (1994). *Workshop on acoustic voice analysis.* Iowa: National Center for Voice and Speech.

Van As, C. J., Hilgers, F. J. M., Verdonck-de Leeuw, I. M., & Koopmans-van Beinum, F. J. (1998). Acoustical analysis and perceptual evaluation of tracheoesophageal prosthetic voice. *Journal of Voice, 12*, 239-248.

Van As, C. J., Koopmans-van Beinum, F. J., Pols, L. C., & Hilgers, F. J. (2003). Perceptual evaluation of tracheoesophageal speech by naive and experienced judges through the use of semantic differential scales. *Journal of Speech Language and Hearing Research, 46*(4), 947-959.

Van As-Brooks, C. J., Koopmans-van Beinum, F. J., Pols, L. C., & Hilgers, F. J. (2006). Acoustic Signal Typing for Evaluation of Voice Quality in Tracheoesophageal Speech. *Journal of Voice, 20*(3), 355-368.

Van Gogh, C. D. L., Festen, J. M., Verdonck-de Leeuw, I. M., Parker, A. J., Traissac, F. R. C. S. L., Cheesman, A. D., et al. (2005). Acoustical analysis of tracheoesophageal voice. *Speech Communication, 47*, 160-168.

Van Gogh, C. D. L., Verdonck-de Leeuw, I. M., Boon-Kamma, A. B., Langendijk, J. A., Kuik, D. J., & Mahieu, H. F. (2005). Feasibility of a screening questionnaire for voice problems after treatment for early glottic cancer. *International Journal of Radiation Oncology * Biology * Physics, 62*(3), 700-705.

Van Gogh, C. D. L., Verdonck-de Leeuw, I. M., Boon-Kamma, B. A., Rinkel, R. N., de Bruin, M. D., Langendijk, J. A., et al. (2006). The efficacy of voice therapy in patients after treatment for early glottic carcinoma. *Cancer, 106*(1), 95-105.

Van Rossum, M. A., de Krom, G., Nooteboom, S. G., & Quené, H. (2002). "Pitch" accent in alaryngeal speech. *Journal of Speech Language and Hearing Research, 45*, 1106-1118.

Van Weel, C. (1993). Functional status in primary care: COOP/WONCA charts. *Disability Rehabilitation, 15*, 96-101.

Verdonck-de Leeuw, I. M., Hilgers, F. J., Keus, R. B., Koopmans-van Beinum, F. J., Greven, AJ., de Jong, J. M., et al. (1999). Multidimensional assessment of voice characteristics after radiotherapy for early glottic cancer. *Laryngoscope, 109*(2), 241-248.

Wakumoto, M., Ohno, K., Imai, S., Yamashita, Y., Akizuki, H., & Michi, K. I. (1996). Analysis of the articulation after glossectomy. *Journal of Oral Rehabilitation, 23*(11), 764-770.

Ward, E. C. & Conroy, A. L. (1999). Validity, reliability and responsivity of the Royal Brisbane Outcome Measure for Swallowing. *Asia Pacific Journal of Speech Language and Hearing, 4*, 109-129.

Weymuller, E., Alsarraf, R., Yueh, B., Deleyiannis, F., & Coltrera, M. (2001). Analysis of the performance characteristics of the UW-QOL & modification of the instrument. *Archives of Otolaryngology—Head and Neck Surgery, 127*(5), 489–493.

Yumoto, E., Sasaki, Y., & Okamuro, H. (1984). Harmonics-to-noise ratio and psychophysical measurement of the degree of hoarseness. *Journal of Speech and Hearing Research, 27*(1), 2–6.

Zuydam, A. C., Lowe, D., Brown, J. S., Vaughan, E. D., & Rogers, S. N. (2005). Predictors of speech and swallowing function following primary surgery for oral and oropharyngeal cancer. *Clinical Otolaryngology, 30*(5), 428–437.

# Chapter 3

# RADIATION AND CHEMOTHERAPY

## Lyndell E. Kelly

# Introduction

Decisions regarding the optimal management of a patient with a head and neck malignancy are best made by a team of specialists from several disciplines. These health care professionals form a dedicated head and neck clinic, typically situated in a centralized tertiary hospital, and develop a great deal of experience through the large numbers of patients they jointly see and their interactions with each other. Routine audits of treatment results help the team to assess whether their results are of an acceptable standard. The head and neck clinic is usually comprised of otolaryngologists/head and neck surgeons, plastic surgeons, maxillofacial surgeons, radiation oncologists, medical oncologists, speech-language pathologists, dieticians, a dentist or prosthodontist, and oncology nurses, with treatment decisions being based on the multidisciplinary contributions of the team members.

Radiation has been securely part of head and neck treatment since the 1960s because of its well-proven ability to cure when used alone or in conjunction with surgery. The place of chemotherapy, however, has been uncertain until recently. Chemotherapy without radiation is unable to increase cure rates of squamous cell carcinomas when used either alone or adjuvant to surgery. The benefit of chemotherapy in head and neck cancers occurs when it is used synchronously with radiation. The development of synchronous chemotherapy and radiation schedules has been one of the greatest advances in oncology in the last 20 years. The acceptance of this treatment into general use in the management of head and neck cancers only occurred in the 1990s. It has taken time for clinicians to accept, firstly, that "untreatable" cancers were being cured, and then that functionally damaging surgery could be avoided with cure rates the same or better by using chemoradiation. There are many things we are still learning. For example, there are multiple regimens accepted throughout the world, varying in both the radiation schedule and chemotherapy drugs used. We are learning that functional deficits that have been regarded as late effects of these regimens are often, but not always, due to tumor destruction of normal tissues. We do not know if effectiveness increases with toxicity and what morbidity is acceptable or even necessary to maximize cure rates. Because of surprising

cures of massive tumors, it is hard to be confident about the decision *not* to treat, that is, to know if someone is incurable and better left without the side effects of chemoradiation while dying. It is often the patient's general condition which determines whether or not this treatment is offered.

To illustrate the wide range of post-treatment scenarios, here are four genuine cases:

1. A 68-year-old man was referred to us by a regional otolaryngologist with a hypopharyngeal tumor. Swallowing had become difficult and he had lost weight. On examination, an exophytic tumor based in his left piriform fossa and completely occluding his supraglottis was found. He was able to breathe through a necrotic hole in the middle of this mass. There were bilateral lymph nodes in level 3 of 2 cm and 3 cm in diameter. After insertion of a gastrostomy tube, he was given chemoradiation which he tolerated very well but remained an inpatient the whole time. Six months after treatment was completed he developed stridor, was given a tracheostomy, and biopsies were taken from the supraglottic and piriform area. The supraglottis had collapsed due to the extent of destruction of the cartilage and muscle by the tumor. There was, and still is, no evidence of residual carcinoma but he remains PEG (percutaneous endoscopic gastrostomy) and tracheostomy dependent.

2. A 47-year-old man was shaving when he found a lump in his left upper neck. He was referred to an otolaryngologist and was diagnosed with a left posterior tongue carcinoma. The primary tumor was 2.5 cm in maximum dimension extending just to the midline from the lateral pharyngeal wall. The level 2 lymph node was 3 cm diameter and mobile. He was given a course of chemoradiation and required a week in the hospital at the end of the course because of dehydration and mucosal pain. Eighteen months later he was back competing in triathlons. He remains tumor-free 4 years later with the only sequel of his treatment moderate xerostomia. His knees have worn out.

3. A 35-year-old woman noticed a lesion on her lateral border of tongue. At resection it was a 4 × 3 cm squamous cell carcinoma invading to a depth of 16 mm. Upper neck dissection showed two nodes in levels 1 and 2 to be involved, one with extracap-

sular spread. Because the lesion was histologically aggressive, she then underwent a course of chemoradiation. Three years later, she is tumor-free but gastrostomy dependent because of restriction of her anterior tongue and a failure of her posterior tongue to meet her soft palate. After multiple videofluoroscopic assessments of swallowing, it now appears that she has fusion of her posterior tongue to her epiglottis, a sequel of ulceration of opposing surfaces and atrophy of posterior tongue muscles. Exercises have been rigorously performed with little benefit. Laser surgery is thought unlikely to release this fusion or to free her base of tongue. It appears she is likely to be PEG dependent indefinitely.

4. In 1999, a 58-year-old man noticed a lump while swallowing and sought advice. He was found to have a T2 N0 SCC of his right piriform fossa. He was offered a pharyngolaryngectomy which was the standard treatment at the time. He refused as his livelihood depended on using his voice. He was given chemoradiation and is still free of tumor with normal appearance, mild xerostomia, a good voice, and normal swallowing.

To understand each modality and the combinations in general use, it will be helpful to learn how they work, their place in the treatment protocols, and the management of side effects. The current chapter will detail for the reader the biological effect of radiotherapy and chemotherapy and their impact on the patient and discuss the various forms of administration (i.e., in isolation, in conjunction with surgery, or combined chemoradiotherapy) used in the head and neck cancer patient.

## Radiation (XRT)

### Types of Radiation Used

The spectrum of electromagnetic radiation extends from radio waves to x and gamma waves in order of increasing energy, increasing frequency, and shortening wavelength: radio waves, microwaves, infrared (heat), visible light, ultraviolet, and x-rays and gamma rays. These waves are composed of packets of energy with negligible mass called *photons*. Ultraviolet, x-rays,

and gamma rays have enough energy to alter a chemical environment, and so are called "ionizing radiation."

A beam can be composed of either photons (x-rays and gamma rays) or particles (electrons and beta rays). X-rays and electrons can be produced electrically (this process will be detailed in the following section), and can be of a variable energy, dependent on the generating machine. In contrast, gamma rays and beta rays result from an intranuclear reaction in a radioactive substance emitting gamma or beta beams of a fixed and unalterable energy for that substance. In medical use, x-rays may be of low energy (50–150 kilovolts), for diagnostic purposes; or of higher energy (100 kV–18 megavolts) for the destruction of selected biological tissue such as neoplasms. In the same way, low-energy gamma beams are used in nuclear medicine for diagnostic purposes (e.g., technetium-90), and higher energy gamma beams are used for therapeutic purposes (e.g., cobalt-60, caesium-90).

In summary, radiation oncologists have several sources of radiation at their disposal; gamma beams from several isotopes, x-ray beams of various energies, beta beams from certain isotopes, and electron beams of various energies. Which beam is used depends on the purpose and depth of penetration required. There has been a trend away from radioactive sources towards artificially created beams because of greater choice of beam from the one machine, the ability to turn the machine off (a radioactive source can only be shielded), and fewer problems with disposal.

## Creation and Measurement of Radiation

Most therapeutic radiation is produced by linear accelerators (LAs), an example of which is shown in Figure 3–1. Initially, a wire filament is heated causing electrons to be ejected. They are then attracted to a positively-charged plate with a central hole, and from there into a long tube where radio waves create electromagnetic fields. The effect on the electrons is that at frequent intervals they are propelled down the tube, gaining energy at the rate of 80–150 kV/cm. The electrons may approach the speed of light, near which energy gain would be translated into increased mass which, while verifying Einstein's formula $e = mc^2$, makes calculations and predictions difficult. This very energetic beam

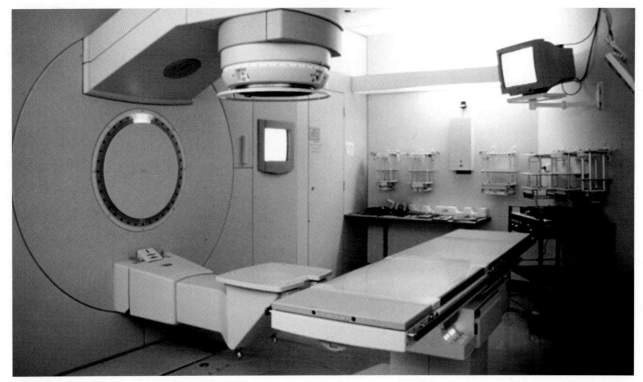

**A.**

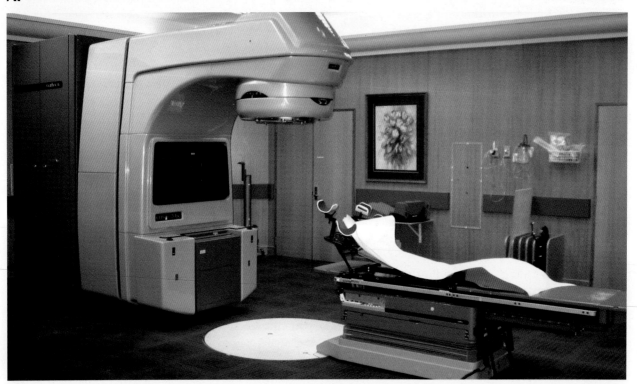

**B.**

**Figure 3–1.** Two linear accelerators in current use. **A.** shows an old machine with brackets around the walls which allow the manual placement of 5 cm thick shielding blocks to define the radiation field shape. This can be hard work for radiation therapists. In the new machine, **B.**, the blocks are inside the machine and are set by a computer to a predetermined shape, eliminating a source of human error and human fatigue.

then ploughs into a heavy metal target (usually tungsten) and rapidly decelerates. The acquired energy is emitted as heat and x-rays. The emerging beam is now composed of x-rays of varying energies, up to a maximum energy level that is dependent on the length of the accelerating tube and the energy the electrons attained. In practice, this is usually 4-18 MV. The beam is then defined and shaped by thick lead shielding. It is aimed at a fixed point (the isocenter) where a patient can be positioned.

Some radiotherapy departments use gamma rays from cobalt-60 instead of an x-ray beam from a linear accelerator. A cobalt machine emits a beam of photons, all of which have 1.3 MV energy. This averages out to similar biological effect as a 4 MV (max) LA beam. The main disadvantage is that the cobalt source deteriorates at the rate of 20% per year, having a half-life of only 5.3 years. This and the difficulty of cobalt disposal have made these machines a rarity in the developed world.

Every radiotherapy department has a corps of physicists and engineers who ensure the machines are in perfect working order and that the output of radiation is no more or less than that expected. For each machine, physicists have calibrated a summary of the beam's absorption in biological tissue (the isodose diagram), as shown in Figure 3-2. Beams of higher energies penetrate further into biological tissue before absorption as shown in Figure 3-3. This is obtained from painstaking measurements of the beam's penetration in a tank of water, which absorbs like body tissue. In the same way as ionization occurs in vivo, an electric current is produced in vitro and can be measured to obtain a figure (in Grays) indicating the strength or absorption of the beam. The dose of radiation, therefore, equates to the ionizing ability of and energy absorption from the beam. Energy deposition of one joule per kilogram of water is called a Gray.

At times it is desirable to use a beam composed not of x-ray photons, but of electrons. The tungsten target is removed from the path of the electrons, the number of electrons is attenuated, and they are then directed towards the isocenter. In biological tissue, electrons do not penetrate as deeply as do photons, and are more quickly absorbed. This is very useful for treating superficial structures and protecting deeper structures such as the spinal cord. Again, more energetic electrons penetrate further than less energetic

ones, allowing an electron beam to be chosen to suit the specific anatomic requirements, as illustrated in Figure 3-4.

Isodose diagrams are superimposed on an outline of the patient's anatomy or CT scan, and the incident dose necessary to give the tumor a given dose is calculated. It is usually better to aim at the tumor from several different directions, sparing more superficial normal tissues and giving the tumor area a summated dose. This can be done by hand with a slide rule if necessary (see Figure 3-5) but modern computer programs allow for more complex and accurate diagrams (see Figure 3-6). For example, Figure 3-7 shows a technique used to treat a tonsil and posterior tongue squamous cell carcinoma with the patient in the supine position. After the patient is immobilized in a shell in the treatment position, a CT scan is done. The radiation oncologist marks on the CT slices the volume requiring the therapeutic dose. Fields are brought in from several directions with as much normal tissue shielding as is safe and the total dose calculated. In this way, an accurate assessment of the risk to normal structures is made, and the delivery of an effective dose to the tumor ensured.

## Biological Effect

When directed into a substance such as water or biological tissue, radiation gradually dissipates as it is absorbed. The depth to which the beam penetrates is greater for more energetic beams. The process by which absorption occurs also varies with beam energy; for high energy beams used in radiation oncology the *Compton effect* predominates. This means that, at an atomic level, an incoming photon may come into the vicinity of an orbiting electron. They interact, with the photon being deflected and slowed to some extent, proceeding on its way with reduced energy, and the electron acquiring enough energy to leave the nucleus and behave in neighboring atoms like an unguided missile, causing ionization, and breaking chemical bonds. A photon beam is therefore described as "indirectly ionizing" because it relies on the ejected electron for its effect. In contrast, a beam of particles such as electrons ionizes directly as a primary event.

The biological impact of the beam is realized at the molecular, cellular, and visceral level leading to notable clinical changes both to normal and malignant tissue.

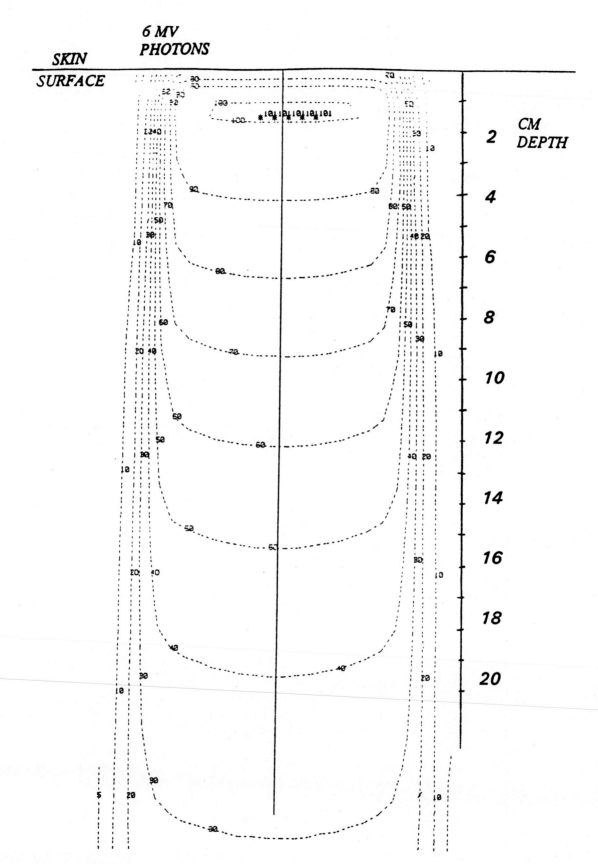

**Figure 3–2.** Isodose diagram of 6 MV photons as they are absorbed in a tank of water (which has similar absorption characteristics to a human body).

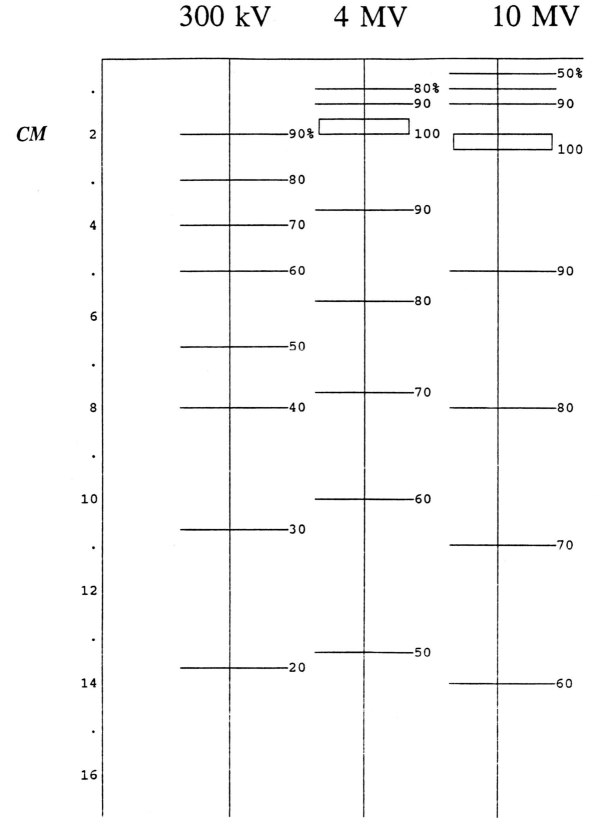

**Figure 3–3.** Comparison of the dose at the depth of photon beams of differing energies. Curves like this allow the choice of the most appropriate beam for a particular site (e.g., a rib metastasis is better treated with 300 kV, a bladder with 10 MV).

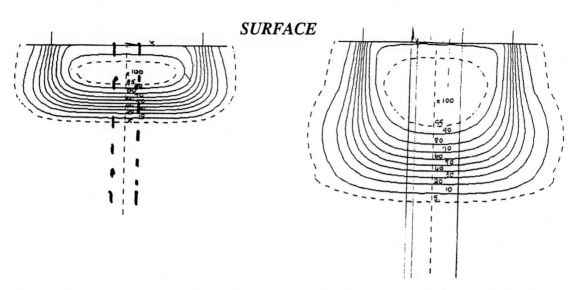

**Figure 3–4.** Comparison of the dose at the depth of electron beams of different energies. The most common use of an electron beam is to treat the lymph nodes overlying the spinal cord but not the spinal cord. The energy of electrons used depends on the thickness of the neck and can be easily determined on a CT scan.

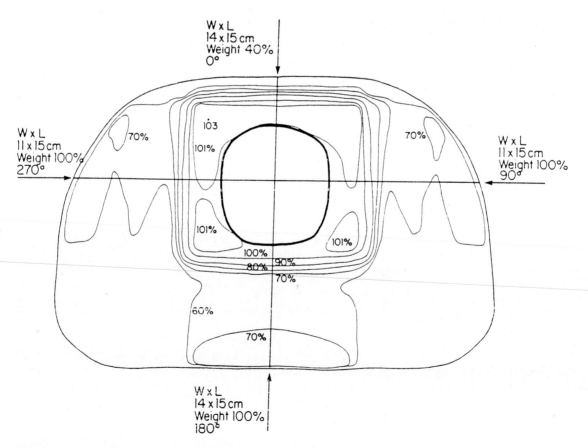

**Figure 3–5.** Simple radiation plan made by summation of beams superimposed on a patient outline. This used to be a simple but only vaguely accurate procedure.

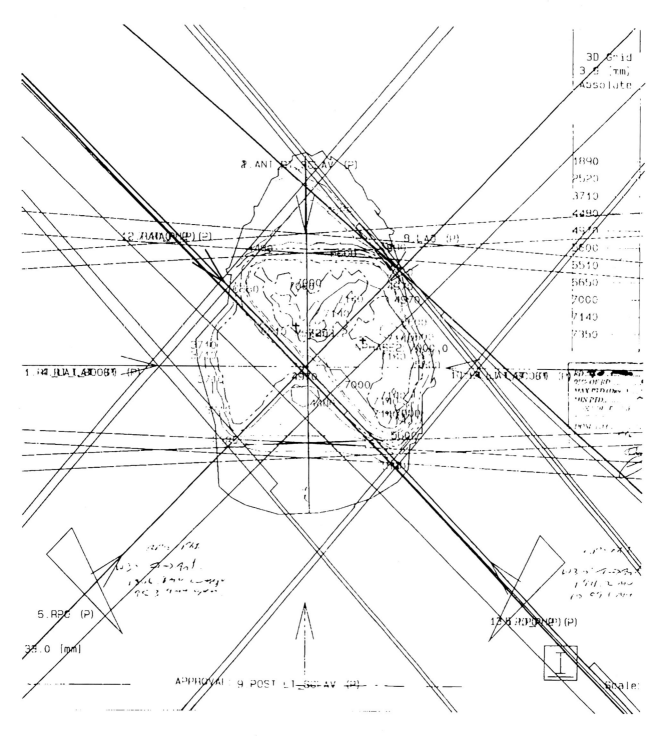

**Figure 3–6.** Isodose diagram for a complicated treatment of a left tonsil carcinoma with a large neck node using multiple oblique beams and lead wedges to limit the dose to the spinal cord.

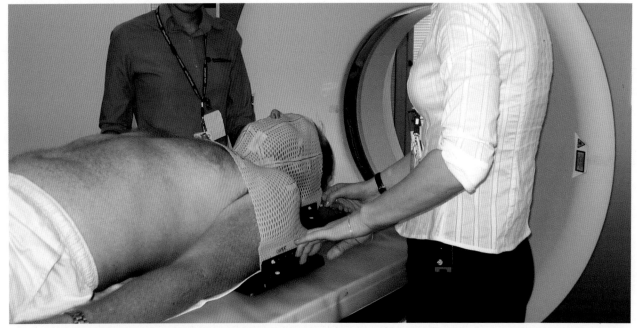

**A.**

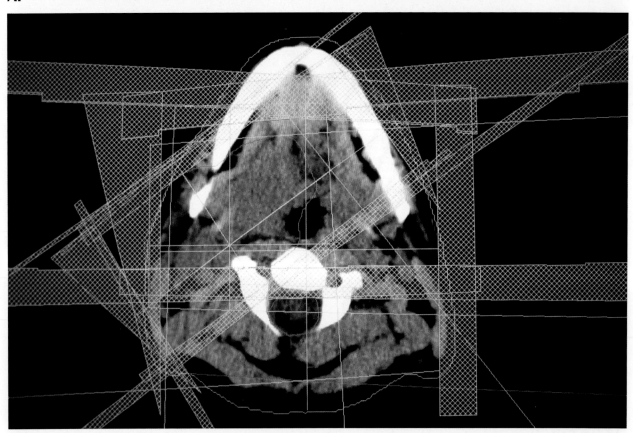

**B.**

**Figure 3–7.** Current treatment plan for a patient with a large oropharyngeal SCC. **A.** The patient has a custom-made plastic shell fitted in which he has a CT scan. **B.** This shows tumor and normal anatomy for the radiation oncologist to outline (here, in red) the volume of concern. Dosimetry is much more precise with allowance by the software for atomic number of, and thence of absorption in, of the anatomic structures. Definition of the volume at risk is much greater. *(continues)*

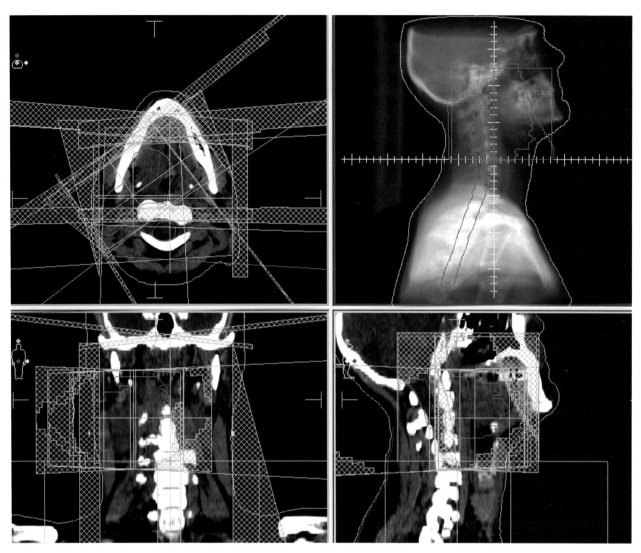

**Figure 3–7.** *(continued)* **C.** The plan can be viewed in any dimension so that coverage of various structures can be assessed. Isodose lines are not shown on these illustrations.

## The Molecular Level

At a molecular level, the chemical with which the electron interacts may be DNA, or it may be a less critical but more abundant molecule such as water. Because 80% of the cell is water, it plays an important role in the overall radiation effect. Water can be ionized to several forms (e.g., $H_2O^+$, $OH^-$, $H^+$, $e-$, $H_3O^+$, etc.). These compounds are called free radicals and are so unstable they exist for about a billionth of a second before reacting with a compound in the vicinity, breaking stable covalent bonds and altering the biochemical environment.

## The Cellular Level

Whether the action of radiation is a direct hit to DNA or is mediated via free radicals, the result can be a breakage of one or both DNA strands. The DNA repair mechanism then swings into action, sometimes repairing the strand well, but often joining chromosomes aberrantly, perhaps cross-linking DNA strands. The cell is still capable of functioning, having lost none of its nuclear material, but at the next mitosis the chromosomes are not able to separate at anaphase. So instead of two new daughter cells we have a dead cell.

## The Visceral Level

This process of cell death occurs in all irradiated tissues. The effect is obvious when there is enough cell death to cause a tissue deficit. In slowly turning over tissues such as skeletal muscle, the atrophic effect may take years to become obvious. But in rapid turnover tissues (skin, mucous membranes, and bone marrow), the effect is evident within a few days. In the few hours after a dose of radiation, normal DNA recovers from radiation damage better than malignant DNA. In order to multiply this difference, a total dose of radiation is given in many fractions. A course usually consists of a small dose given daily four or five times per week for several weeks. As the cumulative dose increases, side effects in normal tissues and damage to the tumor become evident.

## Clinically

The first sign is an inflammatory reaction in the irradiated area, followed by signs of a lack of regenerative activity, such as skin or mucosal ulceration. The severity of this naturally depends on the total dose and the dose per fraction of radiation administered. The effect on the health of the patient depends on the volume being treated and the sensitivity of the structures within that volume. For example, small intestinal reaction tends to occur quickly, causing nausea, vomiting, malabsorption, and diarrhea. In contrast, a larger volume of thigh receiving a higher dose can cause the patient no symptom whatever.

After the course of radiation is finished, the tissue regenerates. Surviving stem cells proliferate and usually the organ recovers sufficiently to continue normal function. However, occasionally tissue atrophy or even necrosis occurs if the dose was too high or if the tissue was unusually sensitive. The late effects of radiation occur after one or more years and are due to three main factors: (a) reduced cell numbers, (b) fibrosis of the interstitial space, caused by the organization of fibrinogen which has leaked out of capillaries, and (c) intimal thickening of arterioles causing reduced blood flow and possible ischemia.

These late effects are worse if the radiation course was given in large-dose fractions; in fact, this last side effect on blood vessels is exploited in stereotactic radiosurgery (discussed later in chapter). Years of trial and error have led to the development of dose limits and schedules, which respect the sensitivity of the different organs. Recent radio-biological advances have made the prediction of radiation effects, a biological effective dose (BED), more reliable. Whether or not a tumor can be cured by radiation depends on the relative sensitivity of the tumor and the tissue surrounding it. Just as normal tissues vary in their ability to repair radiation damage and therefore their sensitivity to radiation, tumors have an innate sensitivity or resistance to XRT. Squamous cell carcinomas of the head and neck are radio-sensitive compared to other histological types of tumors.

## Curative Use of XRT

XRT can be used in the curative setting either alone or in combination with surgery and/or chemotherapy. In oncology the term "radical" means an attempt to cure, in contrast to its surgical connotation of being more extensive than conservative. Before a radical treatment is undertaken and the inevitable side effects inflicted (from either surgery or XRT), it is imperative that the patient is fully assessed to ensure that cure is a realistic goal. The most common curative modality used in oncology is surgery, but there are some conditions where XRT and/or chemotherapy is preferable.

### XRT in Isolation

Radiation is used alone when:

1. Surgery is not possible because of the tumor's location, that is, the involvement of essential structures (e.g., gliomata in critical parts of the brain or spinal cord, cervix carcinoma with extension beyond the cervix, Hodgkin's disease and non-Hodgkin's lymphoma, nasopharynx carcinoma, posterior tongue carcinoma, advanced breast carcinoma, and central lung carcinomas).
2. The results of surgery and XRT are equal in terms of cure, but the functional deficit after XRT is less than that after surgery (e.g., early carcinomas of the larynx, extensive skin carcinoma, and anal carcinoma).
3. The patient's general condition is so poor that surgery is contraindicated (e.g., obese elderly women

with early cervix carcinoma, patients with lung carcinoma and poor respiratory function).

A *curative* course of radiation involves treating the area of gross tumor and likely microscopic tumor to the maximum dose compatible with long-term health of the area. A *radical* dose of XRT is usually the maximum consistent with allowing normal tissue to remain functional. The higher the dose of XRT, the greater the likelihood that all malignant cells have been destroyed. However, the price of cure must be acceptable to the patient, and have a low chance of normal tissue necrosis. At times, tumor bulk or inherent resistance to radiation damage (as in some melanomas) is so great that a curative dose of XRT is certain to cause severe normal tissue damage and is therefore avoided. In this situation a lesser dose may cause temporary shrinkage with minimal normal tissue damage, so palliation but not cure is achieved. The prescribed dose of XRT varies with: tumor type and size, part of the body involved, volume of the body in field, and age and health of the patient.

In the head and neck, macroscopic disease is usually given 60 to 70 Gy in fractions of 1.8 to 2 Gy given 5 days weekly for 6 or 7 weeks. Microscopic deposits can be killed by a lower dose such as 50 to 55 Gy, allowing neck nodes to be treated in 5 weeks. If gross disease is larger than 2 cm, the addition of synchronous chemotherapy is advisable.

Fast-growing tumors such as squamous cell carcinomas of the head and neck may be better treated with faster radiation. There are various ways of doing this. Radiation treatments can be given twice or even three times daily, leaving a gap of at least 6 hours to allow normal tissue repair. If the dose per twice-daily fraction is close to the 1.8-2 Gy normal, the treatment is referred to as "accelerated," but if it is significantly less, such as 1.1-1.6 Gy, the treatment is regarded as "hyperfractionated". A higher total dose of hyperfractionated radiation can be safely given, for example 84 Gy in 70 fractions over 7 weeks (Nguyen & Ang, 2002). Results of speeding up the treatment show improved local control. An English group (Dische et al., 1997) gave three fractions daily to a dose of 54 Gy in 36 fractions over 12 uninterrupted days (labeled CHART—continuous hyperfractionated accelerated radiation therapy) and compared the result to 66 Gy in 33 fractions over 6.5 weeks. The accelerated dose of 54 Gy

was just as effective as, and had fewer late effects than, the higher dose and longer treatment. It is common for chemotherapy to be combined with altered fractionation schedules of radiation in an attempt to optimize the difference between effects on the tumor and on normal tissue.

New techniques of giving radiation have been developed with the aim of improving dose delivery to the tumor and the sparing of normal tissue. Intensity-modulated radiation therapy (IMRT) uses beams with variable dose intensities across the beam and multiple directions all focused on the target. In this technique, it is possible to restrict the dose to particular tissues below the threshold of functional loss; for example, parotid dose can be limited to less than 20 Gy and retain saliva production capacity. The place of IMRT in head and neck cancer is still being explored, mainly because the entire volume is treated in the same time period regardless of dose, that is, 50 Gy and 70 Gy both in 7 weeks, which may reduce the benefit in areas of subclinical disease such as neck nodes.

Stereotactic radiosurgery (SRS) is the term given to very focused radiation designed to destroy the target and replace it with scar tissue. It is used to sclerose blood vessels in arteriovenous malformations in the brain, and to kill benign but debilitating tumors in the brain or base of skull, such as unresectable meningiomas or acoustic neuromas. With the patient immobilized in a fixed head-frame on a linear accelerator couch, the machine is moved in several arcs with the desired sized beams focused on the target. Usually only one fraction is given as the desired outcome is the very side effect that fractionated radiation is designed to avoid, the closure of blood vessels. SRS is now being used to boost central tumor volumes in any part of the body that can be adequately immobilized. A variation of this is the gamma knife which uses multiple cobalt-60 sources that can be shielded, or not, to focus on a particular target.

### XRT and Surgery

XRT has been used as a treatment modality offered either prior to or following surgical intervention.

**XRT Presurgery.** There are some circumstances where shrinkage of the tumor prior to surgery is to the patient's advantage. An example is a large mass in the parotid where surgery would endanger the facial nerve and possibly leave the patient with a facial nerve paralysis. After reduction of the mass, it can be safer to dissect around the nerve, leaving it intact. Surgeons have always been rather nervous of the slower healing that occurs in an irradiated surgical bed. Postoperative infections may be more common and slower to respond to antibiotics. Preoperative radiation-only treatments are now quite rare, with synchronous chemoradiation often replacing both the preoperative radiation and the operation.

**XRT Postsurgery.** Frequently surgery, however extensive, is unable to remove enough normal tissue around the tumor to engender confidence that there are no malignant cells remaining in the region. Alternatively, the operative or pathology findings may indicate the likelihood of cancer cells remaining in the locality, or that regional nodes may be involved. In any situation where there is a suspicion of residual malignant cells, postoperative XRT should be considered, for example, if clinical features and/or histology shows: (a) large or deep primary (such as depth of invasion into the tongue), (b) close surgical margins, (c) extensive nodal involvement, especially with perinodal spread, and/or (d) extensive lymphatic, vascular, or perineural invasion. Postoperative radiation is often the patient's last chance of cure so radiation fields must cover all areas possibly containing malignant cells.

## Side Effects of XRT to the Head and Neck

Radiation is infamous for its side effects. We are always searching for a way of easing the adverse effects. With head and neck radiation, the degree of discomfort depends on the area of mucosa and the proportion of salivary gland mass in the field. Xerostomia occurs early because salivary tissue is very sensitive to radiation, with apoptosis (cell death) occurring after only a few fractions and no recovery at all if the gland receives more than about 25 Gy. Saliva becomes thick and sticky and usually has considerably reduced volume. The patient needs to modify his or her diet when this happens as the lack of lubrication and amylase rules out starches (bread, biscuits, and cake) and meat without gravy. As treatment progresses, the mucosa becomes inflamed, referred to as mucositis, and then

ulcerated as the basal layer of the mucosa is unable to adequately replace dying cells as shown in Figure 3–8. This ulceration is painful. Secondary infection, especially with endotoxic gram-negative bacteria, occurs, adding to the inflammatory stimulus.

Frequent, even hourly, mouthwashes help reduce the dead cell accumulation which provides fertile ground for bacterial and fungal infection. There are commercial preparations available but most patients still favor sodium bicarbonate made up as a weak solution of one teaspoon per liter water. Slow-release narcotics are indicated to keep people able to eat and carry on their daily activities. Antibiotic mouthwashes reduce the gram-negative colonization of damaged mucosa. Gram-negative bacteria have a toxin in their body wall (endotoxin) which is released on their death and contributes to inflammation. Antibiotic lozenges help reduce this extra contribution to the discomfort patients experience (Sutherland & Browman, 2001). However, in clinical practice lozenges are relatively contraindicated because of xerostomia. Patients need to artificially moisten their mouths when a lozenge of any type is in situ to prevent development of an osmotic ulcer. For a full review of measures taken to ease mucositis and their effectiveness see Sutherland and Browman (2001).

Amifostine is a radio-protective agent which has been found to protect normal tissue but not tumor (Wasserman et al., 2005). Although mucositis still occurs in the presence of amifostine, it is less severe and the patients are less likely to require admission for symptom control. Preservation of salivary function and patient comfort has been shown (McDonald, Meyerowitz, Smudzin, & Rubin, 1994). At Johns Hopkins, Baltimore, it is in routine use for almost all head and neck radiation treatments (T. De Weese, personal communication, December, 2003). However, currently the expense of the drug and its administration, and the hassle of adding a 90-minute intravenous infusion to each day's work for each head and neck patient, are factors limiting its use in other centers. A recent European trial of subcutaneous amifostine has found it to be just as effective as intravenous and much more convenient to administer (J. Bourhis, personal communication, November 25, 2005). So it is possible that amifostine will be in wider use in the near future.

If patients are unable to maintain their weight, alternative feeding routes relieve the stress of trying

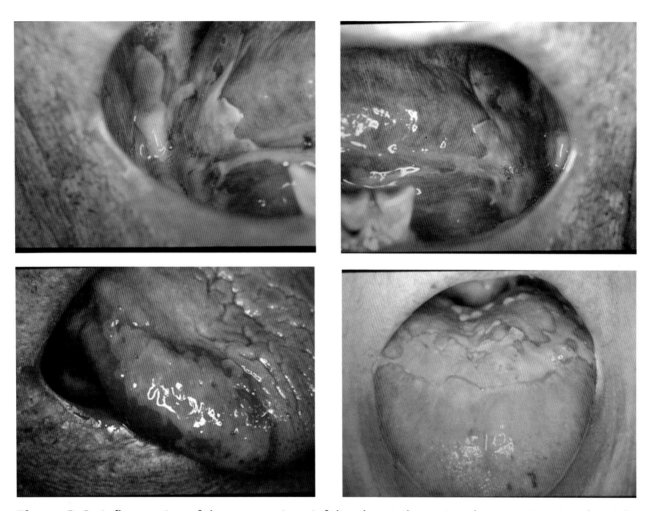

**Figure 3–8.** Inflammation of the mucosa is painful and contributes to reluctance to eat and weight loss. These pictures show various stages of mucositis and ulceration. Healing occurs quickly, usually within 2 or 3 weeks after the completion of radiation. (Photos courtesy of Dr. Sue Mason.)

and failing to maintain body weight. Gastrostomy insertion is indicated for longer term feeding (more than a few weeks), but if symptoms are mild or moderate and if it can be assumed it will be required only a short time, a nasogastric tube can be used.

In a dry mouth, teeth are in great danger of decay. Food and acid stick to the teeth, there is no flushing effect from saliva, and the teeth rapidly decay, particularly around the neck of the teeth (see Figure 3-9). Management of the teeth is an area of controversy. Some centers remove all teeth that will be in irradiated mandible and allow a few weeks for healing before radiation commences. Other centers restore and try to preserve teeth as long as possible (Stevenson-Moore &

Epstein, 1993). The long-term danger is that of osteoradionecrosis of the mandible (ORN) where the mandible is incapable of healing itself or of fighting infection due to a poor blood supply after radiation. If no disturbance occurs to the mucosa or alveolus, this is less likely. But if a tooth abscess develops or a tooth is extracted, ORN can set in. Intravenous antibiotics, hyperbaric oxygen, and surgical debridement are used to try to control the snowballing infection and ischemic death of bone (Bennett, Feldmeier, Hampson, Smee, & Milross, 2005). A large German study stretching back to 1969 showed an incidence of 8.2%, more in men than women, probably reflecting poor dental care and ongoing smoking (Reuther, Schuster, Mende,

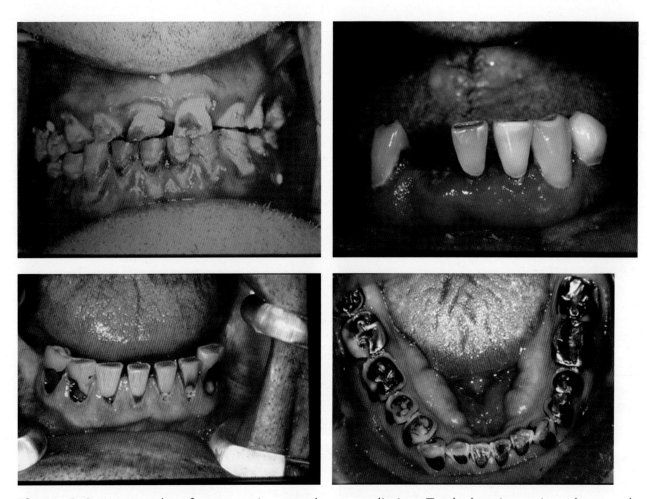

**Figure 3–9.** Late results of xerostomia secondary to radiation. Teeth deteriorate in a dry mouth which develops caries close to the gum line, causing them to snap off. The patient needs to be vigilant with cleaning and fluoride application daily. (Photos courtesy of Dr. Sue Mason.)

& Kubler, 2003). The rate of ORN after radiation is now only about 1% (Narozny et al., 2005), but it is a serious side effect that can go on for years, destroying the mandible and oral function.

In addition and particularly in those who continue to smoke, fibrosis of soft tissues in the neck or pharynx can snowball with hypoxia and TGF-beta-induced inflammation. This may respond to oxypentifylline and vitamin E, maximally vasodilating arterioles to the area and preventing damage from reintroduced oxygen respectively (Delanian & Lefaix, 2004). This treatment is also effective in improving healing if surgery is required after radiation.

After radiation is complete, time is required for bone remodeling to occur before dental prostheses are made. Most centers ask the patient to wait for 12 months before attempting to wear dentures, a time lag which distresses most people and which has recently been found to be longer than necessary (Gerngross et al., 2005).

Most patients finish their XRT in moderate discomfort from their acute side effects, but recover in subsequent weeks and months, with great variability between patients. Some may be left in long-term discomfort, for example from xerostomia, thinning of mucosa, or trismus.

# Chemotherapy

## Chemotherapy Agents and Their Mechanisms of Action

The most alarming feature about cancers is their enormous and uncontrolled reproductive capacity. Most cytotoxic drugs sabotage this. They are categorized by the part of the process where they act. The reader is referred to an oncology textbook for a full description of these agents. Discussion here is limited to some agents used in head and neck SCC therapy:

### Antimetabolic Agents

Antimetabolites are similar in structure to molecules essential for cell function, but are unable to perform when required. Two more commonly used agents within this group include methotrexate and 5-flurouracil (5FU). Methotrexate binds to and inhibits dihydrofolate reductase, the enzyme that maintains intracellular folate in a reduced state. Without reduced folate, one-carbon-groups cannot be carried and synthesized into thymidylate and purines. Methotrexate has activity against SCCs and is most often used for palliation as a weekly injection. The antimetabolic agent 5FU was designed to substitute for uracil into a nucleotide, 5-deoxyuridylate (5-FdUMP), bind thymidylate synthetase, and inhibit synthesis of deoxythymidine triphosphate, one necessary precursor of DNA. 5FU has a wide range of activity and is used in colonic/rectal and lung cancer treatments as well as head and neck SCCs. Side effects of high doses include marrow suppression and, unfortunately, ulceration of mucosal surfaces. Doses and administration schedules vary with tumor cell type.

### Alkylating Agents

These agents have the ability to bind covalently with DNA and disrupt its functioning or replication. Some agents work by forming DNA cross-links. Single- or double-strand breaks can occur directly due to covalent bonding or secondary to an attempt to repair the DNA by the cell. DNA damage by these agents potentiates DNA damage by ionizing radiation. In addition,

synthesis is inhibited of DNA, RNA, and proteins. Two alkylating agents, cisplatin and carboplatin, both consist of platinum bound to diamine groups, which are detached in vivo from the active compound enabling it to bind with guanine bases, forming cross-links, resulting in adducts with DNA. The overall three-dimensional structure of the DNA molecule is changed with the double helix distorted and an unwinding of the DNA. Cellular protein defense strategies are activated to deal with the changed DNA. If damage is too severe, cell apoptosis results. Cisplatin is the most widely used alkylating agent in head and neck cancers and is particularly able to form DNA cross-links. It can be given as a single high dose of $100mg/m^2$ every three weeks or a lower dose daily for 5 days. From 20–75% is excreted in urine in the first 24 hours after administration, the remainder staying in tissues or bound to plasma proteins. Such high concentrations in kidneys are toxic unless glomerular filtration is high and renal tubule reuptake is low. It is therefore imperative to prehydrate and keep urine production high for several hours after administration of a high dose. Fractionating the cisplatin dose into five daily treatments improves renal safety. Most patients experience nausea and vomiting, warranting premedication with tropisetron or ondansetron. Other less common toxicities include neurotoxicity and ototoxicity.

Carboplatin is a less nephrotoxic analog of cisplatin which is a much more stable molecule. Ninety percent of cisplatin is bound to serum protein at 4 hours, in contrast to 24% of carboplatin. Most carboplatin is excreted in urine unchanged, making precautions against nephrotoxicity unnecessary. This advantage is offset by greater marrow toxicity. Because there is no necessity for prehydration before carboplatin, administration is faster, easing the workload in busy oncology units.

### Antimicrotubule Agents

In a normal cell at initiation of mitosis, the nuclear membrane dissolves and the centromeres move to each end of the cell with spindle connecting them to DNA. The spindle, composed of polymers of tubulin, then contracts and draws apart the duplicated chromosomes. Spindle has other purposes within the cell between mitoses—it acts as a skeleton for the cell to maintain solidity. Both of these roles require a dynamic and rapidly responsive material. Tubulin is constantly changing with the polymer ends capable of rapid synthesis or dissolution. Two types of antimicrotubule agents are the vinca alkaloids and taxanes. Vinca compounds bind to the end of tubulin and slow down the response to cell activities, impeding mitosis. Instead of anaphase, DNA remains clumped in the center of the cell, which may then go on to apoptosis. Taxanes are a relatively new class of compounds originally from the bark of the Pacific yew tree. They bind to the interior of the tubulin structure, promote polymerization, and reduce dissolution of tubulin at the normally active ends. The spindle thereby loses the ability to change as the cell requires—it is locked, preventing mitosis and damaging normal function. Taxanes have found use in many malignancies, ovary, breast, sarcomas, lymphomas, and head and neck.

### Antitumor Antibiotics

Topoisomerases form a class of enzymes that control DNA unwinding and rewinding. Before DNA can be repaired or replicated, the double helix must be unwound to allow access to the DNA strand. Topoisomerases are therefore essential for the smooth organization of cellular function and DNA integrity. Anthracyclines are cytotoxic agents, which have been in use for decades, but the precise mechanism of action is still being elucidated. It is now understood that topoisomerases are their main target and that the deterioration in DNA is secondary to this. Accumulation occurs of protein-linked double and single-strand DNA breaks, damage from which the cell may be unable to recover, leading to apoptosis. The most commonly used drug is doxorubicin (Adriamycin). It is widely used today in breast, lung, and sarcoma treatments as well as in some combinations of head and neck treatments. The main toxicities of these drugs are marrow suppression, alopecia, and cardiotoxicity.

## Side Effects of Chemotherapy

In the public mind, chemotherapy has a dreadful reputation. Much of this comes from observations of other patients many years ago. Contemporary chemotherapy is much easier for the patient and much less danger-ous. New drugs such as the serotonin antagonists, ondansetron and tropisetron, have made nausea and vomiting much less severe. Marrow suppression can be overcome by colony-stimulating factors such as filgastrim and patient education has made dangers such as neutropenic sepsis more successfully treatable. Hair loss can be complete or partial. Anthracyclines are the most likely to cause alopecia. Ice packs have been used to reduce blood flow to the scalp for a few hours with partial success. Fatigue is one side effect for which we have no remedy, most people needing to cut down work and social commitments during their course. See Table 3–1 for a summary of these common side effects.

## Curative Use of Chemotherapy

### Chemotherapy in Isolation

Chemotherapy is often curative for cancer types such as leukemia; however, there are few solid malignancies for which chemotherapy is curative when used alone. These are seminomas and nonseminomatous testicular carcinomas, Hodgkin's disease, and non-Hodgkin's lymphomas. There are rare cures with small cell carcinomas of the lung. Curative chemo is more successful in children because pediatric malignancies seem more sensitive to chemotherapy and children are able to tolerate higher doses. In head and neck cancer, chemotherapy alone is best regarded as never curative.

### Chemotherapy with Surgery or Radiation

The role of chemotherapy when combined with surgery or radiation is twofold. It can be given preoperatively as neo-adjuvant therapy in an attempt to make surgery or radiation more likely to encompass the entire disease. Alternatively, it can be given postoperatively or postradiation (as adjuvant therapy) aiming to kill cells that may have disseminated throughout the body. As will be described later in the chapter, chemotherapy can also be given simultaneously with radiation.

During the 1980s, chemotherapy was used in the neo-adjuvant setting, that is, as first treatment after diagnosis. It was thought from experimental data that a gap between chemo and radiation was necessary

**Table 3–1.** Common Side Effects of Chemotherapy Drugs Used in Head and Neck Squamous Cell Carcinomas

| Side Effect | Drug | Cause | Therapy |
|---|---|---|---|
| Nausea, vomiting | Many | Sensitivity of vomiting center | Ondansetron, tropisetron, dexamethasone, metoclopramide, prochlorperazine |
| Mucosal toxicity | 5FU | Loss of cell numbers in mucosa | Wait, reduce dose, local anesthetics |
| Infection | Many; anthracyclines, methotrexate, 5FU, carboplatin | Reduced numbers of marrow stem cells | Broad-spectrum antibiotics, isolation, filgrastim, reduce dose of next course |
| Bleeding | As for infection | As for infection | Platelet transfusion |
| Anemia | As for infection | As for infection | Red blood cell transfusion; ensure iron, folate, and B12 adequate; erythropoietin |
| Nephrotoxicity | Cisplatin | Renal tubule sensitivity | Ensure strong glomerular filtration rate with IV and oral fluids; amifostine |
| Cardiotoxicity | Anthracyclines | Direct toxicity to myocardial cells | Pretreatment and progress assessment of heart stroke volume (echocardiogram); limit total dose of drug |
| Alopecia | Anthracyclines, antitumor antibiotics | Sensitivity of hair follicles | Scalp ice pack or wig; regrowth is usually strong |
| Induced tumors | Many | Mutations in stem cells | Ongoing follow-up of young patients; avoid worst drugs |

in order to keep normal tissues safe (Steel, 1988). Although responses to chemo were impressive, this did not usually translate to an improvement in tumor-free or overall survival. For example, the Department of Veterans' Affairs Laryngeal Cancer Study Group found a response rate of 85% after two cycles of cisplatin and 5-fluorouracil in patients with advanced laryngeal cancer, which translated into a 64% cure rate allowing retention of larynx after three cycles of chemo and subsequent high-dose radiation (Department of Veterans' Affairs Laryngeal Cancer Study Group, 1991). Although the response rate was so high, there were more local recurrences but fewer distant metastases in the group that received chemotherapy compared to laryngectomy. Such results led to the dismissal of chemotherapy in head and neck treatments as nothing more than a good way to bide time before surgery or

radiation (Tannock & Browman, 1986) or to select out the more responsive and better prognosis tumors.

However, both presurgery chemotherapy (Faivre et al., 2005) and preradiation chemotherapy have been advocated again recently. Carcinoma of the nasopharynx sometimes extends through the base of skull. This makes dose limitation, and protection of critical structures such as retinas, brainstem, and the optic nerves, very difficult (or even impossible) when the tumor is adjacent to, or surrounding, these structures. Shrinking the tumor before radiation would seem to be a good idea and, indeed, chemotherapy has been used for this purpose (Rischin et al., 2002). However, the traditional thinking in radiation oncology is that the entire original extent of the tumor should be treated in order to kill surviving edge deposits and prevent local recurrence.

Head and neck sarcomas are rare and respond differently to chemotherapy. As with sarcomas elsewhere, chemo can reduce the size of the primary mass as well as reduce the chance of metastatic spread. So in this disease, chemotherapy is beneficial as neo-adjuvant and adjuvant, that is, preoperatively and postoperatively. For example, esthesioneuroblastomas are often unresectable at first assessment. Chemotherapy is given in the hope that the lesion will shrink enough to allow resection, if necessary, from cranial and facial directions. If it is still unresectable by virtue of involvement of the sphenoid, clivus, and brainstem, etc., radiation is used. If resection proceeds, postoperative radiation is used to kill the remaining microscopic tumor in the region. Other sarcomas such as osteogenic sarcomas are also treated firstly with chemo, then surgery if possible, then radiotherapy if the histology indicates much surviving tumor, followed by ongoing adjuvant chemo to reduce the risk of metastatic deposits surviving.

There are many malignancies where postoperative chemotherapy is advised. These include bowel cancer, breast cancer, and lung cancer where there is a high rate of dissemination in blood vessels. In breast cancer, this has particularly been very successful, with a reduction in breast cancer mortality risk in young women of 38% with the use of adjuvant chemotherapy (Early Breast Cancer Trialists' Collaborative Group, 2005). Apart from the sarcomas, there has been little benefit shown for postoperative chemotherapy in head and neck malignancies, with one exception. Adenocarcinoma of the nasal cavity or paranasal sinuses is uncommon but unresponsive to radiation. It can be treated successfully by resection of as much disease as possible and the remaining disease being treated by topical 5-fluorouracil applied on a nasal pack (Knegt, Ah-See, vd Velden, & Kerrebijn, 2001).

# Chemoradiotherapy

As described in the introduction, this modality is one of the great advances in head and neck cancer treatments and is very recent. In 1987, the Christie in Manchester published results of a randomized controlled trial of their usual small-volume, high-intensity radiation treatment (50 Gy in 15 fractions) with or without high-dose methotrexate (Gupta, Pointon, & Wilkinson, 1987). They found significant improvement in both control of primary and survival with chemotherapy given simultaneously. At the same time, a Munich group put together a regimen of twice daily (accelerated) radiation given in three episodes synchronously with 5-fluorouracil 350 mg/m$^2$/day × 5 and cisplatin 60 mg/m$^2$ on day 1 (Wendt, Hartenstein, Wustrow, & Lissner, 1989) as described in Figure 3–10. Leucovorin was used to potentiate the 5-fluorouracil. Data revealed that 81% had a complete response; local control was 72% and disease-free survival was 60% at 2 years. These results are still regarded as very good.

Another combination was that used by a Chicago team published in 1987 (Murthy et al., 1987). They gave radiation in alternate weeks, that is, weeks 1, 3, 5, 7, 9, and 11, at the rate of 10 Gy per week, the usual weekly dose. Each treatment week, the patient also received cisplatin 60 mg/m$^2$ on day 1, and 5-fluorouracil 800 mg/m$^2$/day over days 1 to 5 (see Figure 3–11). Regional control persisted in 87% of the patients for 2 years but distant metastases developed in 23% of these people. Longer follow-up showed a 5-year disease-free survival of 60% (Taylor et al., 1997). Others have tried this regimen but have difficulty getting further than the third week, that is, week 5, of treatment because of bone marrow suppression and renal damage.

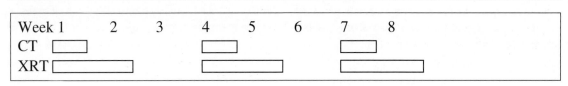

**Figure 3–10.** The schedule of chemotherapy and radiation used by Wendt et al. (1989), with three episodes of accelerated radiation given synchronously with 5FU and cisplatin, separated by two rest periods.

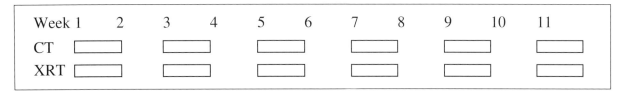

**Figure 3–11.** Schedule of Murthy et al. (1987), giving synchronous radiation and cisplatin-5FU with rest periods in alternate weeks. The overall duration of this regimen is now regarded as disadvantageous.

The large number of randomized controlled trials and the varied treatment regimens between centers can be confusing. In addition, trials with positive results receive more attention than negative trials. An overview of these trials helps us assess results objectively. Pignon, Bourhis, Domenge, and Designe (2000) studied 63 trials of locoregional treatment with or without chemotherapy, examining trials in groups of similar treatments. Not all trials showed a benefit but synchronous chemoradiation overall yielded an improvement of 7% in overall survival at 2 years, and 8% at 5 years. Concomitant or alternating chemoradiation is more effective than induction chemotherapy (2% absolute survival improvement at 2 and 5 years).

## How the Combination Improves the Result

The precise way that cisplatin and carboplatin improve cell kill with radiation is not understood. The evidence is inconclusive as to whether it is an additive or super-additive effect. Research is conflicting about whether the effect is due to sensitization of hypoxic cells, inhibition of sublethal damage repair in tumors, or inhibition of potentially lethal damage repair. It may be that the platinums independently kill tumor cells and the effect is simply additive. Most agree that platinums cause reduced bulk and that allows reoxygenation and repositioning of cells from radio-resistant phases of the cell cycle (especially $G_0$) into more sensitive phases. As the mass reduces in size, more cells receive enough blood to pull them out of the resting phase and into the active proliferation part of the cell cycle where they are more sensitive to radiation damage. We are still arguing about whether high-dose infrequent cisplatin

(Forastiere et al., 2003) or daily low-dose cisplatin (Bartelink, van den Bogaert, Horiot, & van Glabbeke, 2002) is the preferred option to use in an attempt to inflict chemotherapy damage on tumor cells but not normal cells.

## Side Effects

There is no doubt that patients have a tougher time during radiation treatment if chemotherapy is added to their burden (Denis et al., 2003). The side effects of radiation described previously in the chapter (i.e., xerostomia, mucositis, and odynophagia) are rendered more severe by chemotherapy-induced sensitization of normal cells to radiation damage. Additionally, the patient suffers chemotherapy side effects of a more general nature, such as lethargy, weariness, and susceptibility to infection. There is debate about the required dose of chemotherapy agents, with some using the maximum dose tolerable (Adelstein et al., 1997) and others using a low dose still effective at sensitizing cells to radiation (Merlano et al., 1996). For a review of strategies in development to reduce toxicities, see Milas, Mason, Liao, and Ang (2003). It is now thought that the late functional outcome (i.e., pharyngeal/laryngeal function) is less determined by the specific chemoradiation regimen than the site of disease and the amount of destruction caused by the tumor (Logemann et al., 2006).

## Curative Use: Regimens in Current Use

The situation has evolved to the position where there are multiple regimens in use throughout the world, many on the basis of institutional experience alone, as is appropriate in a rapidly changing area of practice. There are regimens selected for use in frail, robust, deaf, renally or hepatically compromised patients. The factors that determine which regimens will eventually rise above the others to become widely acknowledged as best practice are cultural, financial, and personal among oncologists and their organizations. It will take many years and many randomized controlled trials comparing regimens before the better ones are recognizable. Institutional studies are not comparable because of variations in the staging process, tumor stage at presentation of the population, quality of treatment delivery, and support services during and after treatment. A regimen that achieves 50% 5-year disease-free survival at one institution may achieve 25% at another. A well-supervised multi-institutional randomized controlled trial is very expensive and needs financial support of government or industry to be achieved. The following sections outline some of the combinations recognized around the world as valid.

### Calais

The French head and neck cancer study group (GORTEC study 94-01) conducted a randomized controlled trial comparing standard radiation (70 Gy in

7 weeks) with and without three cycles of carboplatin 70 mg/m$^2$/day × 4 and 5-fluorouracil 600 mg/m$^2$/day × 4 (Calais et al., 1999) (see Figure 3–12). Mucosal toxicity was higher in the chemotherapy group, but locoregional control improved at 3 years from 42% to 66% with the addition of chemotherapy and 25% to 48% at 5 years (Denis et al., 2003). This has translated to an improvement in survival at 5 years from 16% to 22% with the addition of chemotherapy.

### Adelstein

A group in Cleveland, Ohio (Adelstein et al., 1997), conducted a randomized controlled trial of standard radiation compared to that plus cisplatin 20 mg/m$^2$/day and 5-fluorouracil 1000 mg/m$^2$/day, given as an infusion over 4 days in weeks 1 and 4 of the program (see Figure 3–13). Although toxicity was greater in the group that received chemotherapy, relapse-free survival projections for 3 years were 52% without chemotherapy and 67% with chemotherapy.

### Merlano

An Italian group (Merlano et al., 1996) came up with an alternating schedule of cisplatin 20 mg/m$^2$/day × 5 and 5-fluorouracil 200 mg/m$^2$/day × 5 in weeks 1, 4, 7,

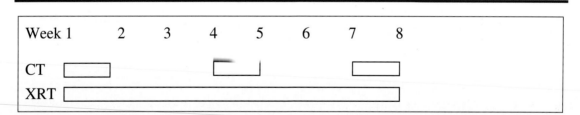

**Figure 3–12.** Schedule of Calais et al. (1999), which uses continuous radiation for 7 weeks and carboplatin-5FU weeks 1, 4, and 7.

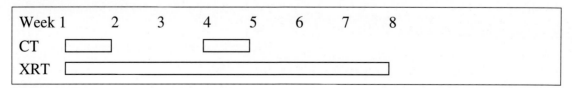

**Figure 3–13.** Schedule of Adelstein et al. (1997), which uses fractionated cisplatin and high-dose 5FU in weeks 1 and 4 of a continuous radiation course.

and 10, sandwiching radiation 10 Gy per week in weeks 2-3, 5-6, and 8-9, as diagrammed in Figure 3-14. In a randomized controlled trial, this was compared to conventional radiation of 70 Gy in 7 weeks. Complete response was improved in the chemoradiation arm 43% vs. 22%. Five-year local control rates were 64% compared to 32%.

## Brizel

In 1998, a randomized controlled trial was published comparing hyperfractionated radiation up to 75 Gy in 60 twice-daily fractions with 70 Gy in 1.25 Gy fractions also given twice daily with a gap after 3 weeks of 7 days. Chemotherapy in this 70 Gy arm was cisplatin and 5-fluorouracil given synchronously with radiation as well as postradiation. Locoregional control was improved by chemotherapy to 70% versus 40%, but at the cost of late necrosis of an extra 5% (Brizel et al., 1998).

## Corry

During the 1990s, radiobiologists began to tell us that repopulation in squamous cell carcinomas is detrimental to the chance of cure if the treatment goes on for too long (e.g., more than 6 weeks). One strategy to

overcome this was to give chemotherapy at the end of the course of radiation in order to reduce reproductive activity of residual cancer cells enjoying a new low population environment (Corry et al., 2000). The Melbourne group used conventional radiation of 70 Gy in 7 weeks with cisplatin 10 mg/m$^2$/day and 5-fluorouracil 360 mg/m$^2$/day for days 1-5 of the last 2 weeks as diagrammed in Figure 3-15. Locoregional failure occurred in 40% at 2 years. Although only a small phase II study with 28 patients, this was a novel approach.

## Dobrowski

The question remained as to whether chemoradiation was more effective than accelerated radiation. In a trial of three arms, Dobrowski and Naude (2000) compared conventional radiation (70 Gy over 7 weeks) to CHART (55.3 Gy in 33 fractions over 17 days) to CHART + mitomycin C chemotherapy. With a median follow-up of 48 months, the local control rates were 31%, 32%, and 48%, respectively, showing that chemotherapy adds something that altered fractionation cannot.

## Olmi

An Italian group compared conventional fractionation to 70 Gy with accelerated hyperfractionated radiation

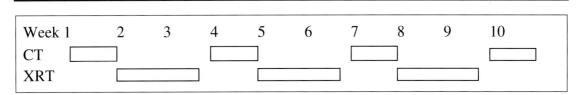

**Figure 3-14.** Schedule of Merlano et al. (1996), using alternating chemotherapy in weeks 1, 4, 7, and 10, and radiation weeks 2-3, 5-6, and 8-9. Doses of both chemotherapy and radiation are moderate.

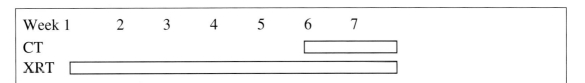

**Figure 3-15.** Schedule of Corry et al. (2000), who used chemotherapy in the last 2 weeks of a conventional radiation course to compensate for the repopulation that cancer cells undergo after about 6 weeks of cell loss. Doses of chemotherapy were moderate.

as 1.6 Gy twice daily to 38.4 Gy, a 2-week rest, and then resume radiation treatment up to 64–67.2 Gy. As a third arm, they used conventional fractionation with carboplatin 75 mg/m²/day and 5-fluorouracil 1000 mg/m²/day both on days 1–4 in weeks 1 and 5, as well as a postradiation week 9 (Olmi, 2003) (see Figure 3–16). Although disease-free survival at 2 years was 23%, 20%, and 42%, respectively, there was no significant difference in overall survival.

### Forastiere

In the United States now, the standard chemoradiation regimen is 70 Gy in 35 fractions given as 2 Gy daily conventional fractionation. This is combined with cisplatin alone, 100 mg/m² on days 1, 22, and 43. This arose from a trial of standard radiotherapy with either neo-adjuvant (induction) cisplatin and 5-fluorouracil chemotherapy, synchronous chemotherapy with cisplatin alone, or no chemotherapy (Forastiere et al., 2003). A group of 518 patients were available for assessment, a very large trial. Toxicity was worse in the synchronous group with worse radiation effects such as pharyngeal mucositis as well as chemo-induced neutropenia, nausea, and vomiting. Severe toxic effects occurred in 81% of the induction chemotherapy group, 82% of the synchronous group, and 61% in those assigned to radiotherapy alone. In the induction chemotherapy group, 72% retained their larynx at 3.8 years, compared to 84% of the synchronous group and 67% of the radiation alone group. Although this synchronous regimen is effective, the toxicity is such that close supervision and good support services are mandatory. Great care must be taken in hot climates

due to dehydration leading to kidney failure—xerostomia negates the thirst stimulus to drink, odynophagia due to radiation effects increases reluctance to ingest anything, and the kidneys have had a dose of cisplatin which is toxic in the setting of dehydration.

### ECLA Regimen

During the 1990s at Royal Brisbane Hospital, we adapted the Chicago alternating regimen (Murthy et al., 1987) to one we could use to achieve a radical dose of radiation in 7 weeks. This has been labeled the early chemo-late acceleration (ECLA) regimen. We wished to separate the toxic effects of chemotherapy and radiation, and to achieve a rapid initial response so that less tumor was hypoxic and therefore less resistant to radiation when the serious, accelerated radiation started in week 5. We have since learned from the TROG trial of accelerated radiation versus conventional (Poulsen et al., 2001), that acute side effects of radiation are more short-lived in accelerated regimens. So this regimen gives chemotherapy as cisplatin 25 mg/m²/day on days 1–5 and 5-fluorouracil 300 mg/m²/day days 1–4 with 2 Gy radiation daily × 5 in weeks 1 and 3 (see Figure 3–17).

The dose of 5-fluorouracil is low in order to provide radiosensitization of the tumor but minimize 5FU's toxic effect on mucosa. Weeks 2 and 4 are rest weeks during which the tumor shrinks and reoxygenation can occur, making the tumor more radiosensitive (Nordsmark et al., 2005). Weeks 5, 6, and 7 are accelerated with twice daily radiation giving 2 Gy to large volumes in the morning and 1.33 Gy to the reduced volume as an evening boost. The total radiation dose is

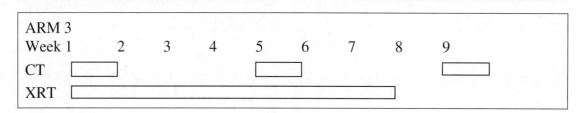

**Figure 3–16.** The third arm of a three-arm trial reported by Olmi et al. (2003), comparing arm 1—conventional radiation to arm 2—accelerated split-course radiation, and to this combination of chemotherapy and radiation. The chemotherapy was given in weeks 1 and 5 of a 7-week conventional radiation course as well as after the radiation was complete in week 9. Local control but not survival was improved.

70 Gy to gross tumor and 50 Gy to microscopic tumor. Most patients are able to eat well during weeks 2 and 4, and weeks 5 and 6. By week 5, patients have recovered from chemotherapy side effects and are experiencing a great reduction in symptoms caused by the tumor bulk. Mucositis is usually not significant until the beginning of week 7 and has largely abated by week 10. Toxicity with this regimen is moderate and local control rates in 66 patients with at least 12 months' follow-up are good, being 72% at 5 years, which is equal to other more toxic regimens. *Disease-specific*

survival at 5 years is 53% (the difference between 72% and 53% indicating those who died of disseminated metastases while maintaining local control). Figures 3–18 and 3–19 show the presenting tumors of two patients treated more than 10 years ago. Both remain well and free of a tumor at the time of writing.

### *Intra-arterial*

In order to spare normal tissues, some centers have developed intra-arterial chemotherapy using the expert-

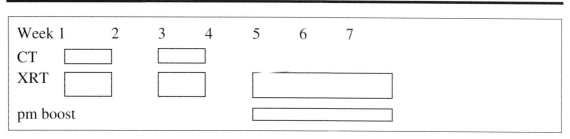

**Figure 3–17.** Early chemo-late acceleration schedule used by the author and colleagues. Chemotherapy is given in weeks 1 and 3 with rest periods weeks 2 and 4. This is followed by accelerated (twice daily) radiation in weeks 5, 6, and 7.

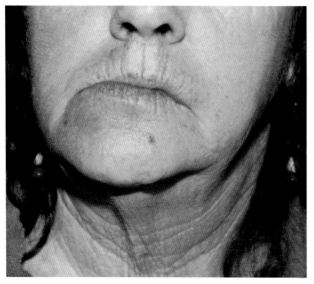

**A.**

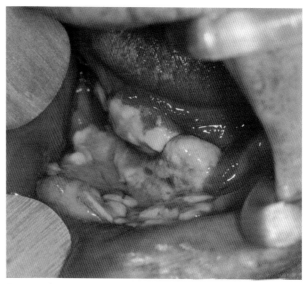

**B.**

**Figure 3–18. A.** This woman had SCC of the floor of mouth extending from the ventral tongue to the subcutaneous tissues of the chin, hence the asymmetry. **B.** She was cured with chemoradiation in 1994 after refusing radical surgery.

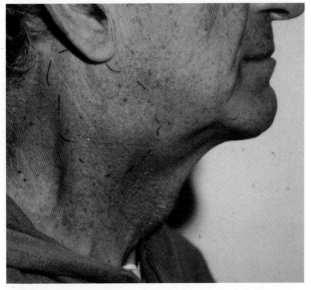

**A.**

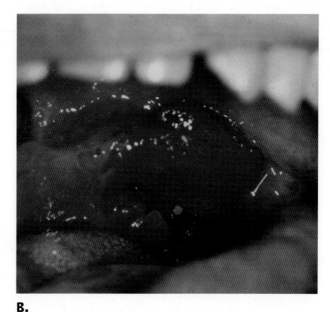

**B.**

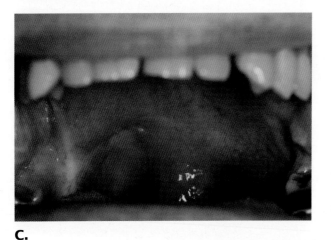

**C.**

**Figure 3–19.** The first patient who had the ECLA regimen in 1992 showing **A.** an 8 × 6 cm lymph node in level 2 of the right neck and **B.** a T4 SCC of the right tonsil extending across the midline to involve the entire soft palate. He refused surgery so received chemo-XRT. **C.** shows his oropharynx 8 months later with no sign of tumor. In 2001, he required hyperbaric oxygen after a molar tooth was extracted, leading to osteoradionecrosis. This treatment was successful. He remains well in 2006.

ise of interventional radiologists who can navigate through the femoral artery to the tumor bed arteries. There they deliver a high dose of cisplatin (150 mg/m$^2$) while protecting the rest of the body with thiosulfate intravenously (Samant et al., 1999). This is repeated on days 1, 8, 15, and 22 during a course of conventional radiation to 68.4 Gy. Complete response was 88%, but projected 5-year disease-free survival was 50%, and overall survival 23%. Mucositis was still a significant toxicity in 40% of patients, an improvement over most treatments.

## Chemoradiation and Surgery

### Preoperative Application

If a tumor is advanced and marginally resectable, preoperative tumor shrinkage with chemoradiation can allow a better functional outcome of surgery. In a Japanese study of oral cavity carcinoma (Kirita et al., 1999), they used 40 Gy in 2 Gy fractions with either cisplatin or carboplatin-based combinations. Surgery was undertaken 2 to 6 weeks after completion and consisted of resection of residual primary and immediate reconstruction. Complete response was 60% and partial response was 38% for the primary, and 16% and 37% for the lymph nodes. At operation, no tumor was found histologically in 50% of patients and 40% had only microscopic residual disease. Toxicity was low with no patient experiencing severe toxicity. Studies such as this raise the question of whether the dose of chemotherapy and of radiation needs to be "as high as is survivable" and if more is always better.

### Postoperative Application

If, after resection, the histology report indicates that the tumor is unusually aggressive, chemoradiation may be more effective at sterilizing residual cancer cells than radiation alone. This has been confirmed in both a European and an American trial (Bernier et al., 2005). Chemoradiation is indicated if at resection the cancer is found to have spread outside the capsule of one or more lymph nodes or to involve resection margins.

# Chemotherapy and Radiotherapy: Role in Palliative Care

Often the patient with head and neck cancer is weakened by the tumor, loss of function, and/or many years of alcohol or tobacco abuse. It may be that he or she is unable to withstand the toxicity of chemotherapy and/or the high doses of radiation. Alternatively, a patient may have significant pain or functional or cosmetic deficits in the head and neck, but be incurable because of disseminated metastases. In such cases, modified, less toxic treatment regimens can be given to provide relief and tumor control for a time.

Radiation alone can achieve this. Fractionation schedules in use include 6 Gy fractions given twice weekly for 3 weeks. Long-term damage from the large fraction size is irrelevant with a short life expectancy. An alternative protocol of 14 Gy can be given in four fractions over 2 days. This was found to result in improved quality of life (EORTC QLQ C30) in about half the participants (Corry et al., 2005).

If the patient has disseminated metastases or lives far from a radiation treatment center, administration of chemotherapy can be advantageous, hopefully obtaining an effect on SCC wherever it is in the body. Weekly intravenous methotrexate is an old palliative regimen that gives short-term responses with minimal morbidity. We frequently use the first half of the ECLA regimen for palliation, delivering cisplatin, 5-fluorouracil, and 20 Gy in 3 weeks. Good tumor restraint can be achieved. If a tumor or the patient is assessed as borderline-treatable, the first 3 weeks of this regimen can be used as a diagnostic test to assess the general condition and the sensitivity of the tumor to treatment. Tumor shrinkage allows for improved oral or pharyngeal function and reduced pain so that we sometimes progress to radical treatment after an initial palliative foray. Pain relief and the palliation of symptoms are as important in this area of oncology as in others.

# Conclusion

Head and neck malignancies are among the most curable cancers because of their sensitivity to radiation and chemotherapy, and their low rate of disseminated spread. Because a long life expectancy is possible, the quality of the patient's treatment and rehabilitation is all the more important. Members of the head and neck clinic are rewarded by achieving successful outcomes for most patients, and also through their involvement with an enthusiastic and dedicated team of medical and allied health professionals.

## Further Reading

DeVita, V. T., Jr., Hellman, S., & Rosenberg, S. A. (Eds.). (2005). *Cancer: Principles and practice of oncology.* Philadelphia: Lippincott Williams and Wilkins.

## References

Adelstein D. J., Saxton, J. P., Lavertu, P., Tuason, L., Wood, B. G., Wanamaker, J. R., et al. (1997). A phase III randomized trial comparing concurrent chemotherapy and radiotherapy with radiotherapy alone in resectable Stage III and IV squamous cell head and neck cancer: Preliminary results. *Head and Neck, 19,* 567-575.

Bartelink, H., van den Bogaert, W., Horiot, J. C., & van Glabbeke, M. (2002). Concomitant cisplatin and radiotherapy in a conventional and modified fractionation schedule in locally advanced head and neck cancer: A randomised phase II EORTC trial. *European Journal of Cancer, 38,* 667-673.

Bennett, M. H., Feldmeier, J., Hampson, N., Smee, R., & Milross, C. (2005). Hyperbaric oxygen therapy for late radiation tissue injury. *Cochrane Database of Systematic Reviews, 3,* CD005005.

Bernier, J., Cooper, J. S., Pajak, T. F., van Glabbeke, M., Bourhis, J., Forastiere, A., et al. (2005). Defining risk levels in locally advanced head and neck cancers: A comparative analysis of concurrent postoperative radiation plus chemotherapy trials of the EORTC (#22931) and RTOG (#9501). *Head and Neck, 27,* 843-850.

Brizel, D. M., Albers, M. E., Fisher, S. R., Scher, R. L., Richtsmeier, W. J., Hars, V., et al. (1998). Hyperfractionated irradiation with or without concurrent chemotherapy for locally advanced head and neck cancer. *New England Journal of Medicine, 338,* 1798-1804.

Calais, G., Alfonsi, M., Bardet, E., Sire, C., Germain, T., Bergerot, P., et al. (1999). Randomized trial of radiation therapy versus chemotherapy and radiation therapy for advanced-stage oropharynx carcinoma. *Journal of the National Cancer Institute, 91,* 2081-2086.

Corry, J., Peters, L., D'Costa, I., Milner, A. D., Fawns, H., Porceddu, S., et al. (2005, November). The "QUAD SHOT"—A phase II study of palliative radiotherapy for incurable head and neck cancer. *Radiotherapy and Oncology, 77,* 137-142.

Corry, J., Rischin, D., Smith, J. G., D'Costa, I. A., Hughes, P., Sexton, M. A., et al. (2000). Radiation with concurrent late chemotherapy intensification ("chemoboost") for locally advanced head and neck cancer. *Radiotherapy & Oncology, 54,* 123-127.

Delanian, S., & Lefaix, J. L. (2004). The radiation-induced fibroapoptotic process: Therapeutic perspective via the antioxidant pathway. *Radiotherapy & Oncology, 73,* 119-131.

Denis, F., Garaud, P., Bardet, E., Alfonsi, M., Sire, C., Germain, T., et al. (2003). Late toxicity results of the GORTEC 94-01 randomized trial comparing radiotherapy with concomitant radiochemotherapy for advanced-stage oropharynx carcinoma: Comparison of LENT/SOMA, RTOG/EORTC, and NCI-CTC scoring systems. *International Journal of Radiation, Oncology, Biology & Physics, 55,* 93-98.

Department of Veterans' Affairs Laryngeal Cancer Study Group. (1991). Induction chemotherapy plus radiation compared with surgery plus radiation in patients with advanced larynx cancer. *New England Journal of Medicine, 324,* 1685-1690.

Dische, S., Saunders, M., Barrett, A., Harvey, A., Gibson, D., & Parmar, M. (1997). A randomized multicentre trial of CHART versus conventional radiotherapy in head and neck cancer. *Radiotherapy and Oncology, 44,* 123-136.

Dobrowski, W., & Naude, L. (2000). Continuous hyperfractionated accelerated radiotherapy with/without mitomycin C in head and neck cancers. *Radiotherapy and Oncology, 57,* 119-204.

Early Breast Cancer Trialists' Collaborative Group. (2005). Effects of chemotherapy and hormonal therapy for early breast cancer on recurrence and 15-year survival: An overview of the randomized trials. *Lancet, 365,* 1687-1717.

Faivre, S., Marti, A., Rixe, O., Janot, F., Julieron, M., Gatineau, M., et al. (2005). Preoperative sequential chemotherapy in locally advanced squamous cell carcinoma of the head and neck. *Head and Neck, 27,* 311-319.

Forastiere, A. A., Goepfert, H., Maor, M., Pajak, T. F., Weber, R., Morrison, W., et al. (2003). Concurrent chemotherapy and radiotherapy for organ preservation in advanced laryngeal cancer. *New England Journal of Medicine, 349,* 2091-2098.

Gerngross, P. J., Martin, C. D., Ball, J. D., Engelmeier, R. L., Gilbert, H. D., Powers, J. M., et al. (2005). Period between completion of radiation therapy and prosthetic rehabilitation in edentulous patients: A retrospective study. *Journal of Prosthodontics, 14,* 110-121.

Gupta, N. K., Pointon, R. C. S, & Wilkinson, P. M. (1987). A randomized clinical trial to contrast radiotherapy with radiotherapy and methotrexate given synchronously in head and neck cancer. *Clinical Radiology, 38,* 575-581.

Kirita, T., Ohgi, K., Shimooka, H., Yamanaka, Y., Tatebayashi, S., Yamamoto, K., et al. (1999). Preoperative concurrent chemoradiotherapy plus radical surgery for advanced squamous cell carcinoma of the oral cavity: An analysis of long-term results. *Oral Oncology, 35,* 597-606.

Knegt, P. P., Ah-See, K.W., vd Velden, L. A., & Kerrebijn, J. (2001). Adenocarcinoma of the ethmoidal sinus complex: Surgical debulking and topical fluorouracil may be the optimal treatment. *Archives of Otolaryngology, Head and Neck Surgery, 127*, 141–146.

Logemann, J. A., Rademaker, A. W., Pauloski, B. R., Lazarus, C. L., Mittal, B. B., Brockstein, B., et al. (2006). Site of disease and treatment protocol as correlates of swallowing function in patients with head and neck cancer treated with chemoradiation. *Head and Neck, 28*(1), 64–73.

McDonald, S., Meyerowitz, C., Smudzin, T., & Rubin, P. (1994). Preliminary results of a pilot study using WR-2721 before fractionated irradiation of the head and neck to reduce salivary dysfunction. *International Journal of Radiation, Oncology, Biology, & Physics, 29*, 747–754.

Merlano, M., Benasso, M., Corvo, R., Rosso, R., Vitale, V., Blengio, F., et al. (1996). Five-year update of a randomized trial of alternating radiotherapy and chemotherapy compared with radiotherapy alone in treatment of unresectable squamous cell carcinoma of the head and neck. *Journal of the National Cancer Institute, 88*, 583–589.

Milas, L., Mason, K. A., Liao, Z., & Ang, K. K. (2003). Chemoradiotherapy: Emerging treatment improvement strategies. *Head and Neck, 25*, 152–167.

Murthy, A. K., Taylor, S. G., Showel, J., Calderelli, D. D., Hutchinson, J. C., Holinger, L. D., et al. (1987). Treatment of advanced head and neck cancer with concomitant radiation and chemotherapy. *International Journal of Radiation, Oncology, Biology, & Physics, 13*, 1807–1813.

Narozny, W., Sicko, Z., Kot, J., Stankiewicz, C., Przewozny, T., & Kuczkowski, J. (2005). Hyperbaric oxygen therapy in the treatment of complications of irradiation in head and neck area. *Undersea and Hyperbaric Medicine, 32*, 102–110.

Nguyen, L. N., & Ang, K. K. (2002). Radiotherapy for cancer of the head and neck: Altered fractionated regimens. *Lancet Oncology, 3*, 693–701.

Nordsmark, M., Bentzen, S. M., Rudat, V., Brizel, D., Lartigau, E., Stadler, P., et al. (2005). Prognostic value of tumor oxygenation in 397 head and neck tumors after primary radiation therapy. An international multi-centre study. *Radiotherapy and Oncology, 77*, 18–24.

Olmi, P., Crispino, S., Fallai, C., Torri, V., Rossi, F., Bolner, A., et al. (2003). Locoregionally advanced carcinoma of the oropharynx: Conventional radiotherapy vs. accelerated hyperfractionated radiotherapy vs. concomitant radiotherapy and chemotherapy—A multi-

center randomized trial. *International Journal of Radiation, Oncology, Biology, & Physics, 55*, 78–92.

Pignon, J. P., Bourhis, J., Domenge, C., & Designe, L. (2000). Chemotherapy added to locoregional treatment for head and neck squamous-cell carcinoma: Three meta-analyses of updated individual data. *Lancet, 355*, 949–955.

Poulsen, M. G., Denham, J. W., Peters, L. J., Lamb, D. S., Spry, N. A., Hindley, A., et al. (2001). Osteoradionecrosis of the jaws as a side effect of radiotherapy of head and neck tumor patients—A report of a thirty year retrospective review. *International Journal of Oral and Maxillofacial Surgery, 32*, 289–295.

Reuther, T., Schuster, T., Mende, U., & Kubler, A. (2003). Osteoradionecrosis of the jaw as a side effect of radiation of head and neck tumour patients—report of a thirty year retrospective review. *International Journal of Oral and maxillofacial Surgery, 32*, 289–295.

Rischin, D., Corry, J., Smith, J., Stewart, J., Hughes, P., & Peters, L. (2002). Excellent disease control and survival in patients with advanced nasopharyngeal cancer treated with chemoradiation. *Journal of Clinical Oncology, 20*, 1845–1852.

Samant, S., Kumar, P., Wan, J., Hanchett, C., Vieira, F., Murry, T., et al. (1999). Concomitant radiation therapy and targeted cisplatin chemotherapy for the treatment of advanced piriform sinus carcinoma: Disease control and preservation of function. *Head and Neck, 21*, 595–601.

Steel, G. G. (1988). The search for therapeutic gain in the combination of radiotherapy and chemotherapy. *Radiotherapy and Oncology, 11*, 31–53.

Stevenson-Moore, P., & Epstein, J. B. (1993). The management of teeth in irradiated sites. *Oral Oncology, 29B*, 39–43.

Sutherland, S. E., & Browman, G. P. (2001). Prophylaxis of oral mucositis in irradiated head-and-neck cancer patients: A proposed classification scheme of interventions and meta-analysis of randomized controlled trials. *International Journal of Radiation, Oncology, Biology, & Physics, 49*, 917–930.

Tannock, I. F., & Browman, G. (1986). Lack of evidence for a role of chemotherapy in the routine management of locally advanced head and neck cancer. *Journal of Clinical Oncology, 4*, 1121–1126.

Taylor, S. G., Murthy, A. K., Griem, K. L., Recine, D. C., Kiel, K., Blendowski, C., et al. (1997). Concomitant cisplatin/5FU infusion and radiotherapy in advanced head and neck cancer: 8-year analysis of results. *Head and Neck, 19*, 684–691.

Wasserman, T. H., Brizel, D. M., Henke, M., Monnier, A., Escwege, F., Sauer, R., et al. (2005). Influence of intravenous amifostine on xerostomia, tumor control, and survival after radiotherapy for head-and-neck cancer: 2-year follow-up of a prospective, randomized, phase III trial. *International Journal of Radiation, Oncology, Biology, & Physics, 63,* 985–990.

Wendt, T. G., Hartenstein, R. C., Wustrow, T. P. U., & Lissner, J. (1989). Cisplatin, fluorouracil with leukovorin calcium enhancement, and synchronous accelerated radiotherapy in the management of locally advanced head and neck cancer: A phase II study. *Journal of Clinical Oncology, 7,* 471–476.

# Chapter 4

# ORAL, OROPHARYNGEAL, AND NASOPHARYNGEAL CANCER: INTERVENTION APPROACHES

Ludwig E. Smeele

## Introduction

In this chapter, the anatomy of the oral cavity, oropharynx, and nasopharynx are briefly reviewed. The epidemiology and the biology of cancer in these regions are described, as well as the treatment modalities according to the various anatomical subsites and stages of extension.

## Oral Cavity and Oropharynx

### Anatomy

The *oral cavity* includes the vermillion border of the lips and extends through the mouth posteriorly to the anterior pharyngeal arches, the circumvallatae papillae on the dorsal surface of the tongue, and to the posterior rim of the hard palate. The oral cavity is further subdivided into anatomical areas: lips, tongue, floor of mouth, upper and lower alveolar processes, buccal mucosa, and palate.

The *oropharynx* is generally described as a chamber with four walls: anteriorly the base of tongue, posteriorly the pharyngeal wall, laterally the tonsillar fossae, and cranially the soft palate.

### Cancer of the Oral Cavity and Oropharynx

Worldwide, the predominant type of cancer in the oral cavity is squamous cell carcinoma and it comprises 85–95% of all malignant tumors in this area. In the oropharynx, undifferentiated carcinoma is the second most common carcinoma after squamous cell carcinoma. Other histological types are salivary gland cancer, malignant lymphoma, sarcomas, secondary cancers (metastases), and primary melanoma of the mucus membranes. Non-Hodgkin's lymphoma is more often found in the oropharynx due to the more abundant lymphoid tissues (tonsils, base of tongue) than in the oral cavity.

## Epidemiology

In most studies the incidence of oral cavity cancer is specified for the predominant histological type, squamous cell carcinoma. Its incidence varies around the world. It ranks 6 among all cancers around the world, but 58% of cases are seen in Asia. In Karachi, Pakistan, it is the second most common cancer in both males and females (Bhurgri, 2005). Other areas with an increasing incidence are Brazil and Eastern Europe. In Western Europe and the United States the incidence is 5 in males and 2.5 in females (per 100,000 per year). For cancers of the oropharynx, the incidence is somewhat less: 2.5 for males and 0.8 for females respectively (Franceschi, Bidoli, Herrero, & Munoz, 2000; Hamada, Bos, Kasuga, & Hirayama, 1991; Khawaja, Shafiq, Nusrat, & Khawaja, 2005; Plesko, Macfarlane, Evstifeeva, Obsitnikova, & Kramarova, 1994).

## Etiology

The use of alcohol and tobacco is strongly related to oral and oropharyngeal cancer. For both alcohol and tobacco it was found that the risk of developing cancer increases with increasing use of either of the two substances. Alcoholic drinks with a high content of ethanol are associated with an increased risk. The toxic effect of the simultaneous use of alcohol and tobacco has often been reported; in populations that are exposed to both risk factors the effect is probably multiplying (Blot et al., 1988; Franceschi et al., 2000; Kabat & Wynder, 1989; Mashberg, Boffetta, Winkelman, & Garfinkel, 1993; Merletti, Boffetta, Ciccone, Mashberg, & Terracini, 1989; Schlecht et al., 1999).

Cessation of smoking results in a decreased risk and this is proportional to the amount of time a person has stopped his or her habits. Contrary to this, cessation of the use of alcohol does not seem to decrease the risk (Franceschi, Levi, Dal Maso, et al., 2000). In Southeast Asia and Taiwan oral cancer is mainly related to the use of betel nut and gutka (Nair, Bartsch, & Nair, 2004). It may lead to oral submucous fibrosis, a premalignant condition.

Consumption of meat (raw, cooked, or salted) may carry an increased cancer risk. A diet containing fruits and vegetables may have a protective effect (De Stefani, Oreggia, Ronco, Fierro, & Rivero, 1994; Levi et al.,

1998; Negri et al., 2000). Viral infections are often mentioned as causative factors. Epstein-Barr virus is not related to oral cancer, contrary to human papillomavirus (HPV), but a causal relation is difficult to prove. Most HPV-related tumors are found in the oropharynx and present as tonsillar carcinomas (Badaracco, Venuti, Morello, Muller, & Marcante, 2000; Khabie et al., 2001; Mao et al., 1996; Mellin, Friesland, Lewensohn, Dalianis, & Munck-Wikland, 2000; Paz, Cook, Odom-Maryon, Xie, & Wilczynski, 1997).

## Clinical Presentation

The oral cavity and most of the oropharynx are easily accessible for inspection. Self-examination and investigation by a health care professional require only the use of a focused light source. Despite this fact, many patients present late. In hindsight, this is often related to the relatively mild early symptoms. Poor socioeconomic status, with a poor health awareness and/or limited access to the health care system, may also play a role. Patients may present with symptoms of local tumor growth, or with a neck lump, or both (see Figures 4-1, 4-2, 4-3, and 4-4). Distant metastases is rarely seen as a first symptom. The main presenting symptoms are summarized in Table 4-1.

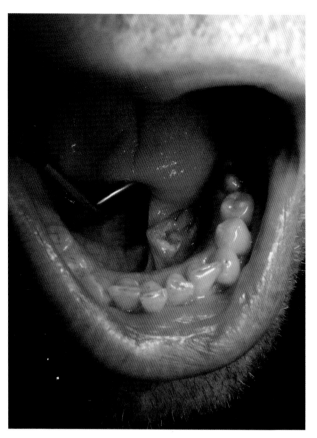

**Figure 4–2.** Squamous cell carcinoma of the anterior floor of the mouth.

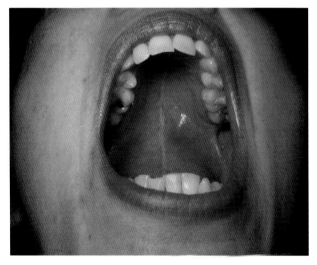

**Figure 4–1.** Mucoepidermoid carcinoma of the soft palate presenting as a submucous swelling.

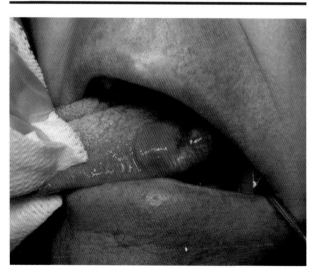

**Figure 4–3.** Squamous cell carcinoma of the lateral border of the oral tongue.

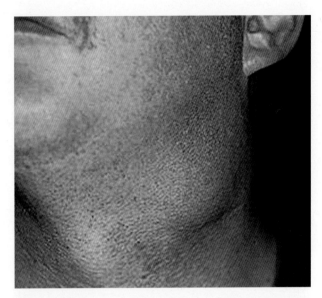

**Figure 4–4.** Metastases of a tonsillar carcinoma presenting as a neck lump.

**Table 4–1.** Symptoms of Oral and Oropharyngeal Cancer

| Symptoms |
| --- |
| Pain |
| Radiating pain (earache, sore throat) |
| "Lump in the throat" sensation |
| Bleeding |
| Swallowing complaints |
| Loose teeth; ill-fitting dentures |
| Ulcers |
| White or red patches |
| Neck swelling |

## Involved Subsites

In developed countries, the subsites in the oral cavity most typically involved include the lateral borders of the tongue and the floor of mouth. In contrast in devolving countries, the buccal mucosa and palate are mentioned as sites of predilection. This pattern relates to the different carcinogens involved: typically cigarette smoking and alcoholic beverages versus betel nut

chewing. The oropharyngeal subsites that are affected most frequently are the tonsillar fossa and soft palate. The base of tongue is less often affected and tumors originating from the posterior wall are relatively rare (Day et al., 1993).

## Regional and Distant Metastases

For the purpose of classification, the nodal structures in the neck are divided into five levels on each side and a sixth level medially (Figure 4-5) (Robbins et al., 2002). Lymphatic spread of tumor cells generally follows a certain pattern that is related to the primary site. Tumor deposits from the lips and the anterior oral cavity are found in the submental (level Ia) and submandibular (level Ib) nodes, whereas tumors from the posterior oral cavity tend to spread to the subdigastric nodes (level IIa). All subsites from the oropharynx tend to metastasize to level IIa as well. Well-lateralized tumors produce unilateral metastases but midline lesions or lesions close to the midline may cause bilateral metastases. In advanced disease, affected lymph nodes may become very large and cause skin ulceration, and/or more levels may become involved.

Cancer originating from the oral cavity and oropharynx may ultimately spread to other organs and cause distant metastases. The single predictive factor for this to occur is the status of involved neck nodes. Bilateral neck nodes, nodes in the lower neck, large neck nodes, and extranodal spread are associated with distant metastases. The organs most frequently involved are the lungs, the liver, and the bones (Ampil et al., 1995; Alvi & Johnson, 1997; Barbone et al., 1996; de Bree, Deurloo, Snow, & Leemans, 2000).

## Premalignant Lesions

Leukoplakia and erythroplakia are premalignant lesions that are identifiable as white or red patches of mucosa. Some of these lesions are related to a causative factor, such as mechanical irritation from a dental filling or smoking. If the lesion disappears after elimination of such a factor, it is no longer a "true" leukoplakia or erythroplakia. "True" leukoplakias or erythroplakias may ultimately transform into carcinomas.

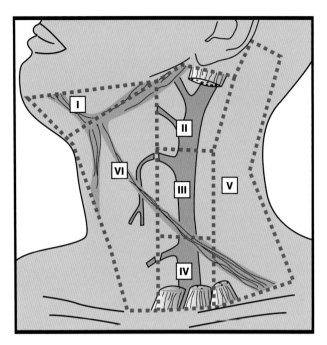

**Figure 4–5.** Diagrammatic representation of distribution of neck nodes into levels I–VI.

## Diagnosis and Staging

Before any cancer therapy is applied, a systematic policy of making a diagnosis and staging of the tumor should be performed. The diagnosis is generally established after histological evaluation of a biopsy is performed. As the oral cavity is easily accessible, a biopsy is usually done in the outpatient clinic under local anaesthesia. General anaesthesia is often required for oropharyngeal tumors. Staging is done in a systematic way according to the UICC (Union International Contre le Cancer) TNM System (Sobin & Wittekind, 2002) (Table 4–2).

### Staging of the Primary Site

The primary tumor is usually staged after physical examination; in selected cases this may be performed with the patient under general anaesthesia. Modern imaging techniques enhance the sensitivity greatly. Nuclear magnetic resonance (NMR) and computed tomography (CT) scans offer important data on local

**Table 4–2.** TNM Staging of Oral and Oropharyngeal Cancer

| Primary Tumor | T0 | Not detectable |
|---|---|---|
| | T1 | Diameter 2 cm or less |
| | T2 | Diameter more than 2 cm and not larger than 4 cm |
| | T3 | Diameter 4 cm or more |
| | T4a | Invasion of deeper structures (bone, muscle) |
| | T4b | Invasion of deep, unresectable structures (carotid artery, skull base) |
| Lymph Nodes | N0 | No detectable nodes |
| | N1 | Single ipsilateral node, diameter 3 cm or less |
| | N2a | Single ipsilateral node, diameter more than 3 cm and not larger than 6 cm |
| | N2b | Multiple ipsilateral nodes, none larger than 6 cm |
| | N2c | Bilateral nodes, none larger than 6 cm |
| | N3 | Diameter more than 6 cm |
| Distant Metastasis | M0 | Not detectable |
| | M1 | Any distant metastasis |

*Source:* Sobin & Wittekind, 2002

advancement of the tumor (Bootz, Lenz, Skalej, & Bongers, 1992; Campbell et al., 1995; Crecco et al., 1994). Invasion of mandibular bone may be detected with conventional radiography and technetium (Tc) scanning (Luyk, Laird, Ward-Booth, Rankin, & Williams, 1986; Van den Brekel et al., 1998; Zieron, Lauer, Remmert, & Sieg, 2001).

## Staging of the Neck

Palpation of the neck is often performed as a routine investigation, but its sensitivity is not adequate for staging. Modern imaging has a lot to offer in this area. Sensitivity is increased with the application of CT and NMR imaging (Curtin et al., 1998; Leslie, Fyfe, Guest, Goddard, & Kabala, et al., 1999; Wide et al., 1999). Ultrasound in combination with fine needle aspiration cytology (USFNAC) combines high sensitivity (25-75%) with 100% specificity and in most head and neck cancers it has become the standard instrument for staging of neck nodes (van den Brekel et al., 1993; Stuckensen, Kovacs, Adams, & Baum, 2000; Takes et al., 1996; Takes et al., 1998).

## Staging of Distant Sites

A plain chest film is the first step in evaluating intrapulmonary metastases. In selected cases, a chest CT, Tc scan, or CT of the abdomen may be performed (Ampil et al., 1995; de Bree et al., 2000; Ong, Kerawala, Martin, & Stafford, 1999).

## Treatment for Oral and Oropharyngeal Cancers

As a rule of thumb it can be said that early cancer may be treated with a single modality (surgery, laser, radiation) and advanced disease with multimodality protocols (surgery, radiation, and chemotherapy). Specifically, though, the surgical treatment options include photodynamic therapy, local excision, and composite resection with primary reconstruction. Nonsurgical management includes radiation, given as brachytherapy or external beam irradiation, or combined radiotherapy-chemotherapy treatment. Indications for each treatment for different tumor types are often overlapping (see Tables 4-3 and 4-4) and in each individual case the advantages and disadvantages of each should be taken into consideration. Oncologic outcome, but also comorbidity and post-treatment

**Table 4-3.** Classification of Neck Dissection

| | |
|---|---|
| Radical | Clearance of all neck levels, SCM, IJV, and nIX sacrificed |
| Modified Radical | Clearance of all neck levels, SCM, and/or IJV and/or nIX spared |
| Selective | Clearance of selected neck levels, SCM, IJV, and nIX all spared |

Note. SCM = sternomastoid muscle, IJV = internal jugular vein, nIX = accessory nerve.

**Table 4-4.** Curative Treatment Options for Oral Cancer

| Stage | Treatment Options |
|---|---|
| T1, T2N0 <5 mm infiltrating | Photodynamic therapy or surgical excision |
| T1N0 >5 mm infiltrating | Surgical excision or brachytherapy |
| T2N0 >5 mm infiltrating | Surgical excision with elective neck dissection |
| Any T, N+ | Local excision with therapeutic neck dissection or composite resection with reconstruction and postoperative (chemo-) radiation |
| T3, T4 any N | Composite resection with reconstruction and postoperative (chemo-) radiation |
| Unresectable | Chemoradiation |

quality of life, should play a role in decision choices. Consequently the relevant options need to be discussed with the patient and his or her relatives prior to finalizing treatment decisions.

## Photodynamic Therapy for Oral Cancers

Photodynamic therapy is a relatively new treatment modality that only has application in the management of oral cancers. In the curative setting, it is applicable to early stage disease with a maximum depth of infiltration of 5 mm. A photo sensitizer is administrated intravenously prior to the treatment. Depending on the type of sensitizer used, an adequate biodistribution is achieved within a few days or less. The tumor area is then treated with a blue laser. It is very important that healthy tissue is shielded during the procedure (Figures 4-6 and 4-7). In order to achieve this, the patient is best put under general anesthesia in order to achieve good exposition of the tumor area, including a margin of healthy tissue. The advantage of this modality is healing without fibrosis. In areas like the floor of mouth this may be of benefit regarding tongue mobility.

## Local Excision

Small (less than 4 cm) tumors of the anterior oral cavity are easily accessible for a wide local excision. If the tumor involves or is adjacent to the alveolar ridges or the gums, a margin of bone with or without teeth may be included in the resection. Closure of the defect is achieved by either (a) primary wound closure—where closure is achieved by suturing the wound edges together, (b) secondary healing—where the wound is left open: its surface will be covered by the ingrowth of new tissue from its edges, or (c) use of a split thickness skin graft—a very thin layer of epidermis that is taken from a remote donor site where scars are easily concealed, such as the thigh, and transferred to the wound where it is sutured in place and covered with some form of a dressing. In the upper jaw, the nasal cavity or the paranasal sinus is often opened. In these cases, closure may be achieved with an obturator, an acrylic plate similar to a dental prosthesis that can be removed by the patient for regular cleaning.

Only small (less than 2 cm) tumors of the anterior oropharynx may be accessible for a wide local excision. Eligible subsites are the anterior pharyngeal arches, the tonsils, and the soft palate. Either primary wound closure or secondary healing achieves closure of the defect.

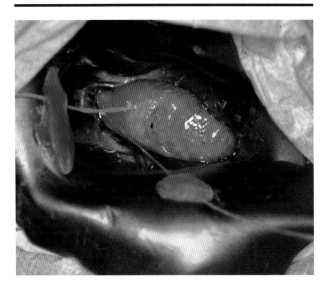

**Figure 4-6.** Photodynamic therapy of early tongue cancer, prior to illumination with a laser. The tumor is isolated from the surrounding tissue by drapes and black wax.

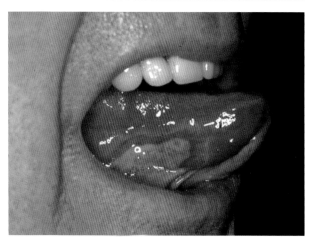

**Figure 4-7.** The same patient as in Figure 4-6, 4 weeks after photodynamic therapy, showing healing of the treated area without scar formation.

### Composite Resection with Primary Reconstruction

Not all T3 and T4 tumors and those T2 lesions that are located in the posterior oral cavity can be resected adequately through the mouth. In such cases a composite resection is performed; this implies an open neck approach. Because the neck is entered during such a procedure, a neck dissection is always performed (Table 4-5). To optimize access to the tumor, the mandible is divided, or if involved by tumor tissue, partly resected. Primary healing of the surgical defect is mandatory and can only rarely be achieved by closure of existing tissues. Therefore, a tissue transfer is done with pedicled flaps or a free vascularized flap. A pedicled flap is vascularized by its own natural set of blood vessels (the "pedicle"), which are dissected free but left intact. The length of this pedicle limits the range of transfer because these vessels may not be stretched; otherwise, this may interrupt blood flow. A pectoralis major flap, elevated from the chest wall, is the most often used pedicled flap. In a free vascularized flap, the pedicle is also dissected from its surroundings, but it is then divided. The blood vessels, at least one artery and one vein, are then sutured to blood vessels (the "anastomosis") in the recipient area, after which the circulation of blood is reestablished. The advantage of a free flap is that tissue can be transferred between remote sites, (e.g., from the lower leg to the head and neck area.) From a functional standpoint, a free vascularized flap offers better opportunities. As this procedure requires a microvascular anastomosis in the neck it is technically more demanding. The advantage, however, is that mucosa may be replaced with thin fasciocutaneous tissue and mandibular bone may be replaced directly with bone. This may enhance oral functions like speech, chewing, and swallowing greatly (Figures 4-8, 4-9, 4-10, 4-11, and 4-12). For more advanced tumors of the oropharynx, or if other subsites are involved, a composite resection is mandatory. Usually, the mandible is divided or partially resected.

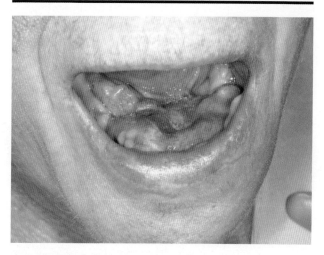

**Figure 4–8.** A patient with advanced oral cancer with invasion of the mandibular bone.

**Table 4–5.** Curative Treatment Options for Oropharyngeal Cancer

| Stage | Treatment Options |
| --- | --- |
| T1, T2N0 | Surgery, or brachytherapy, or external beam irradiation |
| T3, T4N0 | Composite resection with reconstruction and postoperative (chemo-) radiation or external beam irradiation |
| T1, T2N+, nodes <3 cm | External beam irradiation |
| T1, T2N+, nodes >3 cm | Composite resection with reconstruction and postoperative (chemo-) radiation |
| T3, T4N+, nodes <3 cm | Composite resection with reconstruction and postoperative (chemo-) radiation or external beam irradiation |
| T3, T4N+, nodes >3 cm | Composite resection with reconstruction and postoperative (chemo-) radiation |
| Unresectable | Chemoradiation |

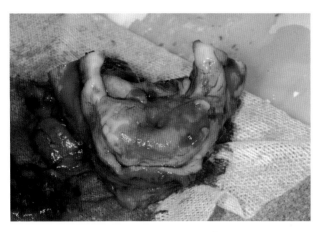

**Figure 4–9.** Surgical specimen of resected tumor and surrounding tissues.

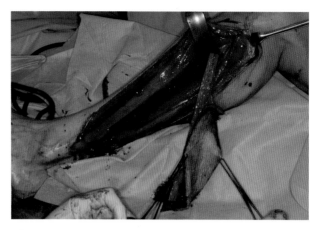

**Figure 4–10.** Harvest of a vascularized osteo-cutaneous fibula flap to aid in reconstruction of the defect.

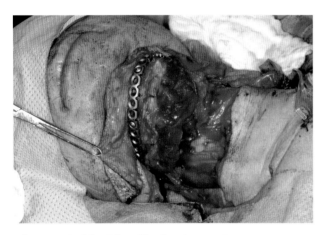

**Figure 4–11.** The fibular is cut into segments and fixated to the remaining mandible with a plate and screws.

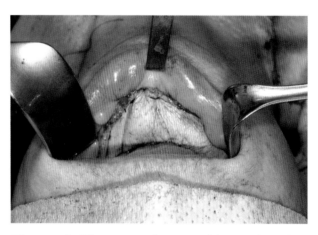

**Figure 4–12.** Intraoral view of lower leg skin island, sutured into the floor of mouth.

## *Brachytherapy and External Beam Radiotherapy*

In selected cases, primary irradiation of the tumor is a valuable option. In brachytherapy, radioactive sources are implanted into the tissues. In doing so, a high dose can be delivered to the tumor area and the surrounding tissues are spared. Small tumors of the mobile tongue can be treated this way. This treatment may be combined with external beam irradiation. Disadvantages of primary irradiation of the oral cavity are acute and late toxicity. In the acute phase, mucositis and necrosis occur, while in the late phase, xerostomia, dental decay, and necrosis of bone are encountered. All subsites of the oropharynx are, in principle, suitable for brachytherapy, but the technique is technically demanding and is therefore only applied in specialized centers. External beam irradiation is in fact a first choice treatment option for early stage disease. Disadvantages of primary irradiation of the oropharynx are acute and late toxicity. As for oral cancers, mucositis and necrosis occur early during treatment with xerostomia, dental decay, and necrosis of bone encountered in the long term.

External beam radiotherapy is also applied postoperatively in cases of oral or oropharyngeal cancers with positive surgical margins, multiple positive lymph nodes, and extranodal spread.

### Chemoradiation

In advanced cases of oral or oropharyngeal cancer the tumor may become unresectable. There are two subtypes: a tumor may be *anatomically* or *functionally* unresectable. If resection of the tumor would involve vital structures (e.g., the carotid artery), it is anatomically unresectable. If a tumor is technically resectable, but the operation would produce an unacceptable mutilation (e.g., a total removal of the tongue), it is considered functionally unresectable. In these cases, chemoradiation protocols (chemotherapy combined with external beam radiotherapy) have been developed (for further discussion of these see Chapter 3). Most protocols use cisplatin in a daily low dose, given intravenously, during the radiation. Alternatively, the course of radiotherapy is interrupted three or four times and a high dose is given intra-arterially after cannulation of the feeding vessels to the tumor.

Another indication for chemoradiation is after surgery. Selected cases with unfavorable tumor characteristics (positive surgical margins, multiple positive lymph nodes, and extranodal spread) may benefit from the addition of chemotherapy to the postoperative radiotherapy schedule.

### Treatment Results

Oncologic outcome is related to many issues. Among these, patient factors (age, sex, comorbidity, socioeconomic factors), tumor factors (stage, subsite, regional metastases), and treatment factors (surgical margins, irradiation fields) are found. The most favorable oncologic outcome for the patient is complete curation of the disease (survival). In head and neck squamous cell cancer, outcome is often expressed as duration of locoregional control (no recurrence at the primary site and the neck nodes) because treatment is only directed to these areas. It should be kept in mind that some locoregional recurrences can be treated, which may lead to curation in up to 30% of recurrent cases. Successful treatment of the cancer, however, may be jeopardized by the tendency of developing new (secondary) cancers in the head and neck area or at other sites.

Patients who are diagnosed with *oral cancer* generally have a chance for survival of around 50% (Prince & Bailey, 1999; Sessions et al., 2000; Sessions et al., 2002). The 3-year local control rate for patients with oral cancer treated with surgery and postoperative radiotherapy varies from 66% to 87% (Langendijk et al., 2003).

Locoregional control for early stage *oropharyngeal carcinoma* treated with irradiation is around 80% (Selek et al., 2004). Within the oropharynx, base of tongue lesions have a worse outcome than other subsites, but T-stage remains a very important factor for prognosis (Levendag et al., 2004; Mendenhall, Morris, Amdur, Hinerman, & Mancuso, 2003; Sundaram, Schwartz, Har-El, & Lucente, 2005; Zhen et al., 2004). Survival has been reported to vary between 68% for early disease and only 27% for advanced disease (Mak-Kregar et al., 1995).

## Nasopharynx

### Anatomy

The nasopharynx is the most cranial part of the pharynx. Its roof is defined by the skull base, which contains the sphenoid sinus and the cavernous sinuses on each side of it. The lateral walls contain both eustachian tube orifices and medially to these, fossa of Rosenmüller. Anteriorly both nasal cavities are found and its floor is made up of the soft palate.

### Cancer of the Nasopharynx

Carcinoma is the most common type of cancer in the nasopharynx. Two subtypes are distinguishable: squamous cell carcinoma and undifferentiated carcinoma. Apart from these, non-Hodgkin's lymphoma, salivary gland tumors, sarcomas, chordoma, and mucosal melanoma are found.

### Epidemiology

The population affected by nasopharyngeal carcinoma is younger than the population affected by head and neck carcinomas at other sites. Also striking is a predilection for certain geographical areas: it is almost endemic in Hong Kong and southern China, and its incidence is elevated in Chinese immigrants in the United States, in Inuit and Alaskan people, and in countries bordering the Mediterranean Sea. In northern Europe and the United States, only sporadic cases are seen (Chan, Teo, & Huang, 2004; Dodge, Mills, & Yang, 2005; Wei & Sham, 2005).

## Etiology

In view of the geographical distribution of the disease and its strong association with positive Epstein-Barr virus serology, it is clear that the etiology is a complex interaction between genetic and environmental factors. The mechanism of this interaction is far from understood. In any case the risk factors involved in other head and neck cancers (smoking and alcohol) play no role here (Chan et al., 2004; Dodge et al., 2005; Spano et al., 2003; Wei & Sham, 2005).

## Clinical Presentation

Interestingly, many patients present with a neck swelling rather than with symptoms of the primary tumor (Figures 4-13, 4-14, and 4-15). Only in very advanced cases nasal blockage or cranial nerve dysfunction occur. Symptoms are summarized in Table 4-6.

## Involved Subsites

Typically nasopharyngeal carcinoma arises in the mucosa of the roof of the nasopharynx or in the adjacent areas in the fossa of Rosenmüller. Advanced disease will involve the skull base and the parapharyngeal space. Through these passageways cranial nerve involvement and intracranial extension may take place.

## Regional and Distant Metastases

Regional lymph node involvement is a strong feature of nasopharyngeal carcinoma. Bulky, bilateral nodal involvement is found in many cases; enlarged nodes

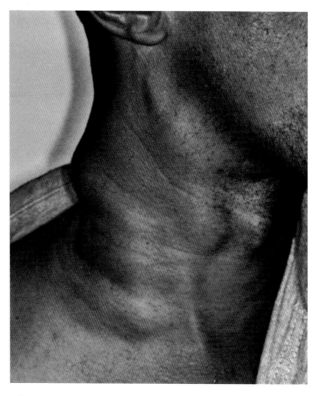

**Figure 4–13.** Metastases from a primary nasopharyngeal carcinoma presenting as multiple neck lumps.

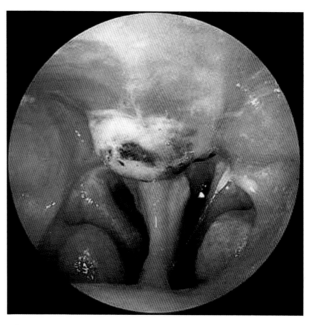

**Figure 4–14.** Endoscopic view of primary carcinoma at the roof of the nasopharynx.

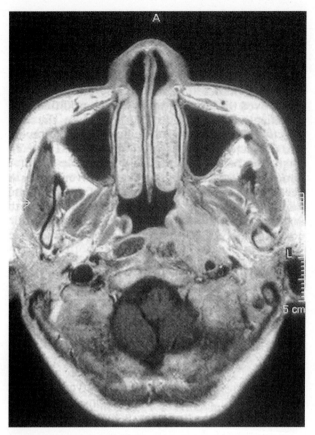

**Figure 4–15.** MRI scan of nasopharyngeal carcinoma showing parapharyngeal space extension.

**Table 4–6.** Symptoms of Nasopharyngeal Cancer

| |
|---|
| Neck swelling |
| Nasal blockage |
| Bleeding from nose or throat |
| Eustachian tube dysfunction causing aural symptoms |
| Headache |
| Cranial nerve palsy (nerves III, IV, V, VI) |

may be found in the subdigastric areas and in the upper and middle portions of the posterior triangle (Chow, Payne, Keane, Panzarella, & Izard, 1997; Teo, Chan, Lee, Leung, & Johnson, 1999). Distant metas-

tases occur most frequently to the bones, but also the lungs and the liver may become affected. The incidence of distant metastases is related mainly to the amount of involved neck nodes (Leung et al., 2005; Spano et al., 2003).

## Diagnosis and Staging

Physical examination should start with palpation of the neck and endoscopic inspection of the nasopharynx. A biopsy taken under local anesthesia can often be done at the first consultation. As nasopharyngeal cancer is not a type of head and neck cancer that can be managed by surgery, the issue of occult nodal metastases does not play a major role in electing a treatment. Contrary to the staging of squamous cell carcinoma at other sites in the head and neck area, there is little controversy regarding which imaging techniques are most appropriate. Staging of nasopharyngeal cancer is outlined in Table 4–7. For staging of the primary site, NMR and CT scans are suitable for evaluating the nasopharynx and adjacent structures. Staging of the neck occurs simultaneously with staging the primary site by NMR and/or CT. If there is doubt upon the nature of enlarged nodes, metastases may be confirmed by USFNAC. With respect to staging of distant sites, a Tc bone scan, chest film, and CT or ultrasound of the abdomen may confirm or rule out distant metastases.

## Treatment Options for Nasopharyngeal Cancer

Carcinoma of the nasopharynx is treated with radiotherapy and chemotherapy as primary modalities. Surgery is only performed in selected cases of recurrence in the nasopharynx or in the neck. Radiotherapy is the mainstay of treatment for carcinoma of the nasopharynx because it is a uniquely radiosensitive tumor. The irradiation field is a very large area that includes the primary site as well as the neck bilaterally. Morbidity from this treatment is a major concern. Chemotherapy is effective in treating advanced carcinoma of the nasopharynx when given concomitant to the radiotherapy. The agents used most widely are

**Table 4–7.** TNM Staging of Nasopharyngeal Cancer

| Primary Tumor | T0 | Not detectable |
|---|---|---|
| | T1 | Nasopharynx |
| | T2a | Extension into nasal cavity/oropharynx |
| | T2b | Parapharyngeal extension |
| | T3 | Extension into bony structures/paranasal sinuses |
| | T4 | Intracranial/orbital extension, cranial nerve palsy |
| Lymph Nodes | N0 | No detectable nodes |
| | N1 | Unilateral node(s) <6 cm, above supraclavicular fossa |
| | N2 | Bilateral node(s) <6 cm, above supraclavicular fossa |
| | N3a | Nodes, larger than 6 cm |
| | N3b | In supraclavicular fossa |
| Distant Metastasis | M0 | Not detectable |
| | M1 | Any distant metastasis |

*Source:* Sobin & Wittekind, 2002

cisplatin, bleomycin, epirubicin, and 5-fluorouracil. The chemotherapy is given intravenously, as a bolus, or as a continuous infusion.

## Treatment Results

Oncologic outcome is related to patient factors (age, sex, comorbidity, socioeconomic factors), tumor factors (stage, regional metastases), and treatment factors (irradiation fields, chemotherapy schemes). The most favorable oncologic outcome for the patient is complete curation of the disease (survival). In nasopharyngeal cancer, outcome is often expressed as duration of locoregional control (no recurrence at the primary site and the neck nodes) separate from the incidence of distant metastases. Some local recurrences may be treated with surgical excision and neck recurrences may be treated with a neck dissection. The 5-year overall and disease-free survival rates of patients treated with radiotherapy alone were 59% and 52%, respectively (Yeh, Tang, Lui, Huang, & Huang, 2005). The addition of chemotherapy in selected advanced cases may be of benefit regarding locoregional control and preventing the development of distant metastases (Langendijk, Leemans, Buter, Berkhof, & Slotman, 2004).

## Conclusion

Cancers of the oral cavity and oropharynx are mainly squamous cell carcinomas, whereas in the nasopharynx undifferentiated carcinoma is also encountered. To establish a definitive diagnosis, a tissue sample ("biopsy") is mandatory. Imaging techniques such as ultrasound, CT scans, and MRI scans provide information about the extent of the disease. For small cancers of the oral cavity and oropharynx, one-modality treatment is offered, mostly surgery or irradiation. For larger stages of disease, both are usually applied. If the extent of the disease is such that no operation can be done, chemotherapy and irradiation are applied. In the nasopharynx, irradiation is performed for small cancers and it is combined with chemotherapy in larger tumors.

## References

Alvi, A., & Johnson, J. T. (1997). Development of distant metastasis after treatment of advanced-stage head and neck cancer. *Head Neck, 19*(6), 500–505.

Ampil, F. L., Wood, M. J., Chin, H. W., Hoasjoe, D. K., Aarstad, R. F., & Hilton, D. L. (1995). Screening bone scintigraphy in the staging of locally advanced head and neck cancer. *Journal of Cranio-maxillo-facial Surgery, 23*(2), 115–118.

Badaracco, G., Venuti, A., Morello, R., Muller, A., & Marcante, M. L. (2000). Human papillomavirus in head and neck carcinomas: Prevalence, physical status and relationship with clinical/pathological parameters. *Anticancer Research, 20*(2B), 1301–1305.

Barbone, F., Franceschi, S., Talamini, R., Barzan, L., Franchin, G., Favero, A., et al. (1996). A follow-up study of determinants of second tumor and metastasis among subjects with cancer of the oral cavity, pharynx, and larynx. *Journal of Clinical Epidemiology, 49*(3), 367–372.

Bhurgri, Y. (2005). Cancer of the oral cavity—trends in Karachi South (1995–2002). *Asian Pacific Journal of Cancer Prevalence, 6*(1), 22–26.

Blot, W. J., McLaughlin, J. K., Winn, D. M., Austin, D. F., Greenberg, R. S., Preston-Martin, S., et al. (1988). Smoking and drinking in relation to oral and pharyngeal cancer. *Cancer Research, 48*(11), 3282–3287.

Bootz, F., Lenz, M., Skalej, M., & Bongers, H. (1992). Computed tomography (CT) and magnetic resonance imaging (MRI) in T-stage evaluation of oral and oropharyngeal carcinomas. *Clinical Otolaryngology, 17*, 421–429.

Campbell, R. S., Baker, E., Chippindale, A. J., Wilson, G., Mclean, N., Soames, J. V., et al. (1995). MRI T staging of squamous cell carcinoma of the oral cavity: Radiological-pathological correlation. *Clinical Radiology, 50*(8), 533–540.

Chan, A. T., Teo, P. M., & Huang, D. P. (2004). Pathogenesis and treatment of nasopharyngeal carcinoma. *Seminars in Oncology, 31*(6), 794–801.

Chow, E., Payne, D., Keane, T., Panzarella, T., & Izard, M. A. (1997). Enhanced control by radiotherapy of cervical lymph node metastases arising from nasopharyngeal carcinoma compared with nodal metastases from other head and neck squamous cell carcinomas. *International Journal of Radiation Oncology, Biology, Physics, 39*(1), 149–154.

Crecco, M., Vidiri, A., Palma, O., Floris, R., Squillaci, E., Mattioli, M., et al. (1994). T stages of tumors of the tongue and floor of the mouth: Correlation between MR with gadopentetate dimeglumine and pathologic data. *American Journal of Neuroradiology, 15*(9), 1695–1702.

Curtin, H. D., Ishwaran, H., Mancuso, A. A., Dalley, R. W., Caudry, D. J., & McNeil, B. J. (1998). Comparison of CT and MRI in staging neck metastases. *Radiology, 207*, 1233–1240.

Day, G. L., Blot, W. J., Austin, D. F., Bernstein, L., Greenberg, R. S., Preston-Martin, S., et al. (1993). Racial differences in risk of oral and pharyngeal cancer: Alcohol, tobacco, and other determinants. *Journal of the National Cancer Institute, 85*(6), 465–473.

de Bree, R., Deurloo, E. E., Snow, G. B., & Leemans, C. R. (2000). Screening for distant metastases in patients with head and neck cancer. *Laryngoscope, 110*(3 Pt 1), 397–401.

De Stefani, E., Oreggia, F., Ronco, A., Fierro, L., & Rivero, S. (1994). Salted meat consumption as a risk factor for cancer of the oral cavity and pharynx: A case-control study from Uruguay. *Cancer Epidemiology Biomarkers and Prevention, 3*(5), 381–385.

Dodge, J. L., Mills, P. K., & Yang, R. C. (2005). Nasopharyngeal cancer in the California Hmong, 1988–2000. *Oral Oncology, 41*(6), 596–601.

Franceschi, S., Bidoli, E., Herrero, R., & Munoz, N. (2000). Comparison of cancers of the oral cavity and pharynx worldwide: Etiological clues. *Oral Oncology, 36*(1), 106–115.

Franceschi, S., Levi, F., Dal Maso, L., Talamini, R., Conti, E., Negri, E., et al. (2000). Cessation of alcohol drinking and risk of cancer of the oral cavity and pharynx. *International Journal of Cancer, 85*(6), 787–790.

Franceschi, S., Levi, F., La Vecchia, C., Conti, E., Dal Maso, L., Barzan, L., et al. (1999). Comparison of the effect of smoking and alcohol drinking between oral and pharyngeal cancer. *International Journal of Cancer, 83*(1), 1–4.

Hamada, G. S., Bos, A. J., Kasuga, H., & Hirayama, T. (1991). Comparative epidemiology of oral cancer in Brazil and India. *The Tokai Journal of Experimental and Clinical Medicine, 16*(1), 63–72.

Kabat, G. C., & Wynder, E. L. (1989). Type of alcoholic beverage and oral cancer. *International Journal of Cancer, 43*(2), 190–194.

Khabie, N., Savva, A., Kasperbauer, J. L., McGovern, R., Gostout, B., & Strome, S. E. (2001). Epstein-Barr virus DNA is not increased in tonsillar carcinoma. *Laryngoscope, 111*(5), 811–814.

Khawaja, M. I., Shafiq, M., Nusrat, R., & Khawaja, M. R. (2005). Preventing the oral cavity cancer epidemic. *Asian Pacific Journal of Cancer Prevention, 6*(3), 420.

Langendijk, J. A., de Jong, M. A., Leemans, C. R., de Bree, R., Smeele, L. E., Doornaert, P., et al. (2003). Postoperative radiotherapy in squamous cell carcinoma of the oral cavity: The importance of the overall treatment time. *International Journal of*

*Radiation Oncology, Biology, Physics, 57*(3), 693-700.

Langendijk, J. A., Leemans, C. R., Buter, J., Berkhof, J., & Slotman, B. J. (2004). The additional value of chemotherapy to radiotherapy in locally advanced nasopharyngeal carcinoma: A meta-analysis of the published literature. *Journal of Clinical Oncology, 22*(22), 4604-4612.

Leslie, A., Fyfe, E., Guest, P., Goddard, P., & Kabala, J. E. (1999). Staging squamous cell carcinoma of the oral cavity and oropharynx: A comparison of MRI and CT in T- and N-staging. *Journal of Computer Assisted Tomography, 23*(1), 43-49.

Leung, T. W., Tung, S. Y., Sze, W. K., Wong, F. C., Yuen, K. K., Lui, C. M., et al. (2005). Treatment results of 1070 patients with nasopharyngeal carcinoma: An analysis of survival and failure patterns. *Head Neck, 27*(7), 555-565.

Levendag, P., Nijdam, W., Noever, I., Schmitz, P., van de Pol, M., Sipkema, D., et al. (2004). Brachytherapy versus surgery in carcinoma of tonsillar fossa and/or soft palate: Late adverse sequelae and performance status: Can we be more selective and obtain better tissue sparing? *International Journal of Radiation Oncology, Biology, Physics, 59*(3), 713-724.

Levi, F., Pasche, C., La Vecchia, C., Lucchini, F., Franceschi, S., & Monnier, P. (1998). Food groups and risk of oral and pharyngeal cancer. *International Journal of Cancer, 77*(5), 705-709.

Luyk, N. H., Laird, E. E., Ward-Booth, P., Rankin, D., & Williams, E. D. (1986). The use of radionuclide bone scintigraphy to determine local spread of oral squamous cell carcinoma to mandible. *Journal of Maxillofacial Surgery, 14*, 93-98.

Mak-Kregar, S., Hilgers, F. J., Levendag, P. C., Manni, J. J., Lubsen, H., Roodenburg, J. L., et al. (1995). A nationwide study of the epidemiology, treatment and survival of oropharyngeal carcinoma in The Netherlands. *European Archives of Otorhinolaryngology, 252*(3), 133-138.

Mao, E. J., Schwartz, S. M., Daling, J. R., Oda, D., Tickman, L., & Beckmann, A. M. (1996). Human papilloma viruses and p53 mutations in normal pre-malignant and malignant oral epithelia. *International Journal of Cancer, 69*(2),152-158.

Mashberg, A., Boffetta, P., Winkelman, R., & Garfinkel, L. (1993). Tobacco smoking, alcohol drinking, and cancer of the oral cavity and oropharynx among U.S. veterans. *Cancer, 72*(4), 1369-1375.

Mellin, H., Friesland, S., Lewensohn, R., Dalianis, T., & Munck-Wikland, E. (2000). Human papillomavirus (HPV) DNA in tonsillar cancer: Clinical correlates, risk of relapse, and survival. *International Journal of Cancer, 89*(3), 300-304.

Mendenhall, W. M., Morris, C. G., Amdur, R. J., Hinerman, R. W., & Mancuso, A. A. (2003). Parameters that predict local control after definitive radiotherapy for squamous cell carcinoma of the head and neck. *Head Neck, 25*(7), 535-542.

Merletti, F., Boffetta, P., Ciccone, G., Mashberg, A., & Terracini, B. (1989). Role of tobacco and alcoholic beverages in the etiology of cancer of the oral cavity/oropharynx in Torino, Italy. *Cancer Research, 49*(17), 4919-4924.

Nair, U., Bartsch, H., & Nair, J. (2004). Alert for an epidemic of oral cancer due to use of the betel quid substitutes utkha and pan masala: A review of agents and causative mechanisms. *Mutagenesis, 19*(4), 251-262.

Negri, E., Franceschi, S., Bosetti, C., Levi, F., Conti, E., Parpinel, M., et al. (2000). Selected micronutrients and oral and pharyngeal cancer. *International Journal of Cancer, 86*(1), 122-127.

Ong, T. K., Kerawala, C. J., Martin, I. C., & Stafford, F. W. (1999). The role of thorax imaging in staging head and neck squamous cell carcinoma. *Journal of Cranio-maxillo-facial Surgery, 27*(6), 339-344.

Paz, I. B., Cook, N., Odom-Maryon, T., Xie, Y., & Wilczynski, S. P. (1997). Human papillomavirus (HPV) in head and neck cancer: An association of HPV 16 with squamous cell carcinoma of Waldeyer's tonsillar ring. *Cancer, 79*(3), 595-604.

Plesko, I., Macfarlane, G. J., Evstifeeva, T. V., Obsitnikova, A., & Kramarova, E. (1994). Oral and pharyngeal cancer incidence in Slovakia 1968-1989. *International Journal of Cancer, 56*(4), 481-486.

Prince, S., & Bailey, B. M. (1999). Squamous carcinoma of the tongue: Review. *British Journal of Oral and Maxillofacial Surgery, 37*(3), 164-174.

Robbins, K. T., Clayman, G., Levine, P. A., Medina, J., Sessions, R., Shaha, A., et al. (2002). Neck dissection classification update: Revisions proposed by the American Head and Neck Society and the American Academy of Otolaryngology-Head and Neck Surgery. *Archives of Otolaryngology—Head & Neck Surgery, 128*(7), 751-758.

Schlecht, N. F., Franco, E. L., Pintos, J., Negassa, A., Kowalski, L. P., Oliveira, B. V., et al. (1999). Interaction between tobacco and alcohol consumption and the risk of cancers of the upper aero-digestive tract in Brazil. *American Journal of Epidemiology, 150*(11), 1129-1137.

Selek, U., Garden, A. S., Morrison, W. H., El-Naggar, A. K., Rosenthal, D. I., & Ang, K. K. (2004). Radiation therapy for early-stage carcinoma of the oropharynx. *International Journal of Radiation Oncology, Biology, Physics, 59*(3), 743-751.

Sessions, D. G., Spector, G. J., Lenox, J., Haughey, B., Chao, C., & Marks, J. (2002). Analysis of treatment results for oral tongue cancer. *Laryngoscope, 112*(4), 616-625.

Sessions, D. G., Spector, G. J., Lenox, J., Parriott, S., Haughey, B., Chao, C., et al. (2000). Analysis of treatment results for floor-of-mouth cancer. *Laryngoscope, 110*(10 Pt 1), 1764-1772.

Sobin, L. H., & Wittekind, C. (Eds.). (2002). *UICC TNM Classification of Malignant Tumors* (6th ed.). Heidelberg, Germany: Springer Verlag.

Spano, J. P., Busson, P., Atlan, D., Bourhis, J., Pignon, J. P., Esteban, C., et al. (2003). Nasopharyngeal carcinomas: An update. *European Journal of Cancer, 39*(15), 2121-2135.

Stuckensen, T., Kovacs, A., Adams, S., & Baum, R. (2000). Staging of the neck in patients with oral cavity squamous carcinomas: A prospective comparison of PET, US, CT and MRI. *Journal of Cranio-maxillo-facial Surgery, 28*, 319-324.

Sundaram, K., Schwartz, J., Har-El, G., & Lucente, F. (2005). Carcinoma of the oropharynx: Factors affecting outcome. *Laryngoscope, 115*(9), 1536-1542.

Takes, R. P., Knegt, P. P. M., Manni, J. J., Meeuwis, C. A., Spoelstra, H. A. A., de Boer, M. F., et al. (1996). Regional metastases in head and neck cancer: The value of ultrasound guided fine needle aspiration biopsy. *Radiology, 198*, 819-823.

Takes, R. P., Righi, P., Meeuwis, C. A., Manni, J. J., Knegt, P., Marres, H. A. M., et al. (1998). The value of ultrasound with ultrasound guided fine needle aspiration cytology compared to CT in the detection of regional metastases in the clinically negative neck. *International Journal of Radiation Oncology, Biology, Physics, 40*(5), 1027-1032.

Teo, P. M., Chan, A. T., Lee, W. Y., Leung, T. W., & Johnson, P. J. (1999). Enhancement of local control in locally advanced node-positive nasopharyngeal carcinoma by adjunctive chemotherapy. *International Journal of Radiation Oncology, Biology, Physics, 43*(2), 261-271.

van den Brekel, M. W. M., Castelijns, J. A., Stel, H. V., Golding, R. P., Meyer, C. J., & Snow, G. B. (1993). Modern imaging techniques and ultrasound-guided aspiration cytology for the assessment of neck node metastases. *European Archives of Otorhinolaryngology, 250*, 11-17.

van den Brekel, M. W. M., Runne, R. W., Smeele, L. E., Tiwari, R. M., Snow, G. B., & Castelijns, J. A. (1998). Assessment of tumour invasion into the mandible: The value of different imaging techniques. *European Radiology, 8*, 1552-1557.

Wei, W. I., & Sham, J. S. (2005). Nasopharyngeal carcinoma. *Lancet, 365*(9476), 2041-2054.

Wide, J. M., White, D. W., Woolgar, J. A., Brown, J. S., Vaughan, E. D., & Lewis-Jones, H. G. (1999). MRI in the assessment of cervical node metastases in oral squamous carcinoma. *Clinical Radiology, 54*, 90-94.

Yeh, S. A., Tang, Y., Lui, C. C., Huang, Y. J., & Huang, E. Y. (2005). Treatment outcomes and late complications of 849 patients with nasopharyngeal carcinoma treated with radiotherapy alone. *International Journal of Radiation Oncology, Biology, Physics, 62*(3), 672-679.

Zhen, W., Karnell, L. H., Hoffman, H. T., Funk, G. F., Buatti, J. M., & Menck, H. R. (2004). The National Cancer Data Base report on squamous cell carcinoma of the base of tongue. *Head & Neck, 26*(8), 660-674.

Zieron, J. O., Lauer, I., Remmert, S., & Sieg, P. (2001). Single photon emission tomography: Scintigraphy in the assessment of mandibular invasion by head and neck cancer. *Head & Neck, 23*, 979-984.

# Chapter 5

# SPEECH AND SWALLOWING FOLLOWING ORAL, OROPHARYNGEAL, AND NASOPHARYNGEAL CANCERS

Cathy L. Lazarus, Elizabeth C. Ward, and Edwin M. Yiu

## CHAPTER OUTLINE

## Introduction

While the previous chapter (Chapter 4) detailed the various surgical and nonsurgical treatment options for patients with oral, oropharyngeal, and nasopharyngeal cancers, the current chapter reviews the evaluation and management of the resultant speech and swallowing disorders following treatment for these populations. As discussed in Chapter 4, cancer of the oral and oropharyngeal region may be treated surgically, or with primary radiotherapy +/– chemotherapy. In comparison, due to the radiosensitive nature of the tumor type, nasopharyngeal cancers are managed primarily using radiotherapy +/– chemotherapy. For each of these populations, the *location of the cancer*, the *treatment modality*, and the *extent of treatment* (i.e., the extent of surgery, radiotherapy dose) have specific implications for speech and swallowing, the subsequent management of the presenting disorders, and final patient outcomes. The content of the current chapter will commence with a discussion of the speech and swallowing changes noted following both main types of treatment modality. The subsequent sections will detail the assessment and rehabilitation techniques applicable for these populations and patient outcomes.

## Speech and Swallowing Following Surgical Management of Oral and Oropharyngeal Cancer

Surgical management of oral and oropharyngeal cancer can have a major impact on speech and swallowing (Cerenko, McConnel, & Jackson, 1989; Conley, 1962; Fujiu, Logemann, & Pauloski, 1995; Hamlet, Jones, Mathog, Bolton, & Patterson, 1988; Hamlet, Mathog, Patterson, & Fleming, 1990; Hamlet, Patterson, & Flemming, 1989; Logemann, 1985; Logemann & Bytell, 1979; Pauloski et al., 1994). The following sections detail the specific nature of the deficits that present in this population, as well as discuss the impact of the extent and type of reconstruction and the additional negative impact of postoperative radiotherapy.

## Speech Disorders Following Surgical Management

Speech impairment after oral and oropharyngeal cancer treatment can include reduced intelligibility and articulation errors, including omissions, substitutions, and distortions of stop, affricate, and fricative consonants and vowels (Dios, Feijoo, Ferriero, & Alvarez, 1994; Greven, Meijer, & Tiwari, 1994; Hamlet et al., 1990; Hamlet et al., 1989; Heller, Levy, & Sciubba, 1991; Hufnagle, Pullon, & Hufnagle, 1978; Imai & Michi, 1992; Morrish, 1988; Nicoletti et al., 2004; Pauloski et al., 1998; Rentschler & Mann, 1980). Speech intelligibility is often reduced after total glossectomy (Rentschler & Mann, 1980). However, total and subtotal glossectomy patients often spontaneously compensate for the lack of lingual tissue by placing a narrowing or contact at a nearby site. Specifically, back-velar tongue sounds (i.e., /k/, /g/) are substituted with stop consonants produced in the pharynx by constricting the residual tongue base to the pharyngeal wall and tip-alveolar stop consonants (i.e., /t/, /d/) are produced by using a slightly altered bilabial seal, which differentiates these phonemes from the bilabial stops /b/, /p/ (Lazarus, Davis, Logemann, & Hurst, 1983; Morrish, 1988; Skelly, Spector, Donaldson, Brodeur, & Paletta, 1971). Resonance is often hypernasal when surgery involves resection of the soft palate. In this case, palatal obturator prostheses (see later in chapter) should be considered to improve resonance as well as prevent nasal reflux of material for swallowing.

## Swallowing Disorders Following Surgical Management

Following surgical management, swallowing disorders have been observed in both the oral and pharyngeal phases of swallowing. Disorders can include increased oral transit times, with reduced ability to manipulate and propel the bolus of food or liquid into the pharynx, increased oral residue, reduced oral tongue and tongue base range of motion (ROM) and strength, reduced pharyngeal contraction, increased pharyngeal residue, reduced hyolaryngeal motion, reduced airway entrance closure, and aspiration (Fujiu et al., 1995;

Furia et al., 2000; Hamlet et al., 1989; Lazarus, Logemann, & Gibbons, 1993; Pauloski, Logemann, Fox, & Colangelo, 1995; Pauloski et al., 1993; Pauloski et al., 1994; Logemann et al., 1993). On the CD (see Chapter 5: MBS files: "Partial Tongue Resection" and "Floor of Mouth Reconstruction") examples of modified barium swallow (MBS) assessments have been provided for the reader to exemplify this typical postsurgical pattern of deficits.

Patients with oral tongue resections typically demonstrate oral phase swallowing problems. However, pharyngeal phase swallowing disorders can occur after anterior oral cavity resections, particularly if the floor of mouth muscles are cut or resected, resulting in altered hyolaryngeal excursion, tongue base and pharyngeal wall motion, and cricopharyngeal opening during swallowing (Pauloski et al., 1995). Patients having undergone posterior oral cavity resection often have the tongue base, faucial arch, and lateral pharyngeal wall resected. These patients often demonstrate delayed triggering of the pharyngeal motor response, reduced tongue base posterior motion, and reduced pharyngeal contraction for swallowing.

## Nature and Extent of Surgery

The extent of surgical resection and type of reconstruction can have an impact on speech and swallow function. Larger surgical resections, including oral tongue or tongue base, are associated with worse speech function, in terms of understandability and correct

phoneme productions (Nicoletti et al., 2004; Pauloski et al., 1998). Similarly, larger reconstruction procedures have been found to have a negative impact on speech and swallowing (Nicoletti et al., 2004). Primary closure (where remaining tissues from around removed tumor are sutured together—see Figure 5-1) for oral and oropharyngeal resections has resulted in better speech and swallow function than flap reconstruction procedures (Nicoletti et al., 2004; McConnel et al., 1998; Pauloski et al., 1998). However, free flap reconstructions, such as the radial forearm flap (see Figure 5-2), are often thinner and more flexible than local and regional flaps, and can result in less tethering of the residual tongue for improved speech and swallowing (Urken, Moscoso, Lawson, & Biller, 1994).

## Impact of Additional Postoperative Radiotherapy

Postoperative radiotherapy (XRT) can have a negative impact on speech and swallow functioning and can result in worsened performance (Nicoletti et al., 2004; Pauloski et al., 1994). For many patients who resume oral intake postsurgery, the subsequent course of postoperative radiotherapy, with its negative acute side effects such as tissue edema and mucositis (see Chapter 3 for a full discussion of XRT side effects) leads to a temporary decline in function. This can be upsetting for some patients and they need to be counseled to anticipate this temporary setback. While some of the acute reactions to XRT such as the

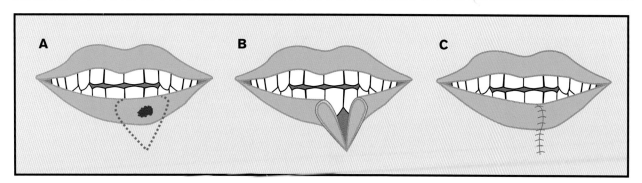

**Figure 5–1.** Schematic representation from **A.** to **C.** of the process of a primary lip closure after surgical removal of a tumor of the lip.

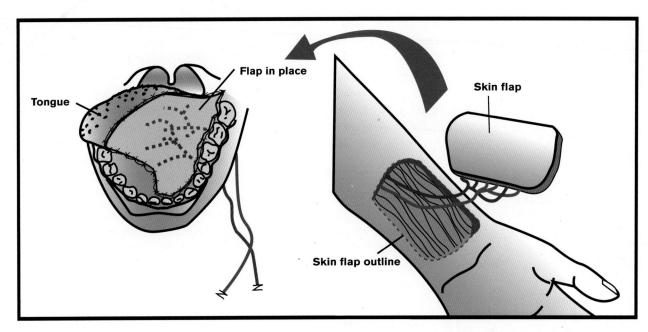

**Figure 5–2.** Schematic representation of a radial forearm reconstruction after surgical removal of a tumor of the tongue.

mucositis, edema, and associated pain/discomfort typically last only a few weeks post-treatment, other consequences such as xerostomia and discomfort from thinning of the oral mucosa may persist in the long term and have an ongoing negative impact to swallowing function.

The long-term impact of radiotherapy is a further decline in patient function, with both swallow and speech function found to be worse over time in irradiated oral cancer patients as compared to those treated with surgery alone (Pauloski et al., 1994) (see Chapter 3 for a discussion of the long-term physiological changes associated with XRT). Pauloski, Rademaker, Logemann, and Colangelo (1998) found poorer swallow functioning in a group of oral cancer patients treated with surgery and postoperative radiotherapy as compared to a similar group of surgically treated patients without postoperative radiotherapy. In particular, the irradiated patients were found to have longer oral transit times, lower oropharyngeal swallow efficiency, increased pharyngeal residue, and reduced cricopharyngeal opening duration. Speech was also found to be worse in the irradiated patients, with fewer correctly produced phonemes.

## Speech and Swallowing Following Radiotherapy and Chemoradiotherapy

Primary radiotherapy with adjuvant or concurrent chemotherapy has become a common treatment modality for head and neck cancer treatment, with comparable cure rates when compared to surgical resection (Kraus et al., 1994; Mendenhall et al., 2000; Sessions, Leonx, Spector, Chao, & Chaudry, 2003; Vokes, Moran, Mick, Weichselbaum, & Panje, 1989). For patients with nasopharyngeal cancer, radiotherapy is indeed the standard treatment (Wei & Sham, 2005). However, since nasopharyngeal tumor is located at the base of the skull, critical structures including the brainstem, cranial nerves, middle and inner ears, and parotid glands are particularly susceptible to the effects of radiotherapy (Wei & Sham, 2005). Therefore, side effects including cranial nerve palsy (Lin, Jen, & Lin, 2002) and dysphagia (Chang et al., 2003; Nguyen et al., 2004) are common. Chemoradiotherapy, also known as "organ preservation treatment," is designed to preserve the anatomy of the organ when used to treat larger, often unresectable tumors of the oral cavity and oropharynx. However, organ *function* is not necessarily spared, with voice, speech, and swallowing often affected.

## Voice and Speech Disorders Following Radiotherapy or Chemoradiotherapy

Voice and speech have been found to be impaired following organ preservation treatment. Patients have been reported to demonstrate dysphonia, abnormal vocal fold vibratory movement, and abnormal aerodynamic and acoustic measures (Carrara-de Angelis, Feher, Barros, Nishimoto, & Kowalski, 2005; Fung et al., 2001). Incorrect production of consonant phonemes has also been observed (Mittal et al., 2001). For those patients who become dysphonic or aphonic following radiotherapy +/− chemotherapy to the pharynx and larynx regions, vigorous voice exercises are not indicated, as irritation to the tissues of the larynx, including the vocal folds, often occurs. This type of vigorous vocal fold adduction exercise will only contribute to further mucosal irritation and possible development of benign vocal fold lesions. Voice typically returns within a few months of radiotherapy treatment and quality can be modified by altering pitch, loudness, breath support, and breath phrasing.

## Swallowing Disorders Following Radiotherapy or Chemoradiotherapy

The swallowing impairment associated with radiotherapy +/− chemotherapy can involve both oral and pharyngeal phases of swallowing, with pharyngeal phase impairment occurring when pharyngeal structures are included in the radiation treatment field. Swallowing problems can include reduced lingual manipulation and propulsion of the bolus, reduced lingual strength, delayed triggering of the pharyngeal motor response, impaired tongue base motion, pharyngeal contraction, hyolaryngeal motion, laryngeal closure (vestibular and glottic), and cricopharyngeal opening (Carrara-de Angelis et al., 2005; Eisbruch et al., 2004; Eisele, Koch,

Tarazi, & Jones, 1991; Ekberg & Nylander, 1983; Hughes et al., 2000; Kendall, McKenzie, Leonard, & Jones, 1998; Koch et al., 1995; Kotz, Abraham, Beitler, Wadler, & Smith, 1999; Lazarus, 1997; Lazarus et al., 1996; Lazarus et al., 2000). The extent, rate, timing, and coordination of pharyngeal structural movement is often impaired, resulting in reduced bolus clearance through the pharynx and aspiration, which may often be silent (Eisbruch et al., 2004; Eisele et al., 1991; Ekberg & Nylander, 1983; Kendall et al., 1998; Koch et al., 1995; Kotz et al., 1999; Lazarus, 1997; Lazarus et al., 1996; Lazarus et al., 2000; Logemann, 1985; Smith, Logemann, Colangelo, Rademaker, & Pauloski, 1999). These characteristics can be observed on the MBS assessments of patients managed with radiation +/− chemotherapy included on the DVD (see Chapter 5; MBS files; "Chemoradiotherapy for SCC at Base of Tongue," and "Post Chemoradiotherapy—Aspiration").

Xerostomia (reduced saliva flow) is a common side effect of radiotherapy which often worsens over time and can affect a patient's perception of swallowing ability (Kuo et al., 1993; Liu, Fleming, Toth, & Keene, 1990; Logemann et al., 2001; Pow, McMillan, Leung, Wong, & Kwong, 2003). Xerostomia can cause increased difficulty with bolus manipulation and propulsion and can result in delayed triggering of the pharyngeal swallow (Hamlet et al., 1997; Hughes et al., 1987). Trismus (discussed further in Chapter 7) can also result from radiotherapy, with restriction in jaw movement for mouth opening and lateral motion (Ichimura & Tanaka, 1993). Range of motion exercise for the jaw is routinely provided at the onset of radiotherapy treatment to prevent trismus from occurring (Logemann, 1983).

The effects of radiotherapy often result in worsening of swallow function over time (Lazarus, 1993; Smith, Kotz, Beitler, & Wadler, 2000), due to vascular changes that can result in reduced blood supply to the muscles and eventual tissue fibrosis (Law, 1981; Ben-Yosef & Kapp, 1992; Bentzen, Thames, & Overgaard, 1989; Brown, Fixsen, & Plowman, 1987; Watkin et al., 2001). Therefore, although no prospective or retrospective studies have examined the effects of exercise programs either during or after chemoradiotherapy, it has become common practice for patients to be given prophylactic exercises to minimize the effects of fibrosis on swallowing in irradiated patients (Cooper, Fu,

Marks, & Silverman, 1995; Lazarus, 2000). Studies are currently underway investigating the effects of preventative swallow exercise programs in this population.

## Impact of New Radiotherapy Delivery Techniques

Novel ways to provide radiotherapy treatment have been recently developed, including intensity modulated (IMRT) and tissue/dose compensation (TDC) radiotherapy techniques (see Chapter 3 for further discussion). These newer techniques are designed to reduce the radiation dosage to normal surrounding tissues and reduce overall toxicity (Eisbruch et al., 2004; Kwong et al., 2004; Mittal et al., 2001). Some benefit has been found in swallowing and speech function with these techniques. Mittal et al. (2001) found improved oral intake, lower pharyngeal residue, improved oropharyngeal swallowing efficiency, and greater range of bolus type with TDC as compared to standard radiotherapy. These authors also found improved articulation with TDC. Eisbruch and colleagues (2004) found a moderate affect on swallowing with IMRT. Kwong et al. (2004) found that the parotid glands are spared, facilitating continuous improvement in salivary flow in nasopharyngeal cancer patients treated with IMRT.

## Management of Patients with Oral, Oropharyngeal, and Nasopharyngeal Tumors

### Pretreatment Counseling and Assessment

The speech-language pathologist (SLP) plays a critical role in defining the speech and swallowing disorders following oral cancer treatment. Management of patients with newly diagnosed oral, oropharyngeal, and nasopharyngeal tumors should begin prior to treatment. It is important to include carers and significant others in the counseling process as they can provide invaluable support and encouragement during the treatment process. Pretreatment counseling allows the SLP to determine how well the patient understands the upcoming treatment, once determined. It also allows

the SLP to discuss the patient's role in rehabilitation, with focus on optimal rehabilitation of function following brief but frequent, daily practice of speech and swallow exercises. Pretreatment counseling includes discussion regarding the role of the SLP, specifically, assessing speech and swallowing, the latter with the clinical and instrumental evaluation, providing speech and swallow therapy, and involvement in construction of palatal augmentation prostheses (discussed later in this chapter), as appropriate.

The SLP also assesses the patient's speech and swallowing pretreatment. Pretreatment speech assessment typically involves a brief clinical evaluation of the current function of the articulators, voice quality, and also a discussion of the patient's communication needs and goals (e.g., currently employed and anxious about reestablishing good communication skills versus retired and expressing little concern regarding a decline in articulatory precision). In relation to swallowing, typically a clinical swallow evaluation is conducted with an instrumental assessment (e.g., MBS) performed as needed, particularly if the patient is experiencing difficulty swallowing.

The clinical swallow evaluation includes an oral-motor examination to assess the range of motion, rate, strength, precision, and coordination of the vocal tract, structural and muscular movements of the lips, tongue, velum, larynx, jaw, and respiratory muscles for speech, and precision of nonspeech tasks (in isolation and rapid repetition). The evaluation provides information concerning the overall timing of the oropharyngeal swallow (i.e., oropharyngeal transit time), tongue function for swallowing, and an estimate of laryngeal motion during the swallow (Logemann, 1998). Intraoral inspection provides information on location and extent of oral residue, an indication of reduced lingual control and/or reduced lingual strength. It also allows for potential identification of aspiration, if observable by coughing, throat-clearing or a wet-gurgly voice quality (Logemann, 1998; Logemann, Veis, & Colangelo, 1999). However, aspiration may be undetectable and silent, requiring instrumental examination (Lundy et al., 1999; Smith et al., 1999).

Instrumental examination can include flexible endoscopic examination of swallowing (FEES), flexible endoscopic examination of swallowing with sensory testing (FEESST) or fluoroscopic assessment, a modified barium swallow (MBS) procedure (Aviv, Thomson, Sunshine, & Close, 1998; Langmore, Schatz, & Olson, 1988; Logemann, 1993) (for further discussion of these techniques see Chapter 2). Both FEES and FEESST involve transnasal insertion of an endoscopic tube into the pharynx at the level of the tongue base, and therefore this exam provides no information on the oral preparatory and oral phases of swallowing. Hence, considering that oral stage deficits are common in this population, it is not ideal for a comprehensive assessment of swallowing function. The technique does however allow visualization of the pharynx and larynx, does not involve any radiation exposure, and can be used at bedside (Langmore et al., 1988), so it has application for determining aspiration risk. In contrast, the MBS procedure allows for visualization of oral and pharyngeal structures, bolus flow through the oral cavity and pharynx, and identification of physiologic swallow disorders (Logemann, 1993; Martin-Harris, Michel, & Castell, 2005). This exam also provides information on the effects of therapeutic techniques, such as postures, swallow maneuvers, and sensory enhancements on swallow function (Logemann, 1993, 1998; Martin, Logemann, Shaker, & Dodds, 1993).

Manometry can also be used to examine oral and pharyngeal pressure generation and upper esophageal sphincter function during the swallow (Castell & Castell, 1993; McConnel, 1988). Manometry alone does not provide visualization of structures or structural movement. However, it can be paired with fluoroscopy to provide information on oral and pharyngeal structural movement simultaneous with pressure information (Lazarus, Logemann, Song, Rademaker, & Kahrilas, 2002; McConnel, 1988).

## Post-Treatment: Evaluation and Management of Speech and Swallowing Following Surgical Intervention

The SLP is typically consulted to evaluate a patient's speech and swallowing approximately 5–7 days after surgery. A speech evaluation is typically performed approximately 14 days postoperatively if a free flap reconstruction technique has been used, as a longer period of time is needed to ensure adequate healing, particularly at anastomotic sites of reconnected nerves,

arteries, and veins. The SLP should always confirm with the referring physician that adequate healing has occurred prior to evaluating and treating patients who have undergone surgical management. This will ensure that suture lines will not be compromised with active exercise. Speech and swallow therapy are typically provided daily during a patient's hospital stay, initially weekly following discharge and bimonthly thereafter.

### *Postoperative Evaluation: Speech*

The clinical examination should include a thorough oral-motor evaluation, as described previously. An intraoral exam should reveal the flap location and size, unless surgically placed within the oropharynx and not easily visible (see Figure 5–3). Range, rate, strength, precision, and coordination of the vocal tract musculature should be assessed, as described previously. Speech should be assessed at the isolated, CVC word, and phrase levels, with particular focus on the ability to produce lingual-palatal contacts for stop consonants and precision of fricatives and affricate phonemes, as tongue-palate contact and tongue control and shaping may be reduced after surgery.

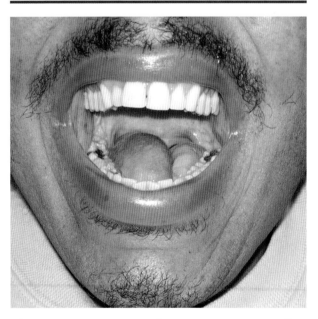

**Figure 5–3.** An oral cancer patient after hemiglossectomy and radial forearm free flap reconstruction.

## Postoperative Rehabilitation: Speech

If a mandibulotomy was performed during the surgery, lip closure may be reduced, with imprecision for bilabial sounds /b/, /p/, and /m/. Reduced lip closure can also result in leakage of material out the front of the mouth. In either case, speech exercises to improve precision of bilabial phonemes and lip range of motion and strengthening (resistance) exercises should be given to improve articulatory precision as well as improve lip seal for swallowing (Logemann, 1983).

Jaw range of motion exercises should also be given post-healing if a mandibulotomy or partial mandibulectomy was performed during surgery, as bite force, range of motion, and overall masticatory ability can be reduced after surgery (Marunick & Mathog, 1990).

Exercises include jaw opening, lateral movement, and a rotary movement for chewing (Logemann, 1983). Use of the Therabite device (Atos Medical, www.atos medical.com) (see Figure 5–4) can also have a beneficial effect on jaw range of motion, particularly following radiotherapy.

Tongue range of motion, control, and strengthening exercises should be given once healing is complete, even for patients who have undergone small resections of the tongue (Logemann, 1983; Logemann, Pauloski, Rademaker, & Colangelo, 1997).

■ *Tongue range of motion exercises* should include slow repetitions during maximum movement on protrusion, elevation (including tip and back dorsum of the

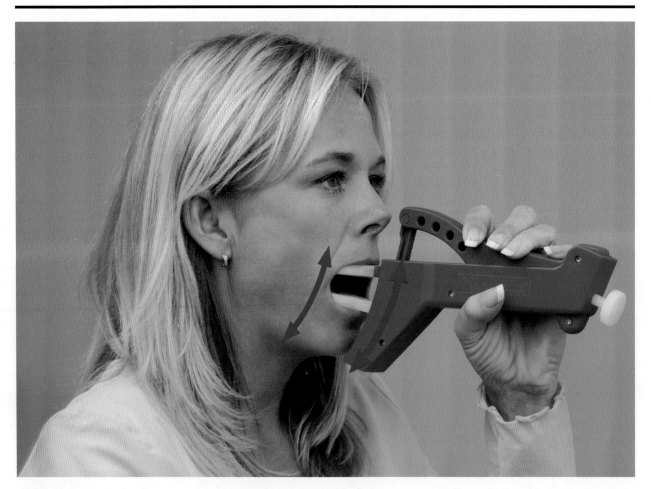

**Figure 5–4.** A patient using the Therabite system. Red arrows demonstrate the anatomical correct opening curve of the device. (Photo courtesy of Atos Medical, www.atosmedical.com.)

tongue), and lateral motion. Tongue base range of motion exercises should also be included (i.e., tongue base motion posteriorly toward the posterior pharyngeal wall), as tongue base motion is critical for bolus clearance through the upper pharynx during swallowing; and is often reduced following oral cancer surgery (Logemann, 1998; McConnel, 1988; Pauloski & Logemann, 2000). It is difficult to determine whether a patient is performing this tongue base range of motion exercise correctly, as it cannot be visualized. Palpation of the submental region can give a crude estimate as to the presence and extent of tongue base retraction. However, a better way to ensure that a patient is performing this exercise correctly is by instructing the patient under x-ray. This will ensure that the instructions are having the desired effect, namely, the greatest degree of posterior lingual movement. Veis, Logemann, and Rademaker (2000) examined the effects of three instructions to improve tongue base posterior motion on x-ray. These included (a) "pull your tongue back as far as you can," (b) "pull your tongue back like you are yawning," and (c) "pull your tongue back like you are gargling." These authors found that the third instruction resulted in the greatest extent of movement in most participants; however, the other two occasionally resulted in maximum posterior movement. Ideally, when examined on x-ray, a patient will make complete contact to the posterior pharyngeal wall when performing this exercise.

- *Tongue control exercises* can include manipulation of licorice in the lateral directions as well as up and back, as if propelling a bolus (Logemann, 1983). This exercise should also include sealing the licorice against the anterior and lateral upper alveolar ridge to work on lingual control, strength, and vertical range of motion (Logemann, 1983).

- *Tongue strengthening exercises* include active resistance against a tongue depressor with the tongue in the anterior, lateral, and upward direction (Logemann, 1983). Active resistance exercises have been found to

increase tongue strength and lingual mass in healthy young, elderly, and disordered populations (Kays, Hind, Hewitt, Gangnon, & Robbins, 2004; Lazarus, Logemann, Huang, & Rademaker, 2003; Robbins, Gangnon, Theis, Kays, & Hind, 2005).

Speech exercises should be given following oral cancer surgery, even with small tongue resections, as imprecise articulation can result. Patients should be instructed to practice errored phonemes in all vocalic positions in words and phrases, focusing on the clearest possible production, since normal articulation may not be a realistic goal after surgery. Once clearer productions are being made, therapy should work on carryover into conversation, working on paragraph reading, taping of monologues, and conversation. Some patients compensate well following oral cancer surgery, even with limited tongue range of motion. A sample of speech following oral cancer surgery can be heard on the CD (see Chapter 5: Video: Conversational Speech—Oral Cancer Patient). This same patient's tongue range of motion can be seen on a second video clip on the CD (see Chapter 5: Video: Tongue Range of Motion).

### Postoperative Evaluation: Swallow

An instrumental assessment of swallowing, typically the MBS procedure, is usually indicated postoperatively since patients frequently experience difficulty in both the oral and pharyngeal phases of swallowing after surgery. Once the swallowing disorders are identified, therapeutic strategies can be implemented in x-ray to assess their effects on swallow safety and efficiency. An example of a patient (post-XRT for a base of tongue tumor) implementing a double swallow with breath hold technique during MBS assessment is available for viewing on the CD (see Chapter 5: MBS Files: Double Swallow with Breath Hold).

### Postoperative Management: Swallow

Following instrumental assessment, the SLP makes recommendations regarding oral vs. non-oral means of nutrition, diet type, specific techniques to be used during meals, and specific swallow exercises to be practiced. These strategies include (a) postures, (b) maneuvers, and (c) sensory enhancements, such as modification of bolus viscosity, volume, and thermal/tactile stimulation. Patients are typically instructed to practice their exercises on a short, frequent, daily basis for maximum gain in function.

Postures are compensatory techniques that improve bolus flow and can prevent aspiration (Logemann, 1983, 1998; Logemann, Rademaker, Pauloski, & Kahrilas, 1994; Rasley et al., 1993). The main postural compensatory techniques which have application in this population include:

■ *Head tilt.* Tilting the head to the unoperated side can improve bolus flow and transit through the oral cavity and pharynx (Logemann, 1983). This posture is often useful for patients having undergone hemiglossectomy or lateral composite resection. This posture can be combined with the head back posture to facilitate bolus clearance through the oral cavity.

■ *Head rotation.* This posture can improve bolus clearance through the pharynx by closing off the operated/irradiated side of the pharynx (Logemann, 1983). This posture is also useful to improve opening within the cricopharyngeal region, as well as improve airway protection if glottic closure is reduced (Logemann, 1983; Ohmae, Ogura, Kitahara, Karaho, & Inouye, 1998).

■ *Head back.* The head back posture is useful to facilitate transit of a bolus through the oral cavity and is used in those patients with intact pharyngeal phase functioning (Logemann, 1983). Typically, patients are instructed in an airway protection maneuver (i.e., super supraglottic swallow) when using this posture, since material can enter the pharynx fairly quickly. This posture is often used with patients after subtotal and total glossectomy who experience difficulty propelling material from the oral cavity. Patients having undergone total glossectomy typically are limited to some type of liquid diet; however, some individuals with palatal augmentation prostheses can handle pureed and very soft foods as well (Davis, Lazarus, Logemann, & Hurst, 1987).

■ *Side lying.* Side lying is used when pharyngeal clearance is reduced, resulting in residue that enters the airway after the swallow (Logemann, 1983). Residue will still be present after the swallow when this maneuver is used, but will remain on the lateral pharyngeal wall and will be cleared on subsequent dry swallows.

■ *Chin tuck.* The chin tuck posture is useful for those patients with delayed triggering of the pharyngeal motor response, as material can catch within the vallecular space prior to triggering (Shanahan, Logemann, Rademaker, Pauloski, & Kahrilas, 1993; Welch, Logemann, Rademaker, Pauloski, & Kahrilas, 1993). Using this posture also results in added airway protection, with the tongue base situated in a more posterior position and the arytenoids situated closer to the epiglottic base, narrowing the airway entrance (Shanahan et al., 1993; Welch et al., 1993). However the application of the chin tuck posture is not applicable for all oral cancer patients. Particularly those with anterior tongue resections, gravity tends to cause material to slip to the front of the mouth, making it more difficult to propel material into the pharynx. However, this posture is often useful for those with tongue base resections, as the residual tongue is situated closer to the pharyngeal wall, potentially improving bolus clearance through this region.

In addition to postural changes, sensory enhancement techniques are useful for those patients who demonstrate delayed triggering of the pharyngeal motor response and can include thermal/tactile stimulation of the swallow (i.e., rubbing the base of the faucial arches with a size 00 cold laryngeal mirror) (Lazzara, Lazarus, & Logemann, 1986; Rosenbek, Roecker, Wood, & Robbins, 1996). The cold and tactile stimulation serves as an alerting mechanism for the central nervous system. The usefulness of this technique in the head and neck cancer population has not been examined and the effects may be less robust than those seen in the neurologically impaired population. This may be because the delay in the triggering of the pharyngeal motor response may be due to peripheral changes at the level of the mucosa, rather than more centrally mediated, as in the neurologically impaired population. Sensory enhancements can include modification of taste, temperature, as well as carbonation (Bisch, Logemann, Rademaker, Kahrilas, & Lazarus, 1994; Bülow, Olsson, & Ekberg, 2003; Logemann, Pauloski, Lazarus, Fujiu, & Kahrilas, 1995).

Sensory enhancements also include bolus modifications, including volume and viscosity. Systematic shifts in the extent, timing, degree, and coordination of pharyngeal structural movement occur with bolus volume and viscosity in healthy individuals (Bisch et al., 1994; Hiss, Strauss, Treole, Stuart, & Boutilier, 2004; Logemann et al., 2000; Logemann, Pauloski, Rademaker, & Kahrilas, 2002; Robbins, Hamilton, Lof, & Kempster, 1992; Sonies, Parent, Morrish, & Baum, 1988; Perlman, Schultz, & VanDaele, 1993). Larger bolus volumes increase the extent and duration of hyolaryngeal motion and increase the width and duration of cricopharyngeal sphincter opening in healthy individuals. A similar shift and improvement in hyolaryngeal motion and cricopharyngeal opening can occur in surgically treated oral cancer patients with bolus volume. Total glossectomy patients can benefit from a "dump and swallow," where the pharynx is filled with liquid (i.e., larger volumes) and the patient repeatedly swallows while maintaining glottic and supraglottic closure during the swallow. This can be combined with a head back posture to facilitate bolus transit through the oral cavity and pharynx (Logemann, 1983). Viscosity can have a major effect on swallowing. Specifically, thin liquids tend to slip into the anterior and lateral sulci during oral manipulation following partial glossectomy due to reduced tongue control, but can be propelled through the oral cavity more easily than thicker bolus viscosities. Thicker boluses are also more difficult to propel through the pharynx, particularly after tongue base resection.

Swallow maneuvers are designed to alter the physiology of the swallow, specifically, the pharyngeal motor response. The maneuvers that can be beneficial in this patient population include:

- *Supraglottic and super supraglottic swallow.* The supraglottic swallow technique is designed to improve airway closure before and during the swallow at the level of the glottis (Logemann, 1993; Martin et al., 1993). Patients are instructed to hold their breath, swallow, and cough. In comparison, the super supraglottic swallow is designed to improve airway closure before and during the swallow at the level of the airway entrance (i.e., laryngeal vestibule) and glottis (Logemann, 1993; Martin et al., 1993). The super supraglottic swallow involves a tighter breath hold than that used with the supraglottic swallow and is designed to achieve arytenoid to epiglottic base contact for closure of the laryngeal vestibule, reducing the risk of penetration of material into this region and aspiration after the swallow. The patient is instructed to hold his or her breath very tightly while bearing down with the abdominal muscles (for a tighter breath hold), swallow, and cough.

- *Effortful swallow.* This maneuver is designed to improve tongue base posterior motion during the swallow and improve pressures to clear the bolus past the tongue base (Fujiu & Logemann, 1996; Hind, Nicosia, Roecker, Carnes, & Robbins, 2001; Lazarus et al., 2002; Logemann, 1993; Logemann, 1998; Pouderoux & Kahrilas, 1995). It is helpful for those patients who demonstrate reduced tongue base posterior motion disorder that can result in residue on the tongue base, valleculae, and upper pharyngeal wall. Patients are instructed to squeeze hard with the tongue and throat muscles during the swallow when performing this maneuver. This maneuver is often combined with the chin tuck posture, which places the tongue closer to the pharyngeal wall to maximize bolus clearance past the tongue base.

- *Mendelsohn swallow maneuver.* The Mendelsohn maneuver is designed to increase the extent and duration of laryngeal elevation and anterior motion during the swallow, thereby increasing the width and duration of cricopharyngeal opening during the swallow (Kahrilas, Logemann, Krugler, & Flanagan, 1991). This maneuver can also improve the coordination of the pharyngeal events occurring during the pharyngeal swallow (Lazarus et al., 1993). The patient is instructed to swallow normally, and in the middle of the swallow, when the larynx is felt to elevate, the patient is instructed to maintain laryngeal elevation for an extra 2 seconds by squeezing hard with the throat muscles and tongue. This maneuver is useful for patients having undergone anterior or posterior oral tongue resections, as well as those having undergone tongue base resection, as all may demonstrate problems with laryngeal motion following surgery.

- *Tongue-hold maneuver.* The tongue-hold maneuver (also called the Masako maneuver) is designed to increase the extent of anterior motion of the posterior pharyngeal wall (Fujiu & Logemann, 1996). The tongue is anchored between the teeth (or gums in edentulous patients), which places the tongue base in a more anterior position. This results in greater anterior motion of the posterior pharyngeal wall, improving tongue base to pharyngeal wall contact and clearance of material past this region for swallowing (Fujiu & Logemann, 1996). This technique obviously cannot be used for patients with anterior tongue resections, but is useful for those patients who have anterior lingual tissue but demonstrate reduced tongue base posterior motion. This exercise is designed to be a range of motion exercise for the pharyngeal constrictors and should be practiced with saliva or very small (½ cc) amounts of water. This exercise should not be practiced with food or liquid boluses, since anchoring of the tongue tip might result in reduced bolus control and aspiration.

## Intraoral Prosthetics

For some patients, in addition to behavioral rehabilitation the use of intraoral prosthetic devices can facilitate speech and swallowing function. The SLP works collaboratively with the maxillofacial prosthodontist to construct the prosthesis. For patients undergoing oral cancer surgery, construction of the prosthesis typically begins 4-6 weeks postoperatively. For those patients undergoing radiotherapy, construction typically begins at least 6-8 weeks after completion of treatment. When patients are seen by the SLP with the maxillofacial prosthodontist, additional speech and swallow exercises are provided and should be practiced with the prosthesis in place to maximize its use

for swallowing and speech. Figure 5-5 provides an algorithm for management of the surgically treated oral cancer patient.

There are three types of intraoral prosthetics including: (a) palatal lift, (b) palatal obturator, and (c) palatal augmentation (also known as "drop" or "lowering").

- *A palatal lift* aids in velopharyngeal closure by lifting the soft palate that is not functioning due to neurologic impairment.
- *A palatal obturator* seals off the velopharyngeal port for those patients who undergo soft palate resection, preventing material from entering the nasopharynx and improving intraoral pressure (Light, 1995).
- *A palatal augmentation prosthesis* lowers the palatal vault for those patients who have undergone oral cancer resection (see Figure 5-6). This type of prosthesis allows the remaining lingual tissue to contact the prosthesis for improved tongue control, anchoring, and propulsion of material through the oral cavity (Davis et al., 1987; Logemann, Kahrilas, Hurst, Davis, & Krugler, 1989; Wheeler, Logemann, & Rosen, 1980). A palatal augmentation prosthesis can benefit patients who have had a significant portion of the oral tongue resected, resulting in improved bolus transport through the oral cavity, reduced oral residue, and reduced aspiration (Davis et al., 1987; Wheeler et al., 1980). Palatal augmentation prostheses are also useful after small tongue resections, as they not only improve tongue control but can improve articulatory precision. Mixed success with regards to speech has been found with prosthesis usage in patients with posterior tongue resection (Colangelo et al., 1996). For patients with total glossectomy, the palatal augmentation prosthesis is typically fairly large because the augmentation portion needs to be near the remaining muscles comprising the floor of the mouth in order to assist with bolus control and clearance through the oral cavity. A sample of a fairly large palatal augmentation prosthesis, constructed for a patient who has undergone 70% glossectomy, can be seen in Figure 5-7.

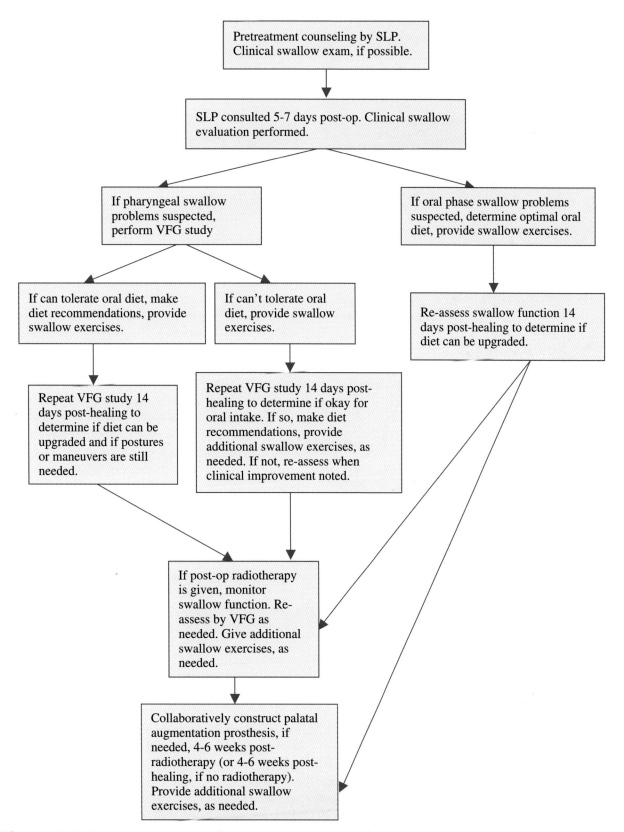

**Figure 5–5.** Optimal care algorithm for management of surgically treated oral cancer patients. From "Management of swallowing disorders in head and neck cancer patients: Optimal patterns of care," by C. L. Lazarus, 2000, *Seminars in Speech and Language*, *31*, 293–309. (From *Seminars in Speech and Hearing*, *21*(4), p. 303. Reprinted with permission of the publisher.)

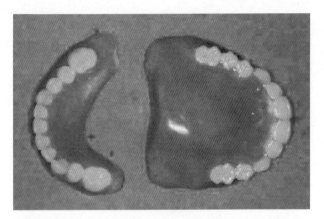

**Figure 5–6.** Palatal augmentation prosthesis with moderate augmentation.

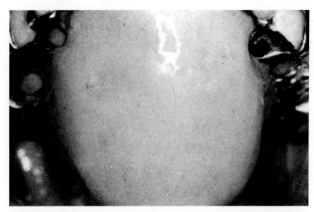

**Figure 5–7.** Palatal augmentation prosthesis with large augmentation.

## Post-Treatment: Evaluation and Management of Speech and Swallowing Following Radiotherapy or Chemoradiotherapy

For those patients who will undergo radiotherapy with or without chemotherapy, prophylactic swallow exercises are provided to reduce the chance of a swallowing impairment during and after chemoradiotherapy. These exercises are designed to maintain the range of motion, strength, coordination, and timing of oral and pharyngeal structural movement for swallowing and include: (a) tongue range of motion, (b) jaw range of motion, (c) tongue base range of motion (i.e., base of tongue retraction range of motion exercise, effortful swallow, and tongue-hold maneuver), (d) laryngeal range of motion (i.e., Mendelsohn maneuver), and (e) laryngeal closure, including supraglottic and glottic (i.e., super supraglottic swallow). Patients are instructed to practice these exercises daily, as they are able, with typically five repetitions per exercise. However, patients frequently are unable to practice their exercises as chemoradiotherapy treatment progresses, since they often feel tired and weak from their treatment. In this case, patients are strongly encouraged to practice their jaw ROM exercises to reduce the risk of trismus. Once chemotherapy treatment is finished, patients are strongly encouraged to continue daily practice of their exercises since swallowing, as mentioned earlier, can

become impaired over time due to radiotherapy fibrosis effects.

Tongue strength is often impaired after primary radiotherapy in patients with oral and pharyngeal cancers, since the oropharynx and tongue base are often in the treatment field (Lazarus et al., 2000; Lazarus, 2005). Tongue strength has been found to be reduced long after completion of radiotherapy treatment for oral or pharyngeal cancer (Lazarus, 2005). Thus, exercises targeting tongue strength are often prescribed. However, these exercises are typically given following radiotherapy treatment, rather than preventatively as are other swallow exercises, as tumor presence can result in lingual pain and preclude active resistance exercise during radiotherapy.

Should patients exhibit dysphagia during the course of chemoradiotherapy, physicians typically refer to the SLP to conduct a clinical swallow examination. This assessment often leads to an instrumental examination. Once the oropharyngeal swallow physiology has been defined, management strategies are identified and implemented. Patients treated with primary radiotherapy with or without chemotherapy can pose a challenge to clinicians. For those patients whose swallow function is normal following irradiation, coaxing them to perform daily swallow exercises can be difficult. For those patients who become dysphagic following radiotherapy, the severity of the swallowing problem can preclude oral intake, despite intensive and prolonged swallow rehabilitation.

## Outcomes

Studies have examined speech and swallow function over time in the surgically treated and irradiated head and neck cancer patients (Pauloski et al., 1994; Pauloski et al., 1998). Both swallowing and speech have been found to improve over time except for patients who undergo postoperative radiotherapy, where function either remains stable or worsens. One study has prospectively examined swallow function and tongue strength in oral and oropharyngeal cancer patients treated with radiotherapy with or without chemotherapy and found improvement in tongue strength, swallow function, and diet over the course of 12 months (Lazarus et al., in press). However, only some of these patients received swallow treatment, and the type, frequency, and duration of the treatment was not controlled in this study. Only one study to date has examined the effects of exercise on swallow and speech function in the treated head and neck cancer patient. Logemann, et al. (1997) found that surgically treated oral cancer patients who practiced tongue range of motion exercises were found to perform better on both speech and swallowing tasks than those not given exercises. Oropharyngeal swallow efficiency (OPSE), a global measure of swallow function that describes the interaction of the speed of bolus movement and the safety and efficiency of the mechanism in clearing material from the oropharynx (Rademaker, Pauloski, Logemann, & Shanahan, 1994), was found to be higher in patients who performed lingual range of motion exercises. Future studies need to prospectively examine the effects of specific exercise programs on speech and swallow function in the treated head and neck cancer patient. The type, dosage, and duration of treatment also need to be evaluated.

## References

Aviv, J. E., Thomson, J. E., Sunshine, S., & Close, L. G. (1998). Fiberoptic endoscopic evaluation of swallowing with sensory testing (FEESST) in healthy controls. *Dysphagia, 13*, 87-92.

Ben-Yosef, R., & Kapp, D. S. (1992). Persistent and/or late complications of combined radiation therapy and hyperthermia. *International Journal of Hyperthermia, 8*, 733-745.

Bentzen, S. M., Thames, H. D., & Overgaard, M. (1989). Latent-time estimate for late cutaneous and subcutaneous radiation reactions in a single follow-up clinical study. *Radiotherapy and Oncology, 15*, 267-274.

Bisch, E. M., Logemann, J. A., Rademaker, A. W., Kahrilas, P. J., & Lazarus, C. L. (1994). Pharyngeal effects of bolus volume, viscosity, and temperature in patients with dysphagia resulting from neurologic impairment and in normal subjects. *Journal of Speech and Hearing Research, 37*, 1041-1049.

Brown, A. P., Fixsen, J. A., & Plowman, P. N. (1987). Local control of Ewing's sarcoma: An analysis of 67 patients. *The British Journal of Radiology, 60*, 261-268.

Bülow, M., Olsson, R., & Ekberg, O. (2003). Videoradiographic analysis of how carbonated thin liquids and thickened liquids affect the physiology of swallowing in subjects with aspiration on thin liquids. *Acta Radiologica, 44*, 366-372.

Carrara-de Angelis, E., Feher, O., Barros, A. P. B., Nishimoto, I. N., & Kowalski, L. P. (2005). Voice and swallowing in patients enrolled in a larynx preservation trial. *Archives of Otolaryngology-Head & Neck Surgery, 129*(7), 733-738.

Castell, J. A., & Castell, D. O. (1993). Modern solid state computerized manometry of the pharyngoesophageal segment. *Dysphagia, 8*, 270-275.

Cerenko, D., McConnel, F., & Jackson, R. (1989). Quantitative assessment of pharyngeal bolus driving forces. *Otolaryngology-Head & Neck Surgery, 100*, 57-63.

Chang, Y. C., Chen, S. Y., Lui, L. T., Wang, T. G., Wang, T. C., Hsiao, T. Y., et al. (2003). Dysphagia in patients with nasopharyngeal cancer after radiation therapy: A videofluoroscopic swallowing study. *Dysphagia, 18*(2), 135-143.

Colangelo, L. A., Paoloski, B. R., Logemann, J. A., Stein, D. W., Beery, Q. C., Heiser, M. A., et al. (1996). Effects of intraoral prostheses on speech in oropharyngeal cancer patients. *American Journal of Speech-Language Pathology, 5*, 43-55.

Conley, J. J. (1962). The crippled oral cavity. *Plastic and Reconstructive Surgery, 30*, 469-478.

Cooper, J. S., Fu, K., Marks, J., & Silverman, S. (1995). Late effects of radiation therapy in the head and neck region. *International Journal of Radiation Oncology, Biology, Physics, 31*, 1141-1164.

Davis, J. W., Lazarus, C., Logemann, J. A., & Hurst, P. S. (1987). Effect of maxillary glossectomy prosthesis on articulation and swallowing. *Journal of Prosthetic Dentistry, 57,* 715-720.

Dios, P. D., Feijoo, J. F., Ferriero, M. C., & Alvarez, J. A. (1994). Functional consequences of partial glossectomy. *Journal of Oral and Maxillofacial Surgery, 52,* 12-14.

Eisbruch, A., Schwartz, M., Rasch, C., Vineberg, K., Damen, E., Van As, C. J., et al. (2004). Dysphagia and aspiration after chemoradiotherapy for head-and-neck cancer: Which anatomic structures are affected and can they be spared by IMRT? *International Journal of Radiation Oncology, Biology, Physics, 60,* 1425-1439.

Eisele, D. W., Koch, D. G., Tarazi, A. E., & Jones, B. (1991). Aspiration from delayed radiation fibrosis of the neck. *Dysphagia, 6,* 120-122.

Ekberg, O., & Nylander, G. (1983). Pharyngeal dysfunction after treatment for pharyngeal cancer with surgery and radiotherapy. *Gastrointestinal Radiology, 8,* 97-104.

Fujiu, M., & Logemann, J. A. (1996). Effect of a tongue-holding maneuver on posterior pharyngeal wall movement during deglutition. *American Journal of Speech-Language Pathology, 5,* 23-30.

Fujiu, M., Logemann, J. A., & Pauloski, B. R. (1995). Increased postoperative posterior pharyngeal wall movement in patients with anterior oral cancer: Preliminary findings and possible implications for treatment. *American Journal of Speech-Language Pathology, 4,* 24-30.

Fung, K., Yoo, J., Leeper, A., Hawkins, S., Neenfeman, H., Doyle, P. C., et al. (2001). Vocal function following radiation for non-laryngeal versus laryngeal tumors of the head and neck. *Laryngoscope, 111,* 1920-1924.

Furia, C. L., Carrara-de Angelis, E., Martins, N. M., Barros, A. P., Carneiro, B., & Kowalski, L. P. (2000). Videofluoroscopic evaluation after glossectomy. *Archives of Otolaryngology-Head & Neck Surgery, 126,* 378-383.

Greven, A. J., Meijer, M. F., & Tiwari, R. M. (1994). Articulation after total glossectomy: A clinical study of speech in six patients. *European Journal of Disorders of Communication, 29,* 85-93.

Hamlet, S., Faull, J., Klein, B., Aref, A., Fontanesi, J., Stachler, R., et al. (1997). Mastication and swallowing in patients with postirradiation xerostomia. *International Journal of Radiation Oncology, Biology, Physics, 37,* 789-796.

Hamlet, S., Jones, L., Mathog, R., Bolton, M., & Patterson, R. (1988). Bolus propulsive activity of the tongue in dysphagic cancer patients. *Dysphagia, 3,* 18-23.

Hamlet, S., Mathog, R., Patterson, R., & Fleming, S. (1990). Tongue mobility in speech after partial glossectomy. *Head & Neck, 12,* 210-217.

Hamlet, S., Patterson, R., & Fleming, S. (1989). Recovery of tongue function for speech and swallowing in partial glossectomy patients. *Journal of the Acoustical Society of America, 86,* 113.

Heller, K. S., Levy, J., & Sciubba, J. J. (1991). Speech patterns following partial glossectomy for small tumors of the tongue. *Head & Neck, 13,* 340-343.

Hind, J. A., Nicosia, M. A., Roecker, E. B., Carnes, M. L., & Robbins, J. (2001). Comparison of effortful and non-effortful swallows in healthy middle-aged and older adults. *Archives of Physical Medicine and Rehabilitation, 82,* 1661-1665.

Hiss, S. G., Strauss, M., Treole, K., Stuart, A., & Boutilier, S. (2004). Effects of age, gender, bolus volume, bolus viscosity and gestation on swallowing apnea onset relative to lingual bolus propulsion onset in normal adults. *Journal of Speech, Language, and Hearing Research, 47,* 572-583.

Hufnagle, J., Pullon, P., & Hufnagle, K. (1978). Speech considerations in oral surgery. (Part II. Speech characteristics of patients following surgery for oral malignancies). *Oral Surgery, 46,* 354-361.

Hughes, C. V., Baum, B. J., Fox, P. C., Marmary, Y., Yeh, C., & Sonies, B. C. (1987). Oral-pharyngeal dysphagia: A common sequela of salivary gland dysfunction. *Dysphagia, 1,* 173-177.

Hughes, P. J., Scott, P. M., Kew, J., Cheung, D. M. C., Leung, S. F., & Ahuja, A. T. (2000). Dysphagia in treated nasopharyngeal cancer. *Head & Neck, 22,* 393-397.

Ichimura, K., & Tanaka, T. (1993). Trismus in patients with malignant tumours in the head and neck. *The Journal of Laryngology and Otology, 107,* 1017-1020.

Imai, S., & Michi, K. (1992). Articulatory function after resection of the tongue and floor of mouth: Palatometric and perceptual evaluation. *Journal of Speech and Hearing Research, 35,* 68-78.

Kahrilas, P. J., Logemann, J. A., Krugler, C., & Flanagan, E. (1991). Volitional augmentation of upper esophageal sphincter opening during swallowing. *American Journal of Physiology-Gastrointestinal Physiology, 260*(23), G450-456.

Kays, S., Hind, J., Hewitt, A., Gangon, R., & Robbins, J. (2004). *Effects of lingual exercise on swallowing-related outcomes after stroke.* Poster presented at the annual meeting of the American Speech-Language-Hearing Association, Philadelphia, PA.

Kendall, K. A., McKenzie, S. W., Leonard, R. J., & Jones, C. (1998). Structural mobility in deglutition after single modality treatment of head and neck carcinomas with radiotherapy. *Head & Neck, 20,* 720-725.

Koch, W. M., Lee, D. J., Eisele, D. W., Miller, D., Poole, M., Cummings, C. W., et al. (1995). Chemoradiotherapy for organ preservation in oral and pharyngeal carcinoma. *Archives of Otolaryngology–Head & Neck Surgery, 121,* 974-980.

Kotz, T., Abraham, S., Beitler, J., Wadler, S., & Smith, R. V. (1999). Pharyngeal transport dysfunction consequent to an organ-sparing protocol. *Archives of Otolaryngology–Head & Neck Surgery, 125,* 410-413.

Kraus, D. H., Pfister, D. G., Harrison, L. B., Shah, J. P., Spiro, R. H., Armstrong, J. G., et al. (1994). Larynx preservation with combined chemotherapy and radiation therapy in advanced hypopharynx cancer. *Otolaryngology Head and Neck Surgery, 111,* 31-37.

Kuo, W., Wu, C. C., Lian, S. L., Ching, F. Y., Lee, K. W., & Juan, K. H. (1993). The effects of radiation therapy on salivary function in patients with head and neck cancer. *Kaohsiung Journal of Medical Science, 9,* 401-409.

Kwong, D. L., Pow, E. H., Sham, J. S., McMillan, A. S., Leung, L. H., Leung, W. K., et al. (2004). Intensity-modulated radiotherapy for early-stage nasopharyngeal carcinoma: A prospective study on disease control and preservation of salivary function. *Cancer, 101*(7), 1584-1593.

Langmore, S. E., Schatz, K., & Olson, N. (1988). Fiberoptic endoscopic examination of swallowing safety: A new procedure. *Dysphagia, 2,* 216-219.

Law, M. P. (1981). Radiation-induced vascular injury and its relation to late effects in normal tissues. In J. T. Lett & H. Adler (Eds.). *Advances in Radiation Biology* (Vol. 9, pp. 37-73). New York: Academic Press.

Lazarus, C. L. (1993). Effects of radiation therapy and voluntary maneuvers on swallow function in head and neck cancer patients. *Clinics in Communicative Disorders, 3,* 11-20.

Lazarus, C. L. (1997). *The effects of radiotherapy on tongue strength and swallowing in oral and oropharyngeal cancer patients.* Unpublished doctoral dissertation, Northwestern University, Evanston, IL.

Lazarus, C. L. (2000). Management of swallowing disorders in head and neck cancer patients: Optimal patterns of care. *Seminars in Speech and Language, 31,* 293-309.

Lazarus, C. L. (2005, November) *Effects of radiotherapy on tongue strength in cancer patients.* Poster presented at the annual meeting of the American Speech-Language-Hearing Association meeting, San Diego, CA.

Lazarus, C. L., Davis, J., Logemann, J. A., & Hurst, P. (1983). *Effects of a maxillary reshaping prosthesis on speech and swallowing.* Paper presented at the annual meeting of the American Speech-Hearing Association (ASHA) convention, Cincinnati, OH.

Lazarus, C., Logemann, J. A., & Gibbons, P. (1993). Effects of maneuvers on swallowing function in a dysphagic oral cancer patient. *Head & Neck, 15,* 419-424.

Lazarus, C. L., Logemann, J. A., Huang, C. H., & Rademaker, A. W. (2003). Effects of two types of tongue strengthening exercises in young normals. *Folia Phoniatrica, 55,* 199-205.

Lazarus, C., Logemann, J. A., Pauloski, B. R., Colangelo, L. A., Kahrilas, P. J., Mittal, B. B., et al. (1996). Swallowing disorders in head and neck cancer patients treated with radiotherapy and adjuvant chemotherapy. *Laryngoscope, 106,* 1157-1166.

Lazarus, C. L., Logemann, J. A., Pauloski, B. R., Rademaker, A. W., Helenowski, I., Vonesh, E., et al. (in press). Effects of radiotherapy with or without chemotherapy on tongue strength and swallowing in oral cancer patients. *Head & Neck.*

Lazarus, C. L., Logemann, J. A., Pauloski, B. R., Rademaker, A. W., Larson, C. R., Mittal, B. B., et al. (2000). Swallowing and tongue function following treatment for oral and oropharyngeal cancer. *Journal of Speech, Language, and Hearing Research, 43,* 1011-1023.

Lazarus, C., Logemann, J. A., Song, C. W., Rademaker, A. W., & Kahrilas, P. J. (2002). Effects of voluntary maneuvers on tongue base function for swallowing. *Folia Phoniatrica, 54,* 171-176.

Lazzara, G., Lazarus, C., & Logemann, J. A. (1986). Impact of thermal stimulation on the triggering of swallowing reflex. *Dysphagia, 1,* 73-77.

Light, J. (1995). A review of oral and oropharyngeal prostheses to facilitate speech and swallowing. *American Journal of Speech Language Pathology, 4,* 15-21.

Lin, Y. S., Jen, Y. M., & Lin, J. C. (2002). Radiation-related cranial nerve palsy in patients with nasopharyngeal carcinoma. *Cancer, 95*(2), 404-409.

Liu, R. P., Fleming, T. J., Toth, B. B., & Keene, H. J. (1990). Salivary flow rates in patients with head and neck cancer 0.5 to 25 years after radiotherapy. *Oral*

*Surgery, Oral Medicine, and Oral Pathology, 70,* 724-729.

Logemann, J. A. (1983). *Evaluation and treatment of swallowing disorders.* San Diego, CA: College Hill.

Logemann, J. A. (1985). Aspiration in head and neck surgical patients. *Annals of Otology, Rhinology and Laryngology, 94,* 373-376.

Logemann, J. A. (1993). *Manual for the videofluorographic study of swallowing* (2nd ed.). Austin, TX: Pro-Ed.

Logemann, J. A. (1998). *Evaluation and treatment of swallowing disorders* (2nd ed.). Austin, TX: Pro-Ed.

Logemann, J., & Bytell, D. (1979). Swallowing disorders in three types of head and neck surgical patients. *Cancer, 81,* 469-478.

Logemann, J. A., Kahrilas, P. J., Hurst, P., Davis, J., & Krugler, C. (1989). Effects of intraoral prosthetics on swallowing in patients with oral cancer. *Dysphagia, 4,* 118-120.

Logemann, J., Pauloski, B., Lazarus, C., Fujiu, M., & Kahrilas, P. (1995). Effects of a sour bolus on oropharyngeal swallow measures in patients with neurogenic dysphagia. *Journal of Speech and Hearing Research, 38,* 556-563.

Logemann, J. A., Pauloski, B. R., Rademaker, A. W., & Colangelo, L. A. (1997). Speech and swallowing rehabilitation for head and neck cancer patients. *Oncology, 5,* 651-659.

Logemann, J. A., Pauloski, B. R., Rademaker, A. W., Colangelo, L. A., Kahrilas, P. J., & Smith, C. H. (2000). Temporal and biomechanical characteristics of oropharyngeal swallow in younger and older men. *Journal of Speech, Language, and Hearing Research, 43,* 1264-1274.

Logemann, J. A., Pauloski, B. R., Rademaker, A. W., & Kahrilas, P. J. (2002). Oropharyngeal swallow in younger and older women: Videofluoroscopic analysis. *Journal of Speech, Language, and Hearing Research, 45,* 434-445.

Logemann, J. A., Pauloski, B. R., Rademaker, A. W., McConnel, F. M. S., Heiser, M. A., Cardinale, S., et al. (1993). Speech and swallow function after tonsil/base of tongue resection with primary closure. *Journal of Speech and Hearing Research, 36,* 918-926.

Logemann, J. A., Rademaker, A. W., Pauloski, B. R., & Kahrilas, P. J. (1994). Effects of postural change on aspiration in head and neck surgical patients. *Otolaryngology-Head & Neck Surgery, 4,* 222-227.

Logemann, J. A., Smith, C. H., Paoloski, B. R., Rademaker, A. W., Lazarus, C. L., Colangelo, L. A., et al. (2001). Effects of xerostomia on perception and performance of swallow function. *Head & Neck, 23,* 317-321.

Logemann, J. A., Veis, S., & Colangelo, L. (1999). A screening procedure for oropharyngeal dysphagia. *Dysphagia, 14,* 44-51.

Lundy, D. S., Smith, C., Colangelo, L., Sullivan, P., Logemann, J. A., Lazarus, C. L., et al. (1999). Aspiration: Etiology and implications. *Otolaryngology-Head & Neck Surgery, 120,* 474-478.

Martin, B. J. W., Logemann, J. A., Shaker, R., & Dodds, W. J. (1993). Normal laryngeal valving patterns during three breath-hold maneuvers: A pilot investigation. *Dysphagia, 8,* 11-20.

Martin-Harris, B., Michel, Y., & Castell, D. O. (2005). Physiologic model of oropharyngeal swallowing revisited. *Otolaryngology-Head & Neck Surgery, 133,* 234-240.

Marunick, M. T., & Mathog, R. H. (1990). Mastication in patients treated for head and neck cancer: A pilot study. *Journal of Prosthetic Dentistry, 63,* 566-573.

McConnel, F. M. S. (1988). Analysis of pressure generation and bolus transit during pharyngeal swallowing. *Laryngoscope, 98,* 71-78.

McConnel, F. M. S., Pauloski, B. R., Logemann, J. A., Rademaker, A. W., Colangelo, L., Shedd, D., et al. (1998). Functional results of primary closure vs flaps in oropharyngeal reconstruction. *Archives of Otolaryngology-Head & Neck Surgery, 124,* 625-630.

Mendenhall, W. M., Stringer, S. P., Amdur, R. J., Hinerman, R. W., Moore-Higgs, G. J., & Cassisi, N. J. (2000). Is radiation therapy a preferred alternative to surgery for squamous cell carcinoma of the base of tongue? *Journal of Clinical Oncology, 18,* 35-42.

Mittal, B. B., Kepka, A., Mahadevan, A., Kies, M., Pelzer, H., List, M. A., et al. (2001). Tissue/dose compensation to reduce toxicity from combined radiation and chemotherapy for advanced head and neck cancers. *International Journal of Cancer-Radiation Oncology Investigations, 96,* 61-70.

Morrish, E. C. (1988). Compensatory articulation in a subject with total glossectomy. *British Journal of Disorders of Communication, 23,* 13-22.

Nicoletti, G., Soutar, D., Jackson, M. S., Wrench, A. A., Robertson, G., & Robertson, C. (2004). Objective assessment of speech after surgical treatment for oral cancer: Experience from 196 selected cases. *Plastic and Reconstructive Surgery, 113,* 114-125.

Nguyen, N. P., Moltz, C. C., Frank, C., Vos, P., Smith, H. J., Karlsson, U., et al. (2004). Dysphagia following chemoradiation for locally advanced head and neck cancer. *Annals of Oncology, 15*(3), 383-388.

Ohmae, Y., Ogura, M., Kitahara, S., Karaho, T., & Inouye, T. (1998). Effects of head rotation on pharyngeal function during normal swallow. *Annals of Otolaryngology, Rhinology and Laryngology, 107*, 344-348.

Pauloski, B. R., & Logemann, J. A. (2000). Impact of tongue-base and posterior-pharyngeal wall biomechanics on pharyngeal clearance in irradiated postsurgical oral and oropharyngeal cancer patients. *Head & Neck, 22*, 120-131.

Pauloski, B. R., Logemann, J. A., Colangelo, L. A., Rademaker, A. W., McConnel, F. M. S., Heiser, M. A., et al. (1993). Speech and swallow function after anterior tongue and floor of mouth resection with distal flap reconstruction. *Journal of Speech and Hearing Research, 36*, 267-276.

Pauloski, B. R., Logemann, J. A., Colangelo, L. A., Rademaker, A. W., McConnel, F. M. S., Heiser, M. A., et al. (1998). Surgical variables affecting speech in treated patients with oral and oropharyngeal cancer. *Laryngoscope, 108*, 908-916.

Pauloski, B. R., Logemann, J. A., Fox, J. C., & Colangelo, L. A. (1995). Biomechanical analysis of the pharyngeal swallow in postsurgical patients with anterior tongue and floor of mouth resection and distal flap reconstruction. *Journal of Speech and Hearing Research, 39*, 110-123.

Pauloski, B. R., Logemann, J. A., Rademaker, A. W., McConnel, F. M. S., Stein, D., Beery, Q., et al. (1994). Speech and swallowing function after oral and oropharyngeal resections: One-year follow-up. *Head & Neck, 16*, 313-322.

Pauloski, B. R., Rademaker, A. W., Logemann, J. A., & Colangelo, L. (1998). Speech and swallowing in irradiated and non-irradiated postsurgical oral cancer patients. *Otolaryngology-Head & Neck Surgery, 118*, 616-624.

Perlman, A. L., Schultz, J. G., & VanDaele, D. J. (1993). Effects of age, gender, bolus volume, and bolus viscosity on oropharyngeal pressure during swallowing. *Journal of Applied Physiology, 75*, 33-37.

Pouderoux, P., & Kahrilas, P. J. (1995). Deglutitive tongue force modulation by volition, volume and viscosity in humans. *Gastroenterology, 108*, 1418-1426.

Pow, E. H., McMillan, A. S., Leung, W. K., Wong, M. C., & Kwong, D. L. (2003). Salivary gland function and xerostomia in southern Chinese following radiotherapy for nasopharyngeal carcinoma. *Clinical Oral Investigations, 7*(4), 230-234.

Rademaker, A. W., Pauloski, B. R., Logemann, J. A., & Shanahan, T. K. (1994). Oropharyngeal swallow efficiency as a representative measure of swallowing function. *Journal of Speech and Hearing Research, 37*, 314-325.

Rasley, A., Logemann, J. A., Kahrilas, P. J., Rademaker, A. W., Pauloski, B. R., & Dodds, W. J. (1993). Prevention of barium aspiration during videofluoroscopic swallowing studies: Value of change in posture. *American Journal of Roentgenology, 160*, 1005-1009.

Rentschler, G. J., & Mann, M. B. (1980). The effects of glossectomy on intelligibility of speech and oral perceptual discrimination. *Journal of Oral Surgery, 38*, 348-354.

Robbins, J., Gangnon, R., Theis, S., Kays, S. A., & Hind, J. (2005). The effects of lingual exercise on swallowing in older adults. *Journal of American Geriatrics Society, 53*, 483-489.

Robbins, J., Hamilton, J. W., Lof, G. L., & Kempster, G. B. (1992). Oropharyngeal swallowing in normal adults of different ages. *Gastroenterology, 103*, 823-829.

Rosenbek, J. C., Roecker, E. B., Wood, J. L., & Robbins, J. (1996). Thermal application reduces the duration of stage transition in dysphagia after stroke. *Dysphagia, 11*, 225-233.

Sessions, D. G., Leonx, J., Spector, G. J., Chao, C., & Chaudry, O. A. (2003). Analysis of treatment results for base of tongue cancer. *Laryngoscope, 113*, 1252-1261.

Shanahan, T. K., Logemann, J. A., Rademaker, A. W., Pauloski, B. R., & Kahrilas, P. J. (1993). Chin-down posture effect on aspiration in dysphagic patients. *Archives of Physical Medicine and Rehabilitation, 74*, 736-739.

Skelly, M., Spector, D. J., Donaldson, R. C., Brodeur, A., & Paletta, F. X. (1971). Compensatory physiologic phonetics for the glossectomy. *Journal of Speech and Hearing Disorders, 36*, 101-114.

Smith, C. H., Logemann, J. A., Colangelo, L. A., Rademaker, A. W., & Pauloski, B. R. (1999). Incidence and patient characteristics associated with silent aspiration in the acute care setting. *Dysphagia, 14*, 1-7.

Smith, R. V., Kotz, T., Beitler, J. J., & Wadler, S. (2000). Long-term swallowing problems after organ preservation therapy with concomitant radiation therapy and intravenous hydroxyurea. *Archives of Otolaryngology-Head & Neck Surgery, 126*, 384-389.

Sonies, B. C., Parent, L. J., Morrish, K., & Baum, B. J. (1988). Durational aspects of the oral-pharyngeal phase of swallow in normal adults. *Dysphagia, 3*, 1-10.

Urken, M. L., Moscoso, J. F., Lawson, W., & Biller, H. F. (1994). A systematic approach to functional reconstruction of the oral cavity following partial and total glossectomy. *Archives of Otolaryngology-Head & Neck Surgery, 120,* 589-601.

Veis, S., Logemann, J. A., & Rademaker, A. W. (2000). Effects of three techniques on tongue base posterior motion. *Dysphagia, 15,* 142-145

Vokes, E. E., Moran, W. J., Mick, R., Weichselbaum, R. R., & Panje, W. R. (1989). Neoadjuvant and adjuvant methotrexate, cisplatin, and fluorouracil in multimodal therapy of head and neck cancer. *Journal of Clinical Oncology, 7,* 838-845.

Watkin, K. L, Diouf, I., Gallagher, T. M., Logemann, J. A., Rademaker, A. W., & Ettema, S. L. (2001). Ultrasonic quantification of geniohyoid cross-sectional area and tissue composition: A preliminary study of age and radiation effects. *Head & Neck, 23,* 467-474.

Wei, W. I., & Sham, J. S. (2005). Nasopharyngeal carcinoma. *Lancet, 365*(9476), 2041-2054.

Welch, M., Logemann, J. A., Rademaker, A. W., Pauloski, B. R., & Kahrilas, P. J. (1993). Changes in pharyngeal dimensions affected by chin tuck. *Archives of Physical Medicine and Rehabilitation, 74,* 178-181.

Wheeler, R. L., Logemann, J. A., & Rosen, M. S. (1980). Maxillary reshaping prostheses: Effectiveness in improving speech and swallowing in postsurgical oral cancer patients. *Journal of Prosthetic Dentistry, 43,* 313-319.

# Chapter 6

# LARYNGEAL AND HYPOPHARYNGEAL CANCER: INTERVENTION APPROACHES

## Alfons J. M. Balm

# Introduction

Carcinomas of the larynx and hypopharynx originate at closely related anatomical sites, yet are characterized by different etiological traits, symptomatology, and prognosis. In relation to prognosis, laryngeal cancer is associated with better outcomes than hypopharyngeal carcinoma due to a number of factors. Overall, laryngeal cancers are detected much earlier than hypopharyngeal carcinomas, since tumor growth on or near the vocal folds causes the early warning symptom of hoarseness. In comparison, the diagnosis of a hypopharyngeal carcinoma can be significantly delayed by late symptoms of vague, unspecific swallowing complaints and referred otalgia (earache). The significant delays in diagnosis, consequently, have a negative influence on clinical outcome.

Greater visibility by either indirect laryngoscopy or endoscopy also leads to improved early detection of laryngeal cancer, an important factor contributing to prognosis. Hypopharyngeal carcinomas, especially those located in the postcricoidal area and pyriform sinus, are difficult to detect by regular mirror and/or endoscopic view and need an examination under general anesthesia for proper visualization. Not infrequently, hypopharyngeal carcinomas are diagnosed during the workup for a neck node metastasis of unknown primary origin, a clinical condition that is very rarely seen in laryngeal cancer (except for small supraglottic carcinomas of the laryngeal side of the epiglottis).

The issue of regional and distant metastases is the third factor differentiating between the prognosis of cancer of the larynx and hypopharynx. Metastases result when cancer cells spread from the primary tumor site to other tissue sites via the lymphatic system. Laryngeal cancers, particularly glottic carcinomas, have reduced propensity for regional metastases due to scarce availability of regional lymph drainage. In comparison to hypopharyngeal tumors, which arise and extend into tissues with lymphatic drainage, the incidence of ipsilateral and contralateral occult metastases is high (50%) (Jones, Phillips, Helliwell, & Roland, 1993).

Both carcinomas have carcinogenic influences of heavy smoking and alcohol abuse in common, with the last habit being the more characteristic for patients with hypopharyngeal carcinoma (Rothman, Cann, Flanders, & Fried, 1980; Takezaki et al., 2000). Generally

speaking, patients with hypopharyngeal carcinoma are therefore more often characterized with negative social conditions than patients with laryngeal carcinoma. In women aged 30 to 50 years, postcricoid/pyriform sinus carcinoma can be related to the Plummer-Vinson syndrome: the combination of dysphagia, hypopharyngeal and esophageal webs, weight loss, and iron deficiency (Adams & Maisel, 2005). In the United States more than 10,000 new cases of laryngeal cancer are diagnosed per year and the number of new hypopharyngeal cancers is around 3,000 per year. Since differences between smoking and drinking habits of men and women changed dramatically for the last 50 years, the female:male ratio of 5:1 has become less prominent than before (Jemal et al., 2004).

For the last few decades the treatment options for laryngeal and hypopharyngeal cancer have demonstrated a trend toward organ sparing management approaches over surgery intervention. For laryngeal cancer, endoscopic $CO_2$ laser treatment and radiotherapy have become the treatment modalities of first choice in early stages. In hypopharyngeal carcinoma, total laryngectomy as the first treatment option has been replaced by organ sparing (chemo-) irradiation protocols.

This current chapter will focus on the various treatment strategies currently implemented for different tumor sizes at each of the laryngeal and hypopharyngeal regions. Discussion will include both organ sparing and surgical management practices, including discussion of radiotherapy (+/− chemotherapy), laser surgery, common partial laryngeal surgical techniques (supraglottic laryngectomy, partial vertical hemilaryngectomy, supracricoid hemilaryngectomy), total laryngectomy and (partial) pharyngectomy, and neopharynx construction by free and pedicled tissue transplant (pharyngolaryngectomy). Finally, the chapter will discuss current palliative management for large laryngeal and hypopharyngeal cancers.

# Laryngeal Tumor Sites

The larynx is vertically divided into three subsites, listed in ranking order of estimated tumor frequencies: glottis, supraglottis, and subglottis. The different anatomic areas where the laryngeal tumors arise are shown in Figure 6–1. The *glottis* is made up by the vocal folds, anterior commissure, and posterior commissure. The *supraglottis* comprises the suprahyoid epiglottis (tip, lingual [anterior, ventral], and laryngeal [posterior, dorsal]) surfaces, the laryngeal aspect of the aryepiglottic fold, arytenoid, infrahyoid epiglottis, and the false cords. The *subglottis* starts 0.5 cm below the free edge of the true vocal fold and ends at the level of the inferior border of the cricoid. In those cases where all three levels are involved, the tumor is depicted as a transglottic carcinoma. In a retrospective survey of 1507 patients with laryngeal cancers referred to our institution in the period 1977–2004, we found 65.7% glottic carcinomas, 31.4% supraglottic carcinomas, 1.8% subglottic carcinomas, and 1.1% carcinomas at unspecified subsites of the larynx.

Glottic carcinomas cause early symptoms of hoarseness and are usually diagnosed at a very early stage. The majority of this subtype consists of T1 carcinomas and as a result of the scarcity of lymphatics, the risk for neck node metastasis is less than 5% (Ghouri, Zamora, Sessions, Spitznagel, & Harvey, 1994). Invasive glottic carcinomas may involve the laryngeal musculature and paraglottic space, leading to immobility of the vocal fold. This mobility impairment determines the T3 stage of the disease (Union International Contre le Cancer [UICC] TNM Classification, Sobin & Wittekind, 2002). Once the tumor has invaded the paraglottic space, there are few anatomical barriers, leading to sub- and supraglottic tumor extension outside the laryngeal cartilaginous framework. These lesions are classified as T4 tumors. Figure 6–2 is an illustration of a T4 larynx tumor.

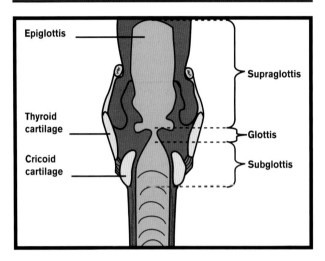

**Figure 6–1.** Anatomical (sub) sites of the larynx.

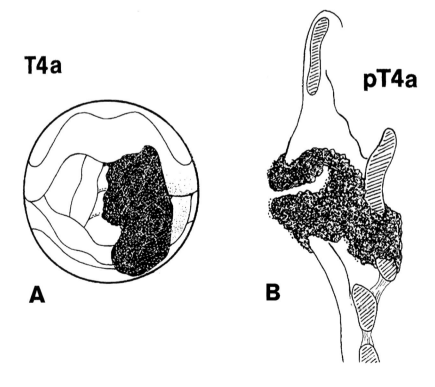

**Figure 6–2.** Schematic drawing of a T4 glottic carcinoma. Tumor invades beyond the larynx **A.** and invades thyroid cartilage **B.** (From C. Wittekind, R. V. P. Hutter, F. L. Greene, M. Klimpfinger, & L. H. Sobin (Eds.), 2005, *The UICC TNM Atlas Illustrated Guide to the TNM Classification of Malignant Tumors: V ed.*, Figures 68a and 68b. Heidelberg, Germany: Springer Verlag. Reprinted with permission of theauthor.)

The majority of supraglottic carcinomas arise at the laryngeal side of the epiglottis, followed by the false cord and the lingual side of the epiglottis. These tumors spread more easily to the neighboring anatomical areas than glottic carcinomas and may spread to the pre-epiglottic space, enabling detection by CT scan of the larynx. These lesions are designated as T3 tumors (Sobin & Wittekind, 2002). There is a higher chance for neck node metastases to be located in the upper jugular node site (level II) and middle jugular nodes (level III) in supraglottic carcinomas compared to glottic carcinomas, since more lymphatics are present (Shah, 1990). In some cases a neck node metastasis is the first symptom of a supraglottic cancer. Figure 6–3 shows the various anatomical levels at which neck node metastasis may arise.

Subglottic carcinomas are rare and usually spread to the pretracheal (Delphian) node and paratracheal nodes in 2-5% of the cases (Harrison, 1971).

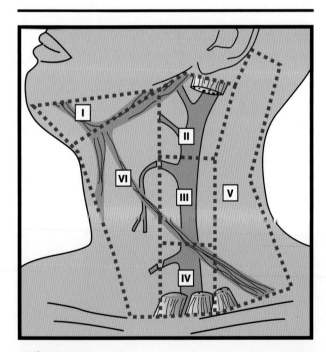

**Figure 6–3.** The six levels in the neck, which define the anatomic boundaries of (selective) lymph node dissections. Level I: submental and submandibular nodes, level II: upper jugular nodes, level III: middle jugular nodes, level IV: lower jugular nodes, level V: posterior triangle nodes, level VI: anterior compartment group.

## Hypopharyngeal Tumor Sites

In relation to hypopharyngeal cancers, a retrospective institutional survey of 366 patients with tumors of this region referred between 1977 and 2004 revealed that the majority (72.6%) presented with piriform sinus carcinomas, with far fewer patients presenting with tumors originating at the posterior pharyngeal wall (12%), postcricoid carcinomas (8%), and carcinomas at unspecified subsites of the hypopharynx (7.6%). The different anatomic areas where the hypopharyngeal tumors arise are shown in Figure 6–4. Anatomically, the *piriform sinus* extends from the pharyngo-epiglottic fold to the upper end of the oesophagus, laterally bounded by the thyroid cartilage and medially by the hypopharyngeal surface of the aryepiglottic fold and the arytenoid and cricoid cartilages. The *posterior pharyngeal wall* extends from the superior level of the hyoid bone (or floor of the vallecula) to the level of the inferior border of the cricoid cartilage and from the apex of one piriform sinus to the other. The *postcricoid area* extends from the level of the arytenoid cartilages and connecting folds to the inferior border of the cricoid cartilage, forming the anterior wall of the hypopharynx.

Hypopharyngeal carcinomas metastasize primarily to the upper (level II), middle (level III), and lower

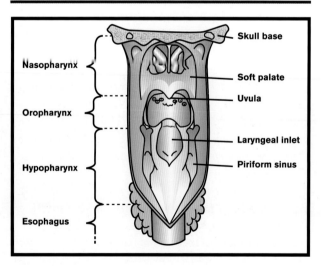

**Figure 6–4.** Anatomical (sub) sites of the pharynx.

(level IV) jugular nodes (see Figure 6–3), but regional spread to the retropharyngeal and parapharyngeal nodes may also occur. Since these latter nodes are difficult to assess by palpation and/or ultrasound examination, they are only detected by CT or MRI scan images.

## Diagnosis, Classification, and Staging

Both the larynx and hypopharynx are not easily accessible for physical examination and require clinical skill and specific equipment for thorough examination.

## Direct Examination

The appropriate diagnostic process of laryngeal carcinoma starts with mirror examination by an experienced otolaryngologist. This type of examination, using either a direct or indirect light source, still gives the best color and depth perception of the larynx. To avoid eliciting the gag reflex, application of local anesthesia (Xylocaine 1%) sprayed on the oropharyngeal mucosa may be helpful. An intense gag reflex or difficult patient requires an evaluation with a flexible laryngoscope transferred though the nasal cavity. Although the technical advances have made it much more convenient for both physician and patient to start with an endoscopic examination, one has to keep in mind that this type of examination is not replacing the overview by indirect laryngoscopy.

Assessment of the local tumor extension is of course the main objective of laryngeal examination, with special emphasis on the vocal fold mobility and extension to the different subsites of the larynx. In glottic carcinomas, special attention should be focused on the extension into the anterior commissure, ventricle, and arytenoids. In supraglottic carcinomas the examiner should pay special attention to the extension to the vocal folds, piriform sinus, and vallecula. For a proper judgment of base of tongue invasion, palpation can be very helpful. It remains often difficult to discriminate a supraglottic carcinoma originating in the aryepiglottic fold from a medial wall piriform sinus carcinoma. In these cases an examination under general anesthesia will give the final answer. Assessment of subglottic carcinomas by mirror examination is often difficult, particularly regarding the distal extension of the tumor.

It is strongly advised to record the dynamic laryngeal function by videostroboscopy, using a 90° telescope, in every laryngeal carcinoma. Particularly in vocal fold carcinoma, stroboscopy is an essential tool for proper assessment of the mucosal wave and the mobility of the vocal fold (see Figure 6–5), which often determines the difference between irradiation or $CO_2$ laser treatment of the larynx.

In contrast to laryngeal carcinoma, hypopharyngeal carcinomas are often extremely difficult to assess by mirror and/or endoscopic examination in the office. Proper view is not only hampered by the specific hidden location of the tumors in the piriform sinus and postcricoidal area, but also by pooling of secretions in the hypopharynx due to impaired swallowing. Nonspecific complaints of dysphagia and/or referred earache should therefore always be followed by an examination under general anesthesia (Klop, Balm, Keus, Hilgers, & Tan, 2000).

Every patient suspected of a laryngeal and hypopharyngeal malignancy should be examined under general anesthesia using a rigid laryngoscope. Telescopes can be passed through the laryngoscope for a more precise assessment of the extensions of the disease, and in particular to assess the subglottic extension and to visualize the anterior commisure. In cases of early glottic cancers, microscopic evaluation of the tumor allows better visualization of the larynx.

## Imaging

Laryngeal and hypopharyngeal carcinomas can be visualized radiologically by CT scan and MRI. The interpretation of images should be preferably done by an experienced head and neck radiologist. The optimal slice thickness is 4 mm, with imaging in an axial plane. Intravenous injection of contrast improves the delineation of the tumor process. Scans with unintended movement artifacts are not acceptable for judgment of tumor extension. Attention is focused on the supra- and subglottic extension and infiltration into the

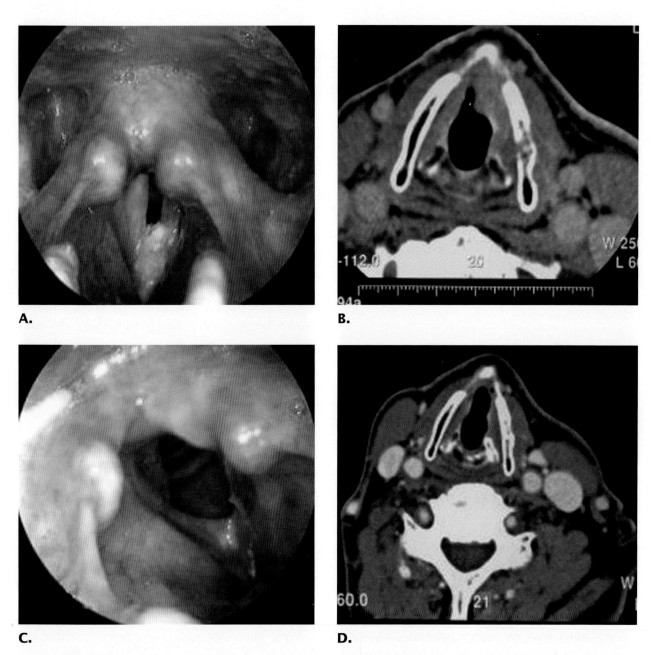

A.  B.

C.  D.

**Figure 6–5.** Stroboscopic view **A.** and CT scan **B.** of a T1 glottic carcinoma of the left vocal cord. This patient has been successfully treated by $CO_2$ laser excision **C., D.**

ventricle, pre-epiglottic space, and cartilage invasion (see Figure 6-6). Comparative studies between MRI and CT scanning of the larynx show a higher sensitivity for MRI imaging using T1 and T2 weighed images, but the specificity is lower (Dutch Head and Neck Cooperative Group, 2000).

Volumetry is increasingly used for the prediction of local control; however, this measurement needs special technical CT scan equipment and expertise of the individual head and neck radiologist (Pameijer, Mancuso, Mendenhall, Parsons, & Kubilis, 1997; Hermans, 1998). It is not yet routine procedure for tumor

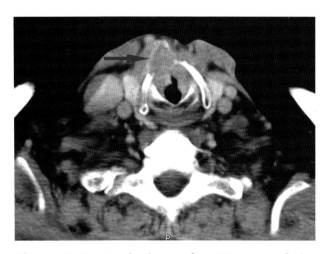

**Figure 6–6.** Axial plane of a CT scan of the larynx demonstrating destruction of the thyroid cartilage and invasion of the surrounding tissues by an infiltrating glottic carcinoma. This patient has undergone a total laryngectomy followed by postoperative irradiation.

staging, but with the technical advances being made in imaging machines, routine volumetry may be possible in the not too far future. Cutoff points for local control in T2 and T3 (supra-) glottic carcinomas range from 3.5–6 cc.

## Histology

As part of the diagnostic process, a tissue biopsy is conducted under general anesthesia to confirm the malignant nature of the disease. There are many histologies found among the laryngeal carcinomas; however, approximately 90% of the epithelial carcinomas are squamous cell carcinomas. Verrucous carcinomas comprise 1–2% of all laryngeal cancers (Orvidas, Olsen, Lewis, & Suman, 1998). One tenth of malignant tumors are represented by adenocarcinoma, salivary gland carcinoma, sarcoma, and malignant lymphoma. Dysplasia grade III or carcinoma in situ of the laryngeal epithelium harbors a risk of 24–46% of conversion into an infiltrating carcinoma and is treated by $CO_2$ laser resection or evaporization (Dorman & Lambie, 1994; Stenersen, Hoel, & Boysen, 1991).

Tumor tissue is classified as either well differentiated, moderately well differentiated, or undifferentiated (Shanmugaratnam, 1991). This classification is determined by the keratinization of epithelial cells; histological specimens with the presence of keratin pearls are called "well differentiated." Prognosis is generally better for well differentiated tissue.

## Tumor Classification and Staging

The rules for tumor classification and staging were formulated by the European UICC and the American Joint Committee on Cancer (UICC TNM Classification: Sobin & Wittekind, 2002). Tumor classification and staging serves many purposes, including serving as an aid to treatment planning, contributing insight into the prognosis of the various tumors, and facilitating the evaluation of treatment strategies. The international adoption of standard classification and staging criteria allows a directly comparable exchange of information among treatment centers, with all oncologists effectively communicating in the "same language."

The T (extent of the primary tumor), N (the absence or presence and extent of regional lymph node metastases), M (the absence or presence of distant metastases) classification system is based on unidimensional dimensions of the tumor expressed in centimeters of diameter (e.g., 2-4 cm) or referenced to anatomical boundaries (see Tables 6-1 and 6-2). The final TNM classification is based on evidence acquired before treatment, implementing results of physical examination, imaging, endoscopy, biopsy, and other relevant examinations. Tables 6-1 and 6-2 outline the criteria for the T and N classification of tumors occurring at the various laryngeal sites and for hypopharyngeal cancers respectively. A "pTNM" classification implies the tumor dimensions after resection.

Stage grouping (Stage I to IV) of tumors means a sampling of specific TNM classifications per stage, which have similar prognostic values in common. TNM staging rules and stage grouping are summarized in Table 6-3. Imaging of the neck is an essential part of larynx and hypopharynx carcinoma staging, with staging under general anesthesia preferably guided by preoperative CT scanning of the larynx and hypopharynx and ultrasound guided fine needle aspiration of the

**Table 6–1.** UICC TNM Classification of Larynx Carcinoma Subsites

### Supraglottis

| | |
|---|---|
| T1 | One subsite, normal mobility |
| T2 | Mucosa of more than one adjacent subsite of supraglottis or glottis, or adjacent region outside the supraglottis; without fixation |
| T3 | Cord fixation or invades postcricoid area, pre-epiglottic tissues, paraglottic space, thyroid cartilage erosion |
| T4a | Through thyroid cartilage; trachea, soft tissues of neck: deep/extrinsic muscle of tongue, strap muscles, thyroid, esophagus |
| T4b | Prevertebral space, mediastinal structures, carotid artery |

### Glottis

| | |
|---|---|
| T1 | Limited to vocal cord(s), normal mobility<br>(a) one cord<br>(b) both cords |
| T2 | Supraglottis, subglottis, impaired cord mobility |
| T3 | Cord fixation, paraglottic space, thyroid cartilage erosion |
| T4a | Through thyroid cartilage; trachea, soft tissues of neck: deep/extrinsic muscles of tongue, strap muscles, thyroid, esophagus |
| T4b | Prevertebral space, mediastinal structures, carotid artery |

### Subglottis

| | |
|---|---|
| T1 | Limited to subglottis |
| T2 | Extends to vocal cord(s) with normal/impaired mobility |
| T3 | Cord fixation |
| T4a | Through cricoid or thyroid cartilage; trachea, deep/extrinsic muscle of tongue, strap muscles, thyroid, esophagus |
| T4b | Prevertebral space, mediastinal structures, carotid artery |

### All Sites

| | |
|---|---|
| N1 | Ipsilateral single >3 cm |
| N2 | (a) Ipsilateral single >3 to 6 cm<br>(b) Ipsilateral multiple ≤6 cm<br>(c) Bilateral, contralateral ≤6 cm |
| N3 | >6 cm |

*Source:* Sobin & Whittekind, 2002

**Table 6–2.** UICC TNM Classification of Hypopharynx Carcinoma

### Hypopharynx

| | |
|---|---|
| T1 | 2 cm and limited to one subsite |
| T2 | >2 to 4 cm or more than one subsite |
| T3 | >4 cm or with hemilarynx fixation |
| T4a | Thyroid/cricoid cartilage, hyoid bone, thyroid gland, esophagus, central compartment soft tissue |
| T4b | Prevertebral fascia, carotid artery, mediastinal structures |
| N1 | Ipsilateral single ≤3 cm |
| N2 | (a) Ipsilateral single >3 to 6 cm<br>(b) Ipsilateral multiple ≤6 cm<br>(c) Bilateral, contralateral ≤6 cm |
| N3 | >6 cm |

*Source:* Sobin & Whittekind, 2002

**Table 6–3** Stage Grouping for Larynx and Hypopharynx Carcinoma

| Stage | T | N | M |
|---|---|---|---|
| Stage 0 | T1s | N0 | M0 |
| Stage 1 | T1 | N0 | M0 |
| Stage II | T2 | N0 | M0 |
| Stage III | T1, T2 | N1 | M0 |
| | T3 | N0, N1 | M0 |
| Stage IVA | T1, T2, T3 | N2 | M0 |
| | T4a | N0, N1, N2 | M0 |
| Stage IVB | T4b | Any N | M0 |
| | Any T | N3 | M0 |
| Stage IVC | Any T | Any N | M1 |

neck (USFNAC—ultrasound guided fine needle aspiration cytology). Pathological lymph nodes are characterized by a roundish appearance of the neck node, irregular uptake of contrast and a diameter of ≥10 mm (van den Brekel et al., 1990; Friedman, Roberts, Kirshenbaum, & Colombo, 1993). The sensitivity of CT scan for the detection of neck node metastases ranges from 80% to 83% respectively, whereas these values for MRI range from 70% to 82% (van den Brekel et al., 1993; Curtin et al., 1998). Ultrasound fine needle aspiration cytology is the method of choice for staging of the N0 neck with sensitivities ranging from 42-73% and specificities of 100% (van den Brekel et al., 1993; Takes et al., 1998).

Multidisciplinary discussions on staging and treatment are well served by a proper documentation of the tumor extensions by schematic drawings, photographs, and/or video films. Airway obstructing tumors require a specific expertise of the anesthesiologist with respect to endoscopic intubation. Controlled debulking of an obstructing tumor process can be performed by the carbon dioxide laser (Laccourreye et al., 1999). If properly timed, this careful management may prevent emergency tracheotomy.

## Treatment

The following sections deal with the different treatment options of laryngeal and hypopharyngeal cancer. In general, glottic carcinomas (in particular the early T1 and T2 disease) are biologically less aggressive than supraglottic carcinoma and hypopharyngeal carcinoma. Where possible, treatment options will be discussed in relation to separate tumor stages for educational purposes. In principle, for both laryngeal and hypopharyngeal cancer the three basic oncological treatment options are at disposal of the treating physician: ($CO_2$ laser) surgery, radiotherapy, and chemotherapy.

## Treatment of Glottic Carcinoma

Depending on the extent of glottic cancer, different management is chosen to optimize outcome.

### T1 Glottic Carcinomas

T1a glottic carcinomas can be successfully managed with radiotherapy (Mendenhall, Million, & Bova, 1984; Pelliteri, Kennedy, Vrabec, Beiler, & Hellstrom, 1991; Rosier et al., 1998), with local cure rates reaching 90% in specialized head and neck cancer centers. The chance for neck node metastases is very low in T1 glottic lesions (0-2.5%), and consequently there is often no need for elective treatment of the neck (Ghouri et al., 1994; Yang, Andersen, Everts, & Cohen, 1998). Radiotherapy is usually given to a total dose of 66 Gy in 33 fractions of 2 Gy or 60 Gy in 25 fractions of 2.4 Gy.

Alternatively they can be managed using $CO_2$ laser treatment. The reported local control rates for endoscopic $CO_2$ laser treatment are sometimes even better than radiotherapy and reach values of around 94% in some series (Gallo et al., 2002). However, it has to be realized that the majority of these lesions are selected T1a carcinomas, whereas in the group of irradiated patients T1b patients are included as well.

Results on voice analyses differ from series to series. Most studies suggest the risk for deterioration of voice quality after $CO_2$ laser treatment is increased, except for one publication which demonstrated a better voice for the endoscopically treated patients compared with irradiated patients (Goor et al., 2003). However, since there are no randomized series comparing the results of radiotherapy and endoscopic laser surgery, it is still difficult to assess the exact clinical value of $CO_2$ laser surgery for early glottic cancer. The cost and time saving advantages of endoscopic laser treatment over radiotherapy, however, are considerable (one operation session of approximately 1 hour versus 5 weeks of radiotherapy). Currently in most centers, laser treatment for local recurrences remains optional. Radiotherapy is possible as salvage intervention post-laser treatment.

Recurrence of T1a glottic carcinoma after radiotherapy can be salvaged by frontolateral (vertical) partial (hemi-) laryngectomy with good local cure rates (Sewnaik, Meeuwis, van der Kwast, & Kerrebijn, 2005). This operation is primarily used for tumors limited to the membranous vocal fold, but may also be used in cases where extension into the anterior commissure (T1b) and to the arytenoids has occurred. The extension of the tumor dictates whether the surgical laryngofissure is positioned in the midline or 2-3 mm paramedian. The operation aims at removal of both true and false cords and the subglottic tissues are resected to the superior border of the cricoid cartilage (see Figure 6-7). In case of contralateral extension, the vertical dissection plane is through the opposite true and false cords and subglottic tissue. If there is impaired mobility and invasion of the thyroid cartilage, partial laryngectomy is usually contraindicated.

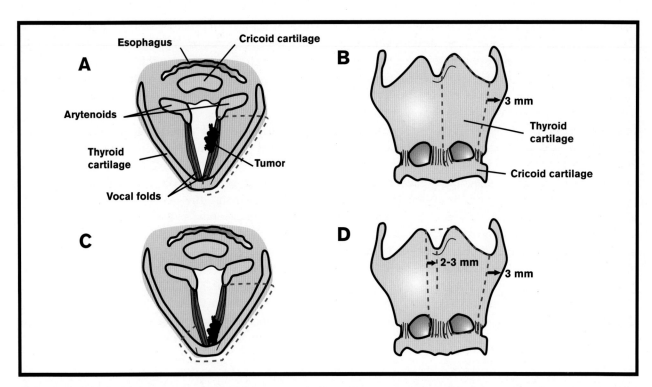

**Figure 6–7.** Schematic drawing of a vertical hemilaryngectomy for removal of recurrent T1a glottic carcinoma (midline laryngofissure) **A., B.** and for T1b glottic carcinoma (paramedian laryngofissure **C., D.**

For T1b glottic carcinomas similar treatment options can be applied, but adequate $CO_2$ endoscopic laser treatment is strongly dependent on the expertise of the individual surgeon.

## T2-T3 Glottic Carcinomas

For function sparing reasons, radiotherapy is the treatment of choice for T2-T3 glottic carcinoma. The local control rates range from 75-90% for T2 glottic carcinoma (Le et al., 1997; Spector et al., 1999) and drops to 45-75% for glottic lesions with impaired vocal fold mobility (Wiggenraad, Terhaard, Hordijk, & Ravasz, 1990). Usually 70 Gy in 7 weeks is given. Endoscopic laser surgery is possible for these tumors, but literature data of large series are scarce. The chance of occult neck node metastases in T2N0 glottic carcinomas is <10%, and does not justify an elective treatment of the neck (Bocca et al., 1984; Yang et al., 1998). In contrast, in T3 glottic carcinoma occult neck node metastases may occur in 30% of the patients (Kligerman et al., 1995; Terhaard et al., 1992). Every neck in a T2 and T3

patient should be staged properly by USFNAC and cytologically proven metastases can be irradiated resulting in a regional control rate of 75-90% (Bataini et al., 1988; Chow, Payne, Keane, Panzarella, & Izard, 1997). For lymph nodes with a diameter exceeding 3 cm, a selective neck dissection is advised, removing nodes at levels II-IV (see Figure 6-3 and Table 4-3 in Chapter 4 for a classification of neck dissections). In these circumstances surgery precedes the radiotherapy for the primary tumor and neck (Verschuur, Keus, Hilgers, Balm, & Gregor, 1996). For patients with poor prognostic signs (e.g., extracapsular rupture), a concomitant boost of radiotherapy is given at the level of the lymph nodes.

Recurrences after radiotherapy are usually salvaged by total laryngectomy with a locoregional control rate of 50-80% for T2 carcinoma (McLaughlin et al., 1996; Schwaab et al., 1994) and 50% for T3 lesions (Lundgren et al., 1988; Terhaard, Karim, et al., 1991). During a total laryngectomy the entire larynx including the hyoid bone, epiglottis, thyroid cartilage, cricoid cartilage, and the first two or three tracheal rings is removed.

After removal of these structures, the pharyngeal walls that were previously connected to the larynx are sutured back together to reestablish the digestive tract. The tracheal end that was attached to the larynx is bowed forward and sutured into the neck where it forms a permanent (tracheo) stoma. During the total laryngectomy procedure, a tracheoesophageal puncture may be created to allow later or immediate placement of a voice prosthesis (this aspect will be later discussed in more detail in Chapter 9). Also, during the total laryngectomy, the surgeon may carry out a myotomy of the cricopharyngeal sphincter, a neurectomy of the pharyngeal plexus, or nonmuscle closure, all of which are intended to improve postoperative voice quality and will be discussed in more detail in Chapter 9. Figure 6-8 shows a schematic drawing of the anatomical situation before and after total laryngectomy. A total laryngectomy has implications for voice production (discussed in Chapter 8 and 9), swallowing (described in Chapter 10), pulmonary function (discussed in Chapter 12), and olfaction (described in Chapter 13), and it implies the need for daily stoma care and the use of a variety of appliances (discussed in Chapter 11).

Vertical hemilaryngectomy as a salvage procedure can be performed in selected cases with a higher chance of recurrence than in T1 recurrent glottic carcinoma.

## T3-T4 Glottic Carcinomas

In T3-T4 glottic laryngeal carcinoma initial treatment is aimed at laryngeal preservation as well. Conventional radiotherapy results in a local control rate of 41-57% (Barton, Keane, Gadella, & Maki, 1992; Terhaard et al., 1992). In a large series of 971 patients, conventional radiotherapy (five fractions per week during 6.5 weeks) was compared with accelerated radiotherapy (six fractions during 5.5 weeks) and resulted in an improvement of the locoregional control of 14% in the group of patients treated according to the accelerated scheme (Overgaard, Sand Hansen, & Overgaard, 1997). In 1991, The Department of Veterans' Affairs (VA) Laryngeal Cancer Study Group reported on a landmark larynx

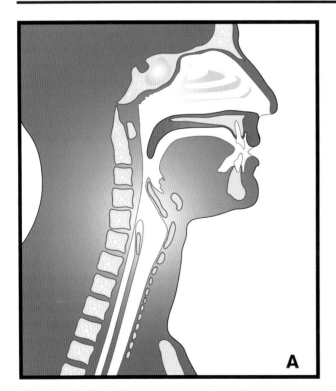
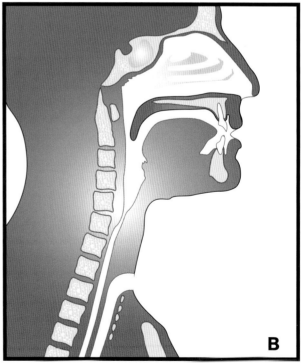

**Figure 6–8.** Schematic drawing of the anatomical situation before **A.** and after **B.** total laryngectomy removing the entire larynx and hyoid bone. The surgery results in a complete separation of air and food passage.

preservation trial for advanced laryngeal cancer in the *New England Journal of Medicine*. Three hundred and thirty-two patients were randomized to undergo the standard treatment of laryngectomy and postoperative radiotherapy or induction chemotherapy with cisplatin and fluorouracil, followed by radiotherapy (and no surgery) for patients responding to induction chemotherapy. Patients with no response to chemotherapy or who had residual disease after radiotherapy were offered "salvage laryngectomy." The larynx could be preserved in 64% of the patients and after two years 41 patients were alive with a functioning larynx (VA, 1991).

To answer the question whether radiotherapy alone could achieve similar results as the VA trial, in 2003 the Radiotherapy Oncology Group and Head and Neck Intergroup reported on a randomized trial comparing induction chemotherapy followed by radiotherapy, concurrent chemotherapy and radiotherapy, and radiotherapy alone (Forastière, 2003). Survival rates did not differ among the studied groups, but the 172 patients treated with concurrent chemotherapy and radiotherapy had a higher rate of survival with a functioning larynx (84%) than the patients in the two other groups. The acute toxicity was higher in the groups with chemotherapy; however, swallowing dysfunction was similar in all three groups (Forastière, 2003).

Accurate staging of patients with advanced laryngeal cancer by a multidisciplinary team is of utmost importance and it should be realized that patients undergoing concurrent chemotherapy and radiotherapy have a higher local recurrence rate and chance of chronic aspiration for which salvage laryngectomy is required.

## Treatment of Supraglottic Carcinomas

Weighing the functionality against the expected outcome of treatment is an important issue in the decision-making process of laryngeal cancer treatment, and supraglottic cancer in particular. The different treatment options are discussed in view of the different T stages of the tumor.

### T1 Supraglottic Carcinomas

For curative treatment of T1 supraglottic carcinoma, all three modalities of radiotherapy, endoscopic laser surgery, and surgery can be employed. There are several studies published on the results of radiotherapy for T1 lesions, but in contrast to the T1 glottic literature, these investigations are smaller with less than 100 patients in the participant groups investigated. Results for local control range from 83% to 96% for the last 15 years (Nakfoor et al., 1998; Spriano et al., 1997; Terhaard, Snippe, et al., 1991). The radiotherapy schedule is more or less similar to that of T1 glottic carcinoma: 66–70 Gy in fractions of 2 Gy. With endoscopic laser surgery, good local control rates can be achieved. In a series of 39 and 40 patients local control rates were respectively 79% and 89% (Eckel & Thumfart, 1992; Iro et al., 1998).

In comparison to the organ sparing regimes, international experience with the use of surgery, specifically a supraglottic laryngectomy (horizontal partial laryngectomy) for the management of T1 supraglottic cancers, is larger. Local cure rates of up to 97% following supraglottic laryngectomy are reported (Adamopoulos et al., 1997; Spriano et al., 1997). For surgery, strict inclusion criteria should be applied. First of all, involvement of the anterior commissure, thyroid cartilage, and extension into the ventricle and arytenoids should be excluded by CT scan imaging. Arytenoidectomy leads to serious aspiration and makes decannulation after surgery sometimes impossible. In patients with a decreased lung function (FEV1/FVC < 50%) surgery is contraindicated. The procedure can be performed in formerly irradiated patients; however, extreme caution is recommended because of an expected rise of postoperative complications. In the age category of 65–70 the indication for surgery needs careful consideration by the multidisciplinary team in light of the possibility of recurrent aspiration pneumonias. Rehabilitation in this group of patients remains difficult.

Lesions of the laryngeal side of the epiglottis are ideal for a supraglottic laryngectomy if the base of the tongue is free of disease. The horizontal incision through the thyroid cartilage is at the level of one half of the vertical dimension in men and upper one third in women. The incision is conducted horizontally through the ventricle and just anterior to the arytenoid. The upper line of resection runs through the base of the tongue (see Figure 6-9). Whether or not the hyoid bone is removed is dependent on the preference of the individual surgeon. Closure consists of approximation of the musculature of the base of the tongue to the peri-

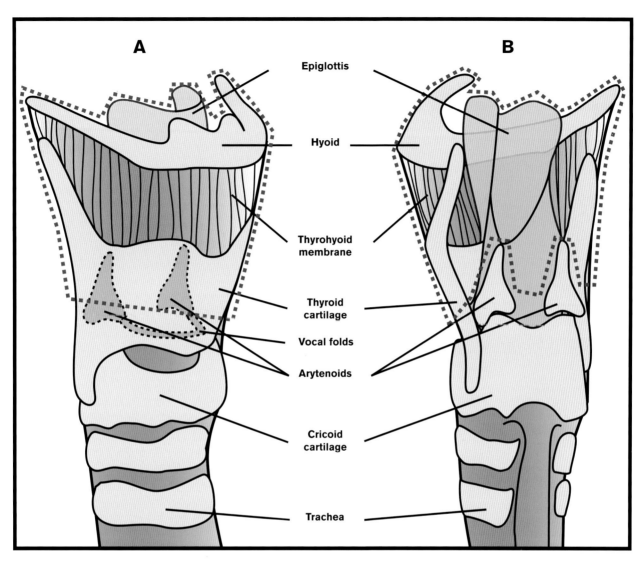

**Figure 6–9.** Schematic drawing of the tissues that are removed during a horizontal supraglottic laryngectomy in anterolateral view **A.** and posterolateral view **B.** The red dotted lines indicate the width of excision.

chondrium and remaining strap muscles. A tracheotomy and nasogastric tube insertion are routinely performed. Preoperatively, permission for total laryngectomy is requested in every patient, just in case unforeseen tumor extensions are detected perioperatively.

The supracricoid partial laryngectomy with a cricohyoepiglottopexy allows for resection of both vocal folds, both false cords, the thyroid cartilage, paraglottic spaces, and possibly one arytenoid (see Figure 6–10). It can be used for selected T2 and T3 carcinomas of the glottis and T1b carcinomas.

Postoperative radiotherapy is indicated by positive resection margins and increases the risk for aspiration and swallowing problems due to edema of the arytenoids, although not confirmed by every author. The chance of regional metastases is higher in supraglottic cancer than in glottic carcinoma, due to the increased amount of draining lymphatics. With the use of modern imaging techniques in 15% of cases occult neck node metastases are found in T1 well-differentiated carcinomas, but this percentage is more than tripled in T3 carcinomas (Dutch Head and Neck Cooperative

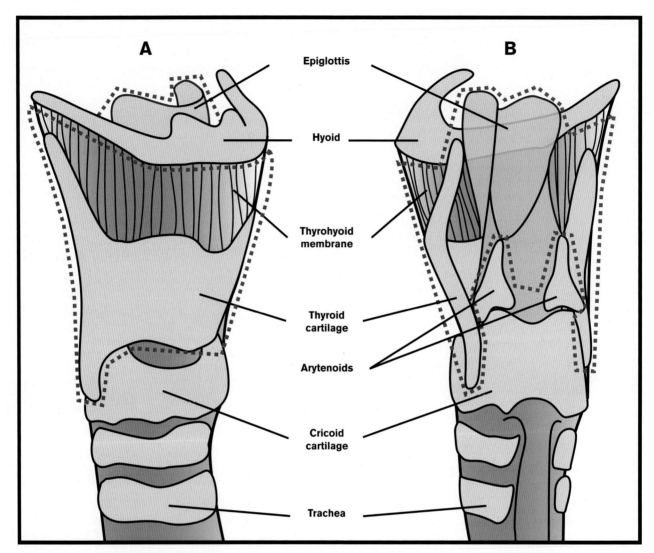

**Figure 6–10.** Schematic drawing of the tissues that are removed during a horizontal supracricoid laryngectomy in anterolateral view **A.** and posterolateral view **B.**

Group, 2000). Primary radiotherapy can cure lymph node metastases with a diameter of <3 cm (Mendenhall et al., 1984). Neck node metastases with a larger diameter need to be treated surgically with a selective neck dissection of levels II–IV, preceding the radiotherapy for the primary tumor if indicated (Verschuur et al., 1996). The neck dissection has to be performed in such a fashion that the contents of the neck dissection are left attached to the thyrohyoid membrane. Indications for postoperative radiotherapy to the neck are histologically confirmed multiple neck node metastases and extracapsular rupture (Snow, Annyas, van Slooten, Bartelink, & Hart, 1982).

## T2-T3 Supraglottic Carcinomas

Treatment options for T2 and T3 supraglottic larynx carcinoma are more or less identical to those of T1 carcinomas; however, the higher chance of regional metastases (50%) is of importance in the discussion whether the neck should be simultaneously treated surgically. If an N0 neck is staged properly by USFNAC there is no need for an elective neck dissection and the tumor can be treated either by radiotherapy or endoscopic laser surgery. In case of cytologically proven neck node metastases, selective neck dissection is indicated in continuity with a supraglottic laryngectomy or after endoscopic laser surgery. In these patients the contralateral negative neck should be dissected as well.

### T3-T4 Supraglottic Carcinomas

Treatment options for T3 and T4 supraglottic carcinoma are similar to those described previously for T3-T4 glottic carcinomas.

## Subglottic Carcinomas

Subglottic carcinoma is rare and literature on treatment results of this tumor entity is scarce. The rarity of the disease makes it almost impossible to discuss treatment options of the various tumor stages. Studies deal mainly with the treatment results of subglottic tumor extensions of glottic carcinoma, and demonstrate the negative prognostic impact of this finding (Klintenberg et al., 1996; Le et al., 1997; Warde et al., 1998). In that respect, the presence of subglottic carcinoma is almost always part of a T2 or T3 glottic carcinoma. Consequently, the management options for subglottic cancers are the same as those applied for T2-T3 glottic carcinomas as discussed previously. In subglottic carcinomas, tumor metastases typically are located in the paratracheal lymph nodes. In elective dissections 26% occult metastases are found (Timon, Toner, & Conlon, 2003).

## Treatment of Hypopharyngeal Carcinoma

Hypopharyngeal carcinomas are less frequently occurring than laryngeal carcinomas. For years, surgery was the treatment of choice, despite the fact that overall survival remained low, at around 25%. During the last decade focus of treatment has shifted to the organ sparing treatment regimens for hypopharyngeal carcinoma. A classical randomized study in 1996 (immediate surgery followed by postoperative radiotherapy versus induction chemotherapy followed by radiotherapy in the case of complete response, or surgery in case of no response), demonstrating 35% functional larynx preservation after induction chemotherapy, was the start of a more conservative approach towards the treatment of hypopharyngeal carcinoma (Lefèbvre, 1996).

### T1-T2 Hypopharyngeal Carcinoma

T1 and T2 hypopharyngeal carcinomas, originating in the piriform sinus and posterior pharyngeal wall can well be treated by either radiotherapy or organ sparing surgery. Best results are achieved by hyperfractionation (two times per day 1.2 Gy) with a local control rate of 89% for T1 lesions and 77% for T2 (Garden, Morrison, Clayman, Ang, & Peters 1996). Also good local control rates of 69% have been reported on T3 tumors with hyperfractionation (Fein, 1993; Garden, Morrison, Ang, & Peters, 1995). The literature on randomized trials comparing different radiation schemes in hypopharyngeal carcinoma is scarce. The publications on large randomized series mainly deal with oropharyngeal carcinoma and subgroup analyses for hypopharyngeal carcinomas are often lacking. Reports on the results of laser surgery are limited as well, but in selected cases a 5-year disease-free survival rate of 71% was achieved in Stage I and II disease. However, 95% of the 29 cases were postoperatively irradiated (Rudert & Hoft, 2003).

Supracricoid hemi pharyngoplaryngectomy can be performed for the removal of T2 piriform sinus carcinomas, followed by radiotherapy (Laccourreye, Lacau St Guily, Brasnu, Fabre, & Menard, 1987; Laccourreye et al., 1993). Resection includes a vertical hemilaryngectomy with removal of half of the epiglottis and partial pharyngectomy (piriform sinus). Although the recurrence rate was reportedly low, this function sparing technique of partial pharyngectomy has not widely been accepted and puts the patients at risk for chronic aspiration and a permanent tracheostomy. In localized T1 lesions of the posterolateral pharyngeal wall, lateral pharyngectomy can be done with minimal transient disturbance of the swallowing act.

### T3-T4 Hypopharyngeal Carcinoma

Patients presenting with large T3 and T4 cancers comprise the bulk of the hypopharyngeal tumor population. Local cure rates of primary radiotherapy alone (27%) or surgery alone (53%) for advanced T3 and T4 lesions (see Figure 6–11 for an illustrated drawing of a T4 piriform sinus tumor) are lower than for patients undergoing surgery followed by radiotherapy (71%) (Mendenhall, Parsons, Devine, Cassisi, & Million, 1987). Surgery for the more advanced lesions almost always implies the combination of a total laryngectomy and

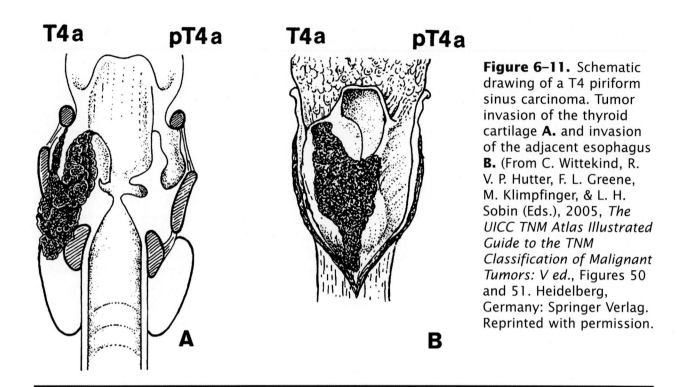

**Figure 6–11.** Schematic drawing of a T4 piriform sinus carcinoma. Tumor invasion of the thyroid cartilage **A.** and invasion of the adjacent esophagus **B.** (From C. Wittekind, R. V. P. Hutter, F. L. Greene, M. Klimpfinger, & L. H. Sobin (Eds.), 2005, *The UICC TNM Atlas Illustrated Guide to the TNM Classification of Malignant Tumors: V ed.*, Figures 50 and 51. Heidelberg, Germany: Springer Verlag. Reprinted with permission.

partial pharyngectomy and "en bloc" (modified) radical neck dissection.

Reconstruction of the hypopharynx after total laryngectomy and total or near total pharyngectomy can be completed by the use of regional flaps or free revascularized tissue transfers. A pharyngolaryngectomy includes surgical removal of both the larynx and hypopharynx, including the posterior pharyngeal wall thereby creating a circumferential defect, which requires a tube formed reconstruction either by using a pedicled flap or a free revascularized flap. If a laryngectomy is combined with a partial pharyngectomy (i.e., in T3 piriform sinus carcinoma), the remaining strip of posterior pharyngeal wall mucosa may be limited to a small strip of 1–3 cm of tissue. Under these circumstances the expression of "near total pharyngectomy" is applied.

A pectoralis major myocutaneous flap serves as an excellent tool for the closure of partial pharyngeal defects. As long as a strip of 3 cm normal pharyngeal mucosa is retained, the pectoralis flap can be used for closure of the defect (Schuller, 1985). For circumferential defects the pectoralis major flap is less optional. Options for reconstruction of this defect include free

jejunal interposition (Giovanoli, Frey, Schmid, & Flury, 1996), radial forearm flap (Azizzadeh et al., 2001), lateral thigh flap (Hayden & Deschler, 1999), and the gastric pull-up (Cahow & Sasaki, 1994). The jejunal free flap has a consistent vascular anatomy and offers an excellent soft tissue coverage with an elastic secreting mucosa. However, harvesting requires a two team approach with entering of the abdominal cavity. Myocutaneous flaps, like the pectoralis major flap, are often too bulky to provide acceptable contour speech and deglutition in case of circumferential pharyngeal defect reconstruction. The fasciocutaneous radial forearm flap has become a nice alternative and the choice for many microvascular surgeons, since it offers a reliable long vascular pedicle of the radial artery in combination with pliability of a thin flap. The flap is easy to harvest and results in limited donor site morbidity. The lateral thigh free flap is based on the third perforator of the profunda femoris artery and requires more microvascular expertise for harvesting. The flap is as pliable as the radial forearm flap, but the large skin island makes this flap more suitable for creation of an extended circumferential lining following pharyngolaryngectomy. In case of esophageal extension of a hypopharyngeal carcinoma, free revascularized flaps cannot be used. In those cases pharyngolaryngectomy should be combined with an esophagectomy and a gastric pull-up. This means replacement of the esophagus and pharynx by transposition of the entire tubed stomach through the posterior mediastinum. The operation is performed in one stage by two teams and only one anastomosis, placed superiorly to the remnant pharyngeal mucosa, is required. Choices for the type of reconstruction depend on the preference and experience of the individual surgeon. Jejunal interposition allows excellent reconstruction with good short- and long-term swallowing outcomes (Ward, Bishop, Frisby, & Stevens, 2002) but preserved autonomic peristaltic movements may lead to interrupted prosthetic voicing and continued secretions may cause a wet voice (Hilgers et al., 1996; McAuliffe, Ward, Bassett, & Perkins, 2000).

In contrast to laryngeal carcinomas, the incidence of ipsilateral and contralateral occult metastases is high (50%) in hypopharyngeal cancers, necessitating assessment and treatment of the N0 neck (Jones et al., 1993). It is evident that nodal levels II and III (see Figure 6–3) are the areas primarily involved. If postoperative radiotherapy is planned, the neck dissection, like in laryngeal cancer, can be limited to levels II–IV, assuming that appropriate staging has been performed by USFNAC (Lohuis et al., 2004). There's also a high chance of involvement of the contralateral neck nodes, which should be covered by extension of the radiation fields.

Concurrent chemo-irradiation improves the locoregional control in patients with advanced Stage III and IV disease compared to radiotherapy alone and can be used as organ sparing therapy in advanced hypopharyngeal carcinomas (Pignon, Bourhis, Domenge, & Designe, 2000). However, the long-term toxicity with swallowing complaints and aspiration should not be underestimated.

## Palliative Treatment

Patients with unresectable, recurrent, or metastatic disease are eligible for palliative treatment, aiming at sustaining an acceptable quality of life. Patients with laryngeal and hypopharyngeal carcinoma may fall victim to various types of locoregional recurrences, but after total laryngectomy they may develop a typical recurrence around the tracheostoma, a so-called *stomal recurrence*. Patients with subglottic extension and preoperative tracheotomy are at higher risk of developing this disease (Zbaren, Greiner, & Kengelbacher, 1996). In general, this type of recurrence cannot be treated curatively by surgical resection.

Palliative treatment is either focused on the tumor recurrence or on non-tumor related problems (pain, wound problems, feeding, respiration). The palliative measures for treatment of tumor recurrences consist of chemotherapy and/or radiotherapy. The efficacy of this type of treatment is limited and cure will almost never be achieved. Percentages of >50% tumor regression (including both partial and complete responses) range from 10–40% (Doyle, Hanks, & MacDonald, 1998) and the median survival does not exceed 7 months (Dutch Head and Neck Cooperative Group, 2004). For patients selected for palliative chemotherapy, the initial treatment regime is to use intravenous administration of methotrexate, which can often be given on an outpatient basis. The side effects are acceptable and less intense than those associated with a combination of cytotoxic agents like cisplatin and 5-fluorouracil. Palliative radiotherapy leads to relief of symptoms in the majority of patients (Erkal, Mendenhall, Amdur, Villaret, & Stringer, 2001) and in case of limited life expectancy, a hypofractionation scheme of 20 Gy in 2–4 fractions can be used. For patients with a longer life expectancy, 30 Gy in 10 fractions can be applied. Palliative radiotherapy is frequently used for pain relief caused by distant metastases. Bone metastases are often very painful and a palliative dose of radiotherapy may help to improve quality of life.

## Conclusion

Laryngeal carcinoma is in principle a curable disease, provided that the disease is recognized early. There are several treatment options available like $CO_2$ laser excision for T1 glottic cancer and radiotherapy and/or partial laryngectomy for the T1–T3 stages. Total laryngectomy is reserved for primary T4 tumors and as surgical salvage for recurrent disease. Hypopharyngeal cancer is much more aggressive and most patients (approximately three quarters) manifest Stage III disease. For the last decade treatment has focused on organ sparing radiotherapy or concurrent chemoradiation. For recurrent disease a total laryngectomy with (partial) pharyngectomy is needed often in combination with pharyngeal reconstruction using free revascularized or pedicled flaps.

# References

Adamopoulos, G., Yotakis, I., Apostolopoulos, K., Manolopoulos, L., Kandiloros, D., & Feridikis, E. (1997). Supraglottic laryngectomy series report and analysis of results. *Journal of Laryngology and Otology, 111*, 730-734.

Adams, G. L., & Maisel, R. H. (2005). Malignant tumours of the larynx and hypopharynx. In *Cummings Otolaryngology: Head and Neck Surgery* (Vol. 3, 4th ed., p. 2225). Philadelphia: Mosby.

Azizzadeh, B., Yafai, S., Rawnsley, J. D., Abemayor, E., Sercarz, J. A., Calcaterra, T. C., et al. (2001). Radial forearm free flap pharyngoesophageal reconstruction. *Laryngoscope, 111*, 807-810.

Barton, M. B., Keane, T. J., Gadella, T., & Maki, E. (1992). The effect of treatment time and treatment interruption on tumour control following radical radiotherapy of laryngeal cancer. *Radiotherapy and Oncology, 23*, 137-143.

Bataini, J. P., Bernier, J., Asselain, B., Lave, C., Jaulerry, C., Brunin, F., et al. (1988). Primary radiotherapy of squamous cell carcinoma of the oropharynx and pharyngolarynx: Tentative multivariate modelling system to predict the radiocurability of neck nodes. *International Journal of Radiation Oncology, Biology, Physics, 14*, 635-642.

Bocca, E., Calcato, C., de Vincentiis, I., Marullo, I., Motta, G., & Ottaviani, A. (1984). Occult metastases in cancer of the larynx and their relationship to clinical and histological aspects of the primary tumour: A four-year multicentric research. *Laryngoscope, 94*, 1086-1090.

Cahow, C. E., & Sasaki, C, T. (1994). Gastric pull-up reconstruction for pharyngo-laryngo-esophagectomy. *Archives of Surgery, 129*, 425-429.

Chow, E., Payne, D., Keane, T., Panzarella, T., & Izard, M. A. (1997). Enhanced control by radiotherapy of cervical lymph node metastases arsing from nasopharyngeal carcinomas compared with nodal metastases from other head and neck squamous cell carcinoma. *International Journal of Radiation Oncology, Biology, Physics, 39*,149-154.

Curtin, H. D., Ishwaran, H., Mancuso, A. A., Dalley, R. W., Caudry, D. J., & McNeil, B. J. (1998). Comparison of CT and MR imaging in staging of neck metastases. *Radiology, 207*, 123-130.

Dorman, E. B., & Lambie, N. K. (1994). Dysplasia and carcinoma-in-situ of the larynx. In R. Smee & G. P. Bridger (Eds.), *Laryngeal Cancer: Proceedings of the 2nd World Congress on Laryngeal Cancer* (pp. 276-281). Amsterdam: Elsevier.

Doyle, D., Hanks, G. W. C., & MacDonald, N. (1998). *Oxford textbook of palliative medicine* (2nd ed.). United Kingdom: Oxford University Press.

Dutch Head and Neck Cooperative Group (NWHHT). (2000). *Guideline Larynx Carcinoma.* Utrecht, The Netherlands: NWHHT.

Dutch Head and Neck Cooperative Group (NWHHT). (2004). *Guideline Oral Cavity and Oropharynx Carcinoma.* Alphen aan den Rijn, The Netherlands: van Zuiden.

Eckel, H. E., & Thumfart, W. F. (1992). Laser surgery for the treatment of larynx carcinomas: Indications, techniques, and preliminary results. *Annals of Otology, Rhinology and Laryngology, 101*, 113-118.

Erkal, H. S., Mendenhall, W. M., Amdur, R. J., Villaret, D. B., & Stringer, S. P. (2001). Squamous cell carcinomas metastatic to cervical lymph nodes from an unknown head and neck mucosal site treated with radiation therapy with palliative intent. *Radiotherapy and Oncology, 59*, 319-321.

Fein, D. A. (1993). Pharyngeal wall carcinoma treated with radiotherapy: Impact of treatment technique and fractionation. *International Journal of Radiation Oncology, Biology, Physics, 26*, 751-757.

Forastière, A. A. (2003). Concurrent chemotherapy and radiotherapy for organ preservation in advanced laryngeal cancer. *New England Journal of Medicine, 349*, 2091-2098.

Friedman, M., Roberts, N., Kirshenbaum, G. L., & Colombo, J. (1993). Nodal size of metastasis squamous cell carcinoma of the neck. *Laryngoscope, 103*, 854-856.

Gallo, A., de Vincentiis, M., Manciocco, V., Simonelle, M., Fiorella, M. L., & Shah, J. P. (2002). $CO_2$ laser cordectomy for early-stage glottic carcinoma: A long-term follow-up of 156 cases. *Laryngoscope, 112*, 370-374.

Garden, A. S., Morrison, W. H., Ang, K. K., & Peters, L. J. (1995). Hyperfractionated radiation in the treatment of squamous cell carcinomas of the head and neck: Comparison of two fractionation schedules. *International Journal of Radiation Oncology, Biology, Physics, 31*, 493-502.

Garden, A. S., Morrison, W. H., Clayman, G. L., Ang, K. K., & Peters, L. J. (1996). Early squamous cell carcinoma of the hypopharynx: Outcomes of treatment with radiation alone to the primary disease. *Head & Neck, 18*, 317-322.

Ghouri, A. F., Zamora, R. L., Sessions, D. G., Spitznagel, E. L., Jr., & Harvey, J. E. (1994). Prediction of occult neck disease in laryngeal cancer by means of logistic regression statistical model. *Laryngoscope, 104*, 280-284.

Giovanoli, P., Frey, M., Schmid, S., & Flury, R. (1996). Free jejunum transfers for functional reconstruction after tumour resections in the oral cavity and the pharynx: Changes of morphology and function. *Microsurgery, 17*, 535-544.

Goor, K. M., Mahieu, H. F., Leemans, C. R., Peeters, A. J., Langendijk, J. A., & van Agthoven, M. (2003). $CO_2$-laser decortication: An efficient alternative to radiotherapy in the treatment of T1a carcinomas of the glottis. *Nederlands Tijdschrift voor Geneeskunde, 147*, 1177-1181.

Harrison, D. F. (1971). The pathology and management of subglottic cancer. *Annals of Otology, Rhinology and Laryngology, 80*, 6-12.

Hayden, R. E., & Deschler, D. G. (1999). Lateral thigh free flap for head and neck reconstruction. *Laryngoscope, 109*, 1490-1494.

Hermans, R. (1998). *Value of computed tomography as treatment outcome predictor of head and neck cancer treated with irradiation.* Unpublished thesis, Catholic University, Leuven.

Hilgers, F. J., Hoorweg, J. J., Kroon, B. B., Schaefer, B., de Boer, J. B., & Balm, A. J. (1996). Prosthetic voice rehabilitation with the Provox system after extensive pharyngeal resection and reconstruction. In *Experta Medica International Congress Series* (Vol. 1112, pp.111-120). New York: Elsevier.

Iro, H., Waldfahrer, F., Altendorf-Hofmann, A., Weidenbecher, M., Sauer, R., & Steiner, W. (1998). Transoral laser surgery of supraglottic cancer. Follow-up of 141 patients. *Archives of Otolaryngology-Head & Neck Surgery, 124*, 1245-1250.

Jemal, A., Tiwari, R. C., Murray, T., Ghafoor, A., Samuels, A., Ward, E., et al. (2004). American Cancer Society. Cancer Statistics, CA: *A Cancer Journal for Clinicians, 54*, 8-29.

Jones, A. S., Phillips, D. E., Helliwell, T. R., & Roland, N. J. (1993). Occult node metastases in head and neck squamous carcinoma. *European Archives of Otorhinolaryngology, 250*, 446-449.

Kligerman, J., Olivatto, L. O., Lima, R. A., Freitas, E. Q., Soares, J. R., Dias, F. L., et al. (1995). Elective neck dissection in the treatment of T3/T4N0 squamous cell carcinoma of the larynx. *American Journal of Surgery, 170*, 436-439.

Klintenberg, C., Lundgren, J., Adell, G., Tutor, M., Norberg-Spaak, L., Edelman, R., et al. (1996). Primary radiotherapy of T1 and T2 glottic carcinoma-nanalysis of treatment results and prognostic factors in 223 patients. *Acta Oncologica, 35*, 81-86.

Klop, W. M., Balm, A. J., Keus, R. B., Hilgers, F. J., & Tan, I. B. (2000). Diagnosis and treatment of 39 patients with cervical lymph node metastases of squamous cell carcinoma of unknown primary origin, referred to Netherlands Cancer Institute/Antoni van Leeuwenhoek Hospital, 1979-1998. *Nederlands Tijdschrift voor Geneeskunde, 144*, 1355-1360.

Laccourreye, H., Lacau St Guily, J., Brasnu, D., Fabre, A., & Menard, M. (1987). Supracricoid hemilaryngopharyngectomy: Analysis of 240 cases. *Annals of Otology, Rhinology and Laryngology, 96*, 217-221.

Laccourreye, O., Lawson, G., Muscatello, L., Biacabe, B., Laccoureye, L., & Brasnu, D. (1999). Carbon dioxide laser debulking for obstructing endolaryngeal carcinoma: A 10-year experience. *Annals of Otology, Rhinology and Laryngology, 108*, 490-494.

Laccourreye, O., Merite-Drancy, A., Brasnu, D., Chabardes, E., Cauchois, R., Menard, M., et al. (1993). Supracricoid hemilaryngopharyngectomy in selected pyriform sinus carcinoma staged as T2. *Laryngoscope, 103*, 1373-1379.

Le, Q. T., Fu, K. K., Kroll, S., Ryu, J. K., Quivey, J. M., Meyler, T. S., et al. (1997). Influence of fraction size, total dose, and overall time on local control of T1-T2 glottic carcinoma. *International Journal of Radiation Oncology, Biology, Physics, 39*, 115-126.

Lefèbvre, J. (1996). Larynx preservation in pyriform sinus cancer: Preliminary results of a European Organization for Research and Treatment of Cancer phase III trial. *Journal of the National Cancer Institute, 88*, 890-899.

Lohuis, P. J., Klop, W. M., Tan, I. B., van den Brekel, M. W., Hilgers, F. J., & Balm, A. J. (2004). Effectiveness of therapeutic (N1, N2) selective neck dissection (levels II to V) in patients with laryngeal and hypopharyngeal squamous cell carcinoma. *American Journal of Surgery, 187*, 295-299.

Lundgren, J. A., Gilbert, R. W., van Nostrand, A. W., Harwood, A. R., Keane, T. J., & Briant, T. D. (1988). T3N0M0 glottic carcinoma—A failure analysis. *Clinical Otolaryngology and Allied Sciences, 13*, 455-465.

McAuliffe, M., Ward, E. C., Bassett, L., & Perkins, K. (2000). Functional speech outcomes following laryngectomy and pharyngolaryngectomy. *Archives of Otolaryngology-Head & Neck Surgery, 126,* 705-709.

McLaughlin, M. P., Parsons, J. T., Fein, D. A., Stringer, S. P., Cassisi, N. J., Mendenhall, W. M., et al. (1996). Salvage surgery after radiotherapy failure in T1-T2 squamous cell carcinoma of the glottic larynx. *Head & Neck, 18,* 229-235.

Mendenhall, W. M., Million, R. R., & Bova, F. J. (1984). Analysis of time-dose factors in clinically positive neck nodes treated with irradiation alone in squamous cell carcinoma of the head and neck. *International Journal of Radiation Oncology, Biology, Physics, 10,* 639-643.

Mendenhall, W. M., Parsons, J. T., Devine, J. W., Cassisi, N. J., & Million, R. R. (1987). Squamous cell carcinoma of the pyriform sinus treated with surgery and/or radiotherapy. *Head & Neck Surgery, 10,* 88-92.

Nakfoor, B. M., Spiro, I, J., Wang, C. C., Martins, P., Montgomery, W., & Fabian, R. (1998). Results of accelerated radiotherapy for supraglottic carcinoma: A Massachusetts General Hospital and Massachusetts Eye and Ear Infirmary experience. *Head & Neck, 20,* 379-384.

Orvidas, L. J., Olsen, K. D., Lewis, J. E., & Suman, V. J. (1998). Verrucous carcinoma of the larynx: A review of 53 patients. *Head & Neck, 20,* 197-203.

Overgaard, J., Sand Hansen, H., & Overgaard, M. (1997). Conventional radiotherapy as primary treatment of squamous cell carcinoma of the head and neck. A randomized multicenter study of 5 versus 6 fractions per week—Report from the DAHANCA 7 trial. *International Journal of Radiation Oncology, Biology, Physics, 39,* 188.

Pameijer, F. A., Mancuso, A. A., Mendenhall, W. M., Parsons, J. T., & Kubilis, P. S. (1997). Can pretreatment computed tomography predict local control in T3 squamous cell carcinoma of the glottic larynx treated with definitive radiotherapy? *International Journal of Radiation Oncology, Biology, Physics, 37,* 1011-1021.

Pellitteri, P. K., Kennedy, T. L., Vrabec, D. P., Beiler, D., & Hellstrom, M. (1991). Radiotherapy: The mainstay in the treatment of early glottic carcinoma. *Archives of Otolaryngology—Head & Neck Surgery, 117,* 297-301.

Pignon, J, P., Bourhis, J., Domenge, C., & Designe, L. (2000). Chemotherapy added to locoregional treatment for head and neck squamous-cell carcinoma: Three meta-analyses of updated individual data. MACH-NC Collaborative Group. Meta-Analysis of Chemotherapy on Head and Neck Cancer. *Lancet, 355,* 949-955.

Rosier, J. F., Gregoire, V., Counoy, H., Octave-Prignot, M., Rombaut, P., Scalliet, P., et al. (1998). Comparison of external radiotherapy, laser microsurgery and partial laryngectomy for the treatment of T1N0M0 glottic carcinomas: A retrospective evaluation. *Radiotherapy and Oncology, 48,* 175-183.

Rothman, K. J., Cann, C. I., Flanders, D., & Fried, M. P. (1980). Epidemiology of laryngeal cancer. *Epidemiologic Reviews, 2,* 195-209.

Rudert, H. H., & Hoft, S. (2003). Transoral carbon dioxide laser resection of hypopharyngeal carcinoma. *European Archives of Otorhinolaryngology, 260,* 198-206.

Schuller, D. E. (1985). Reconstructive options for pharyngeal and/or cervical esophageal defects. *Archives of Otolaryngology, 111,* 193-197.

Schwaab, G., Mamelle, G., Lartigau, E., Parise, O., Jr., Wibault, P., & Luboinski, B. (1994). Surgical salvage treatment of T1/T2 glottic carcinoma after failure of radiotherapy. *American Journal of Surgery, 168,* 474-475.

Sewnaik, A., Meeuwis, C. A., van der Kwast, T. H., & Kerrebijn, J. D. (2005). Partial laryngectomy for recurrent glottic carcinoma after radiotherapy. *Head & Neck, 27,* 101-107.

Shah, J, P. (1990). Patterns of cervical lymph node metastasis from squamous cell carcinoma of the upper aerodigestive tract. *American Journal of Surgery, 160,* 405-409.

Shanmugaratnam, K. (1991). *Histological typing of tumours of the upper aerodigestive tract and ear.* Geneva: WHO.

Snow, G. B., Annyas, A. A., van Slooten, E. A., Bartelink, H., & Hart, A. A. (1982). Prognostic factors of neck node metastasis *Clinical Otolaryngology and Allied Sciences, 7,* 185-192

Sobin, L. H., & Wittekind, C. (Eds.). (2002). *UICC TNM Classification of Malignant Tumors* (6th ed.). Heidelberg, Germany: Springer Verlag.

Spector, J. G., Sessions, D. G., Chao, K. S., Hanson, J. M., Simpson, J. R., & Perez, C. A. (1999). Management of stage II (T2N0M0) glottic carcinoma by radiotherapy and conservation surgery. *Head & Neck, 21,* 116-123.

Spriano, G., Antognoni, P., Piantanida, R., Varinelli, D., Luraghi, R., Cerizza, L., et al. (1997). Conservative management of T1-T2N0 supraglottic cancer: A retrospective study. *American Journal of Otolaryngology, 18*(5), 229-305.

Stenersen, T. C., Hoel, P. S., & Boysen, M. (1991). Carcinoma in situ of the larynx: An evaluation of its natural clinical course. *Clinical Otolaryngology and Allied Sciences, 16,* 358-363.

Takes, R. P., Righi, P., Meeuwis, C. A., Manni, J. J., Knegt, P., Marres, H. A., et al. (1998). The value of ultrasound with ultrasound-guided fine-needle aspiration biopsy compared to computed tomography in the detection of regional metastases in the clinically negative neck. *International Journal of Radiation Oncology, Biology, Physics, 40,* 1027-1032.

Takezaki, T., Shinoda, M., Hatooka, S., Hasegawa, Y., Nakamura, S., Hirose, K., et al. (2000). Subsite-specific risk factors for hypopharyngeal and esophageal cancer (Japan). *Cancer Causes Control, 11,* 597-608.

Terhaard, C. H., Hordijk, G. J., van den Broek, P., de Jong, P. C., Snow, G. B., Hilgers, F. J., et al. (1992). T3 laryngeal cancer: A retrospective study of the Dutch Head and Neck Oncology Cooperative Group: Study design and general results. *Clinical Otolaryngology, 1,* 393-402.

Terhaard, C. H., Karim, A. B., Hoogenraad, W. J., Tjho-Heslinga, R., Keus, R. B., Mehta, D. M., et al. (1991). Local control in T3 laryngeal cancer treated with radical radiotherapy, time dose relationship: The concept of nominal standard dose and linear quadratic model. *International Journal of Radiation Oncology, Biology, Physics, 20,* 1207-1214.

Terhaard, C. H., Snippe, K., Ravasz, L. A., van der Tweel, I., & Hordijk, G. J. (1991). Radiotherapy in T1 laryngeal cancer: Prognostic factors for locoregional control and survival, uni- and multivariate analysis. *International Journal of Radiation Oncology, Biology, Physics, 21,* 1179-1186.

The Department of Veterans' Affairs [VA] Laryngeal Cancer Study Group. (1991). Induction chemotherapy plus radiation compared with surgery plus radiation in patients with advanced laryngeal cancer. *New England Journal of Medicine, 324,* 1685-1690.

Timon, C. V., Toner, M., & Conlon, B. J. (2003). Paratracheal lymph node involvement in advanced cancer of the larynx, hypopharynx, and cervical oesophagus. *Laryngoscope, 113,* 1595-1599.

van den Brekel, M. W. M., Castelijns, J. A., Stel, H. V., Golding, R. P., Meyer, C. J., & Snow, G. B. (1993). Modern imaging techniques and ultrasound-guided aspiration cytology for the assessment of neck node metastases. *European Archives of Otorhinolaryngology, 250,* 11-17.

van den Brekel, M. W., Stel, H. V., Castelijns, J. A., Nauta, J. J., van der Waal, I., Valk, J., et al. (1990). Cervical lymph nose metastases: Assessment of radiologic criteria. *Radiology, 177,* 379-384.

Verschuur, H. P., Keus, R. B., Hilgers, F. J., Balm, A. J., & Gregor, R. T. (1996). Preservation of function by radiotherapy of small primary carcinomas preceded by neck dissection for extensive nodal metastases of the head and neck. *Head & Neck, 18,* 277-282.

Ward, E. C., Bishop, B., Frisby, J., & Stevens, M. (2002). Swallowing outcomes following total laryngectomy and pharyngolaryngectomy. *Archives of Otolaryngology-Head & Neck Surgery, 128,* 1-6.

Warde, P., O'Sullivan, B., Bristow, R. G., Panzarella, T., Keane, T. J., Gullane, P. J., et al. (1998). T1/2 glottic cancer managed by external beam radiotherapy: The influence of pretreatment haemoglobin on local control. *International Journal of Radiation Oncology, Biology, Physics, 41,* 347-353.

Wiggenraad, R. G., Terhaard, C. H., Hordijk, G. J., & Ravasz, L. A. (1990). The importance of vocal cord mobility in T2 laryngeal cancer. *Radiotherapy and Oncology, 18,* 321-327.

Yang, C. Y., Andersen, P. E., Everts, E, C., & Cohen, J. I. (1998). Nodal disease in purely glottic carcinoma: Is elective treatment worthwhile? *Laryngoscope, 108,* 1006-1008.

Zbaren, P., Greiner, R., & Kengelbacher, M. (1996). Stoma recurrence after laryngectomy: An analysis of risk factors. *Otolaryngology-Head & Neck Surgery, 114,* 569-575.

# Chapter 7

# SPEECH AND SWALLOWING FOLLOWING LARYNGEAL AND HYPOPHARYNGEAL CANCER

Kylie Perkins, Kelli L. Hancock, and Elizabeth C. Ward

# Introduction

Changes to the management of cancer of the laryngeal and hypopharyngeal region have emerged over the last decade. These changes largely have been shaped by innovations in surgical techniques, the development of alternative radiation fractionation schedules, and the combination of radiotherapy and chemotherapy regimens. As discussed in the previous chapter, various treatment approaches now may be considered for the management of the same type of cancer—for example, the use of either radiotherapy or $CO_2$ laser treatment for T1 glottic carcinomas. Consequently, in order to determine the optimal management approach, in each case clinical teams need to carefully consider both survival and functional outcomes. Specifically, optimal treatment selection should depend not only on the

location and extent of the tumor, existing comorbidities, the philosophy of the clinician/institution, and the wishes of the patient, but also the potential effects of the treatment on the patient's swallowing and voice.

Despite the current advances in the management of head and neck cancer, there is still no optimal approach that cures cancer and preserves the critical functions of voice and swallowing. To this end, it is important to understand the specific nature and severity of the complications that will present depending on the site of origin, staging and size of the tumor, and the treatment approach. Studies comparing quality of life and functional outcomes following different treatment approaches for head and neck cancer are emerging in the literature. Following on from Chapter 6, which outlined the various approaches currently implemented for managing tumors of the laryngeal and/or hypopharyngeal region, the current chapter aims to provide the clinician with information regarding the voice and swallowing outcomes for patients undergoing these various treatments. Specifically, the initial sections of this chapter will discuss the changing role of the SLP at various stages of the patient care continuum (pre-, during, and post-treatment), and then detail those assessment tools and rehabilitation techniques that have particular relevance for this population. The remainder of the chapter will be dedicated to describing the particular clinical issues associated with managing patients who undergo nonsurgical management (radiotherapy +/− chemotherapy) and surgical management (vertical partial hemilaryngectomy, supraglottic laryngectomy, supracricoid laryngectomy, near total laryngectomy). The more complex clinical management associated with patients undergoing laryngectomy +/− pharyngectomy is detailed elsewhere in Chapters 8 through 13.

## The Continuum of Care

Speech-language pathologists (SLPs) are integral members of the multidisciplinary team involved in the care of the patient with head and neck cancer. This care spans from the point prior to diagnosis and pretreatment planning, continues throughout treatment, and progresses to post-treatment rehabilitation, discharge, and long-term care. Successful treatment of head and neck cancer and rehabilitation of voice and swallowing are facilitated by close cooperation of a cohesive multidisciplinary team working with the patient, family/caregivers, and significant others throughout this care continuum. At each stage, the importance of interdisciplinary collaboration cannot be understated.

## Pretreatment

In most centers, multidisciplinary clinics comprised of clinicians from each of the involved professional groups/disciplines meet to examine the patient, present results of investigations, propose management approaches, and decide on the appropriate treatment plan. This forum offers the SLP an early opportunity to be involved in clinical decision making regarding patient management. To support participation in the

team discussions, it is an advantage for SLPs to have an understanding of:

■ The medical processes leading to diagnosis (e.g., esophagoscopy, laryngoscopy, fine needle aspiration—discussed further in Chapter 1).

■ The indicators for different treatment modalities including staging and TNM classification of cancer of the larynx and hypopharynx (see Chapter 6).

■ The status of the disease and expectation for improvement or deterioration in function (curative or palliative intent).

■ Their own individual team and institution policies and preferences.

■ The current research evidence relating to the acute and late adverse reactions associated with the different treatment approaches, and their impact on voice and swallowing. Specific information regarding the field of treatment (if undergoing radiotherapy) or the extent of resection (if undergoing surgery) is useful for the SLP to predict outcomes and potential complications.

■ Patient factors influencing treatment including: cognition, socioeconomic status, new learning ability, cultural influences, availability of support, motivation, and patient choice.

Pretreatment education and counseling regarding the role of the SLP, possible functional sequelae of the recommended treatment modality, and details of what to expect during treatment can enhance a patient's understanding of his or her condition. It also offers an opportunity for assimilation of the information presented and a forum to ask questions relating to treatment, expected recovery pattern, and rehabilitation of voice and swallowing function.

Prior to treatment it is also important to establish a baseline of function through noninstrumental and instrumental evaluations of voice and swallowing (outlined later in chapter). These assessments will characterize and determine the extent of any preexisting voice or swallowing dysfunction in addition to forming the basis of intervention programs. Difficulty swallowing and voice change are often presenting features of head and neck cancer. Indeed, in a study of 352 patients with various stages of oral, pharyngeal, and laryngeal cancer, approximately half the population reported swallowing difficulty prior to treatment (Pauloski et al., 2000). Results also supported the clinical impression that patients presenting with more advanced disease are more likely to perceive swallowing problems prior to treatment. Even for patients with functional swallows, instrumental assessment confirmed changes to swallow physiology pretreatment that differed from normal controls, including longer oral and pharyngeal transit times, greater amounts of oral and pharyngeal residue, shorter cricopharyngeal opening durations, and lower swallowing efficiencies demonstrated in the group with head and neck cancer (Pauloski et al., 2000). Currently, the exact mechanism underlying swallowing dysfunction prior to treatment remains unclear, yet both size and location of the tumor (oral and pharyngeal tumors present with worse pretreatment swallowing function than patients with laryngeal tumors) are known to influence function pretreatment. Further study is required to determine the impact of additional factors such as tumor infiltration, pain, and ulceration.

In the presence of pretreatment swallowing compromise, intervention is most likely to commence prior to initiation of treatment or surgery. In particular, this may involve implementing appropriate postural changes such as having the chin down for reduced posterior motion of the tongue base or reduced laryngeal closure and introducing a modified diet that enables the patient to optimize nutritional intake yet minimize aspiration risk. Prior to treatment it can also be useful to train patients how to complete certain swallowing exercises or maneuvers that may be integral to rehabilitation in the weeks to come (e.g., demonstrating the supraglottic swallow prior to supraglottic laryngectomy or commencing tongue base exercises prior to supracricoid laryngectomy). In contrast, although the presence of pretreatment dysphonia is also a consequence of the cancer, treatment of the dysphonia at this stage is not warranted.

## Treatment/Acute Phase Postsurgery

While the patient is undergoing treatment (if undergoing radiotherapy +/− chemotherapy) or during the acute phase postsurgery, the SLP continues to evaluate voice and swallowing while implementing appropriate intervention. Maintenance of effective, safe, and adequate nutritional intake is a priority target, and is achieved in collaboration with other members of the multidisciplinary team (e.g., medical, nursing, dietitian). Intervention to facilitate communication during this period is also essential, particularly for patients postsurgery (+/− tracheostomy) when verbal communication is compromised. At this stage, SLPs need to be familiar with the expected patterns of recovery and any contraindications to active assessment/intervention (e.g., surgical healing, pain).

## Post-Treatment and Long-Term Care

The growing trend for early discharge and shortened length of hospital stay impacts on postoperative management. Most patients leave the hospital without adequately establishing oral intake, frequently resulting in intensive long-term therapy to be conducted on an outpatient basis. Post-treatment management includes an objective evaluation of voice and swallowing to provide the basis for the development and implementation of an individualized and targeted intervention plan. The results of instrumental and noninstrumental voice and swallowing evaluations (discussed later in this chapter) may also help to identify the need for referral to other services, e.g., physiotherapy, prosthodontist. In some cases the SLP may be required to coordinate the transfer of speech pathology management to another setting. Provision of information regarding the site of the tumor and the mode and intent of treatment should accompany specific details regarding treatment outcomes including functional status, prognosis for recovery, results of instrumental and noninstrumental procedures, and recommendations for intervention. The transition from hospital to home can be unsettling for some patients. Therefore, provision of support and education from all members of the multidisciplinary team is required. In addition, liaison with relevant community agencies will support a seamless continuation of care after discharge.

The SLP's role also extends to encompass the needs of the head and neck cancer patient requiring palliative care. In this setting the SLP's role primarily entails provision of support, education, and strategies to optimize communication and swallowing function in collaboration with the patient, caregivers, and other members of the multidisciplinary team. Consultation is ongoing to enable a timely response to changes in the patient's status, which have implications for swallowing and communication. Pollens (2004) provides a comprehensive outline of the roles and responsibilities of the SLP in a palliative care setting which are relevant to managing the patient with head and neck cancer requiring palliation. These include:

- provision of consultation to patients, families, and members of the hospice team in the areas of communication, cognition, and swallowing function
- development of strategies in the area of communication skills in order to support the patient's role in decision making, to maintain closeness, and to assist the client in fulfillment of end of life goals
- provision of assistance to optimize function related to dysphagia symptoms in order to improve patient comfort and eating satisfaction, and promote positive feeding interactions for family members
- communication with members of the interdisciplinary hospice team, to provide and receive input related to overall patient care

The SLP may be involved in specific aspects of the patient's care such as ethical decision making regarding the implementation of non-oral feeding, provision of strategies to enhance communication effectiveness, or development of alternative means of communication. Pollens (2004) described a shift in focus towards an enhanced emphasis on comfort and choice when managing dysphagia in a palliative care setting. Clinical evaluation of swallowing is more likely to be the most appropriate technique for evaluation of dysphagia and monitoring decline in swallowing function that typically occurs in this patient group. Instrumental evaluation of swallowing is often contraindicated as the patient's condition may preclude participation in such procedures. The SLP in consultation with the multidisciplinary team needs to consider whether the results of an instrumental evaluation of swallowing are likely to influence an alteration in management.

## General Principles for the Assessment and Management of Swallowing Following Laryngeal and Hypopharyngeal Cancer

The management of patients with head and neck cancer is a specialist clinical skill. Accurate assessment and intervention calls upon knowledge of normal and abnormal aerodigestive physiology for voice, swallowing, respiration, and airway protection, coupled with the ability to recognize altered anatomy as it relates to these functions in order to anticipate the swallowing complications associated with (a) the presence of the tumor and (b) the treatment approach implemented. The following sections detail those assessment and intervention techniques that have application in the diagnosis and rehabilitation of patients with laryngeal or hypopharyngeal cancer. Providing basic instructional information regarding the assessment techniques and treatment approaches is beyond the scope of the current chapter and this textbook. For those readers unfamiliar with the assessment or treatment techniques detailed below they are directed to any of the many textbooks dedicated to dysphagia management such as Logemann (1997), Groher (1997), Huckabee and Pelletier (1999), and Cichero and Murdoch (2006) which outline this type of information in greater detail.

## Assessment of Swallowing

Swallowing is a complex series of sequential neuromuscular events that are integrated into a smooth and continuous process (Gaziano, 2002). This process is often described in four discrete stages: oral preparatory, oral, pharyngeal, and esophageal. The act of swallowing commences with the entry of food into the oral cavity. Food is chewed and collected together by the tongue to form a cohesive bolus. Once formed this bolus is transferred posteriorly by the tongue. The base of tongue contacts the posterior pharyngeal wall. This action initiates the pharyngeal stage of the swallow. Four necessary motor activities are required to complete the swallow including: (1) closure of the airway to prevent food from entering the lungs, (2) closure of the velopharyngeal port to prevent food from entering the nose, (3) opening of the upper esophageal sphincter to enable the bolus of food to pass unobstructed into the esophagus, and (4) application of pressure to push the food through the pharynx and esophagus (Mittal et al., 2003). Mittal et al. (2003) describe swallowing in terms of a sequential generation of pressure at different stages in the swallowing process to ensure safety and efficiency. Initial pressure generation is applied by the tongue body and then by the base of the tongue and pharyngeal walls and, finally, by esophageal contraction to drive the bolus into the stomach.

For patients with laryngeal and hypopharyngeal cancers, both the presence of the tumor and its management will impact on the process of the normal swallow in some way, through either neuromuscular changes associated with the presence of the tumor, altered functional properties of the existing tissues and structures (following radiotherapy +/− chemotherapy), or due to surgical removal of key anatomical structures involved in swallowing. Evaluating this impact requires a combination of both instrumental and noninstrumental evaluations. Over the course of patient management, swallowing assessments of differing purposes—screening, clinical monitoring, and comprehensive diagnostic clinical and instrumental evaluations—will be implemented. Largely, the nature of the dysphagia assessment is dictated by the stage of patient care (i.e., admission, monitoring during treatment, outcome evaluation, review), the patient's medical condition (e.g., level of pain, stage of healing), and the intent of the assessment (establish baseline functioning, maintain safe adequate nutrition and hydration, evaluate the impact of intervention techniques, or identify treatment targets). Chapter 2 has previously outlined clinical and instrumental assessments of swallowing. In the current section these assessment techniques will be discussed with particular relevance to their application with patients with laryngeal and hypopharyngeal cancer.

## Dysphagia Screening Tool

Implementation of a formal dysphagia screening protocol may serve to identify head and neck cancer patients at risk for dysphagia. Although there are currently no standardized screening tools specifically for the head and neck population, there are several tools which are used with the stroke population that may have application for this group. A formal screening protocol may comprise a check sheet/flowchart and simple water swallow (e.g., 3 oz water test). Ideally, such a protocol should be implemented at the patient's point of entry into the organization where he or she is undergoing diagnostic procedures and treatment. A formal screening process would ensure that screens were done on patients across the entire spectrum of severity rather than just screening based on intuitive criteria. A screening protocol could also be administered at intervals during and after treatment to monitor for the presence of dysphagia in the acute phase of patient management and during long-term review. While not essential, a dysphagia screening protocol can serve to initiate early referral for evaluation and management. Early identification of patients presenting with a previous history of dysphagia or potential compromise of pulmonary, hydration, or nutrition status results in a referral to a SLP for clinical evaluation and progression to instrumental evaluation where indicated. This process has the potential to support the head and neck cancer patient's general health status as well as limiting a patient's experience of dysphagia symptoms.

## Case History and Clinical Evaluation

The standard clinical evaluation, comprising a case history and a clinical bedside examination (oromotor examination and swallowing trials), can be implemented at any stage of the patient's care. In particular for the head and neck cancer population, the initial case history should be comprehensive and explore all previous medical and surgical history, current medical diagnosis, proposed treatment, relevant background including learning needs and cultural preferences, previous swallowing difficulties, current swallowing status, appetite, nutritional status including method of intake, the use of any strategies or compensatory techniques to facilitate swallowing, medications and their potential side effects, respiratory status (including presence of a tracheostomy), patients' perception of their swallowing ability, taste, and smell, and the presence of other related disorders such as reflux.

Within the clinical bedside examination, the oromotor component should be conducted as per standard procedures. However for this population, particular note should be made regarding the range of movement of the articulators, particularly the jaw. Attention should also be given to the condition of the oral mucosa.

Observation and evaluation of swallowing food and liquid again follows routine procedures used for all dysphagic patients. The limitation of the clinical bedside examination to identify the physiological basis of the swallowing disorder, particularly pharyngeal stage disorders, is acknowledged. Therefore it should not be used as the only tool in the pretreatment baseline assessment or postsurgery/treatment when determining rehabilitation targets. However, there are stages during the continuum of care when clinical assessments alone are adequate to monitor status and ensure the patient is safely managing an oral diet. At these times in particular, the clinical assessment can be augmented with cervical auscultation and $O_2$ saturation measurement where indicated.

## Instrumental Assessment

The incorporation of instrumental evaluation of dysphagia in routine clinical practice enhances a clinician's understanding of the physiologic and anatomic basis for the dysphagia, enabling diagnosis and information critical to direct intervention. The two major forms of instrumental assessment typically considered for the evaluation and management of dysphagia for patients with laryngeal and hypopharyngeal cancer are the modified barium swallow (MBS) and the fiberoptic endoscopic evaluation of swallowing (FEES). Information obtained from the MBS and FEES should be considered complementary and ideally both should be conducted in order to provide a more thorough understanding of swallowing physiology in the head and neck cancer patient with oropharyngeal dysphagia. Manometry (or videomanometry) is another particularly useful assessment tool, though currently it is less commonly applied in clinical settings. Mittal et al. (2003) describe various methods for measuring swallowing function in patients with head and neck cancer treated with surgery, radiotherapy, and chemotherapy. They make specific mention of MBS, FEES, and manometry, but also make reference to the temporal and durational measurements that can be obtained from the MBS in addition to the more commonly used descriptions of swallowing function. These values are especially important when making pre- and post-treatment comparisons and/or when comparing one treatment with another.

The incorporation of these instrumental techniques and their measures into routine clinical practice enhance

our understanding of the physiologic and anatomic basis for the presenting dysphagia and allow clinicians to evaluate the effectiveness of therapy techniques. As outlined in Chapter 2, a MBS allows the clinician to examine oral, pharyngeal, laryngeal, and cervical esophageal swallowing physiology and provide information on the presence and etiology of aspiration, timing and efficiency of bolus movement, the timing and extent of structural movement, and the patient's response to alterations in bolus volume, consistency, and viscosity. Observations regarding the patient's sensory awareness of and response to residue, penetration, and aspiration can be made. The suitability of specific behavioral therapy techniques (postural changes, increased sensory input, swallow maneuvers, and alterations to the feeding process such as the method and rate of presentation of a bolus) can be identified and the impact of these interventions can be evaluated (see also figures in Chapters 2 and 7 and MBS files in Chapter 7 on CD).

FEES is also well suited for this population (Dworkin, Hill, Stachler, Meleca, & Kewson, 2006). Although this technique does not allow examination of the oral stage of the swallow, it provides an equally valid assessment of pharyngeal stage function and aspiration risk as obtained from the MBS. It has the added benefit of allowing the clinician to directly visualize surface anatomy (particularly important if flaps or grafts have been used), observe secretions and secretion management, gauge the extent of mucosal abnormalities such as erythema and edema, as well as assess the effect of altered anatomy on bolus flow and airway protection that cannot be observed via a MBS (see figures in Chapters 2 and 7, and FEES in Chapter 7 on CD). It can also be repeated regularly with no risk to the patient, allowing the clinician to obtain important information on physiological functioning as rehabilitation progresses.

Following both nonsurgical and surgical management of laryngeal and hypopharyngeal cancer there is a high possibility of absent or altered sensation for the structures involved in swallowing. To better understand the extent of altered sensation, FEES may be extended to include an assessment of laryngopharyngeal sensory thresholds. This is referred to as flexible endoscopic evaluation of swallowing with sensory testing (FEESST) (Aviv et al., 1998). The sensory threshold testing involves delivering pulses of air through an internal port to the laryngopharyngeal mucosa innervated by the superior laryngeal nerve (Aviv et al., 1998) (see Chapter 2).

Although not currently used in routine clinical management, there is the potential in the future for simultaneous videomanometry (see Chapter 2) to play an important role in understanding the swallowing disorders following laryngeal and hypopharyngeal cancer. For most of these patients, swallowing impairment post-treatment (surgery, radiotherapy, or chemoradiotherapy) is associated with increased residue and poor transition of the bolus indicating difficulties establishing the sequential generation of pressure needed to ensure safe and efficient bolus transition. Videomanometry not only permits evaluation of pressure changes at the level of the upper and lower esophageal sphincters and in the body of the esophagus but also measures tongue base to posterior pharyngeal wall pressures. Quantification of this deficit through videomanometry helps to contribute to a more comprehensive understanding of the presenting dysphagia.

### Quality of Life and Outcome Measures

In addition to the clinical and instrumental assessments of dysphagia, it is important for the clinician to measure the patient's outcomes, effectiveness of intervention, and overall well-being and quality of life. Earlier research into dysphagia outcomes was restricted to descriptions of diet consistency as a measure of swallowing outcome. However it is now acknowledged that such limited information is inadequate, as clinical experience with this population will confirm that while patients may report consuming a normal diet, they do so with extreme difficulty, taking considerably longer to complete meals, frequently flushing with liquids to facilitate bolus passage and employing other compensatory techniques to facilitate eating and drinking. They may also have associated deficits such as impaired smell and taste, which contribute to an absence of pleasure, satisfaction, or enjoyment associated with eating. Hence, diet description alone does not address the social and emotional implications of dysphagia nor does it demonstrate the nutritional and health related consequences. Consequently, as outlined in Chapter 2, there are numerous tools available for these purposes, some of which are dysphagia spe-

cific while others are designed to measure overall quality of life. Some of the tools more commonly used in investigations of patients with laryngeal and hypopharyngeal cancer include the Functional Assessment of Cancer Therapy—Head and Neck (FACT-H&N) (List et al., 1996), The University of Washington Quality of Life Head and Neck Questionnaire Revised (UW-QOL-R, version 3) (Weymuller, Alsarraf, Yueh, Deleyiannis, & Coltrera, 2001), the Head and Neck Performance Status Scale (HNPS) (List, Ritter-Sterr, & Lansky, 1990), and the M. D. Anderson Dysphagia Inventory (MDADI) (Chen et al., 2001). See Chapter 2 for descriptions of these and other scales.

## Management of Swallowing

To facilitate the management of dysphagia in the patient with laryngeal and/or hypopharyngeal cancer clinicians must demonstrate:

- the clinical skills and resources necessary to support their role in counseling and patient education
- established interdisciplinary links with medical and dietetic staff to facilitate optimal nutritional support that is maintained throughout the continuum of care
- knowledge and awareness of current evidence to support clinical practice in dysphagia evaluation and treatment
- awareness of associated complications of cancer treatment, such as mucositis, edema, and the need for tracheostomy, which may impact on swallowing
- knowledge of the categories and types of therapy that are of particular benefit for this population
- the skill and knowledge to use a combination of instrumental and noninstrumental methods to accurately define the physiological basis for the swallowing disorder, measure the effectiveness of treatment, and facilitate treatment through the provision of biofeedback
- knowledge of or established networks with local facilities, community services, and agencies which may be required to provide

ongoing support, education, and therapy as the patient progresses through the continuum of care

## Counseling and Patient Education

In order to provide for the education and counseling needs of this patient population the clinician must have a thorough working knowledge of the intended treatment, its consequences, and outcomes. Patient education often involves reiterating the information provided to the patient by the medical team, as the patient and the family attempt to assimilate and cope during this initial stage. It also involves explaining normal voice production, normal swallowing, the various assessments that will be used, and the role of the SLP and how this will change during treatment.

Counseling and patient education continues throughout the continuum of care. Many patients are comforted by ongoing discussions regarding their own progress and the expected pattern of recovery. In particular many find it beneficial to discuss the potential side effects of treatment, including when and why they may occur, prior to their presentation. In this way, changes are not unanticipated, and patients are reassured that what they are experiencing is consistent with the treatment process.

There are numerous resources that are available which may enhance a patient/caregiver's understanding of the condition. Some resources cover general aspects of cancer diagnosis and management and are often institution specific. Others are more specific to head and neck cancer and include information relating to diagnosis and treatment approaches as well as side effects and their management. Several head and neck cancer specific resources, providing information for patients, their relatives, and carers, are available online. An example includes "Support for People with Oral and Head and Neck Cancer" (www.spohnc.org). Dysphagia specific resources include diagrams, figures, or illustrations of normal anatomy as it relates to the functions of voice and swallowing, multimedia (educational CD-ROMs), and models of the head and neck region which support explanations of respiration, voice, and swallowing, as well as brochures/fact sheets with FAQs and responses (see Figure 7–1). It may also be beneficial for those patients with sufficient cognitive status to review images of MBS studies which detail normal swallowing and contrast this with their own MBS or one which demonstrates a similar pattern of oropharyngeal dysphagia to their own.

## Optimal Nutrition Support

The development of a professional relationship with a dietitian is critical in ensuring effective intervention for the patient with dysphagia associated with head and neck cancer. Patients with intermediate and advanced stage disease frequently present with complaints of dysphagia and significant weight loss. This must be addressed during the treatment planning process in order to minimize the potential risk for medical complications as well as lessen the impact on functional and psychosocial aspects of daily living that can be associated with swallowing impairment. In some cases aspiration risk and nutritional compromise are significant enough to warrant implementation of non-oral feeding prior to treatment. Initiation of non-oral feeding prior to treatment has also been advocated for patients identified as high risk. A review of the literature relating to prophylactic percutaneous gastrostomy (PEG) in the head and neck cancer patient suggests that prophylactic PEG insertion in this patient group can improve quality of life during treatment and reduce the likelihood of hospital admissions for dehydration and/or malnutrition. Figure 7–2 shows a PEG in a patient undergoing treatment. There is evidence in the literature which suggests that patients from the following diagnostic groups should be considered for prophylactic PEG insertion during treatment planning stages: those planned for chemoradiotherapy (rather than radiotherapy alone), those with a hypopharyngeal primary, base of tongue, or T4 tumors, and those with a weight loss of more than 7% body mass index prior to commencing treatment (Beaver, Matheny, Roberts, & Myers, 2001; Mekhail et al., 2001; Schweinfurth, Boger, & Feustel, 2001).

Other patients, particularly those who experience severe reaction to radiotherapy (+/− chemotherapy) may also need alternative or supplemental nutrition during treatment when factors such as pain, nausea, and mucositis prevent sufficient oral intake. Surgical resection +/− reconstruction for laryngeal or hypopharyngeal cancer frequently necessitates periods of non-oral feeding postoperatively to permit adequate healing and resolution of edema prior to reintroducing

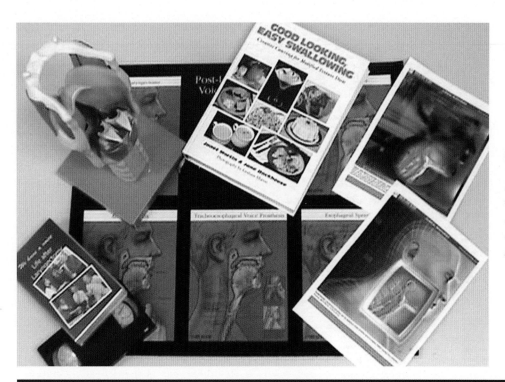

**Figure 7–1.** Example of a range of materials and products which can be used in dysphagia education and counseling.

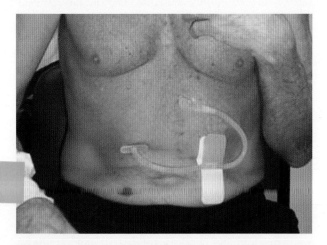

**Figure 7–2.** A PEG in situ, placed prior to chemoradiotherapy to optimize nutritional support during treatment.

oral intake. Surgical approaches which result in alterations to swallowing ability which preclude safe and efficient oral intake and may need prolonged periods of therapy require ongoing nutritional support until such time that a return to oral intake is achieved. A patient's recovery from surgery or response to treatment cannot always be determined in advance and

there will be times when the need for alternative or supplemental non-oral feeding is unexpected. Similarly, patients who experience a decline in swallowing function over time associated with fibrosis/scarring, or a recurrent or progressive disease, may be unable to meet their nutrition and/or hydration requirements and require alternative or supplemental feeding. A SLP's awareness of nutritional evaluation techniques and specific nutrition/hydration requirements as well as management strategies including dietary counseling, education, and monitoring of diet compliance and timely management of symptoms will facilitate the multidisciplinary approach and enhance nutrition intervention in the head and neck cancer patient.

**Tracheostomy Management.** Large tumors of the larynx and/or hypopharynx can compromise airway patency, and may necessitate placement of a tracheostomy tube prior to treatment selection and planning. Tracheostomy may also be necessary for progressive airway obstruction due to residual or recurrent disease. Conversely, radiotherapy (+/− chemotherapy) for hypopharyngeal and laryngeal cancer can result in mucosal inflammation and edema. If severe, edema may cause stenosis interfering with respiration requiring temporary and occasionally long-term tracheostomy. The SLP is involved in educating the patient and family/caregivers regarding tracheostomy and its impact on communication and swallowing.

Surgical approaches to the management of laryngeal and hypopharyngeal cancer frequently require elective placement of a temporary tracheostomy for potential upper airway obstruction created by postsurgical edema and to support provision of postoperative respiratory care (issues relating to tracheostomy management associated with specific surgical procedures are presented in the relevant sections later in this chapter).

A cuffed tracheostomy tube may also be inserted as an attempt to limit aspiration of secretions, food/fluids, and gastric contents. It must be stated, however, that an inflated tracheostomy cuff does not provide effective protection of the airway against aspiration. Secretions can collect above the inflated cuff and pass around it. There is some evidence to support the clinical observation that cuff status influences swallowing physiology in patients with tracheostomy. In a retrospective review of tracheostomy patients, Ding and Logemann (2005) examined specific alterations to swallow physiology under the two conditions of cuff inflated and cuff deflated. Data were available on 623 patients referred for videofluoroscopy, 102 of which had a diagnosis of dysphagia associated with head and neck cancer. Site and size of lesion, treatment status (i.e., pre/post), and mode of treatment data were not presented. Head and neck cancer patients were noted to demonstrate significantly higher frequencies of reduced laryngeal closure, aspiration during the swallow, and aspiration after the swallow. The incidence of aspiration across both conditions for all patients studied was 64.8%. Of these, silent aspiration was reported to be 46.2%. The authors report an association between the lack of reaction to aspiration with an inflated cuff. A significantly greater frequency of reduced laryngeal elevation was observed while the cuff was inflated. The authors emphasized the need to perform investigations of swallowing under the two conditions.

Where indicated, a one-way (speaking) valve may be used to facilitate verbal communication. However, the application of one-way valves in individuals where there is potential for airway obstruction either through tumor or postoperative/treatment induced edema requires consultation with the medical/surgical team.

For this reason, the use of one-way speaking valves in this population is in some cases contraindicated. Evaluation of the effectiveness of a speaking valve on secretion management and/or oropharyngeal swallowing ability in selected head and neck cancer patients with tracheostomy utilizing instrumental procedures such as the MBS or FEES is recommended.

SLPs involved in the care of patients with tracheostomy are encouraged to review the principles of tracheostomy management and its related policies and procedures specific to their institution/employing body. Management of dysphagia and communication with the tracheostomized patient are regarded as an area requiring advanced knowledge and skill often requiring demonstration of competency prior to commencing clinical practice in this area. The reader is referred to Dikeman and Kazandjian (2003) for more detailed information about tracheostomy management.

## Compensatory and Rehabilitative Techniques

Prior to initiation of therapy for dysphagia it is imperative that the anatomic and physiologic basis for the swallowing disorder is defined. This can be achieved through taking a careful case history in conjunction with performing a comprehensive clinical evaluation and should also involve an instrumental evaluation such as a MBS, FEES, and manometry. Close attention during the instrumental evaluation will identify aspiration or aspiration risk, determine the physiology of the oropharyngeal swallow, and ascertain the suitability of specific interventions to improve swallowing. The effectiveness of the selected interventions can be evaluated. This in turn will form the basis for treatment planning. The intervention strategies chosen will be influenced by the patient's general condition, mental status, cognitive ability, cultural influences, and speech and language capacity. Other factors that may influence the effectiveness of intervention include fatigue, motivation, level of cueing and support needed to perform the intervention strategies, and the individual's ability to repeatedly and consistently perform the selected interventions.

There are important differences between those intervention strategies that are termed compensatory and those referred to as rehabilitative. They can be performed alone or in combination.

**Compensatory Treatment Techniques.** Compensatory interventions are strategies that provide an immediate effect by altering the direction of food and liquid flow and modifying the physical relationship of structures, particularly in the pharynx, thereby eliminating symptoms such as aspiration. However, if these strategies are not consistently used, swallowing typically returns to its dysfunctional status. Compensatory treatment procedures do not alter the physiology of the swallow; therefore, they are implemented when minimizing aspiration risk is the primary therapeutic goal (such as pretreatment). Similarly, compensatory treatment procedures are often employed during treatment to facilitate adequate and safe oral nutrition, particularly while active rehabilitation is contraindicated (i.e., due to either the acute effects of radiotherapy or initial postsurgical healing). In the long-term posttreatment, continuation of the use of compensatory techniques (such as dietary modification) should only be advocated once active rehabilitation has ceased and no further gains can be achieved. The compensatory treatment procedures that have application for the head and neck cancer population are outlined in Tables 7–1 and 7–2.

**Table 7–1.** Compensatory Treatment Procedures Commonly Used with Head and Neck Cancer Patients: Postural Changes

| Physiology | Symptom | Posture | Rationale |
|---|---|---|---|
| Inefficient oral transit | Reduced posterior propulsion of bolus by tongue | Head back | Utilizes gravity to clear the oral cavity |
| Delay in triggering the pharyngeal swallow | Bolus past the ramus of the mandible but swallow not triggered | Chin down | Widens valleculae<br>Narrows airway entrance |
| Reduced posterior motion of the tongue base | Residue in valleculae | Chin down | Pushes the tongue base posteriorly towards the posterior pharyngeal wall |
| Unilateral laryngeal dysfunction | Aspiration during the swallow | Head rotated to damaged side | Places extrinsic pressure on thyroid cartilage, increasing adduction |
| Reduced laryngeal closure | Aspiration during the swallow | Chin down | Puts epiglottis in a more protective position<br>Narrows the laryngeal entrance |
| Reduced laryngeal closure | Aspiration during the swallow | Head rotated to damaged side | Increases vocal fold closure by applying extrinsic pressure |
| Reduced pharyngeal contraction | Diffuse residue throughout the pharynx | Lying down on one side (unoperated/stronger side) | Eliminates gravitational effect on pharyngeal residue |
| Unilateral pharyngeal paresis | Residue on one side of the pharynx | Head rotated to the damaged side | Eliminates the damaged side path |
| Unilateral oral and pharyngeal weakness | Residue in oral cavity and pharynx on the same side | Head tilt to stronger side | Directs the bolus down the stronger side |
| Cricopharyngeal dysfunction | Residue in piriform sinuses | Head rotated to damaged side | Pulls cricoid cartilage away from the posterior pharyngeal wall, reducing resting pressure in the upper esophageal sphincter |

**Table 7–2.** Compensatory Treatment Procedures Commonly Used with Head and Neck Cancer Patients: Other

| Approach | Specific Techniques |
|---|---|
| Increasing sensory input/awareness | Increased downward pressure with the spoon when placing food in the mouth<br><br>Increasing bolus taste/flavor, volume, temperature, viscosity:<br>▪ sour bolus<br>▪ carbonation<br><br>Suck swallow—increased vertical tongue/jaw sucking movements with lips closed<br><br>Thermal tactile stimulation<br><br>Self-feeding |
| Changes in the feeding process | Reducing speed of presentation of bolus<br><br>Presenting food differently in the mouth:<br>▪ different pressure<br>▪ different location<br><br>Encouraging dry swallows<br><br>Alternating liquids and solids<br><br>Double swallows/multiple swallows |
| Modifications to the texture and consistency of food and fluids | Altering texture<br><br>Altering viscosity<br><br>Addition of sauce/gravy |

**Rehabilitative Treatment Techniques.** Rehabilitation treatment procedures are interventions that, when used over time, may result in permanent changes to swallow physiology. Specific rehabilitation treatment procedures that have application for patients with laryngeal and hypopharyngeal cancer are detailed in Table 7–3. In some patients rehabilitation can be initiated prior to cancer treatment in an attempt to target specific components of the oropharyngeal swallow that are likely to be affected by nonsurgical and/or surgical approaches. Active rehabilitation can continue early postcancer treatment once the acute reaction to radiotherapy has abated or, for patients who undergo surgery; once healing is sufficient. Patients are encouraged to undertake independent practice and should be advised to complete multiple repetitions (e.g., 5 sets of 10 repetitions) of the rehabilitative exercises 5 to 10 times daily. See CD for footage of a patient completing her daily set of lingual exercises postsurgery (CD: Chapter 7: Video: Daily Exercises). Active rehabilitation should continue for a minimum of 6–8 weeks in order to effect change, though longer periods may be necessary for some patients. Ongoing practice is also required to maintain status.

There is currently considerable research interest in investigating the outcomes of particular treatment strategies for the management of dysphagia. Logemann (2006) provides an update on randomized clinical trials, which includes a brief description of ongoing studies, two of which have specific relevance for the treatment of swallowing disorders in the head and neck cancer population. The first trial compares the effect of the Shaker exercise with a standard therapy exercise program. The other involves a comparison between two treatment protocols in a randomized format for patients treated with head and neck cancer. In both studies, return to oral intake is the primary outcome measure. Results of such as these referred to by Logemann (2006) have the potential to exert huge influence over the type, frequency, and intensity of treatment for the management of oropharyngeal dysphagia in the head and neck cancer population.

**Table 7–3.** Rehabilitation Interventions Commonly Used with Head and Neck Cancer Patients

| Intervention | Rationale | Specific Techniques |
|---|---|---|
| Range of motion, strength, and resistance exercises | To optimize physiological capacity for swallowing | • Range of movement, resistance, and strength drills designed to target the lips, oral tongue (compression, protrusion, and lateral movement drills), base of tongue (yawn/gargle/Masako maneuver), jaw (passive motion/static stretching), larynx (vocal fold adduction exercises, falsetto voice, Shaker exercise), and upper esophageal sphincter (Shaker exercise)<br>• Performed without swallowing food/drink<br>• Instrumentation can be used to provide visual feedback for some tasks (e.g., using lingual pressure bulbs, surface electromyography) to assist and motivate patients |
| Specific swallow maneuvers | To exert voluntary control over specific aspects of swallowing, thereby altering swallow physiology | • Effortful swallow, Mendelsohn maneuver, supraglottic swallow, super supraglottic swallow<br>• Performed while swallowing food/drink<br>• Direct visual feedback during MBS or FEES assessment, or indirectly via instrumentation such as surface electromyography, can assist patients to learn maneuvers |

**Biofeedback.** Research supports the use of biofeedback as a tool for facilitating faster learning and performance of specific maneuvers or exercises to improve swallowing function. Therefore, therapeutic approaches incorporating biofeedback would seem to be a valuable adjunct to a structured dysphagia therapy program. Several biofeedback techniques currently used by SLPs in clinical and research settings include techniques to provide the patients with feedback on swallow physiology (such as FEES and MBS) as well as tools designed to provide feedback on muscular effort and swallowing patterns (surface electromyography [sEMG]), lingual function during swallowing, and swallow-respiratory coordination.

As mentioned earlier in this chapter direct visualization of specific aspects of swallowing can be achieved using FEES. The advantages of FEES as a biofeedback tool in therapy for the patient with head and neck cancer was described by Denk and Kaider (1997). The authors reported that patients readily accepted the biofeedback and were able to learn strategies to reduce aspiration and residue more effectively than patients who did not receive biofeedback. Similarly, the recorded images obtained during the MBS can be reviewed with the patient, family, and/or caregivers to facilitate education regarding swallowing ability. Additionally, selected interventions introduced during the procedure can be explained further and their effectiveness demonstrated. See CD for footage of a patient describing feedback from her MBS assessment (CD: Chapter 7: Video: MBS Feedback). Also, see footage of a patient receiving feedback on supraglottic swallow technique during FEES assessment (Chapter 7: FEES: Supraglottic Swallow).

Biofeedback can also be achieved through the use of surface electromyography (sEMG). Surface electrodes detect information from a number of muscle groups and therefore provide general information on muscle activation. Electrode placement under the chin (submental skin surface, between the mandible anteriorly and hyoid bone posteriorly) can be useful for providing the patient with information regarding the level of effort and the pattern of the swallow (Figure 7–3). Patients report that the signal gained through sEMG is helpful in learning the specific maneuvers and motivates them to continue with the exercises. The Kay Digital Swallowing Workstation and Swallowing Signals Lab (KayPENTAX, www.kaypentax.com) can provide sEMG information along with other physiological data (see Figure 7–4). Some centers may use portable biofeedback units (such as the Neurotrac: Verity Medical Ltd., or the Myotrac: Thought Technology Ltd.) allowing the additional benefit of extending therapy into the home setting. Crary, Carnaby, Groher, and Helseth (2004) undertook a retrospective observational study investigating outcomes for 45 stroke and head and neck cancer patients with chronic dysphagia who participated in a structured intensive therapy program supplemented by sEMG biofeedback. Functional gain was reported post-treatment for the head and neck group; however, the stroke group demonstrated the greater functional change. Specific limitations of the study were highlighted and support given to the need for controlled comparisons to improve our understanding of the efficacy and efficiency of sEMG.

Other tools can also be used to provide biofeedback for other aspects of dysphagia rehabilitation, such as improving lingual strength and function during swallowing and improving the timing of respiratory-swallow coordination. The Iowa Oral Pressure Instrument (see Chapter 10) (IOPI, www.blaisemedical.com) enables quantitative measurement of tongue strength and fatigue and can be used to provide biofeedback of lingual pressures generated in maximum effort tasks and dry swallows. Similarly, the KAY Digital Swallowing Workstation and Swallowing Signals Lab (KayPENTAX, www.kaypentax.com) includes tongue pressure transducers, which enable measurement of lingual pressures during swallowing. These and other physiological signals (such as respiratory patterns, manometric data, etc.) can be viewed and analyzed with both videofluoroscopic and endoscopic data.

## Surgical and Medical Intervention

There are several functionally significant structural lesions which contribute to dysphagia in the head and neck cancer patient and are amenable to selected surgical interventions. Structural lesions such as stenosis/stricture are readily identified during the radiological evaluation and can be managed by dilation (refer to sections on stricture formation in this chapter). Cricopharyngeal dysfunction requires careful evaluation prior to consideration for cricopharyngeal myotomy. This evaluation ideally should comprise pharyngeal manometry with simultaneous visualization of swallowing physiology via MBS or FEES. As with cricopharyngeal myotomy, the use of Botox or dilation is most beneficial when elevated UES resting pressures are observed in combination with normal or elevated pharyngeal pressures. Other surgical interventions include procedures to increase airway closure such as vocal fold medialization or laryngeal suspension. Epiglottic pulldown, suturing the vocal folds together, and total laryngectomy are additional procedures suggested for controlling unremitting aspiration. Surgical intervention for the management of dysphagia in head and neck cancer patients should be considered on a case-by-case basis. There are numerous factors which will influence the surgeon's decision to undertake such procedures. These should only be considered once careful evaluation of swallowing has been completed and extensive discussion with the patient/carers and members of the multidisciplinary team regarding the type of procedure and its implications for the dysphagia.

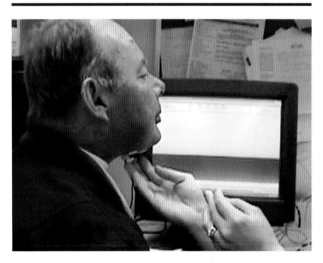

**Figure 7–3.** Submental placement of sEMG electrodes.

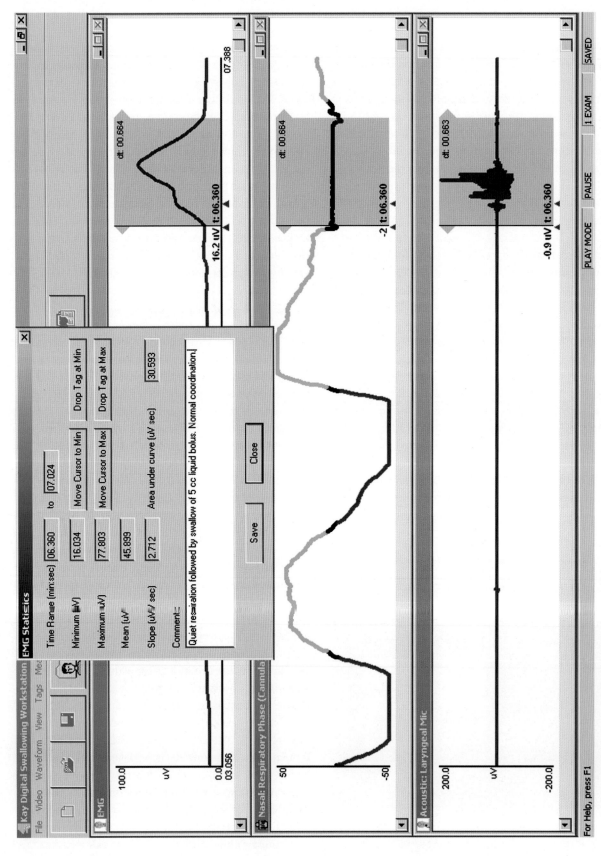

**Figure 7–4.** Images of the simultaneous sEMG, acoustic, and respiratory traces recorded during a swallow using the Kay Digital Swallowing Workstation and Swallowing Signals Lab. Photo provided courtesy of KayPENTAX.

Pharmacological therapy is increasingly proposed for management of specific oropharyngeal swallowing disorders. As yet there is insufficient evidence to support the routine use of medications which may influence particular aspects of dysphagia associated with treatment for head and neck cancer (refer to the sections in this chapter relating to early and late effects of radiotherapy and/or chemotherapy for a brief description of specific drugs and their possible impact on salivary flow and fibrosis).

## General Principles for the Assessment and Management of Voice Following Laryngeal and Hypopharyngeal Cancer

The larynx is a vital structure for normal voice production. The presence of laryngeal or hypopharyngeal cancer and/or its treatment modalities can result in the disruption of voice production and quality, resulting in varying degrees of dysphonia. The purpose of the voice assessment for the patient with laryngeal and hypopharyngeal cancer is to determine the physiological basis for the presenting dysphonia and to describe its presentation with respect to severity and quality and its impact on intelligibility, communication efficiency, and vocal effort. Rehabilitation goals for this population aim for functional voice restoration.

### Assessment of Voice

As for all voice disorders, close interaction with the treating otolaryngologist is critical when assessing voice production and any changes to voice quality in the head and neck cancer patient. There are a number of assessment tools that may be utilized including perceptual and instrumental assessments that facilitate treatment planning and rehabilitation goals. Monitoring outcomes and quality of life measures allow the clinician to accurately document change and determine the impact of the disorder on the patient.

### *Perceptual Assessment*

The completion of a detailed case history is an essential component of an assessment protocol. There are many established case history proformas for general voice populations that can be used with little modification for this population (for examples, see Andrews, 1995). As a starting point the following information should be included: description of the voice problem, onset of the dysphonia, course and variability of the dysphonia, medical history, previous and intended voice use, and the effect of dysphonia on the patient's personal and professional life. In particular, for the patient undergoing surgical management, detailed information of the structures removed during surgery needs to be noted. No two patients receive the exact same procedure and understanding individual variations is important for treatment and outcomes.

Perceptual assessments consider the quality of the voice. For this population, it is important to monitor the parameters of quality (breathiness, harshness), modal pitch and pitch range, vocal intensity and range, resonance, tension/vocal effort, and respiratory support, as well as supralaryngeal factors (i.e., articulation in the case of surgical resection of the pharynx and up into base of tongue). As per a standard perceptual voice assessment, audio recordings are encouraged to allow more accurate pre-/post-treatment comparisons.

### *Instrumental Assessment*

Instrumental assessments include those techniques that allow direct visualization of the vocal folds (endoscopy, stroboscopy) as well as tools that quantify either the aerodynamic function or acoustic quality of voice production (see description of range of assessment techniques outlined in Chapter 2). For this population direct visualization of the laryngeal structures using fiberoptic laryngoscopy is critical in order to accurately determine laryngeal symmetry and functioning, glottic closure, function of residual laryngeal structures (i.e., post-partial laryngeal surgery), and any evidence of constriction, tremor, or spasm. With the use of a flexible scope, voice can be assessed in connected speech. Less ideal is conducting the assessment using a rigid endoscope. Although a rigid endoscope allows direct visualization of the larynx, because the tongue is pulled forward to allow better visualization of the vocal folds, the assessment of vocal and laryngeal activity is limited to sustained vowel sounds.

When a stroboscopic light source is added to a rigid or flexible scope, direct visualization of the vibratory behavior of the vocal folds can be seen. Specifically, patients are instructed to produce a sustained vowel while information on symmetry, regularity of successive vibrations, glottal closure, amplitude of vibrations, and the mucosal wave can be gathered. This form of evaluation is particularly useful to evaluate residual mucosal wave motion for those patients with small glottic cancers managed either with radiotherapy or $CO_2$ laser surgery. Specific stroboscopic changes typically observed in the head and neck population include decreased amplitude of vibration, decreased mucosal wave, and decreased ability to modify vocal fold shape for pitch control.

Other instrumental techniques (detailed further in Chapter 2) can be useful to indirectly measure changes in laryngeal function and voice quality. Techniques such as electroglottography (e.g., Laryngograph, www.laryngograph.com) can provide indirect information on vocal fold vibratory patterns, while other instrumentation such as the Aerophone (KayPENTAX, www.kaypentax.com) allows quantification of aerodynamic functions including laryngeal airway resistance, subglottal pressure, phonatory flow rate, sound pressure levels, and adduction/abduction rate of the vocal folds. Acoustic analysis of the voice can be achieved using a range of commercially available equipment such as the Visipitch or Computerized Speech Lab (CSL) (KayPENTAX, www.kaypentax.com). Parameters useful to monitor over time include measures of cycle to cycle variability of pitch and amplitude, fundamental frequency, phonatory intensity, pitch and intensity range, and signal noise (e.g., noise to harmonic ratio).

## Quality of Life and Outcome Measures

Outcome measures are a useful tool to describe the nature and severity of dysphonia. Many published outcome measures exist which allow the clinician to examine both the severity of the voice impairment and its impact on aspects of the patient's well-being and quality of life. A range of quality of life and specific voice outcome measures are outlined in Chapter 2. The Voice Handicap Index (VHI) (Jacobson et al., 1997) and Voice Related Quality of Life Measure (VR-QOL) (Hogikan & Sethuraman, 1999) are two examples of tools frequently used with this population.

## Management of Voice

As mentioned previously in the chapter, intervention for dysphonia is delayed until post-cancer management, once the patient is stable and ready to commence active rehabilitation. Particularly following surgical management, return to a premorbid voice quality is not possible. Consequently the general goal is to maximize residual laryngeal function.

Considering the often extensive swallowing difficulties that are experienced simultaneously post-treatment, intervention for dysphonia is often a secondary priority for many clinicians and their patients. All patients will experience some degree of dysphonia post-treatment, with more severe deficits associated with the more extensive surgical resections. However, even subtle voice changes may impact negatively on a patient's quality of life; therefore, the clinician is encouraged to discuss vocal rehabilitation goals and possible outcomes with all patients to ensure they are fully informed. Individual patient needs and motivation, access to equipment, and the experience level of the treating SLP are all factors that will impact on the successes of treatment for dysphonia post-head and neck cancer.

Although the current sections have dealt with voice and swallowing rehabilitation separately, optimizing vocal fold function and laryngeal movement are common objectives of both goals (i.e., for airway protection when swallowing, for phonatory pitch and quality during vocalization). Consequently many of the swallowing rehabilitative exercises, particularly laryngeal adduction exercises and the supraglottic swallow technique, will have carryover benefits for voice quality. Recovery of voice needs to be closely monitored particularly when voice production relies on the compensation of remaining laryngeal structures (i.e., following partial laryngeal surgery, to ensure that too much effort or compensation is not applied). In addition, specific voice therapy techniques that aim to improve vocal projection, reduce vocal fatigue, assist vocal fold adduction, and target coordination of respiration and phonation can be applied with this population. Therapy will also include vocal hygiene and misuse education. For some patients introduction of options for amplification can be beneficial. An example of a portable amplification device is shown in Figure 7–5.

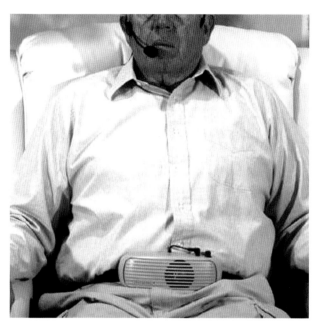

**Figure 7–5.** Portable amplification device. Photo courtesy of Phoenix Hearing Instruments.

Voice therapy may also follow further surgical intervention where there is severe vocal fold scarring and tissue loss (e.g., collagen injection or fat augmentation to facilitate medialization).

## Nonsurgical Management of Laryngeal and Hypopharyngeal Cancer

The use of radiotherapy or chemotherapy alone or in combination as a treatment option for laryngeal and hypopharyngeal cancer forms the basis of what is now commonly referred to as the nonsurgical or organ preservation approach to head and neck cancer. Nonsurgical modalities for the management of laryngeal and hypopharyngeal cancer offer the potential to preserve structures critical for voice and swallowing. However, despite advances in the development of various treatment protocols, a common consequence of nonsurgical modalities is the negative impact on both swallowing and voice production. Growing evidence

suggests that preservation of anatomical structure does not necessarily translate into preservation of function. Consequently, the challenge is to develop future treatments for the effective management of head and neck cancer that limit toxicity and the likelihood of complications associated with treatment.

Current nonsurgical approaches for laryngeal and hypopharyngeal cancer produce unavoidable toxicity to normal cells, with the oral and pharyngeal tissues at significant risk for development of acute and late reactions that can contribute to dysphagia and dysphonia. The following sections will outline some of the main complications associated with radiotherapy, chemotherapy, and combined chemoradiotherapy modalities as well as discuss the nature of the presenting dysphagia and dysphonia and management issues specific to these nonsurgical treatment approaches.

## Radiotherapy

Radiotherapy causes resultant changes to vasculature, muscle, connective tissue, bone, and salivary glands, and consequently can have a negative effect on voice and swallowing function during treatment and in the immediate post-treatment period (referred to as acute reactions) and can continue for months or years after treatment is completed (referred to as chronic or late reactions). The degree to which voice and swallowing are affected will depend on the dose, duration of treatment, and the field of treatment among other factors. The field of treatment is designed for each individual patient and will encompass likely patterns of tumor spread and may include salivary glands, oral tongue, tongue base, soft palate, supraglottic larynx, oropharynx/hypopharynx (unilateral or bilateral), and/or the entire larynx (see Figure 7–6). Normal tissues are inevitably exposed with patients experiencing symptoms of damage during and after the completion of treatment. Unlike the complications associated with chemotherapy alone that are generally of shorter duration and significant for a relatively brief period (a few weeks to a couple of months), the complications associated with radiotherapy are usually more predictable and severe and can result in permanent tissue changes that render the patient at risk for significant long-term complications. It is the tolerance of normal tissues to

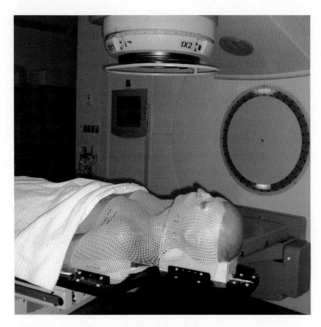

**Figure 7–6.** The field of treatment is identified and mapped prior to treatment, and then a mesh "shell" is used to ensure that the patient is positioned correctly for each session.

radiation that dictates the limit of treatment prescribed. Further details regarding radiation and radiotherapy can be found in Chapter 3.

## Early and Late Effects of Radiotherapy

There is the potential that new methods of delivery of radiation (altered fractionation schedules such as hyperfractionation or accelerated fractionation and intensity modulated radiotherapy [IMRT]—see Chapter 3) and/or the introduction of specific drug protocols in association with delivery of radiation (e.g., radioprotectors and radiosensitizers—see Chapter 3) may help to lessen the side effects of radiotherapy and possibly reduce the impact of radiotherapy on swallowing function. However, these new methods are still being investigated and conclusive research evidence is not available at this time. Regardless of this future potential, all current forms of radiation treatment have a number of significant negative early/acute and late/long-term effects. In particular, the early effects of radiotherapy relevant to voice and swallowing include

dermatitis, oropharyngeal mucositis, xerostomia, infection (most commonly candidiasis), pain, and altered taste. Furthermore, these complications can result in dehydration and compromised nutritional status. More specifically, the SLP may observe voice change, altered sensory awareness, and impaired coordination and timing of swallowing. In addition, severe laryngeal and pharyngeal edema may present as stridor and dyspnea indicating airway obstruction, often requiring tracheostomy. Chronic or long-term complications may include lymphedema, fibrosis and atrophy to vascular and connective tissue, established xerostomia, dental caries, infection, trismus, osteoradionecrosis, and altered taste.

Nordgren et al. (2006) reported on the health related quality of life for patients treated with radiotherapy and/or chemotherapy for oropharyngeal and hypopharyngeal cancer. This prospective, longitudinal, multicenter study presented data obtained at diagnosis and at various post-treatment intervals including 1 and 5 years. Comparisons were made between the two subsites. While both subsites experienced severe treatment related side effects, the longitudinal health related quality of life results for the group of patients with hypopharyngeal cancer demonstrated a worsening of treatment related side effects over the period studied. The side effects described included teeth problems, dry mouth, sensory changes, and sticky saliva.

The following sections will discuss the impact of each of these early and late treatment effects, when they occur, and current management options available to minimize their impact.

**Dermatitis.** Radiation induced damage to basal layers of the skin give rise to a sunburnlike desquamation (see Figure 7–7). Patients usually receive instruction regarding appropriate skin care and avoidance of exposure to potential irritants prior to commencement of treatment. Patients are also instructed to limit direct exposure to sun and wind, and refrain from the transdermal application of fragrances, lotions, and ointments that can interfere with the delivery of the maximal radiation dose. Skin care products that provide comfort and help protect the skin include aloe vera gels and water based lotions.

**Mucositis.** Oropharyngeal mucositis is commonly associated with radiotherapy, chemotherapy, and concurrent chemoradiation for head and neck cancer. Scully,

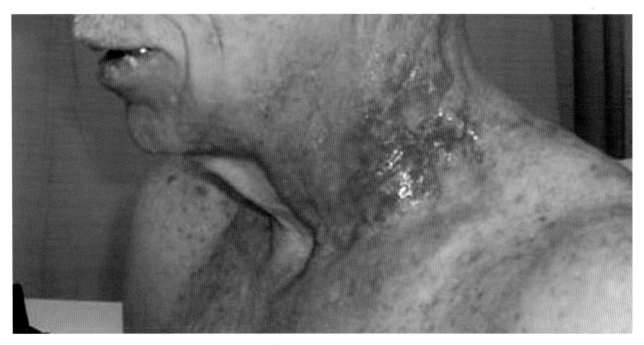

**Figure 7–7.** Early impact of radiation treatment to the neck tissues.

Epstein, and Sonis (2003) describe mucositis as a form of mucosal barrier injury (MBI). Its clinical condition is characterized by oral erythema, ulceration, and pain. The oral mucosa may initially turn whitish followed by erythema and then after a few days more, develop patchy fibrinous exudates (Scully et al., 2003). Recognition of the importance of mucositis and its implications for the management of patients with head and neck cancer is emerging in the literature.

There are variations in the frequency and severity of mucositis and its occurrence can be determined by the field, duration, and total dose of treatment. Mucositis usually develops 2 to 3 weeks after commencement of radiotherapy and persists for 3 to 4 weeks after the completion of treatment. Hyperfractionated radiotherapy may result in increased prevalence, duration, and severity of mucositis. The impact of mucositis associated with radiotherapy is exacerbated by the introduction of concomitant chemotherapy. Several assessment scales are available to establish the severity of the mucositis and guide its management. These grading systems typically incorporate both subjective and objective criteria. The World Health Organization (WHO) Oral Toxicity Scale (OTS) is one example of a validated assessment scale (see Table 7–4).

**Table 7–4.** The World Health Organization (WHO) Oral Toxicity Scale (OTS)

| Grade | Description |
| --- | --- |
| Grade 1 | Soreness +/– erythema |
| Grade 2 | Erythema and ulcers; patient able to swallow solid food |
| Grade 3 | Ulcers with extensive erythema; patient cannot swallow solid food |
| Grade 4 | Mucositis to the extent that alimentation is not possible |

Current approaches to the management of mucositis are both preventative and therapeutic. There are few efficacious interventions for prophylaxis of mucositis and there is currently no universally accepted protocol for its management. Clinically significant mucositis is managed symptomatically. The presence of erythema, ulceration, and pain/discomfort during swallowing which characterize mucositis often necessitates alterations to the texture/consistency of food/fluid and/or the need for non-oral nutrition. Local pain control is often achieved with topical anesthesia. However, the effectiveness of topical pain management is lessened as the severity and duration of mucositis increases. In these cases, alternative methods of pain relief are required. Alternative means of administering pain relief also need to be considered for those patients who are unable to swallow safely or effectively.

Introduction and maintenance of oral hygiene is paramount both during and after treatment. Patients experiencing mucositis are advised to avoid acidic or spicy foods, caffeine, alcohol, and mouthwashes containing alcohol. Coarse textured foods should also be avoided to further limit mucosal irritation. Needless to say, despite the above measures the presence of mucositis in patients receiving nonsurgical treatment for head and neck cancer can result in hospitalization for rehydration, pain control, and alternative feeding.

New approaches for the prevention and management of mucositis that are emerging in the literature and require further study include: anti-inflammatory medications, antimicrobials, biologic response modifiers, and cytoprotective agents (e.g., amifostine). Other approaches include the application of topical protectants/anesthetics and prophylactic oral zinc sulfate.

**Xerostomia.** Xerostomia (reduced saliva production) is a common long-term side effect of both radiotherapy and chemotherapy for head and neck cancer. Xerostomia is caused by a marked reduction in salivary gland secretion. This, coupled with the altered composition and properties of saliva, result in thick, ropey, tenacious secretions, which can interfere with swallowing. The impact of xerostomia on swallowing includes decreased bolus lubrication and therefore greater resistance to bolus movement (Kendall, Leonard, McKenzie, & Jones, 2000) and increased bolus transit time (Mittal et al., 2003). Its presence also has implications for an individual's acceptance and enjoyment of food and may contribute to food aversion and reduced tolerance of specific food textures/consistencies, temperatures, and levels of acidity (see Chapter 13). Logemann et al. (2001) examined the quantity of saliva produced before the onset of treatment and 3 months after treatment in 36 patients who received radiotherapy with or without chemotherapy for oral, pharyngeal, or laryngeal cancers. Patients exhibited a significant decline in saliva weight from their baseline assessment to 3 months after completion of treatment. At 3 months after treatment, significantly more patients perceived

difficulty swallowing, dry mouth, food sticking in the mouth, food sticking in the throat, needing water to assist when swallowing, and a change in taste. Interestingly, the presence of xerostomia appeared to affect the patients' overall sensory perception and comfort in eating more than actual bolus transport for the two bolus consistencies studied.

Symptoms of xerostomia include but are not limited to: dryness, burning sensation, oral discomfort, and increased thirst. The resultant changes to the oral cavity caused by xerostomia include:

- Increased viscosity of saliva and thereby impaired lubrication of oral tissues.
- Buffering and cleansing ability in the mouth is compromised predisposing to dental caries.
- Increased pathogenesis of oral flora.
- Increased plaque formation.

Typically, salivary flow reduces 1 week after the commencement of radiotherapy and xerostomia becomes apparent when doses exceed 10 Gy. Doses exceeding 54 Gy are known to induce irreversible salivary gland dysfunction. Patients often describe xerostomia as one of the most disturbing adverse effects of treatment. This is exacerbated by the fact that currently there are limited therapeutic options for effective management of xerostomia. Currently, patients who experience xerostomia are encouraged to implement routine oral hygiene at regular intervals throughout the day (particularly after meals and before bedtime). This typically includes tooth brushing to remove plaque, use of topical antimicrobial rinses (e.g., chlorhexidine) in addition to rinsing with saline or bicarbonate of soda solution to clean and lubricate the oral tissues, avoidance of food and liquids with a high sugar content, and sipping water to alleviate dryness. Management of xerostomia also includes the use of commercially available oral moisturizers and artificial saliva preparations, which aim to relieve the discomfort associated with xerostomia with varying levels of effectiveness. The administration of sialagogues (e.g., pilocarpine) may also be useful to help stimulate the production of saliva for patients with radiation induced xerostomia. See patient on CD discussing her daily oral care (Chapter 7: Video: Oral Care).

Radioprotectors are drugs that selectively protect normal tissues from radiotherapy. Results of clinical trials involving the use of the radioprotector amifostine have reported a significant reduction in the incidence and severity of radiation induced xerostomia (Brizel, Wasserman, & Henke, 2000). However, clinical use of amifostine remains controversial due to issues regarding amifostine induced toxicity and tumor protection. Wassermann et al. (2005) reported that intravenous amifostine before each fraction of radiation significantly reduced the incidence of moderate to severe xerostomia for 2 years. No significant differences in 2-year locoregional control rates, progression-free survival rates, and overall survival rates were observed between treatment groups in their study. As yet, there have been no objective data published on the impact of amifostine on swallowing. Further research regarding the use of amifostine in patients receiving concurrent chemotherapy for head and neck cancer is required.

**Infection.** Candidiasis of the oropharynx is common in patients receiving radiation for head and neck cancer and its presence may exacerbate the symptoms of mucositis. Topical antifungal agents are often used to treat oral candidiasis. Bacterial infections requiring antibiotic management may occur early in the course of treatment and after completion of treatment.

**Lymphedema.** Radiotherapy alone or in combination with surgery frequently results in lymphedema, which is caused by the development of scar tissue, which interrupts the normal flow of fluid in the lymphatic system. The presence of lymphedema may at first be only slight and is often intermittent, with noticeable variation over the course of the day. If left untreated, the condition may worsen and the swelling become more permanent. The area may become hard and solid as a result of the buildup of fluid and proteins in the tissues (see Figure 7–8). Persistent, extensive, and progressive lymphedema may be managed by external support/compression, or a program of exercise and movement among other treatments directed by the physiotherapist. A high level of motivation and compliance by the patient is a key to successful management and control of lymphedema. It may also occur due to the cancer itself blocking lymphatic system drainage.

**Fibrosis.** Fibrotic changes to soft tissue associated with radiotherapy are considered to be a dose limiting toxicity. As a late or chronic effect of radiotherapy,

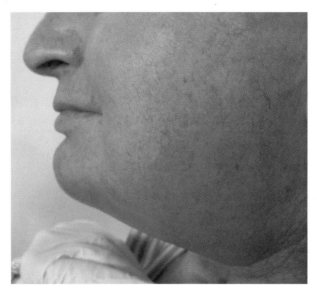

**Figure 7–8.** Long-term lymphedema in cheek and neck tissues post-treatment.

fibrosis can manifest as loss of range of motion and muscle strength, edema, and pain. The severity of radiation induced fibrosis (RIF) is dependent on radiation dose, fraction size, treatment schedule, and volume treated. Radiation induced fibrosis is known to be progressive and can result in delayed changes to the swallowing mechanism.

Typically, a patient re-presents some months or even years post-completion of treatment complaining of gradual worsening of swallowing function, often necessitating clinical evaluation of swallowing followed by instrumental evaluation. Specific changes to the swallowing mechanism associated with fibrosis include fixation of the hyolaryngeal complex, reduced tongue range of motion, reduced glottic closure, and reduced cricopharyngeal relaxation. These changes cause an adverse effect on function and may increase the potential for aspiration and/or influence an individual's ability to meet the nutritional/hydration requirements. RIF does not spontaneously regress and its prevention and management are difficult and challenging. The experience of long-term sequelae of treatment is often a blow to patients who are otherwise tumor free.

The impact of RIF on function has motivated the development and introduction of specific drug protocols for its prevention and management. While the search continues, there are already treatments available to head and neck cancer patients whose management has included radiotherapy alone or in combination with surgery and/or chemotherapy. One such treatment is the combination of pentoxifylline (Trental) and vitamin E (tocopherol) (Delanian, Porcher, Balla-Mekias, & Lefaix, 2003; Haddad, Kalaghchi, & Amouzegar-Hashemi, 2005). Pentoxifylline is a methylxanthine derivative that lowers blood viscosity, increases tissue oxygen levels, and inhibits fibrosis. Oral administration of Trental for individuals post-treatment for head and neck cancer may be difficult. Where such difficulty occurs it may be beneficial to consider approaching a compounding pharmacist for ordering of Trental in an alternative form (such as transdermal application). Preliminary results are encouraging and suggest the possibility of reducing and reversing the fibrotic process but further studies are required. There is a need for long-term investigations of the potential RIF treatments and their possible advantages for long-term speech and swallowing outcomes.

### Stricture Formation.

Fibrosis with stricture formation or stenosis of the hypopharynx and proximal esophagus is also a complication of radiotherapy to the head and neck. Stricture formation may present as dysphagia and weight loss, which persists after completion of radiotherapy, or as dysphagia and weight loss of late onset. Radiation induced stricture is investigated with either a modified or standard barium swallow and/or endoscopy. The severity of stricture may vary from total obliteration of the esophageal lumen to a fibrous membranous ring (Laurell et al., 2003). Incomplete or partial stenosis can be managed with dilation, which may need to be repeated. More severe cases may require surgical excision and reconstruction (see discussion later in this chapter).

### Osteoradionecrosis.

Osteoradionecrosis is a late complication of radiotherapy to the head and neck region most commonly affecting the mandibular bone. It can occur as a complication of external beam radiotherapy or brachytherapy, and as a result of primary radiotherapy, adjuvant treatment, or when used in combination with chemotherapy. Osteoradionecrosis is inconsistently defined in the literature. In general it is referred to as a condition in which irradiated bone becomes devitalized and exposed through the over-lying skin or mucosa, persisting without healing for 3 months (Thorn; Hansen, Specht, & Bastholt, 2000). Common signs and symptoms include pain, secondary infection, drainage, and fistulization to the mucosa or skin (Teng & Futran, 2005). Treatment usually comprises a combination of conservative measures and surgical resection. Hyperbaric oxygen therapy (HBO) has been used as an adjunctive conservative measure to treat osteoradionecrosis; however, it is not universally accepted and its efficacy is in doubt with the emergence of new data which suggest that there is no benefit from HBO in advanced osteoradionecrosis (Teng & Futran, 2005). Recent theories suggest a fibroatrophic process for the development of osteoradionecrosis giving rise to the possibility of using medications, which target this process as an avenue for treatment. Chondronecrosis may also occur as a consequence of radiotherapy. Radiation induced chondronecrosis may cause laryngeal instability, subsequent airway limitation, and possible obstruction necessitating laryngectomy.

### Trismus.

Head and neck cancer patients treated with radiotherapy (alone or combined with another treatment modality) may present with reduced mouth opening, a condition usually referred to as trismus. It is caused by radiation induced fibrosis of the temperomandibular joint and muscles of mastication (Rubin & Doku, 1976). In some head and neck cancer patients trismus may be present at the time of diagnosis due to tumor invasion in the muscles of mastication or the ascending ramus of the mandible, or because of the tumor inducing a reflex spasm of the muscles (Ichimura & Tanaka, 1993). The incidence of trismus reported in different studies varies from 10% (Ichimura & Tanaka, 1993) to 30% (Nguyen et al., 1988). The average maximal interincisal mouth opening (measured between the front teeth) in radiated patients was found to be significantly lower than in their matched controls (3.5 mm +/− 0.07 and 4.6 mm +/− 1.2 respectively) (Steelman & Sokol, 1986). A systematic review of trismus in head and neck oncology revealed that radiotherapy involving the structures of the temperomandibular joint and pterygoid muscles reduces mouth opening with 18% (Dijkstra, Kalk, & Roodenburg, 2004). Quality of life is often diminished in patients with trismus because of pain, altered facial appearance, inability to partake of food or to masticate it properly, speech difficulties, inability to practice effective oral hygiene, and inability to receive proper dental care (Beekhuis & Harrington, 1965). Exercises with tongueblades or a Therabite (Atos Medical AB, Hörby, Sweden) device increase mouth opening significantly, with the effect size being larger for the Therabite device (Dijkstra et al., 2004). Figure 7–9 shows a picture of a patient using the Therabite device, which enables passive stretching of the mouth opening, while guiding anatomically correct opening of the mandible. In a comparative study, the Therabite device combined with unassisted exercise was found to give a significantly higher improvement in mouth opening than unassisted exercise alone, or unassisted exercise combined with tongueblades (Buchbinder, Currivan, Kaplan, & Urken, 1993).

**Taste.** Exposure of oral and pharyngeal mucosa to radiation therapy damages taste receptors and taste discrimination is compromised. Patients may complain of a reduced ability to taste or an absence of taste. The etiology of taste change may be associated with several factors including direct neurotoxicity to taste buds, xerostomia, and infection. Sweet, sour, bitter, and salty tastes can be altered. Patients may notice recovery of taste emerging at approximately 6–8 weeks following completion of treatment. However, some patients will continue to report reduced taste. Zinc sulfate supplements are reported to facilitate recovery of taste. Further discussion of taste and its rehabilitation can be found in Chapter 13.

**Pain.** Other supportive measures include initiation of timely and adequate pain relief. Pain associated with mucositis is often cited by patients as a major reason for limiting oral intake. Effective pain relief timed for maximum effect to coincide with mealtimes can contribute to maintenance of adequate nutrition and hydration.

## Dysphagia and Dysphonia Following Radiotherapy

The timing, dose, and expected field of treatment for radiotherapy as well as the anticipated side effects will impact on speech pathology rehabilitation of voice and swallowing. Acute side effects of treatment that impact on swallowing may become apparent early during the treatment period and are likely to intensify as treatment progresses. Active speech pathology intervention may need to be put on hold during radiotherapy, typically from about the 2nd to 3rd week of treatment up until 3 to 4 weeks after completion of treatment to allow mucositis and other early effects of radiotherapy to dissipate. Intervention during this period may comprise monitoring, introduction, or continuation of specific compensatory techniques, support, and education.

**Dysphagia Following Radiotherapy.** Clinical observation suggests that there is no appreciable difference in the nature of swallowing disorders experienced by patients who undergo radiation as a single modality, or as an adjuvant to surgery or chemotherapy. Wide field radiotherapy to the head and neck region utilizing high radiation volumes and doses can result in alterations to the oral, pharyngeal, and upper esophageal phases of swallowing. Radiation induced edema and fibrosis are the most likely causes of the observed changes, which affect not only the range of movement of structures of the oropharyngeal swallowing mechanism but also impact on sensation.

Numerous studies have demonstrated that swallowing function is compromised as a result of radiotherapy for head and neck cancer. Kendall et al. (2000)

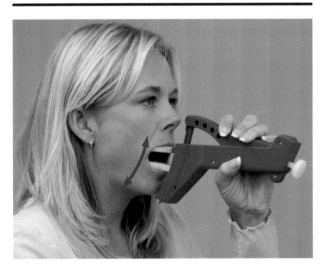

**Figure 7–9.** A patient using the Therabite system. Red arrows demonstrate the anatomical correct opening curve of the device. Photo provided as a courtesy of Atos Medical, www.atosmedical.com.

evaluated swallowing using timing and durational measures obtained from MBS of 20 patients treated with radiotherapy alone for head and neck cancer. Interestingly, none of the 20 patients perceived problems swallowing at the time of assessment. However, statistically significant differences were reported in a number of swallowing parameters in the study group when compared to normal controls. Alterations to swallow parameters included increased pharyngeal transit times observed in patients with base of tongue and pharyngeal tumors. Early maximal hyoid elevation relative to bolus movement and increased maximal duration of hyoid elevation was observed in patients with laryngeal tumors. The authors proposed that radiotherapy patients may adopt this strategy to aid bolus transfer.

Surgical resection of selected pharyngeal/laryngeal tumors with or without reconstruction is often followed by a course of radiotherapy. Dysphagia associated with surgical resection of these tumors may be exacerbated by the early effects of postoperative radiotherapy. Additionally, patients are likely to experience the late impact of radiotherapy on swallowing following completion of treatment and resolution of early (acute) effects. See CD footage for an example of dysphagia following surgery and postoperative radiotherapy (Chapter 7: MBS: Dysphagia Following Surgery and Post-Op XRT).

Specifically, those measures of oropharyngeal swallowing ability that are judged to be abnormal following radiotherapy include increased oropharyngeal transit time, uncoordination of bolus movement through the oropharynx, reduced tongue base contact with the posterior pharyngeal wall, reduced hyoid and laryngeal elevation and movement, reduced closure of the airway entrance, reduced laryngeal closure during the swallow, possible abnormal upper esophageal sphincter function, and persistent pharyngeal residue and aspiration (Mittal et al., 2003). See CD footage for an example of dysphagia postradiotherapy (Chapter 7: MBS: Dysphagia Post-XRT). It is likely that the site of tumor and radiotherapy variables will impact on the incidence and severity of the observed disorders.

Regular contact with the patient during treatment allows the condition to be monitored and the management plan altered with any changes in dysphagia. Some patients are able to continue an oral diet during treatment. Others may be unable to meet their nutrition and hydration requirements orally and require alternative feeding to supplement oral intake or in more severe cases replace oral intake altogether. During this period the SLP can continue to provide support, education, and encouragement. At this time, the goal is to optimize swallowing ability and minimize complications such as aspiration pneumonia. Clinical management largely involves implementing compensatory treatment procedures including:

- postural changes
- techniques to improve sensory input/awareness (modifications to bolus volume, viscosity, and temperature)
- changes to the feeding process (alternating liquids and solids, double swallows)
- modifications to the texture and consistency of food and liquids

Ideally, these should be introduced during the MBS/FEES and their effectiveness evaluated.

In the early stages of treatment, and for those patients who experience minimal acute reaction to radiotherapy, patients can commence specific rehabilitation treatment procedures which include exercises aimed at improving the strength and range of motion of oral and pharyngeal structures (e.g., exercises which target tongue strength and range of motion can facilitate bolus transit and clearance through the oral cavity and pharynx; tongue base exercises will improve tongue base retraction during swallowing and reduce or eliminate vallecular residue). Other interventions include the introduction of selected swallowing maneuvers to exert voluntary control over specific components of the oropharyngeal swallow. These include the supraglottic swallow, the super supraglottic swallow, the effortful swallow, and the Mendlesohn maneuver (refer to Table 7–3).

Individual patient characteristics that require consideration during radiation treatment include the status of oral hygiene and availability of family/social support, as well as the distance to and from the treatment center, and lengthy waiting times between appointments that may predispose a patient to skipping meals/feeds. Clinical observation suggests that those patients who continue to work during treatment, patients with poor family support, or those living in temporary accommodation during treatment (where kitchen facilities/access to supermarkets is inadequate) will experience more difficulty coping with the acute side effects of treatment.

It is possible to monitor swallowing function during treatment through regular administration of a dysphagia screening protocol and progression to a clinical evaluation where indicated. Instrumental techniques may be undertaken during treatment; however, it is important to consider patient comfort and the possible increased risk of mucosal injury when performing a MBS or FEES for those patients experiencing mucositis.

Patients who demonstrate established dysphagia after completion of treatment and resolution of the early/acute effects associated with radiotherapy should be offered structured, intensive therapy utilizing the compensatory and rehabilitative treatment procedures detailed in Tables 7-1, 7-2, and 7-3 respectively. These interventions are best introduced during the instrumental swallowing evaluation and their effectiveness assessed. Some of these interventions (selected swallowing maneuvers) require a period of learning on the part of the patient and their impact may need to be evaluated after the patient is judged to be performing them satisfactorily.

Tissue fibrosis associated with radiotherapy can reduce the mobility of oral and pharyngeal structures involved in bolus preparation, bolus propulsion, airway protection, and upper esophageal sphincter function. These late changes to the oropharyngeal swallowing mechanism are often observed some months or years after completion of treatment. The reader is referred to the earlier section on fibrosis in this chapter for additional detail regarding the impact of this condition. Deterioration in swallowing function and/or late presentation of dysphagia after radiotherapy should be evaluated using a combination of instrumental and noninstrumental procedures. Referral to other professionals may also be required (e.g., dietitian). It is important to note, however, that this presentation may also indicate recurrent or new disease. Under these circumstances the patient would be advised to undergo a reevaluation by the treating doctor. When delayed changes to the oropharyngeal swallowing mechanism are thought to be caused by the late effects of radiotherapy (such as fibrosis and atrophy, established xerostomia, trismus, and altered taste) a structured, individualized rehabilitation program is indicated. The components of this program are likely to comprise selected compensatory and rehabilitation interventions. These patients will continue to require education, counseling, and support as they adjust to the long-term impact of their dysphagia and its effect on their overall quality of life.

**Dysphonia Following Radiotherapy.** While speech is typically not affected in the long term, some patients who receive wide field radiotherapy for laryngeal or hypopharyngeal cancer present with articulatory imprecision, impaired oral coordination, and reduced speech intelligibility that may be associated with edema and mucosal irritation which characterize mucositis.

Patients receiving radiotherapy for laryngeal or hypopharyngeal cancer can experience temporary and permanent alterations in voice and resonance. Patients presenting with tumors that involve the larynx will almost certainly present with dysphonia. This section will focus primarily on treatment for T1 glottic tumors, in particular the impact of radiotherapy, which can be offered as a single mode of treatment for these tumors. Most of the literature reviewed for this section involved comparisons of radiotherapy with endoscopic laser surgery. In the early stage of disease, surgery and radiotherapy produce similar results.

The presence of small glottic tumors (T1) results in asymmetry and reduced elasticity of the affected vocal fold, which leads to slowed vibration of the vocal fold with asynchronous vocal fold movement. The dysphonia, which occurs as a result of the presence of the tumor, can be characterized by varying degrees of hoarseness or breathiness as well as alterations to pitch and intensity. It is expected that the dysphonia will change as the mechanical impact of the tumor is lessened during treatment. Wedman, Heimdal, Elstad, and Olofsson (2002) state that from radiotherapy, the tumor mass is replaced by less pliable tissue. When the larynx is in the field of treatment the resultant dysphonia can occur due to the early (acute) impact of edema. Once these early effects have subsided, residual long-term dysphonia can result due to fibrosis, which may limit laryngeal mobility (Pauloski, Rademaker, Logemann, & Colangelo, 1998). It is the late effects of radiotherapy to the larynx that will determine the long-term impact on voice quality.

Several authors have noted that alterations to vocal fold characteristics and vibratory pattern are not limited to the tumor side alone (Brandenburg, 2001; Wedman et al., 2002), with videostroboscopic evaluation showing a loss of vibration involving both cords. Wedman et al. (2002) studied a small group of patients with T1a glottic carcinoma treated with either radiotherapy or endoscopic laser. Routine videostroboscopic evaluation and voice analysis at conversational level demonstrated no difference between the surgically treated and irradiated groups in their study. Interestingly, the irradiated group showed a more pronounced glottic wave on the side of the tumor when compared to the endoscopically treated patients. These authors inferred that despite the exposure of radiation to both vocal folds, radiotherapy presented a more favorable outcome in terms of the impact of treatment on the mucosal wave.

A more pronounced glottic wave in the irradiated group was also reported by Krengli et al. (2004) who compared voice outcomes in patients treated with radiotherapy or laser cordectomy for T1 glottic cancer. Videostroboscopic analysis showed significant mucosal wave changes in the majority of irradiated patients. Observed changes postradiotherapy included stiff mucosal wave dynamics, hyperventricular fold activity, chronic inflammation, fold tissue inelasticity, and glottal incompetence.

Post-treatment intervention and expected recovery include instruction regarding limitations and expectations of voice outcome. Perceptual and acoustic voice analysis along with videostroboscopic evaluation at post-treatment intervals can provide evidence of voice change over time. A measure of voice outcome (see Chapter 2) should also be utilized at the time of assessment. Results of the perceptual, acoustic, and endoscopic examinations can provide the basis for managing alterations to voice associated with radiotherapy. Intervention for dysphonia can include modifications to pitch, loudness, and vocal effort (as discussed earlier in this chapter). It is important to note that vocal adduction exercises are not indicated while patients are experiencing the acute effects of radiotherapy involving the larynx.

## Chemotherapy and Combined Chemoradiotherapy Protocols

Chemotherapy alone is not traditionally used as definitive treatment for the management of head and neck cancer and its role in the development of swallowing disorders is not clear. However, chemotherapy given in conjunction with radiotherapy has emerged to become an accepted combined modality treatment and now plays a central role in the management of head and neck cancer. Various protocols combining chemotherapy and radiotherapy are in clinical use (see discussion in Chapter 3). Research is continuing to determine the optimal chemotherapy combinations and sequencing of radiotherapy.

## Early and Late Effects of Chemotherapy and Combined Chemoradiotherapy

Patients undergoing chemotherapy for head and neck cancer with or without radiotherapy are at significant risk for the development of complications associated with direct damage to oral/pharyngeal tissues and other complications related to indirect systemic toxicity and compromised immune function.

Chemotherapy for head and neck cancer causes acute reactions that are similar but not identical to the acute reactions associated with radiotherapy. Acute toxicity related to high dose chemotherapy usually resolves following cessation of treatment and healing of damaged tissues. The delivery of radiotherapy concurrent with chemotherapy has been associated with higher rates of severe early and late mucosal and pharyngeal toxicities (Eisbruch, 2004). Hanna et al. (2004) evaluated the efficacy and toxic effects of primary concurrent chemoradiotherapy in patients with advanced head and neck cancer. Statistically significant early treatment related toxic effects reported in this study included neutropenia (a condition in which the neutrophil count is reduced predisposing patients to a higher incidence and severity of infection) and mucositis. Other common complications included nausea, vomiting, dehydration, and compromised nutritional status often resulting in malnutrition. These additional factors can impact on swallowing. The need for intensive supportive care for patients undergoing concurrent chemoradiotherapy was highlighted by the frequency of unplanned hospital admissions for the management of treatment related complications such as dehydration, sepsis, febrile neutropenia, pneumonia, and malnutrition. Certain acute and delayed reactions such as mucositis and the development of radiation induced fibrosis that occur following radiotherapy are intensified when chemotherapy is concomitant with radiotherapy (Delanian & Lefaix, 2004).

**Mucositis.** Mucositis usually emerges approximately 2 weeks after initiation of high dose chemotherapy. Labial mucosa, buccal mucosa, the tongue, floor of mouth, and soft palate are commonly affected. Several cytotoxic agents have been identified as being associated with increased incidence of mucositis. These include methotrexate, 5FU, cisplatin, and carboplatin among others. There is some evidence to support the use of topical cryotherapy to reduce the impact of mucositis caused by agents such as 5FU. Intervention for the prevention and management of mucositis in patients undergoing chemotherapy is generally the same as the management described earlier in this chapter in the section relating to mucositis and radiotherapy.

**Infection.** Bacterial, fungal, and viral infections may arise during treatment with high dose chemotherapy and in the recovery period following cessation of treatment. The presence of oral mucositis in conjunction with a compromised immune system and altered salivary gland function can elevate the risk for infection in patients receiving chemotherapy with or without radiotherapy for head and neck cancer. Inadequate oral hygiene can also increase propensity for infection. It is worth noting that an ill-fitting removable dental/oral appliance can cause trauma to oral mucosa further increasing the risk for infection.

**Xerostomia.** Xerostomia associated with chemotherapy usually appears during treatment and typically resolves within 2–3 months after cessation of treatment. See discussion of xerostomia in the previous radiotherapy section of the chapter.

**Taste.** Patients undergoing chemotherapy often describe an unpleasant taste secondary to diffusion of drugs into the oral cavity. Taste changes can occur during treatment and in the early period following cessation of treatment. The ability to taste generally returns to normal in the weeks to months following treatment. Patients frequently report that altered or absent taste is a major factor limiting appetite during recovery and into the long term. See footage on the CD of a patient discussing this issue (Chapter 7: Video: Coffee).

**Nutritional Compromise.** Head and neck cancer patients are at significant risk of malnutrition due to the presence of the cancer itself and the acute and late reactions to their treatment. Prophylactic as opposed to therapeutic insertion of a percutaneous endoscopic gastrostomy (PEG) may offer more timely commencement of nutritional support and weight maintenance and reduced frequency of unplanned hospital admissions (Lee et al., 1998); however, there are currently no published guidelines for prophylactic PEG insertion in patients undergoing chemotherapy and/or radiotherapy for head and neck cancer. Hanna et al. (2004) report that 73% of patients in their study required placement of a gastrostomy tube for the management of compromised nutritional status during the acute phase of treatment. Weight loss was reportedly a concern during and at least 1 year post-treatment in patients with or without enteral feeding. However, average weight loss was less during and at 1 year post-treatment in those patients who received enteral feeding. In contrast to the findings of Lee et al. (1998), these authors did not report a substantial reduction in the frequency of unplanned hospital admissions in patients who received PEG tube placement. While enteral feeding does not appear to improve survival and locoregional control in head and neck cancer patients, there is some evidence to suggest that initiation of enteral feeding does improve quality of life during treatment when compared to oral intake alone (Senft, Feitkau, Iro, Sailer, & Sauer, 1993). There is also a suggestion in the literature that routine prophylactic PEG insertion may contribute to a "defunctioning" of normal swallowing which may impact negatively on the long-term outcome of swallowing function (Hanna et al., 2004). The issue of prophylactic PEG insertion needs further, comprehensive investigation.

**Generalized Weakness and Fatigue.** Patients undergoing high dose chemotherapy +/− radiotherapy often experience fatigue, which is related to either their disease or the treatment. Functional consequences of fatigue can lead to noncompliance with oral hygiene and may cause patients to skip meals in favor of rest/sleep resulting in weight loss and nutritional compromise. See the video footage on the CD of a patient describing how fatigue impacts on her daily life post-treatment (Chapter 7: Video: Fatigue).

**Stricture Formation.** Chemoradiotherapy for head and neck cancer has been associated with the development of postcricoid hypopharyngeal stenosis/stricture. The pathogenesis of this condition is unclear; however, it is believed that chemoradiation induced mucositis results in ulceration of opposing surfaces of redundant postcricoid mucosa (Hanna et al., 2004; Sullivan et al., 2004). Subsequent healing of the opposing surfaces occurs, leading to circumferential scar formation. The substantially reduced pharyngoesophageal lumen may prevent passage of solid foods. Patients often complain of increased effort and time taken to consume meals and the need to limit their oral intake to liquids. Patients commonly present with significant weight loss necessitating the use of oral supplements and/or the introduction of enteral feeding. Stricture formation may result in the need for endoscopic dilatation. More severe cases may require surgery and reconstruction. Sullivan et al. (2004) outline several additional management strategies which include, but are not limited to, intensive swallowing therapy to increase tongue base retraction and hyolaryngeal elevation.

## Dysphagia and Dysphonia Following Chemoradiotherapy

As discussed previously in the sections relating to radiotherapy, the management of dysphagia in the patient undergoing chemoradiotherapy follows a similar pattern, involving pretreatment counseling and education, baseline evaluation, monitoring and support during treatment with early introduction of prophylactic rehabilitation activities, and continuation during treatment as tolerated. More aggressive rehabilitation can be initiated in the weeks following treatment when acute reactions have largely resolved. However, considering that patients undergoing this treatment modality often present with larger tumors requiring large radiation volume doses, and will experience more severe acute and long-term reactions to treatment, functional outcomes for swallowing are often less than optimal.

### Dysphagia Following Chemoradiotherapy.
Dysphagia is often present prior to commencement of organ preservation treatment in patients with locally advanced tumors. In a recent report by Logemann et al. (2005) it was reported that 15% of their patients

were receiving alternative feeding prior to treatment and 6% were taking 50% or less of their nutrition orally. Interestingly, despite the reported frequency and severity of swallowing disorders, 85% of the 351 swallows contributed for analysis were described as functional prior to treatment. Most of the pretreatment swallowing disorders described occurred in the pharyngeal stage of the swallow and those patients with lesions in the hypopharynx or larynx were most frequently aspirating prior to treatment. This result is consistent with the earlier study by Pauloski and Logemann (2000). Instrumental assessments of swallowing prior to treatment in this population have revealed a range of physiological changes to the swallow (Logemann et al., 2005). These are outlined in Table 7–5.

As stated previously, speech pathology management of patients undergoing combined chemoradiotherapy typically commences prior to treatment and will usually involve provision of education and counseling. Where possible, a baseline evaluation of swallowing should be performed. A comprehensive clinical evaluation should be undertaken with particular attention given to: (a) lingual range of movement, strength, and sensation, (b) jaw range of movement, and (c) laryn-

**Table 7–5.** Impact of Chemoradiotherapy on Swallowing Function

- Reduced tongue base retraction
- Reduced A-P tongue movement
- Reduced vertical tongue movement
- Reduced lateral/anterior tongue stabilization
- Reduced tongue strength
- Reduced tongue control and shaping
- Delayed pharyngeal swallow
- Slowed/delayed laryngeal vestibule closure
- Reduced hyolaryngeal excursion
- Reduced epiglottic inversion
- Bilateral pharyngeal weakness
- Unilateral pharyngeal weakness
- Reduced cricopharyngeal opening
- Cricopharyngeal bar

*Source:* Logemann et al., 2005

geal elevation. Ideally, this should be followed by an instrumental evaluation such as the MBS or FEES. Information gained from the baseline evaluation will determine the most appropriate rehabilitation interventions, which can be introduced prior to commencement of chemoradiotherapy. The early introduction of exercises is a preventative strategy aimed at reducing the incidence of swallowing disorders. These may include: (a) range of motion exercises targeting specific structures included in the field of treatment (jaw, oral, and base of tongue) and (b) swallowing maneuvers (Mendelsohn maneuver, super supraglottic swallow, tongue holding maneuver, effortful swallow).

Treatment itself has a dramatic impact on swallowing function. The exact mechanism that causes dysfunction is not well defined. Direct neuromuscular toxic effects and fibrosis of the oropharyngeal musculature have been identified as possible causes. It has been suggested that severe dysphagia associated with intensive chemoradiation protocols results from a lack of specificity in the sensitization of tissues to radiation by chemotherapy whereby oral, pharyngeal, and laryngeal mucosal cells are sensitized to a similar extent as the cancer cells (Eisbruch, 2004). Patients suffering severe mucositis affecting the oral cavity, oropharynx, and hypopharynx frequently describe pain, thick copious secretions, reduced sensation, and nausea. These factors can contribute to dysphagia in this patient group and increase their potential for aspiration related pneumonia. Acute toxicity is often managed by initiation of alternative feeding and pain relief among other measures.

An individual's response to the treatment and the presence of early/acute effects related to treatment will influence the ability to tolerate continuation of therapy during and immediately after combined chemoradiotherapy. As stated earlier, these will typically include range of motion exercises and the use of appropriate swallow maneuvers (see Tables 7–1, 7–2, and 7–3). It is during this time that the application of compensatory interventions to support oral intake and limit potential for aspiration are most appropriate.

It is, however, the emergence of persistent late toxicity that constitutes one of the major limitations of organ preservation protocols utilized for the treatment of laryngeal and hypopharyngeal cancer. Hanna et al. (2004) cites dysphagia as the most common long-term complication of intensive chemoradiotherapy of the

head and neck. Rademaker, et al. (2003) reported on the characterization of functional eating and drinking ability in patients treated with chemoradiation for head and neck cancer over a 12-month follow-up period. This multicenter, longitudinal study demonstrated that eating ability is severely compromised in head and neck cancer patients immediately after primary chemoradiation treatment for their disease; however, function gradually improved over a 12-month period. Clinical experience suggests, however, that this is not always the case with a large proportion of patients experiencing deterioration in function over time. This discrepancy highlights the need for objective evaluation before and at intervals after treatment. The inclusion of specific outcome and quality of life measures is particularly relevant in assessment protocols for this population.

Mittal et al. (2003) provided a critical review of the relevant literature regarding swallowing dysfunction following treatment for head and neck cancer. Observation suggests that the nature of swallowing dysfunction associated with chemoradiotherapy is similar to that observed following radiotherapy. These disorders include increased oropharyngeal transit time, decreased tongue base contact with the posterior pharyngeal wall, reduced hyolaryngeal excursion, increased pharyngeal residue, and abnormal upper esophageal sphincter function. Logemann et al. (2005) observed that the physiological deficits observed post-treatment were the same disorders as seen prior to treatment, but in higher frequencies and greater severity. They also found that in their group more patients had alternative feeding, and the percentage of functional swallows after treatment had reduced to 65% post-treatment. Eisbruch et al. (2002) also suggest that aspiration pneumonia is underreported following intensive radiation or concurrent chemoradiotherapy and support the introduction of routine post-treatment videofluoroscopy to identify patients at risk of pneumonia. Eisbruch et al. (2002) demonstrated several post-treatment alterations to the biomechanics of swallowing that increased potential for aspiration including reduced laryngeal elevation and closure, reduced epiglottic inversion, and reduced base of tongue motion.

In 2004, Eisbruch et al. identified three anatomic structures whose damage possibly caused the swallowing abnormalities observed after two different intensive chemoradiotherapy regimens. These structures identified were termed DARS (dysphagia/aspiration related structures) and comprised the pharyngeal constrictors and glottic and supraglottic larynx. A prospective review of data obtained from MBS studies demonstrated pharyngeal phase abnormalities, which were common to both regimens. The observed abnormalities included weakness and reduced posterior motion of the tongue base, prolonged pharyngeal transit time, reduced coordination of pharyngeal peristalsis, opening of the UES, and laryngeal closure. Additional observations included reduced elevation of the hyoid and larynx and reduced epiglottic inversion during the swallow. The authors proposed that the combination of these disorders in conjunction with the possibility of glottic and supraglottic sensory loss contributed to the high incidence of aspiration in their study. Documented abnormalities from the MBS data were common to both regimens, supporting their conclusion that the identified abnormalities were not protocol specific and could possibly be generalized to other chemoradiotherapy protocols. Logemann et al. (2005) also found that the effects of different chemoradiotherapy protocols in their study were small. They proposed that it is the site of lesion that affects the occurrence of specific swallowing disorders, and that specific chemoradiation protocols have minimal effect on oropharyngeal swallow function. An example of the type of swallow function observed postchemoradiotherapy is available on the CD for viewing (Chapter 7: MBS: Dysphagia Postchemoradiotherapy).

Table 7–6 outlines some of the patient descriptions of the complex nature and impact of their dysphagia postchemoradiotherapy. Due to such extensive deficits, patients are encouraged to participate in individualized and targeted intervention protocols after the completion of nonsurgical treatment for their cancer. The importance of early and intensive rehabilitation to improve and maintain swallowing function is an emerging focus in the literature. Kotz, Costello, and Posner (2004) suggested that targeted treatment plans for oropharyngeal dysphagia associated with chemoradiotherapy for head and neck cancer include the effortful swallow, tongue base retraction exercises, and the super supraglottic swallow as well as the Mendelsohn maneuver and falsetto voice. Future studies are needed to determine whether the results of such programs lead to improved function and quality of life in this patient group. It is unfortunate, however, that some patients do not persist with post-treatment rehabilita-

**Table 7–6.** Patient Descriptions of Dysphagia and Its Impact Postchemoradiotherapy

- Limited texture and consistency of food managed
- Need for increased concentration to achieve the optimum swallowing pattern
- Limited ability to comply with postural changes due to pain/discomfort
- Limited ability to tolerate variable temperatures of food and liquids
- Inability to tolerate significant alterations in bolus volume
- Fatigue
- Altered production and properties of saliva
- Diminished appetite
- Trismus
- Pain and discomfort during swallowing with patient reports of burning sensation or pain with certain foods or food additives
- Need for extensive mouth care routine before and after meals
- Reduced motivation
- Anxiety

tion and/or are noncompliant with recommendations for managing their dysphagia, often resulting in nutritional compromise, aspiration pneumonia, and an overall reduction in quality of life.

**Dysphonia Following Chemoradiotherapy.** There are several studies that have investigated the efficacy of organ preservation protocols for advanced cancer of the head and neck. Organ preservation strategies include definitive radiotherapy, induction chemotherapy followed by radiotherapy, and concurrent chemoradiotherapy. Equivalent cure rates have been reported for both surgical and nonsurgical modes of treatment for advanced stage laryngeal cancer, yet the known toxic effects of combined chemoradiotherapy protocols when compared to surgical alternatives have prompted researchers to ask the question, Is the larynx worth preserving after chemoradiation?

As a result, both voice specific and overall quality of life data are emerging in the literature (Fung et al.,

2005); however, there are few studies which provide objective data regarding laryngeal function associated with larynx preservation. Meleca, Dworkin, Kewson, Stachler, and Hill (2003) undertook a retrospective study of 14 patients treated nonsurgically for Stage III and IV laryngeal cancer. The aims of the study were to use objective and perceptual evaluations to provide insight into the functional outcomes. Data presented included that obtained through acoustic and speech aerodynamic testing, voice perception analysis, and laryngeal function analysis as well as speech and voice proficiency ratings utilizing the Voice Handicap Index (VHI). Results from the acoustic and aerodynamic analyses demonstrated high cycle to cycle vocal fold vibratory instability with substantially higher than normal noise in the voice signal and lower maximum phonation times as well as increased glottal resistance and subglottal pressures. The authors reported that their data reflected increased valving at the supraglottic level, as well as higher pulmonary driven airflow to help overcome glottal incompetence and other tumor induced or treatment related vocal fold biomechanical abnormalities. Expert listeners judged voice and speech quality to be moderately deviant from normal with respect to prosody, vocal quality, and overall speech intelligibility. Videostroboscopic evaluation after completion of nonsurgical therapy was used to comment on laryngeal biomechanics. Moderately abnormal features were described which are outlined in Table 7–7. The authors proposed that these altered

**Table 7–7.** Abnormal Laryngeal Features Noted Postchemoradiotherapy

- Pooling of thick, sticky secretions around the laryngeal inlet
- Impaired vocal fold mobility
- Glottal incompetence
- Irregularities of the vocal fold margins
- Mucositis
- Asymmetric and insufficient amplitude of vocal fold vibration or mucosal waves which were either reduced or absent
- Recruitment of the ventricular vocal folds

*Source:* Meleca et al., 2003

structure and biomechanical abilities of the larynx after nonsurgical treatment are possibly related to:

- Vocal fold neuromuscular weakness which occurs as a result of disease infiltration
- Scarring caused by multiple biopsies prior to diagnosis/treatment
- Mucositis and postradiation fibrosis of laryngeal soft tissues
- Vocal fold ablative changes as a direct result of the radiotherapy

The post-treatment dysphonia was noticed to persist after treatment and often worsened with time. It is assumed that radiotherapy is largely responsible for the observed changes; however, the specific role of chemotherapy in producing permanent alterations to the function and structure of the larynx is not well defined and requires further investigation.

Despite noted changes to laryngeal and vocal fold function, on average Meleca et al. (2003) found that patients perceived only mild levels of quality of life voice difficulties after treatment. Fung et al. (2005) found similar results. Using the Voice Related Quality of Life measure (VR-QOL) they found that patients who underwent laryngeal preservation therapy reported worse VR-QOL scores compared to normal subjects but better VR-QOL when compared with patients who underwent laryngectomy. Additional prospective research including subjective and objective evaluations are required to identify criteria leading to optimal outcomes in terms of function which includes both swallowing and voice as well as overall quality of life. These measures should also serve to evaluate voice outcome following rehabilitation in this patient group and provide insight into the patient's perceived voice change over time and its impact on the quality of life in the long term.

## Surgical Management of Laryngeal and Hypopharyngeal Cancer

The surgical management of laryngeal and hypopharyngeal cancer involves surgery to the larynx, pharynx, or both larynx and pharynx. The ultimate aim of organ preservation or conservation laryngeal/pharyngeal surgery is to remove the cancer while retaining structures associated with respiration, phonation, and swallowing. The conservative surgical procedures discussed in the current chapter include the use of $CO_2$ laser surgery, vertical partial hemilaryngectomy, supraglottic laryngectomy, and supracricoid laryngectomy. While not conservative in the true sense as neither voice nor swallowing is retained, for completeness near total laryngectomy has also been included in this chapter.

Surgical management may be in isolation, following previous radiotherapy, or prior to radiotherapy +/− chemotherapy protocols. The extent of surgical procedures and subsequent variations can be confusing and often misleading. It is, therefore, important that the managing SLP is aware of the specific surgical resection and reconstruction both before and following surgery. This will enhance preoperative and postoperative management allowing for detailed preoperative education, accurate postoperative rehabilitation, and likely predication of outcome. Conservative surgical techniques preserve the associated organ, not necessarily the function. The presence and severity of the voice and swallowing disorder are generally more severe where the resections are more extensive. Therefore, depending on the procedure, the consequences on voice and swallowing range from minor disruptions to potentially life threatening changes. Consequently depending on the surgery, the extent of intervention by speech therapy, patient recovery patterns, and final outcomes will vary between procedures and will be outlined in the sections below. However, regardless of the intervention, assessment and treatment aims to optimize residual function for voice and swallowing.

Surgical resection of pharyngeal/laryngeal tumors with or without reconstruction is often followed by a course of radiotherapy. Dysphagia associated with surgical resection of laryngeal/hypopharyngeal tumors +/− reconstruction may be exacerbated by the early and late effects of postoperative radiotherapy (discussed in prior sections in this chapter). Therefore clinicians also need to prepare their patients for the additional changes to voice and swallowing function that may occur following completion of radiotherapy.

## CO$_2$ Laser Surgery

The use of laser as a surgical tool has increased since its development in the 1960s. In particular the use of $CO_2$ laser has been emerging in the management of malignancies in the head and neck regions since the 1970s (Cabanillas et al., 2004; Werner, Dunne, Folz, & Lippert, 2002). It is now considered a well-established tool in the excision of early glottic cancers as an alternate to XRT, with expanding application for the removal of larger glottic, supraglottic, and hypopharyngeal tumors. As with traditional surgery, the primary aim is to remove the tumor while preserving as much function as possible. Hence the potential for changes to the functions of swallowing and voice are dependant on the defect and laryngeal structures included in the procedure. As a general rule, the resulting dysphagia or dysphonia mirrors that seen by traditional surgical techniques; however, recovery time is frequently observed to be quicker.

There remains debate in the literature as to whether laser or radiotherapy results in the better outcomes for patients. Particularly in relation to voice outcome, there are studies that report no significant difference when the two modes of treatment are compared (Delsupehe, Zink, Lejaegere, & Bastian, 1999) and others which report a better voice outcome after radiotherapy (Krengli et al., 2004; Rydell, Schalen, Fex, & Elner, 1995). Peeters et al. (2004) retrospectively compared self-ratings on overall voice quality and using the Voice Handicap Index (VHI) in a group of patients treated with either radiotherapy or endoscopic laser surgery for T1a glottic cancer. These results were then compared with overall status of functional health. A significant difference between both treatment modalities was reported, with 58% of patients treated with radiotherapy having an abnormal total VHI score compared to only 40% of patients treated with endoscopic laser. No difference, however, was found when the two treatment modalities were compared with respect to functional health status. The contradictory results of current research would suggest that further research is needed and the methodology of these studies be carefully constructed to minimize limitations and bias.

### Swallowing

The use of $CO_2$ laser surgery will result in varying degrees of dysphagia depending upon the defect and laryngeal structures included in the procedure. Typically the functional interruption to the swallowing mechanism mirrors that observed following the traditional surgical approaches outlined further below. In addition, the rehabilitation strategies outlined will also apply. There are a number of advantages for the patients and the SLP managing swallowing following $CO_2$ laser surgery, including (a) a temporary tracheostomy is usually not required, (b) there is more rapid healing time, and (c) consequently reduced duration of nasogastric feeding. Indeed, Cabanillas and colleagues (2004) compared $CO_2$ laser surgery for supraglottic carcinoma to traditional supraglottic laryngectomy. While there was no difference to swallowing capacity in the long term, early recovery of swallowing deficits was faster following $CO_2$ laser surgery.

Both MBS and FEES are useful instrumental tools to assess and monitor aspiration and swallowing function following $CO_2$ laser surgery. In particular FEES is a useful tool to directly observe the altered anatomy, and its recovery, following laser surgery. On the CD there is footage of a patient at 5 days post- and again at 4 weeks post-laser surgery. Note the significant closing of the glottic gap as tissues ulcerate/granulate as healing progresses (Chapter 7: FEES: Laser 5 Days Post) and (Chapter 7: FEES: Laser 4 Weeks Post).

## Voice

$CO_2$ laser surgery may result in varying degrees of dysphonia depending upon the defect and laryngeal structures included in the procedure. $CO_2$ laser surgery may potentially affect normal vocal fold closure, normal glottic vibrations, and resonance characteristics of laryngeal anatomy resulting in dysphonia. Werner and colleagues (2002) report that $CO_2$ laser surgery for small glottic carcinoma typically does not affect long-term vocal function. Further research into voice quality and laryngeal function post-$CO_2$ laser surgery is required.

## Vertical Partial Laryngectomy/Hemilaryngectomy

A vertical partial laryngectomy or hemilaryngectomy is usually performed where there are unilateral laryngeal tumors. The aim of this surgical procedure is to save one true vocal fold to retain voice function. A standard hemilaryngectomy involves the total removal of one half of the larynx including one true vocal fold, one ventricle, and one false vocal fold. The hyoid bone,

epiglottis, and arytenoid cartilage are usually left intact (see Figure 7-10).

Due to the removal of vital laryngeal structures dysphonia and dysphagia are immediate likely consequences following a vertical partial laryngectomy or hemilaryngectomy. Recovery of voice and swallowing function is aided by both surgical reconstruction and subsequent therapy. Once the tumor is removed surgical reconstruction techniques provide tissue bulk for the remaining vocal fold to approximate with, assisting phonation and airway protection. Speech and swallowing outcomes may be further complicated by the need for extended procedures (e.g., the surgical resection involves the arytenoid cartilage or part of remaining vocal fold). Hence prior to commencing therapy the SLP should be fully aware of the extent of surgical resection and reconstruction technique that has occurred for the individual patient.

### Swallowing

A vertical partial laryngectomy or hemilaryngectomy interrupts airway protective mechanisms resulting in a potential dysphagia. The dysphagia is characterized by asymmetrical laryngeal elevation and reduced laryngeal closure and airway protection resulting in a risk of aspiration during the swallow. Postoperatively, dysphagia with short-term aspiration (50–67%) is experienced by most patients (Logemann et al., 1994). Despite this, the majority successfully resume oral intake. Difficulties are often temporary as the reconstructed tissue bulk quickly allows for approximation of the remaining vocal fold achieving adequate laryngeal closure and airway protection.

Immediately following surgery the patient will present with a tracheostomy tube in place to assist breathing and protect the airway. With respect to management of saliva, the SLP should initially be involved in the removal of the tracheostomy tube as per institution specific guidelines. A temporary feeding tube will also be in place until an oral diet can be satisfactory resumed. Provided there are no complications and instruction from the surgical team has been given, oral trials may commence approximately 7–10 days following surgery.

To prevent likely aspiration the patient will need to learn to compensate for the interruption to one aspect of the airway protective mechanism. Temporary

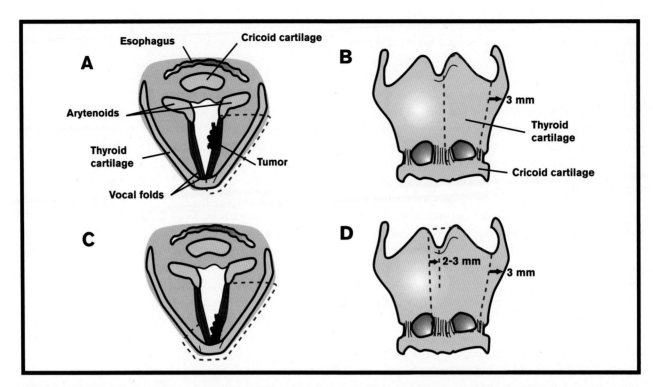

**Figure 7–10.** Illustration indicating the structures removed following vertical hemilaryngectomy for a recurrent T1a glottic tumor (midline laryngofissure) **A., B.,** or a recurrent T1b glottic tumor (paramedian laryngofissure) **C., D.** The dotted red line outlines the structures that are removed.

difficulties for the first few weeks may require the use of the following compensatory strategies to assist laryngeal closure such as chin tuck/tipping head forward, head rotation to operative side, or a combination of the two.

Upon discharge the majority of patients should have commenced oral intake with some returning to a near normal diet within 1 week (Jenkins et al., 1981). However the use of any strategies may need to continue for some weeks and regular follow-up is recommended. Swallowing difficulties further improve as the remaining side of the larynx learns to work harder closing the glottic gap created by surgery.

A standard hemilaryngectomy or vertical partial laryngectomy may be surgically extended to include the arytenoid cartilage posteriorly or the anterior commissure of the larynx or part of the remaining vocal fold anteriorly. The potential for swallowing difficulties is increased and the rehabilitation process is extended. Strategies such as chin tuck and head rotation may need to be employed longer than the first few weeks.

In addition laryngeal adduction exercises and the super supraglottic swallow may be required to further assist airway protection.

## Voice

Dysphonia following a vertical partial laryngectomy or hemilaryngectomy is characterized by breathiness, roughness, and changes to pitch levels and range. The surgical removal of one vocal fold and subsequent reconstruction of the neoglottis impacts on vocal fold closure and the normal glottic vibratory process; listen to the audio files on the CD (Chapter 7: Audio: "Hemilaryngectomy—Sustained Vowel" and "Hemilaryngectomy—Connected Speech").

Immediately postsurgery, voice is characterized by transient hoarseness and excessive breathiness. If the reconstruction technique has provided sufficient tissue bulk for the unoperated vocal fold to approximate with, a functional voice quality can generally be achieved. However vibratory quality of the voice remains compromised. Permanent changes can be experienced (i.e., limited ability to project the voice, or a voice that tires easily).

During the recovery/early postoperative period the voice is very breathy. Monitoring voice quality, providing voice education, and implementing voice care/vocal hygiene strategies are recommended in this early stage. Early intervention aims to increase the patient's awareness of his or her voice and its production, ensure that excessive constriction as a result of overcompensation for anatomical changes does not occur, and lay the foundation for later specific voice therapy programs. Despite a persistent dysphonia many patients are satisfied with the resulting voice quality for daily use and decline further therapy. However permanent changes can prove a concern for professional voice users and a therapy program may be requested.

If required, a more formal voice therapy program may commence once postoperative healing has occurred. Perceptual and instrumental assessment tools should be utilized to assess the resulting dysphonia. In particular, videoendoscopy and videostroboscopy are useful tools to evaluate the degree of incomplete glottic closure, site and quality of vibratory activity, and supraglottic activity during phonation. The general aim of voice therapy is to achieve a functional glottal sound; however, nonglottic sources can also provide satisfactory vibration for appropriate voice quality (Mandell et al., 1999). A supraglottic vibratory source is generally used where excessive breathiness remains. A voice therapy program, tailored to the individual, will likely focus on coordination of respiration and phonation, laryngeal adduction exercises, head and neck relaxation exercises, voice care, and voice projection techniques. The introduction of amplification tools or surgical medialization procedures may also need to be considered.

## Supraglottic Laryngectomy

A supraglottic laryngectomy is usually performed for the surgical treatment of tumors of the supraglottic region. A standard supraglottic laryngectomy involves the surgical resection of structures above the true vocal folds including the false vocal folds, aryepiglottic fold, valleculae, and epiglottis. In most cases part or the complete hyoid bone is also resected. The vocal folds and arytenoid cartilages remain intact (see Figure 7–11).

Due to the removal of vital airway protective mechanisms, dysphagia is a likely consequence following supraglottic laryngectomy. During surgery, surgeons undertake reconstruction to assist future airway protection, elevating the remaining larynx and suturing it under the tongue base. The purpose is to assist laryngeal elevation. While this does help facilitate swallowing recovery, intensive postoperative speech therapy is still needed to assist the successful resumption of oral intake. Functional voice quality is maintained as the true vocal folds are not included in the surgical technique.

Frequently, a standard supraglottic laryngectomy is extended to include other structures (i.e., base of tongue, arytenoid cartilage). Generally where the procedure is extended the rehabilitation process is longer and prognosis for swallowing recovery and airway protection is reduced (Rademaker et al., 1993).

## Swallowing

A supraglottic laryngectomy involves the removal of structures specific to airway protection. The resulting dysphagia is characterized by delayed oral pharyngeal transit time, delayed swallow reflex, reduced laryngeal elevation, and reduced vocal fold adduction. This results in poor pharyngeal clearance and a risk of aspiration of both saliva and fluids. The aspiration risk occurs both before and after the swallow due to the reduced protective ability of the airway and reduced pharyngeal clearance (Logemann et al., 1994; Schweinfurth & Silver, 2000).

Most patients experience dysphagia in the initial postoperative period. The base of tongue, arytenoids, and true vocal folds now provide postsurgical airway protection. While surgical reconstruction assists airway protection by elevating the remaining larynx and suturing it under the tongue base, swallowing difficulties are enhanced if the hyoid bone is involved in the surgical resection (as it provides the suspension mechanism for the larynx). In these cases, laryngeal elevation is reduced and the risk of aspiration is greater. See footage of MBS and FEES assessments of patients in the early stages post-supraglottic laryngectomy (Chapter 7:

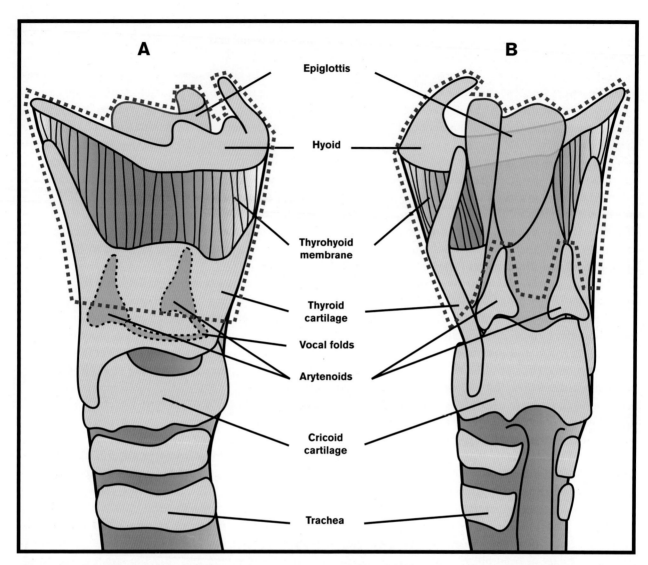

**Figure 7–11.** Illustration indicating the structures removed following supraglottic laryngectomy in anterolateral view **A.** and posterolateral view **B.** The dotted red line outlines the structures that are removed. Note that only the false vocal folds are removed and the true vocal folds remain.

MBS: Supraglottic with Aspiration, Chapter 7: FEES: 7 Days Post-Supraglottic FEES Assessment).

Accurate patient selection for this procedure is paramount and a speech pathology assessment should be considered prior to surgery to determine a patient's ability to relearn the swallowing mechanism. Motivation and the ability to follow and retain directions such as the supraglottic swallow are considering factors. In fact, swallowing therapy can commence prior to surgery and the supraglottic swallow is often introduced at this stage. If the clinician is unsure about a patient's ability to relearn the swallow mechanism then this needs to be discussed with the treating surgeon as this may impact on function following surgery.

Immediately following surgery the patient will present with a tracheostomy tube in place to assist breathing and protect the airway from potential aspiration of saliva. The SLP is involved in the process of determining suitability for removal of the tracheostomy tube. Early introduction of the supraglottic swallow technique without oral intake may assist in the management of secretions, removal of the tracheostomy tube, and strengthening related muscles involved in swallowing.

A temporary feeding tube will also be in place until an oral diet can be satisfactorily resumed. Provided there are no complications and instruction from the surgical team has been given, oral trials may commence approximately 7–10 days following surgery. To prevent likely aspiration the patient must relearn to protect the airway and successfully clear the bolus from the pharynx. Useful strategies include: (a) airway protective strategies such as supraglottic swallow and super supraglottic swallow, (b) rehabilitation exercises such as tongue base exercises, (c) postural changes such as chin tuck and head rotation, and (d) modification of diets and fluids.

The supraglottic swallow not only provides a voluntary airway protective mechanism but also limits pharyngeal residue post-swallow and subsequent aspiration. The super supraglottic swallow assists in closure of the airway entrance by improving tongue base posterior movement and anterior movement of the arytenoids. Tongue base strengthening and range of movement exercises teach the patient to retract the tongue base to make strong contact with the posterior pharyngeal wall to encourage bolus propulsion through the pharynx thus limiting pharyngeal residue (Logemann et al., 1994). Chin tuck and head positioning may also provide some benefits and should be considered in conjunction with a supraglottic swallow. Both MBS and FEES are useful instrumental tools to assess and monitor aspiration and determine the effectiveness of strategies and the appropriate consistency of diet and fluids. FEES is useful as a biofeedback tool when teaching the supraglottic swallow as it allows the patient to directly visualize the area, identifying when he or she achieves closure of the true vocal folds before the swallow and maintain closure during the swallow.

The use of laryngeal closure strategies and modified consistencies may need to continue for some weeks postdischarge and regular follow-up is recommended. On average 1 month is to be expected to relearn the swallow mechanism and resume a satisfactory oral diet without aspiration; however, 3 to 6 months is not unexpected (Jenkins et al., 1981). Success is determined by a number of critical factors including ability to gain airway closure at the level of vocal folds, closure at the level of airway entrance (arytenoid to tongue base), and strong capacity and motivation of the patient to relearn the swallowing mechanism (Rademaker et al., 1993).

Tumor size and location may necessitate a supraglottic laryngectomy be extended either inferiorly or superiorly to include the base of tongue or one or both arytenoids. Surgical extensions superiorly into the base of the tongue increase the risk of aspiration and ongoing swallowing difficulties. Longer rehabilitation programs are required (approximately 6 months) and further strategies may need to be considered such as teaching the super supraglottic swallow maneuver. Range of motion exercises and bolus control exercise may also prove useful (Rademaker et al., 1993). Some patients may never regain adequate tongue base movement to protect the airway from secretions and a total laryngectomy may need to be considered. Extension inferiorly into the piriform sinus and arytenoid cartilage significantly reduces the chance of normal recovery of swallowing without significant aspiration. Jenkins et al. (1981) state that anywhere between 2 and 12 months may be required for safe swallowing without aspiration. If not achieved, alternate feeding or total laryngectomy may be considered.

### Voice

The immediate dysphonia following a supraglottic laryngectomy is temporary in nature and characterized by a hoarse vocal quality. Any initial dysphonia experienced usually resolves in the early postoperative period as swelling to the surgical area reduces. Monitoring voice quality, providing voice education, and introducing voice care strategies are recommended in this early stage. As the true phonatory source (i.e., the vocal folds) is spared in this surgical procedure, long-term changes to voice quality are generally not observed. Subtle changes in voice quality may be experienced as the altered laryngeal anatomy will likely affect resonance characteristics.

## Supracricoid Laryngectomy

The supracricoid partial laryngectomy (SCPL) has emerged as an alternative to total laryngectomy in the management of selected laryngeal cancers. It involves the resection of tissues between the superior surface of the cricoid cartilage and inferior surface of the hyoid bone, specifically the thyroid cartilage, true vocal folds, false vocal folds, part of or complete epiglottis, pre-epiglottic space, and paraglottic space. The cricoid cartilage and one or both of the arytenoid cartilages are spared (see Figure 7–12). Sensory and motor innervation is maintained by retaining both the recurrent and superior laryngeal nerves bilaterally.

A SCPL with cricohyoidepiglottopexy involves the resection of the inferior portion of the epiglottis. The hyoid, tongue base, and epiglottic remnant are sutured to the cricoid cartilage. In contrast, a SCPL with cricohyoidepexy involves the complete resection of the epiglottis with only the hyoid and tongue base being sutured to the cricoid cartilage.

Dysphagia and dysphonia are two predictable morbidities following SCPL. Functional recovery of voice and swallowing is aided by surgical reconstruction where the cricoid cartilage is elevated and sutured to the hyoid bone. A laryngeal sphincter is achieved by the active opposition of the arytenoid cartilage(s) with the tongue base. Postoperatively intensive rehabilitation is beneficial to ensure prompt retraining of voice and swallowing.

Correct patient selection for SCPL is paramount and is frequently the key to good functional results. It is critical that the SLP be involved preoperatively to:

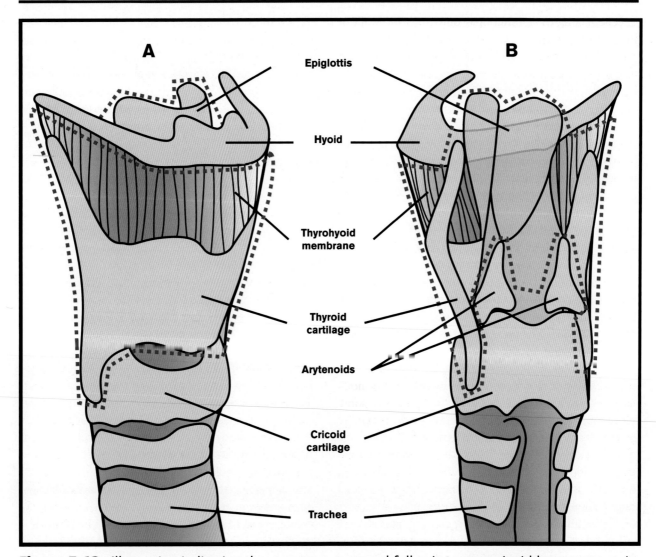

**Figure 7–12.** Illustration indicating the structures removed following supracricoid laryngectomy in anterolateral view **A.** and posterolateral view **B.** Note that the true and false vocal folds are removed.

■ assess the patient's ability to follow a rehabilitation program and advise outcomes to the surgical team

■ assist with counseling and education as patients are frequently prepared for both supracricoid laryngectomy and total laryngectomy

■ commence therapy activities that will enhance the postoperative rehabilitation program (i.e., tongue base retraction exercises)

Considering the severity of the surgical resection, patients who have undergone SCPL have achieved excellent long-term functional outcomes in swallowing and phonation.

## *Swallowing*

Dysphagia is a predicable consequence following SCPL and is characterized by poor airway protection resulting in frank aspiration during the swallow. Significant dysphagia for saliva and fluids is experienced as a SCPL involves the removal of vital airway protective structures (i.e., true vocal folds, false vocal folds, and the complete or part of the epiglottis). Hence the ability to achieve complete laryngeal closure for airway protection is removed. This is demonstrated on both the MBS and FEES footage on the CD (See Chapter 7: MBS/FEES: "Supracricoid MBS at 8 Weeks," "Supracricoid FEES at 10 Weeks' Aspiration Saliva"). Postsurgery, compensation for laryngeal closure is achieved from the approximation of the remaining arytenoids, tongue base, and if present the epiglottic remnant. This creates a neoglottic laryngeal sphincter that aims to provide airway protection. With the hyoid bone sutured to the cricoid cartilage, instant and permanent elevation is provided allowing the tongue base to shield the exposed airway. It is generally thought that retaining one arytenoid, not both, provides a tighter laryngeal sphincter. Reconstruction techniques where both arytenoids are retained often create a wider defect allowing more chronic aspiration.

Immediately following surgery the patient will present with a tracheostomy tube in place to assist breathing and protect the airway from aspiration of saliva. Despite the expectation of aspiration, the tracheostomy tube is frequently removed early following SCPL to enhance recovery of swallowing function. Following decannulation aspiration of secretions is typically observed; however, compensation is generally swift. A temporary feeding tube will also be in place until an oral diet can be satisfactorily resumed. Given the significant postoperative swallowing difficulties experienced, a PEG is often inserted at the time of surgery. Provided there are no complications and instruction from the surgical team has been given, oral trials may commence approximately 10 days following surgery.

Aspiration is expected by all patients when commencing oral trials; however, by the end of the second month the vast majority are on a total oral diet or have commenced resumption of an oral diet in conjunction with alternative/supplemental nutrition. Modifications to diet and fluids will need to be initially considered (i.e., thicken fluids or puree solids). Generally on discharge from hospital patients are no longer aspirating their own saliva and are just commencing a rehabilitation program for swallowing diet and fluids. As a result they require a large amount of outpatient support and monitoring.

The patient will need to specifically learn to push the bolus through the hypopharyngeal region without aspiration. Techniques to facilitate this include: (a) tongue base exercises, effortful swallow, supraglottic swallow, (b) chin tuck, head rotation, and (c) modification of diet and fluids.

The benefits of the supraglottic swallow technique may not be as significant following SCPL as they are for patients following supraglottic laryngectomy; however, it may aid arytenoid approximation and should still be considered as a worthwhile technique. Generally following SCPL, strategies such as the effortful swallow, chin tuck, and different head positioning are more effective as they aid the direction of the bolus. The tongue base now plays a significant role in manipulation of the bolus. Both MBS and FEES are useful instrumental tools to assess and monitor aspiration and determine the effectiveness of strategies and the appropriate consistency of diet and fluids. See footage on CD (Chapter 7: MBS/FEES: "Supracricoid FEES at 10 Weeks" and "Supracricoid MBS at 12 Weeks").

Literature suggests prompt recovery of swallowing function within 30 days. However this is not always the case with long-term recovery taking many months if not years. If chronic aspiration of secretions is detected, the option of a total laryngectomy may need to be considered. Considering the severity of the surgical resection, patients who have undergone SCPL have achieved excellent functional outcomes in swallowing and phonation.

### Voice

Dysphonia following a SCPL is characterized by breathiness, hoarseness, and low volume. Vocal projection is often difficult with the low volume providing functional problems. Patients often describe significant vocal fatigue in the initial stage as they strain to achieve optimal phonation via the neoglottis. However over time, vocal fatigue and strain decrease and there is an improvement in volume and voice quality.

Postoperatively, phonation is achieved via the neoglottis that is created as part of the reconstructive surgery. With the cricoid cartilage sutured to the hyoid bone, the remaining arytenoid(s) are able to approximate with the tongue base to provide a new source of phonation. Complete closure of the neoglottis is not usually achieved in the initial stages although greater approximations are achieved over time.

Immediately following SCPL, voice quality is very breathy. Monitoring voice quality, providing voice education, and implementing voice care/vocal hygiene strategies are recommended at this stage. Early intervention aims to monitor voice in the early stages as early recovery of phonation is more spontaneous and usually evolves in tandem with the improvement of swallowing.

A more formal voice therapy program may commence once postoperative healing has occurred and permission from the surgical team has been gained. Perceptual and instrumental assessment tools should be utilized to assess the resulting dysphonia. Patients need to learn to use a supraglottic vibratory source as both vocal folds are now removed. A voice therapy program following SCPL needs to be tailored to the individual but may include gentle pushing exercises, the implementation of appropriate vocal hygiene strategies, and strategies to assist vocal projection. Despite the significant dysphonia, most patients are generally satisfied with the functional quality of their voice. See endoscopic view and voice sample on CD

(Chapter 7: MBS/FEES: SCPL Voice). Also provided are audio files of sustained vowels and connected speech (Chapter 7: Audio: "Supracricoid—Sustained Vowel" and "Supracricoid—Connected Speech").

## Near Total Laryngectomy

The near total laryngectomy (NTL) procedure was first introduced by Pearson, Woods, and Hartman (1980) as a surgical option for advanced laryngeal cancers with the potential to preserve functional speech and swallowing. It is considered as an alternate to total laryngectomy with tracheoesophageal puncture. Generally, candidates are those considered appropriate for conservation laryngeal surgery but are compromised in terms of health or age or where the tumor extent does not permit conservative surgery but more extreme total laryngectomy is not warranted (Desanta, Pearson, & Olsen, 1989; Gavilan, Herranz, Prim, & Rabanal, 1996). During this procedure, the majority of the larynx is surgically removed leaving a strip of laryngeal musoca including an innovated true vocal fold, arytenoids, and the subgottal wall (see Figure 7–13). Reconstruction techniques utilize the remaining tumor-free tissue to fashion a voice shunt (fistula) between the airway and pharynx. A permanent tracheostoma is created bypassing nasal respiration as per total laryngectomy. Several variations of this surgical procedure exist including reconstruction techniques, extent of resection, and fashioning of the voice shunt.

Swallowing ability returns to normal or near normal following a NTL. The production of voice and its quality undergo significant changes. As aspiration via the voice shunt is an initial risk following this procedure it is recommended that the SLP focus first on regaining swallowing and once achieved then voice production via the voice shunt (Kasperbauer & Thomas, 2004).

### Swallowing

Swallowing function following a near total laryngectomy returns to normal in the long term. However, immediate postoperative aspiration may be experienced. A temporary feeding tube will be in place until an oral diet can be satisfactorily resumed. Provided there are no complications and instruction from the

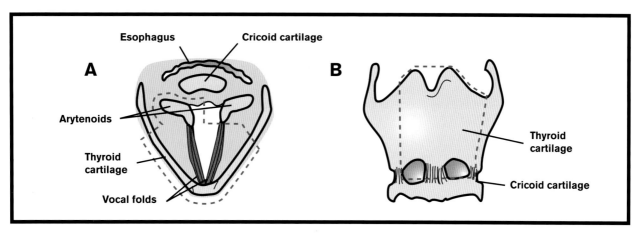

**Figure 7–13.** Illustration of the structures removed following a near total laryngectomy as seen from above **A.** and the front **B.** The dotted red line outlines the structures that are removed.

surgical team has been given, oral trials may commence approximately 10 days following surgery, and typically patients resume adequate oral intake 2 to 3 weeks postsurgery.

Aspiration via the shunt may occur; therefore, the voice shunt needs to be closely observed during assessment to identify if it closes during the swallow process, preventing aspiration. It is not uncommon, however, for patients to experience a slight or occasional leakage via the shunt during the swallow. If this occurs without symptoms, then further surgical procedures are not usually recommended. However if the aspiration is occurring so that there is coughing or risk of aspiration pneumonia then non-oral options or surgical intervention may need to be considered, i.e., closing of shunt. Useful strategies that may prevent or reduce the occurrence of aspiration via a voice shunt include: (a) postural changes, including chin tuck, head turn, (b) modification to bolus size, (c) modification of diets and fluids, particularly use of thicker fluids, and (d) covering stoma and gently exhaling (without voice) when swallowing.

## Voice

The voice undergoes permanent changes following NTL. On exhalation, pulmonary air is diverted via the voice shunt with digital occlusion of the tracheostoma. The remaining laryngeal mucosa forms the new vibratory source. The vibratory source is generally observed around the upper end of the shunt, especially around

the mucosa of the remnant arytenoid (Hanamitsu, Kataoka, Takeuchi, & Kitajima, 1999). The resulting voice quality is generally described as strained or hoarse. Hanamitsu and colleagues (1999) noted the voice quality following NTL to be similar to that of vertical hemilaryngectomy. A functional voice takes some effort to learn; however, once learned the resulting voice can be then produced easily. Unlike a total laryngectomy with tracheoesophageal puncture, no voice prosthesis is required following NTL. Kasperbauer and Thomas (2004) proposed an 80% chance of developing a highly functional voice via the vocal shunt following near total laryngectomy.

The timing of commencing voice therapy following NTL is crucial and requires close collaboration between the surgical team and SLP. Immediately postsurgery the patient will need to rely on alternate means of communication (i.e., writing, gestures, AAC options, mobile phone text writing, PDA/computers). An artificial larynx should also be introduced early as a temporary communication measure. This provides an initial voicing option and later can serve as a backup means of communication if difficulties arise.

The aim of voice therapy is to use the voice shunt for conversational speech. Some patients achieve conversational speech in the first session; however, usually 1 month is required to achieve adequate phonation. Unfortunately though for some patients, it may take months. Hence therapy predominately occurs on an outpatient basis. Learning to direct pulmonary air via the shunt generally commences 2-3 weeks postsurgery.

This allows for sufficient reduction of postsurgical swelling of the shunt, stabilization of swallowing, and removal of the nasogastric tube. Therapy sessions should then focus on learning to occlude the tracheostoma, learning to produce voice via the shunt, refining the quality of the voice produced, and ongoing troubleshooting which are detailed further in the following section.

### Learning to Occlude the Tracheostoma.

Digital occlusion of the tracheostoma on exhalation redirects pulmonary air via the shunt. A tracheostomy or laryngectomy tube should be removed first as it is easier to learn to occlude the stoma with direct skin contact. Inadequate occlusion will result in air leakage from the stoma. Learning to apply the correct pressure, or using a stoma button, can reduce coughing caused from excessive pressure or sensitive skin.

### Learning to Produce Voice.

Therapy should initially target teaching the patient to redirect air for phonation during the production of gentle vowel sounds or single words. Once this is achieved, the SLP can work with the patient, gradually increasing utterance complexity, until conversational speech is achieved. Many patients experience initial or intermittent aphonia. To troubleshoot, ensure that the postsurgical swelling and tightness have reduced, and check the stoma occlusion ensuring pressure is not excessive.

Generally the voice quality following NTL is described as strained or hoarse. However quality may be excessively strained and significant pulmonary effort is used to produce voice. Therapy may focus on ways to reduce this effort (i.e., use a softer voice, revise digital occlusion, reduce the length of utterance, minimize environmental factors such as background noise or excessive muscle tension). The utilization of hands-free appliances traditionally used following total laryngectomy may also be beneficial. The voice quality may also be described as "wet" and frequent dry swallows or instructing the patient to take clearing sips of water may reduce or eliminate this.

### Troubleshooting and Problem Solving.

Patients should be prepared to experience some temporary loss of voice function during radiotherapy, and alternate modes of communication may need to be used during this period. For those patients who, despite extensive therapy, fail to ever produce adequate voice, possible causes may be stenosis or tightening of the shunt. Generally, if voice has not occurred 4-6 months after surgery +/− radiotherapy, dilation of the shunt may be considered. Alternately, closing of the shunt and an artificial larynx, esophageal speech, or tracheoesophageal puncture and voice prosthesis after total laryngectomy are options.

## Conclusion

Multimodality approaches to the management of advanced head and neck cancer have emerged over the last decade. Despite these advances, there is no optimal approach which cures cancer and preserves the critical functions of voice and swallowing. It is known that both surgical and nonsurgical treatment for head and neck cancer adversely affect both voice and swallowing, thereby impacting on quality of life. A review of the current literature suggests an emerging focus on functional status following treatment for head and neck cancer, with the appearance of data on voice and swallowing outcomes being presented alongside logoregional control and survival rates. Objective data outlining the pattern of dysphagia and specific alterations to the anatomy and physiology of swallowing and voice will influence the development of effective intervention programs. In addition, outcome data are needed to assist treatment selection in this patient group.

## References

Andrews, M. L. (1995). *Manual of voice treatment: Pediatrics through geriatrics*. San Diego, CA: Singular Publishing.

Aviv, J. E., Kim, T., Sacco, R. L., Kaplan, S., Goodhart, K., Diamond, B., & Close, L. G. (1998). FEESST: A new bedside endoscopic test of the motor and sensory components of swallowing. *Annals of Otology, Rhinology and Laryngology, 107*, 378-387.

Beaver, M., Matheny, K. E., Roberts, D. B., & Myers, J. N. (2001). Predictors of weight loss during radiation therapy. *Otolaryngology-Head & Neck Surgery, 125*, 645-648.

Beekhuis, G. J., & Harrington, E. B. (1965). Trismus. Etiology and management of inability to open the mouth. *Laryngoscope, 75,* 1234–1258.

Brandenburg, J. H. (2001). Laser cordectomy versus radiotherapy: An objective cost analysis. *Annals of Otology, Rhinology and Laryngology, 110,* 312–318.

Brizel, D. M., Wasserman, T. H., & Henke, M. (2000). Phase III randomized trial of amifostine as a radioprotector in head and neck cancer. *Journal of Clinical Oncology, 18,* 3339–3345.

Buchbinder, D., Currivan, R. B., Kaplan, A. J., & Urken, M. L. (1993). Mobilization regimens for the prevention of jaw hypomobility in the radiated patient: A comparison of three techniques. *Journal of Oral and Maxillofacial Surgery, 51,* 863–867.

Cabanillas, M. D., Rodrigo, J. P., Llorente, L. L., Suarez, M. D., Ortega, M. D., & Suarez, C. (2004). Functional outcomes of transoral laser surgery of supraglottic carcinoma compared with a transcervical approach. *Head & Neck, 26*(8), 653–659.

Chen, A. Y., Frankowski, R., Bishop-Leone, J., Hebert, T., Leyk, S., Lewin, J., & Goepfert, H. (2001). The development and validation of a dysphagia-specific quality-of-life questionnaire for patients with head and neck cancer: The M. D. Anderson dysphagia inventory. *Archives of Otolaryngology-Head Neck Surgery, 127*(7) 870–876.

Cichero, J., & Murdoch, B. (2006). *Dysphagia: Foundation, theory and practice.* Chichester, United Kingdom: Wiley & Sons.

Crary, M. A., Carnaby (Mann), G. D., Groher, M. E., & Helseth, E. (2004). Functional benefits of dysphagia therapy using adjunctive sEMG biofeedback. *Dysphagia, 19,* 160–164.

Delanian, S., & Lefaix, J. L. (2004). The radiation induced fibroatrophic process: Therapeutic perspective via the antioxidant pathway. *Radiotherapy and Oncology, 73,* 119–131.

Delanian, S., Porcher, R., Balla-Mekias, S., & Lefaix, J. L. (2003). Randomised, placebo-controlled trial of combined pentoxifylline and tocopherol for regression of superficial radiation induced fibrosis. *Journal of Clinical Oncology, 21,* 2545–2550.

Delsupehe, K.G., Zink I., Lejaegere, M., & Bastian, R. W. (1999). Voice quality after narrow-margin laser cordectomy compared with laser irradiation. *Otolaryngology-Head and Neck Surgery, 121*(5), 528–533.

Denk, D. M., & Kaider, A. (1997). Videoendoscopic biofeedback: A simple method to improve the efficacy of swallowing rehabilitation of patients after head and neck surgery. *Journal of Otology Rhinology and its Related Specialties, 59*(2), 100–105.

DeSanto, L. W., Pearson, B. W., & Olsen, K, D. (1989). Utility of near-total laryngectomy for supraglottic, pharyngeal, base of tongue and other cancers. *Annals of Otology, Rhinology and Laryngology, 98*(1), 2–7.

Dijkstra, P. U., Kalk, W. W., & Roodenburg, J. L. (2004). Trismus in head and neck oncology: A systematic review. *Oral Oncology, 40,* 879–889.

Dikeman, K. J., & Kazandjian, M. S. (2003) *Communication and swallowing management of tracheostomized and ventilator dependent patients* (2nd ed.). Clifton Park, NY: Thompson Delmar Learning.

Ding, R., & Logemann, J. A. (2005). Swallow physiology in patients with trach cuff inflated or deflated: A retrospective study. *Head & Neck, 27,* 809–813.

Dworkin, J. P., Hill, S. J., Stachler, R. J., Meleca, R. J., & Kewson, D. (2006). Swallowing function outcomes following non surgical therapy for advanced stage laryngeal carcinoma. *Dysphagia, 21*(1), 66–74.

Eisbruch, A. (2004). Dysphagia and aspiration following chemo irradiation of head and neck cancer: Major obstacles to intensification of therapy. *Annals of Oncology, 15,* 363–364.

Eisbruch, A., Lyden, T., Bradford, C. R., Dawson, L. A., Haxer, M. J., Miller, A. E., et al. (2002). Objective assessment of swallowing dysfunction and aspiration after radiation concurrent with chemotherapy for head and neck cancer. *International Journal of Radiation Oncology, Biology, Physics, 53,* 23–28.

Eisbruch, A., Schwartz, M., Rasch, R., Vineburg, K., Damen, E., Van As, C., et al. (2004). Dysphagia and aspiration after chemoradiotherapy for head and neck cancer: Which anatomic structures are affected and can they be spared by IMRT? *International Journal of Oncology, Biology and Physics, 60,* 1425–1439.

Fung, K., Lyden, T. H., Lee, J., Urba, S. G., Worden, F., Eisbruch, A., et al. (2005). Voice and swallowing outcomes of an organ preservation trial for advanced laryngeal cancer. *International Journal of Radiation Oncology, Biology, Physics, 63,* 1395–1399.

Gavilan, J., Herranz, J., Prim, P., & Rabanal, I. (1996). Speech results and complications of near-total laryngectomy. *Annals of Otology, Rhinology and Laryngology, 105,* 729–733.

Gaziano, J. (2002). Evaluation and management of oropharyngeal dysphagia in head and neck cancer. *Cancer Control, 9,* 400–409.

Groher, M. (1997). *Dysphagia: Diagnosis and management* (3rd ed.). Newton, MA: Butterworth-Heinemann.

Haddad, P., Kalaghchi, B., & Amouzegar-Hashemi, F. (2005). Pentoxifylline and vitamin E combination for superficial radiation-induced fibrosis: A phase II clinical trial. *Radiotherapy and Oncology, 77*(3), 324-326.

Hanamitsu, M., Kataoka, H., Takeuchi, E., & Kitajima, K. (1999). Comparative study of vocal function after near total laryngectomy. *Laryngoscope, 109,* 1320-1323.

Hanna, E., Alexiou, M., Morgan, J., Badley, J., Maddox, A., Penagaricano, J., et al. (2004). Intensive chemoradiotherapy as a primary treatment for organ preservation in patients with advanced cancer of the head and neck: Efficacy, toxic effects and limitations. *Archives of Otolaryngology-Head & Neck Surgery, 130,* 861-867.

Hogikan, N. D., & Sethuraman, G. (1999). Validation of an instrument to measure voice-related quality of life (V-RQOL). *Journal of Voice, 13,* 557-569.

Huckabee, M. L., & Pelletier, C. A. (1999). *Management of adult neurogenic dysphagia* (Dysphagia series). San Diego, CA: Singular Publishing.

Ichimura, K., & Tanaka, T. (1993). Trismus in patients with malignant tumours in the head and neck. *Journal of Laryngology and Otology, 107,* 1017-1020.

Jacobson, G., Johnson, A., Grywalski, C., Sibergleit, A., Jacobson, G., Benninger, M. S., & Newman, C. W. (1997). The Voice Handicap Index (VHI): Development and validation. *American Journal of Speech and Language Pathology, 6,* 66-70.

Jenkins, P., Logemann, J., Lazarus, C., & Ossoff, R. (1981, November). *Functional changes after hemilaryngectomy.* Paper presented at ASHA meeting, Los Angeles.

Kasperbauer, J. L., & Thomas, J. E. (2004). Voice rehabilitation after near total laryngectomy. *Otolaryngologic Clinics of North America, 37*(3), 655-677.

Kendall, A. K., Leonard, R. J., McKenzie, S. W., & Jones, C. U. (2000). Timing of swallowing events after single modality treatment of head and neck carcinomas with radiotherapy. *The Annals of Otology, Rhinology and Laryngology, 109,* 767-775.

Kotz, T., Costello, R., & Posner, M. R. (2004). Swallowing dysfunction after chemoradiation for advanced squamous cell carcinoma of the head and neck. *Head & Neck, 26,* 365-372.

Krengli, M., Policarpo, M., Manfredda, I., Aluffi, P., Gambado, G., Maximiliano, P., et al. (2004). Voice quality after treatment for T1a glottic carcinoma. *Acta Oncologica, 43,* 284-289.

Laurell, G., Kraepelien, T., Mavroidis, P., Lind, B. K., Fernberg., J., Beckman, M., et al. (2003). Stricture of the proximal oesophagus in head and neck carcinoma patients after radiotherapy. *Cancer, 97,* 1693-1700.

Lee, J. H., Machtay, M., Unger, L., Weinstein, G. S., Weber, R. S., Chalian, A. A., et al. (1998). Prophylactic gastrostomy tube in patients undergoing intensive irradiation for cancer of the head and neck. *Archives of Otolaryngology-Head & Neck Surgery, 124*(8), 871-875.

List, M. A., D'Antonio, L. L., Cella, D. F., Siston, A., Mumby, P., Haraf, D., & Vokes, E. (1996). The performance status scale for head and neck cancer patients and the functional assessment of cancer therapy-head and neck scale. A study of utility and validity. *Cancer, 77*(11), 2294-2301.

List, M. A., Ritter-Sterr, C. A., & Lansky, S. B. (1990). A performance status scale for head and neck cancer patients. *Cancer, 66,* 564-569.

Logemann, J. A. (1997). *Evaluation and treatment of swallowing disorders.* Austin, TX: Pro-Ed.

Logemann, J. A. (2006). Update on clinical trials in dysphagia. *Dysphagia, 21*(2), 116-120.

Logemann, J. A., Gibbons, P., Rademaker, A. W., Pauloski, B. R., Kahrilas, P. J., Bacon, M., et al. (1994). Mechanisms of recovery of swallow after supraglottic laryngectomy. *Journal of Speech and Hearing Research, 37,* 965-974.

Logemann, J. A., Smith, C. H., Pauloski, B. R., Rademaker, A. W., Lazarus, C. L., Colangelo, L. A., et al. (2001). Effects of xerostomia on perception and performance of swallow function. *Head & Neck, 23,* 317-321.

Logemann, J. A., Williams, R. B., Rademaker, A., Paulowski, B. R., Lazarus, C. L., & Cook, I. (2006). The relationship between observations and measures of oral and pharyngeal residue from video-fluoroscopy and scintigraphy. *Dysphagia, 20*(3), 226-231.

Mandell, D. L., Woo, P., Behin, D., Mojica, J., Minasian, A., Urken, M. L., & Biller, H. F. (1999). Videolaryngostroboscopy following vertical partial laryngectomy. *Annals of Otology, Rhinology and Laryngology, 108,* 1061-1067.

Mekhail, T. M., Adelstein, D. J., Rybicki, L. A., Larto, M. A., Saxton, J. P., & Lavertu, P. (2001). Enteral nutrition during the treatment of head and neck carcinoma. Is a percutaneous endoscopic gastrostomy tube preferable to a nasogastric tube? *Cancer 91*(9), 1785-1790.

Meleca, R. J., Dworkin, J. P., Kewson, D., Stachler, R. J., & Hill, S. (2003). Functional outcomes following non surgical treatment for advanced stage laryngeal carcinoma. *Laryngoscope, 113*(4), 720-728.

Mittal, B. B., Pauloski, B., Haraf, D. J., Pelzer, H. J., Argiris, A, Vokes, E., et al. (2003). Swallowing dysfunction—Preventative and rehabilitation strategies in patients with head and neck cancers treated with surgery, radiotherapy, and chemotherapy: A critical review. *International Journal of Oncology Biology Physics, 57,* 1219-1230.

Nguyen, T. D., Panis, X., Froissart, D., Legros, M., Coninx, P., & Loirette, M. (1988). Analysis of late complications after rapid hyperfractionated radiotherapy in advanced head and neck cancers. *International Journal of Radiation Oncology, Biology, Physics, 14,* 23-25.

Nordgren, M., Jannert, M., Boysen, M., Ahlner-Elmqvist, M., Silander, E., Bjordal, K., & Hammerlid, E. (2006). Health related quality of life in patients with pharyngeal carcinoma: A five year follow up. *Head & Neck, 28,* 339-349.

Pauloski, B. R., & Logemann, J. A. (2000). Impact of tongue base and posterior pharyngeal wall biomechanics on pharyngeal clearance in irradiated post surgical oral cancer patients. *Head & Neck, 22,* 120-131.

Pauloski, B. R., Rademaker, A. W., Logemann, J. A., & Colangelo, L. A. (1998). Speech and swallowing in irradiated and non irradiated post surgical oral cancer patients. *Otolaryngology-Head & Neck Surgery, 118,* 616-624.

Pauloski, B.R., Rademaker, A. W., Logemann, J. A., Lazarus, C. A., Newman, L., Hamner, A., et al. (2000). Swallow function and perception of dysphagia in patients with head and neck cancer. *Head & Neck, 24,* 555-565.

Pauloski, B.R, Rademaker, A. W., Logemann, J. A., Stein, D., Beery, Q., Newman, L., et al. (2000). Pretreatment swallow function in patients with head and neck cancer. *Head & Neck, 22,* 474-482.

Pearson, B., Woods, R., & Hartman, D. (1981). Extended hemilaryngectomy for T3 glottic carcinoma with preservation of speech and swallowing. *The Laryngoscope, 91,* 1950-1961.

Peeters, A. J., van Gogh, C. D., Goor, K. M., Verdonck-de Leeuw, I. M., Langendijk, J. A., & Mahieu, H. F. (2004). Health status and voice outcome after treatment for a T1a glottic carcinoma. *European Archives of Oto-Rhino-Laryngology, 261*(10), 534-540.

Pollens, R. (2004). Role of the speech-language pathologist in palliative hospice care. *Journal of Palliative Medicine, 7,* 694-702.

Rademaker, A. W., Logemann, J. A., Pauloski, B. R., et al. (1993). Recovery of post operative swallowing in patients undergoing partial laryngectomy. *Head & Neck, 15,* 325-224.

Rademaker, A. W., Vonesh, E. F., Logemann, J. A., Paulowski, B. R., Liu, D., et al. (2003). Eating ability in head and neck cancer patients following chemo-radiation: A 12-month follow-up study accounting for dropout. *Head and Neck, 25*(12), 1034-1041.

Rubin, R. L., & Doku, H. C. (1976). Therapeutic radiology—The modalities and their effects on oral tissues. *Journal of the American Dental Association, 92,* 731-739.

Rydell, R., Schalen, L., Fex, S., & Elner, A. (1995). Voice evaluation before and after laser excision vs. radiotherapy of a T1A glottic carcinoma. *Acta Oto-laryngologica. 115*(4), 560-565.

Schweinfurth, J. M., Boger, G. N., & Feustel, G. F. (2001). Preoperative risk assessment for gastrostomy tube placement in head and neck cancer patients. *Head & Neck, 23,* 376-382.

Schweinfurth, J., M., & Silver, S. M. (2000). Patterns of swallowing after supraglottic laryngectomy. *The Laryngoscope, 110,* 1266-1270.

Scully, C., Epstein, J., & Sonis, S. (2003). Oral mucositis: A challenging complication of radiotherapy, chemotherapy, and radiochemotherapy: Part 1, Pathogenesis and prophylaxis of mucositis. *Head & Neck, 25,* 1057-1070.

Senft, M., Feitkau, R., Iro, H., Sailer, D., & Sauer, R. (1993). The influence of supportive nutritional therapy via percutaneous endoscopically guided gastrostomy on the quality of life of cancer patients. *Supportive Care in Cancer, 1,* 272-275.

Steelman, R., & Sokol, J. (1986). Quantification of trismus following irradiation of the temporomandibular joint. *Missouri Dental Journal, 66,* 21-23.

Sullivan, C. A., Jaklitsch, M. T., Hadda, R., Goguen, L. A., Gagne, A., Wirth, L. J., et al. (2004). Endoscopic management of hypopharyngeal stenosis after organ sparing therapy for head and neck cancer. *Laryngoscope, 114*(11), 1924-1931.

Teng, M., & Futran, N. D. (2005). Osteoradionecrosis of the mandible. *Current Opinion in Otolaryngology and Head and Neck Surgery, 13,* 217-221.

Thorn, J. J., Hansen, H. S., Specht, L, & Bastholt, L. (2000). Osteoradionecrosis of the jaws: Clinical characteristics and relation to the field of radiation. *Journal of Oral and Maxillofacial Surgery, 58,* 1088-1093.

Wasserman, T. H., Brizel, D. M., Henke, M., Monnier, A., Eschwege, M. D., Sauer, R., et al. (2005). Influence of intravenous amifostine on xerostomia, tumour control, and survival after radiotherapy for head and neck cancer: Two year follow up of a prospective, randomized, phase III trial. *International Journal of Radiation Oncology, Biology, Physics, 63*(4), 985-990.

Wedman, J., Heimdal, J. H., Elstad, I, & Olofsson, J. (2002). Voice results in patients with T1a glottic cancer treated by radiotherapy or endoscopic measures. *European Archives of Otorhinolaryngology, 259,* 547-550.

Werner, J. A., Dunne, A. J., Folz, B. J., & Lippert, B. M. (2002) Transoral laser microsurgery in carcinomas of the oral cavity, pharynx, and larynx. *Cancer Control, 9*(5), 379-386.

Weymuller, E. A., Alsarraf, R., Yueh, B., Deleyiannis, F. W. B., & Coltrera, M. D. (2001). Analysis of the performance characteristics of the University of Washington Quality of Life Instrument and its modification (UW-QOL-R). *Archives of Otolaryngology–Head & Neck Surgery, 127,* 489-493.

# Chapter 8

# NONSURGICAL VOICE RESTORATION FOLLOWING TOTAL LARYNGECTOMY

Jeff P. Searl and I. Susan Reeves

## Introduction

The history of alaryngeal speech training is longer for artificial larynx (AL; including electrolarynx [EL] and pneumatic devices) and esophageal speech (ES) relative to tracheoesophageal (TE) speech. However, the introduction of TE speech in the early 1980s (Singer & Blom, 1980) has led to a significant shift in postlaryngectomy speech rehabilitation toward TE speech, particularly in countries with predominantly Western medical practices. Despite the rise of TE speech as a viable communication option, it may not be the most appropriate or the preferred choice for all individuals. We agree with Doyle (2005): "Clinicians must fight the urge to dismiss any of the post-laryngectomy communication options presently available (esophageal, electrolarynx or tracheoesophageal puncture speech) without adequate cause" (p. 548).

Gress (2004) indicated that in an ideal situation, patients are informed about the advantages, disadvantages, and prerequisites of AL, ES, and TE speech. However, she recognized that the ideal situation is often not attained in practice for a variety of reasons. The speech-language pathologist (SLP) and surgeon can have a major role in shaping a laryngectomized patient's expectations and attitudes toward any form of alaryngeal speech (Frowen & Perry, 2001). Whether unwittingly or not, the biases that a health care professional has toward AL, ES, and TE speech could serve to restrict the postsurgical speech options that a patient knows about or pursues.

This chapter focuses on the rehabilitation process for AL (predominantly referring EL use) and ES speech, the two main nonsurgical voice restoration options. The third, surgical, voice restoration option, TE speech,

will be covered in detail in Chapter 9. From a clinical perspective, we begin the current chapter from the following premise: AL, ES, and TE speech are not in competition with one another with the goal of crowning one as superior. Rather, the goal is to identify the most appropriate alaryngeal communication option based on a person's abilities, needs, and preferences at a particular point in the recovery.

## Esophageal Speech

### Relevance in the Context of Western Medicine

Prior to the introduction of TE speech in the early 1980s, ES played a prominent role in alaryngeal speech rehabilitation. Electrolarynx speech was another option, but ES was the "gold standard" for many years as a negative bias against AL use persisted (Doyle, 1994; Gates, Ryan, & Lauder, 1982). In addition to the fact that the EL voice was mechanical sounding, there was a prevailing notion that individuals who were offered an AL and had some form of easily acquired verbal communication soon after surgery would have reduced motivation for learning ES, which was considered to be more natural sounding. Over the years, the persistence of many clinicians and laryngectomy patients, as well as improvements in AL devices, has helped to refute the negative bias toward AL by demonstrating how usable this form of speech could be, either as an early postoperative method of communication only or as a long-term communication option (Doyle, 1994; Duguay, 1978; Salmon, 1983). While a negative perception of AL speech may still persist in some locales, significant strides have been made in recognizing the role of good AL speech for the laryngectomized patient. Ironically, with greater acceptance of AL speech and the advent of TE speech as a third option, ES has become the least utilized of the speech modes in many countries with predominantly Western medical practice (Brown, Hilgers, Irish, & Balm, 2003; Hillman, Walsh, Wolf, Fisher, & Hong, 1998; Salmon, 2005).

Despite the reduction in popularity of ES over the last 20-25 years, it can be appropriate, and in some cases preferred, for certain individuals. The issue is identifying these individuals. Esophageal speech does offer advantages over AL and TE speech that can be substantial. Specific advantages and disadvantages per mode are offered in Tables 8-1, 8-2, and 8-3. Table 8-1 addresses issues regarding the speech process, Table 8-2 reviews issues regarding characteristics of the speech itself, and Table 8-3 includes training and other issues. A detailed comparison is not the goal here, but rather a highlighting of key issues.

For some patients, ES may be selected as their primary mode of communication. These may be individuals who: (1) find aspects of TE or AL speech objectionable, (2) do not have the prerequisites for TE or AL speech, or (3) prefer ES because of its advantages. For example, some individuals may object to the reliance on a mechanical device or prosthesis for voice production,

**Table 8-1.** Comparison of Artificial Larynx (AL), Esophageal (ES), and Tracheoesophageal (TE) Speech in Terms of Speech Process Issues

| Speech Process Issues | Artificial Larynx Speech | Esophageal Speech | Tracheoesophageal Speech |
|---|---|---|---|
| Mechanical device/ prosthetic required | Yes | No | Yes |
| Hand occupied during voicing | Yes/no (Yes, unless using a device housed within the dentures, or in a dental bridge, or the newer hands-free EL device) | No | Yes/no (Some are able to use a hands-free speaking valve) |
| Interference with oral movements | Yes/no (Use of an oral adaptor can cause interference) | No | No |
| Good visual acuity required | No (Reduced visual acuity can generally be tolerated although some devices with small dials and buttons may be more problematic) | No | Yes/no (Voice production: No special requirement usually needed) (Prosthesis care: May need caregiver support if visual acuity is reduced) |
| Finger/hand/arm dexterity required | Yes (Requires ability to hold, activate, and manipulate device controls; use of within-the-oral-cavity devices can mitigate this requirement) | No | Yes/no (Voice production: Requires ability to manually occlude stoma unless using a hands-free valve, which itself requires fine motor control for attachment; caregiver could assist) (Prosthesis care: Fine motor control needed unless caregiver assumes the duty) |

**Table 8–2.** Comparison of Artificial Larynx (AL), Esophageal (ES), and Tracheoesophageal (TE) Speech in Terms of Speech Product Issues (i.e., Characteristics of the Alaryngeal Speech/Voice)

| Speech Product Issues | Artificial Larynx Speech | Esophageal Speech | Tracheoesophageal Speech |
|---|---|---|---|
| Voice quality and acceptability[1-4] | Mechanical/unnatural; less preferred than laryngeal; generally less preferred quality than ES or TE | Glottal fry, hoarse, rough, wet, breathy; less preferred than laryngeal and TE | Glottal fry, hoarse, rough, wet, breathy; generally, less deviant than ES and AL, but less preferred than laryngeal |
| Speaking fundamental frequency mean[5-7] | Determined by device used—some are adjustable | Lower than TE and laryngeal speakers | Lower than laryngeal speakers, but generally not as low as ES |
| Intonation/pitch variability[8-10] | Restricted primarily by the device used but some manipulation may be possible | Restricted relative to laryngeal and TE; greater than AL | Restricted relative to laryngeal; greater than ES and AL |
| Speaking intensity mean[3,7,11,12] | Adjustable—potentially louder than ES, TE, and laryngeal speech | Less intense than laryngeal, AL, and TE | Varies from less than, equal to, to greater than laryngeal; greater than ES |
| Speaking rate[10,13,14] | Equal to/possibly faster than laryngeal, ES, and TE | Slower than laryngeal, AL, and TE | Comparable to laryngeal; faster than ES |
| Speech intelligibility[15-17] | Less than laryngeal, TE, and ES in high signal-noise situations; may be higher than TE and ES in noise for some devices/speakers | Less than laryngeal and TE, generally | Less than laryngeal; typically greater than ES and AL (except possibly in noise for the latter) |
| Overall "success" achieving usable speech[4,16,18-21] | Generally, a fairly high success rate (large percentage of users) | Generally considered to have the lowest of the three | Typically higher than ES; comparable to or higher than AL |

Notes. [1]Merwin, Goldstein, & Rothman, 1985; [2]Clark & Stemple, 1982; [3]Tardy-Mitzell, Andrews, & Bowman, 1985; [4]McAuliffe, Ward, Bassett, & Perkins, 2000; [5]Snidecor & Curry, 1960; [6]Weinberg & Bennett, 1972; [7]Robbins, Fisher, Blom, & Singer, 1984; [8]Salmon, 1999; [9]Bennett & Weinberg, 1973; [10]Trudeau, 1994; [11]Blood, 1981; [12]Max, Steurs, & de Bruyn, 1996; [13]Salmon, 2005; [14]Pauloski, 1998; [15]Clark, 1985; [16]Hillman, Walsh, Wolf, Fisher, & Hong, 1998; [17]Blom et al., 1986; [18]Koike et al., 2002; [19]Singer et al., 1981; [20]Mehta et al., 1995; [21]Ward, Koh, Frisby, & Hodge, 2003.

preferring to rely solely on their own body. Others might not have the eyesight, manual dexterity, or a capable caregiver to assume TE valve care.

Some individuals may opt to learn ES to serve as a supplement to either EL or TE speech. For example, a TE or AL user may find it convenient to be able to produce words or short phrases using ES in select circumstances (e.g., quick social niceties such as "Thank you," "Bye-bye," etc.). Still others may learn ES in recognition of the fact that AL and TE speech are sometimes problematic. For example, AL users may find themselves with a broken device and no backup. A TE user with

a malfunctioning indwelling valve may be waiting to see the SLP. Whether it is a matter of days or only hours, all laryngectomy speakers should have a backup means of communicating. Esophageal speech could serve that role.

Scanning Tables 8-1 to 8-3, the principle advantages of ES fall mainly with speech process issues (see Table 8-1). Nothing other than the patient's own body is required and there are no particular requirements as far as visual acuity or hand/arm control. For some individuals, the freedom to use both hands for other tasks while talking is particularly important. Hands-free

**Table 8–3.** Comparison of Artificial Larynx (AL), Esophageal (ES), and Tracheoesophageal (TE) Speech in Terms of the Therapy Process and Other Issues

| Therapy Processes and Other Issues | Artificial Larynx Speech | Esophageal Speech | Tracheoesophageal Speech |
|---|---|---|---|
| Onset of therapy postsurgery | Earliest of the alaryngeal options (within 2–3 days postsurgery) | Later than AL, similar to TE | Later than AL, similar to ES |
| Duration of the therapeutic process to functional speech | Generally shorter than ES and similar in duration to TE | Longest training time of all of the alaryngeal options | Shorter than ES, similar to AL |
| Cost | Less than TE | Less than TE | Most expensive |
| Availability of qualified SLP services | In urban settings and hospitals, SLPs are generally available to provide this service; services in rural areas are less commonly available | Anecdotal reports and personal communications suggest that fewer SLPs are familiar with ES training these days in any setting | In urban settings and larger hospitals, SLPs are generally available to provide this service; services in rural areas for TE care are perhaps less common |
| Ongoing maintenance of device/prosthetic | There is ongoing care of the device and the batteries that power it | No | Daily cleaning of the valve is usually recommended; patient changeable valves and indwelling valves both require a regular schedule of removal and reinsertion |
| Reliance on SLP post-acquisition of speech | No | No | Yes, if using an indwelling valve |

speech is certainly possible with TE speech (see Chapter 9), but requires additional hardware with associated daily care that may be more than what the patient wishes to take on. Recently, hands-free EL approaches, such as the artificial larynx holder for a TruTone™ device (Griffin Laboratories), the JusTalk (JustMed), and the Ultra-Voice Plus (Ultra-Voice) have become available. Again, however, these all involve additional hardware (e.g., chest strap, headset microphone, amplifier), which may be visible to the listener or require care, adjustment, and control by the speaker.

Esophageal speech does not fair nearly so well in terms of speech characteristics. All three communication modes deviate from laryngeal speech. However, TE speech is generally regarded as the most similar to laryngeal speech (Bertino, Bellomo, Miani, Ferrero, & Staffieri, 1996; Eadie & Doyle, 2004; Robbins, Fisher,

Blom, & Singer, 1984; van As, Koopmans-van Beinum, Pols, & Hilgers, 2003). The literature also generally favors TE over ES in terms of intelligibility (Ainsworth & Singh, 1992; Doyle, Danhauer, & Reed, 1988; Max, DeBruyn, & Steurs, 1997) as well as listener and speaker acceptability (Blom, Singer, & Hamaker, 1986; Miani, Bertino, Bellomo, & Staffieri, 1998).

The acoustic, perceptual, and listener preference data should give clinicians reason to ask: why consider ES in light of the advantages of TE speech? Some answers to this question are more obvious and have been alluded to above. Availability of nonsurgical options is necessary for individuals who do not meet the prerequisites for TE use (see Chapter 9) or who do not tolerate the disadvantages associated with TE speech (ongoing costs, intermittent but ongoing reliance on SLP, etc.). Less obvious are indications from the literature that not all people who attempt TE speech are successful at using it. Initial success rates have ranged from approximately 30% to 90%, although most have fallen toward the upper end of this range (Geraghty, Wenig, Smith, & Portugal, 1996; Mehta, Sarkar, Mehta, & Bachher, 1995; Singer, Blom, & Hamaker, 1981). However, not all are successful at it, and the follow-up data suggest that 5% to 30% of individuals with initial success are not using TE speech at 9 months or more (Blom et al., 1986; de Raucourt et al., 1998; Mehta et al, 1995; Ward, Koh, Frisby, & Hodge, 2003). The reasons for this might be many and diligence by the patient and rehabilitation team might mitigate the drop in success over time. However, the consistent reports of less than 100% success and some drop-off in TE usage over time argue for the need to have other alaryngeal speech options available.

However, it is acknowledged that using TE speech acquisition rates to argue for maintaining ES as a viable third alaryngeal speech option is a risky proposition. The rate of successful acquisition of functional ES falls within a range from 5% to 60% (Anderson, 1950; Gates et al., 1982; Hillman et al., 1998; Koike, Kobayashi, Hirose, & Hara, 2002; Schaefer & Johns, 1982). This is generally lower than the long-term follow-up data for TE speech. However, not all individuals can use TE speech and some can learn ES.

There is a final, but valid, consideration. Some patients may simply prefer ES. A report from Quer, Burgues-Vila, and Garcia-Crespillo (1992) relative to this issue is intriguing. They addressed the question: "What type of voice rehabilitation would our patients prefer if they could make a choice between tracheoesophageal and esophageal speech?" (p.190). Twenty-three individuals with good postoperative TE speech were enrolled in ES training. Seventy percent ultimately opted to remove the TE prosthesis in favor of using ES for their daily communication, despite the fact that they considered their TE voice to be better than their ES. This suggests that at least some patients would make a decision on their preferred method based on more than just characteristics of the voice. Clinicians should do the same.

Unfortunately, it seems likely that many laryngectomy patients do not receive much information about ES. Personal communications with SLPs in the United States suggest that fewer and fewer are knowledgeable about ES and even fewer are comfortable training it.

If this trend is real and it continues, the chance that ES is offered as a truly viable communication option will continue to decrease over the years.

# Anatomy and Physiology for Esophageal Speech Production

## Pharyngoesophageal Segment

Prior to total laryngectomy, muscle fibers from the inferior pharyngeal constrictor, cricopharyngeus, and upper esophagus are closely intertwined to form a zone of high pressure at the top of the esophagus referred to as the upper esophageal sphincter, or UES (Gates, 1980; Levitt, Dedo, & Ogura, 1965). Inferior pharyngeal constrictor and cricopharyngeus muscle fiber attachments to the lateral and posterior larynx are severed when the larynx is excised. When closing the deficit, the surgeon attempts to create a region of approximated tissue that serves as a new UES to separate the pharynx and esophagus. The goal is to create an intraluminal zone of tissue which allows passage of food and liquid, and which also is sufficiently approximated at rest to serve as the vibratory source for speech. In the postlaryngectomized individual, this reconstructed zone is most often referred to as the pharyngoesophageal (PE) segment (Diedrich, 1999). The PE tissue is referred to as the neoglottis because it serves as the voice source for ES. The PE segment is located anterior to the cervical vertebrae typically at the level of the fifth or sixth cervical vertebrae although it may be higher or lower than this (Deidrich & Yongstrom, 1966) (see Figure 8–1). PE morphology can vary markedly across individuals, and there does not appear to be a strong correlation between PE segment morphology and speech skill (Diedrich & Yongstrom, 1966; van As, Op de Coul, van den Hoogen, Koopmans-van Beinum, & Hilgers, 2001; van den Berg & Moolenaar-Bijl, 1959).

## The Esophagus as an Air Reservoir in Esophageal Speech

In the nonlaryngectomized speaker, the lungs serve as the reservoir for voice production. Air pressure below the vocal folds is generated to overcome the resistance of the adducted vocal folds to set them into vibration. There is an analogous, but less efficient, situation involved in neoglottal vibration for ES.

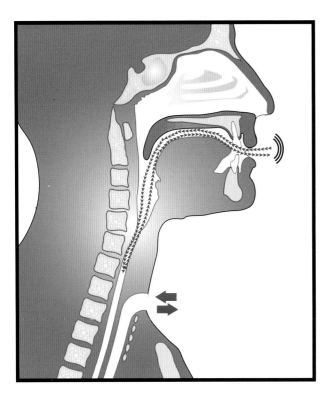

**Figure 8–1.** Schematic representation of esophageal speech production.

The esophagus serves as the air reservoir for ES (methods for loading air into the esophagus are described later in the chapter). When the air pressure within the esophagus is great enough to overcome PE segment resistance, the PE tissue is set into vibration. However, the esophagus is significantly smaller in volume than the lungs, placing restrictions on ES production. Van den Berg and Moolenaar-Bijl (1959) reported that the esophageal volume is ~40 to 80 cc, or roughly 2% of the volume of the lungs (2200 to 4690 cc, per Louden, Lee, & Holcomb, 1988). Additionally, Snidecor and Isshiki (1965) reported that the total volume of air utilized during ES was ~30% of the volume during laryngeal speech. The restricted esophageal air volume can restrict ES speech intensity, phrase duration, and speaking rate.

## Insufflating the Esophagus

There are two main ways to get air into the esophagus for voicing purposes. These are commonly referred to as the "inhalation" and the "injection" methods, respectively. While one method usually predominates for a given speaker, proficient ES speakers often use a combination of insufflation techniques (Berlin, 1963; Moolenaar-Bijl, 1953). The method of air insufflation is not closely correlated with ES speech proficiency (Diedrich & Youngstrom, 1966).

**Inhalation Method.** The inhalation technique relies on the inherent negative air pressure within the esophagus to draw air from the pharynx into the upper esophagus. The esophagus is a semicollapsed tube with negative air pressure at rest ranging from −5 to −10 cmH$_2$O (Dey & Kirchner, 1961). Air from the mouth can be "sucked" into the esophagus by reducing the air pressure within the esophagus even further. Specific instructions for training the technique are offered later. The general approach is to have the individual take a short, rapid inhalation of air through the stoma with a patent oral or nasal passageway. This inhalation causes the thorax to expand and a further pressure drop within the esophagus to −13 to −27 cmH$_2$O (Atkinson, Kramer, Wyman, & Inglefinger, 1957). The esophageal pressure drop creates an even stronger vacuum that can draw air from the mouth and pharynx into the esophagus. The PE tone must be reduced sufficiently to allow air to flow from the pharynx and into the esophagus (Diedrich, 1999). A video clip on the CD (see Chapter 8: Video: Inhalation Method) shows three patients using the inhalation method. The first two are just learning how to produce esophageal speech. The third patient can perform the inhalation method with a bit more ease, although he also demonstrates some unwanted behaviors such as stoma blast (discussed more later in the chapter).

**Injection Methods.** Two types of injection are described. One is the consonant press technique, also cited as consonant injection or plosive injection (Damste, 1958; Duguay, 1999). The second is the glossopharyngeal press, or tongue pumping method (Diedrich & Youngstrom, 1966; Salmon, 1999). Both involve increasing the air pressure in the mouth and pharynx to force air through the PE segment into the esophagus.

The consonant press technique capitalizes on the high intraoral air pressure generated during stops, fricatives, and affricates. Again, details on training are presented subsequently. The general idea is to produce the consonants with greater articulatory effort, compressing the volume of air in the mouth so that air pressure rises. The elevated pressure forces air to flow through the PE segment and into the esophagus. In order to build sufficient intraoral pressure to overcome PE segment resistance, the speaker must maintain tight velopharyngeal closure; otherwise air escape out the nose will thwart the oral air pressure buildup attempt. Sufficiently strong oral articulatory contacts are also needed to compress oral cavity volume. Finally, the tone of the PE segment is again of critical importance as high tone can create enough resistance to prevent the flow of air from the vocal tract into the esophagus. The video clip on the CD (see Chapter 8: Video: Consonant Injection Method) provides examples of three patients performing the consonant press maneuver in single word repetition and syllable series productions.

The glossopharyngeal press technique relies on high intraoral air pressure as well, but is not reliant on consonant production. Rather, the articulators are used to reduce oral cavity volume, causing an air pressure increase during a nonspeech pressing maneuver. This could be done with compression by the lips, cheeks, tongue-to-palate, or a combination of these structures (training instructions are offered below). If the air in the mouth is under sufficient pressure from the pressing actions, it will move through the PE segment and into the esophagus. Four patients attempting a press maneuver are shown in the CD (see Chapter 8: Video: Press Maneuver). These individuals are all at the very beginning stages of learning esophageal speech and demonstrate varying levels of proficiency at completing the press maneuver.

## Returning Air from the Esophagus

As the person exhales through the stoma, intrathoracic air pressure is increased (i.e., elastic recoil of the lungs, return of the diaphragm to its domelike resting state, collapse of the thorax). Primary speculation is that the intrathoracic pressure during pulmonary exhalation exerts pressure on the esophagus, forcing the air within to move upward and through the PE segment, setting it into vibration (Diedrich, 1999; van den Berg, Moolenaar-Bijl, & Damste, 1958). This requires sufficiently low PE segment tone. Additionally, it requires that the lower esophageal sphincter (between the

esophagus and stomach) remain tightly closed to prevent the esophageal air from being squeezed downward into the stomach.

## Factors That May Influence Acquisition of Esophageal Speech

There are a number of prerequisites to learning and producing ES. In addition, there are other issues that may make this process more difficult, but not impossible. Table 8–4 includes some of the factors that have been evaluated empirically or described clinically. Several of these issues are also relevant when considering AL and TE speech.

### Physical Factors

The extent of the surgical resection must be considered when deciding on the feasibility of ES speech. Radical neck dissection does not appear to significantly influence ES acquisition rates (Diedrich & Youngstrom, 1966; Mjones, Olofsson, Danbolt, & Tibbling, 1991; Richardson, 1981). However, with more involved and larger surgical extensions, the clinicians must carefully consider whether ES is the most appropriate option. Resections extending into the tongue could seriously compromise ES training and outcomes. Significant tongue ablation could render injection methods ineffective with the exception of lip or buccal pressing. The inhalation method would still be possible. TE speech may be more appropriate in the case of a laryngectomy plus glossectomy given the more normal sounding, louder voice which does not rely on tongue activity for generating sound. Articulatory compensations would have to be taught for AL, TE, and ES speech when portions, or all, of the tongue are involved in the resection.

Significant pharyngeal resections also can pose a major barrier to successful ES acquisition. Our own clinical experience and reports in the literature suggest that individuals undergoing pharyngolaryngectomy are not likely to develop usable ES, most likely because of the extensive reconstruction that takes place in the hypopharynx and esophagus. Bates, McFeeter, and Coman (1990) reported that only 4% of their group of 46 patients were using ES at 6 months follow-up compared to 54% who used an EL. Ward et al.

**Table 8–4.** Parameters That May Influence Acquisition of Esophageal and Artificial Larynx Speech

| | | Esophageal Speech | | Artificial Larynx Speech |
| --- | --- | --- | --- | --- |
| | | Inhalation Method | Injection Method | |
| Physical | Velopharyngeal competence* | X | XX | X |
| | Ability to seal the oral port (at the lips or tongue-palate) | | XX | |
| | Ability to reduce volume of oral pharyngeal cavity (lips, tongue, cheeks, pharynx) | | XX | |
| | Ability to pass air through the PE segment into the esophagus | XX | XX | |
| | Appropriate PE segment resistance for voicing | XX | XX | |
| | Ability to produce relatively precise oral articulatory movements | XX | XX | XX |
| | Manual dexterity | | | X |
| | Visual acuity | | | X |
| | Hearing acuity | X | X | X |
| | Pulmonary health/respiratory control | X | X | |
| Cognitive/ Psychological | Alertness level, cognitive function (memory, problem solving, decision making, etc.) | X | X | X |
| | Motivation level | X | X | X |
| | Depression, patterns of maladjustment | X | X | X |
| Other Factors | Age? (younger with higher success rate) | ? | ? | |
| | Availability of services; ability to access services | XX | XX | XX |
| | Extent of surgery | X | X | X |
| | Radiation therapy | ? | ? | X |
| | Clinician competence | XX | XX | XX |

Note. XX = very important; X = important but does not preclude; ? = conflicting reports regarding the influence.
*Velopharyngeal (VP) deficits will negatively affect ES and EL speech (also TE); however, a VP deficit will preclude the ability to inject air into the esophagus; PE = pharyngoesophageal.

(2003) reported that 65% of their pharyngolaryngectomy patients used EL speech at one year and 30% used TE as their primary mode of communication. McAuliffe, Ward, Bassett, and Perkins (2000) reported that 77% of their 13 pharyngolaryngectomy patients were judged to be successful TE speakers. Although there may be isolated instances in which a pharyngolaryngectomy patient may be able to acquire ES, the high success rates with EL and TE provide a convincing argument for gravitating away from ES and toward EL or TE as a first choice.

The status of the PE segment is a primary determinant of the success at acquiring ES speech. Problems regarding PE segment resistance can be broadly cast into two categories. First, the PE segment resistance may be insufficient (hypotonic, flaccid) resulting in relatively easy esophageal insufflation, but a breathy voice (Perry & Edels, 1985). This is roughly the equivalent of glottal incompetence in a laryngeal speaker. Second, the PE segment resistance may be excessive such that insufflating the esophagus is problematic and the voice that is generated is strained, inconsistently present, or not generated at all (Gilmore, 1999). Usually the elevated resistance is because of increased tone or spasm of the PE segment (Blom, Singer, & Hamaker, 1985; Winans, Reichbach, & Waldrop, 1974), although strictures and diverticuli in the region also can contribute (Simpson, Smith, & Gordon, 1972). Pre- or postoperatively, esophageal insufflation testing (see Chapter 9) can be used to assess the competence of the PE segment (Blom et al., 1985). Additionally, video-fluoroscopic examination of the pharynx and esophagus at rest, during swallowing, and during voicing could prove useful in identifying PE segment problems (Cheesman, Knight, McIvor, & Perry, 1986; McIvor, Evans, Perry, & Cheesman, 1990; van As et al., 2001; van As-Brooks, Hilgers, Koopmans-van Beinum, & Pols, 2005).

There does not appear to be a consistent link between radiation therapy and ultimate success in acquiring ES (Diedrich & Youngstrom, 1966; Frith, Buffalo, & Montague, 1985; Izdebski, Fontanesi, Ross, & Hetzler, 1988). There may be some changes to PE segment and esophageal wall tissue compliance that could make injection and return of esophageal air difficult for a period of time postradiation therapy (Izdebski, et al., 1988). However, these tissue changes seem to abate over time in most cases. A more likely influence of radiation therapy is induction of acute side effects such as significant pain, tissue dryness, and general fatigue, which could interfere with ES training. Speech therapy may need to be temporarily halted until the side effects resolve.

When producing ES, the integrity of oral, velopharyngeal, and pharyngeal structures is critical, particularly for those attempting injection methods for insufflating the esophagus (i.e., either the consonant press or the glossopharyngeal press). Ability to seal the oral cavity and velopharyngeal port is necessary to generate sufficient intraoral pressure to overcome the resistance of the PE segment. Because the inhalation method does not rely on an increase in intraoral air pressure, the inhalation method is possible with deficits in oral or VP function (although articulatory abilities may still be affected). Careful evaluation via an oral mechanism examination, perceptual observations of speech movements, and various instrumental exams (fluoroscopic, endoscopic, etc.) can all be used to evaluate the integrity of the VP and oral articulatory systems.

Control of the pulmonary air stream during esophageal voicing is important for individuals attempting the inhalation method who must coordinate intake of air through the stoma with oral and/or velopharyngeal maneuvers (Salmon, 1994). For the inhalation method, a sharp inhalation through the stoma creates changes in intrathoracic pressures that help draw air into the esophagus (Deidrich, 1999). Likewise, a controlled pulmonary exhalation may help change intrathoracic pressures such that air is forced up and out of the esophagus to produce esophageal voice. This exhalation must be done in a controlled fashion so that audible noise at the stoma is not generated (Lewin, 2005). The clinician can look carefully at the patient's medical history for indications of impairment. Our clinical experience would indicate that disease processes that influence respiratory activity, such as emphysema or various neuromuscular diseases, can make it more difficult to learn esophageal speech for some patients although there has been little if any investigation of this matter. Observations of the patient breathing at rest and during ES voicing attempts may provide insight into problems with respiratory control for esophageal speech. Observations that might not bode well for ES learning could include the inability to generate a sharp, brief inhalation in a timely fashion, shallow or rapid breathing suggesting a more general respiratory impairment, or inability to manipulate force of exhalation to avoid unwanted noise at the stoma.

Hearing acuity level has also been correlated with ES acquisition rates (Berlin, 1964; Martin, Hoops, & Shanks, 1974). Reductions in hearing acuity have been presumed to negatively affect a person's monitoring of the esophageal voice productions and production of stoma noise (Salmon, 1999). Inquiring about a patient's hearing status is necessary at a minimum and more formal screening or assessment is preferred.

## Cognitive/Psychological Factors

There is some disagreement about the strength of the influence that cognitive and psychological factors have on ES acquisition. Clearly some minimal level of cognitive ability is necessary to participate in the rehabilitation process. Individuals must understand what they are being asked to do, remember to utilize new behaviors, and problem solve throughout the process. Some individuals are able to learn ES fairly intuitively and via imitation rather than through direct instruction. For these individuals, the cognitive demands may be no different than for AL or TE speech. However, when direct instruction is required, learning ES has the potential to be fairly complex. Clinicians must be aware of any cognitive limits in their clients, but our experience has been that cognitive deficits are not a common reason for immediately discounting ES as an option. We make informal observations regarding cognition, but do not routinely assess it for alaryngeal speakers unless the patient's history or behavior in therapy suggests a cognitive impairment

Psychological profiling and consideration of motivational state have received a fair amount of attention relative to ES acquisition (Beamer, 1954; Keith, Ewart, & Flowers, 1974; Sako, Cardinale, Marchetta, & Shedd, 1974). Some have considered degree of motivation to be a principal determinant of ES training outcomes (Gardner, 1971; Gilmore, 1999). On the other hand, Lewin (2005) suggested that lack of motivation is usually not much of a concern in alaryngeal speech rehabilitation because individuals generally are interested in communicating orally. These two positions are not in direct opposition to one another, but rather one suggests that the ES trainee must be motivated while the other suggests that they likely are. Various observations or pieces of information may provide insight into a client's motivation and desire including: demeanor during therapy, responses to direct probes about the interest in learning ES, the amount of practice completed outside of therapy, and perhaps other indications likely to be associated with high/low motivation for oral communication (e.g., gainful employment with high verbal demands, socially active, etc.). Of course the clinician must be cognizant that motivation is sometimes not easy to "see" and so frank discussions with the patient may be in order if the clinician is concerned.

### Other Factors

Age of the individual deserves comment. Salmon (1988) has suggested that younger rather than older adults are

perhaps better candidates for learning ES. Mjones et al. (1991) reported that age was the only factor in their study that was correlated significantly with intelligibility of ES. These authors are likely to agree, however, that clinicians should not let age alone deter them from attempting any of the alaryngeal speech options, including ES. There certainly are many instances in which older adults are able to successfully acquire ES.

Clinician competence and availability of services for ES training is expected to become an increasing problem over the next several years. We have no specific literature to cite in this regard. However, personal communications with a number of experts in alaryngeal speech support the notion that fewer SLPs are well versed in alaryngeal speech in general. Those that are most often train TE and AL speech. As the generation of master clinicians well versed in ES training retires, there will be fewer options for patients and SLPs interested in learning about ES.

## Esophageal Speech Rehabilitation Processes and Techniques

### Preoperative Discussion Regarding Esophageal Speech

Preoperative counseling by the SLP typically covers many issues including the three primary alaryngeal communication options (Glaze, 2005; Salmon, 1999). As part of this discussion, we give the patient general information about ES, describing in rudimentary terms how voice can be produced and what it might sound like. Simple anatomical drawings to supplement this brief discussion (such as Figure 8–1) would be appropriate to show diversion of the trachea to the neck, separation of the upper and lower airway, and the PE segment region and esophagus. We avoid detailed discussion of the alaryngeal options unless they indicate specific interest in knowing more. In our experience many do, but their ability to process and recall the information is often limited because of the magnitude of the issues with which they are dealing. We may play them a brief audio-video sample of each of the three options, including esophageal speech, but we do not dwell on it. If however the patient or significant other request, we have at the ready additional samples to play. The CD includes three audio clips and two video clips of esophageal speakers conversing and reading (see Chapter 8: Video: Esophageal Speaker Demos for Education). These samples give some indication of the range of proficiency that might be expected for individuals who are using ES as their primary mode of communication. Throughout, we try to be unbiased in our discussion so that patients have a chance to consider all the alaryngeal speech options (Doyle, 1994). However, if the patient clearly has some issue(s) that exclude, or make one option highly unlikely, we do not avoid discussing this with the patient.

## Postoperative Training

The SLP should not initiate ES training without first obtaining clearance from the patient's doctor. Sufficient healing must take place in the pharynx, esophagus, and neck so that the elevated pressures likely to occur during ES speech therapy do not strain suture lines. Typically, ES training can begin as early as 7–10 days after the surgery assuming no unusual medical or surgical complications arise. In the earliest days after surgery we advocate the start of therapy focused on EL training, just as others have (Duguay, 1999; Gardner, 1971).

Clinicians may opt for different approaches to the initial training of ES. For example, Graham (2005) suggests a very direct approach involving a fairly high degree of patient education and insight even early on in therapy. Graham (2005) provides an excellent description of the methods of instruction that she employs, including a detailed hierarchy of tasks and stimuli. In contrast, others such as Duguay (1999) and Shanks (J. C. Shanks, personal communication, July 18, 2003) have advocated for more indirect and semi-direct methods of instruction, at least as a starting point in therapy, reverting to more direct instruction only when needed. We tend to favor the latter, but do not discount the value of direct instruction. In general, however, we have found it efficient to utilize more indirect and semi-direct approaches as the starting point for therapy, and so we begin with these. In the following section, the therapy process is presented in two segments: beginning stages and developing usable esophageal speech. While the therapeutic process may not be as orderly or as segmented as the writing suggests, we have found this to be a useful means for

conceptualizing the training. Information on further refining esophageal speech is available from Shanks (1994) and Haroldson (1999), among others.

**Beginning Stages of Esophageal Speech Training.** Throughout the postoperative training, there are several general considerations for the SLP. The therapy atmosphere must be relaxed and not rushed; tension and a sense of urgency are generally counterproductive to learning ES. Multiple repetitions are important regardless of the therapeutic approach chosen; ES is a motor behavior that takes time and practice to learn. A given therapeutic approach will not work for every client and so there must be a willingness to shift tactics as needed. Finally, the SLP should not get in the way of a good thing by overinstructing or asking patients to overanalyze their behaviors, particularly early in therapy.

*Getting First Sounds.* The first goal for the client is to produce esophageal voice consistently on demand. The client ultimately should be able to produce esophageal voice on every attempt. This may strike some SLPs as unrealistic given the usual penchant for setting behavioral goals at something less than 100%. However, the individual with a laryngectomy must know that he or she has a voice whenever it is wanted or needed. We do not expect 100% consistency on the first day, but that is our early goal. Berlin (1963) reported that individuals who ultimately developed good ES were able to generate voice 100% of the time between days 10–14 of therapy (in that study, subjects were seen 2–3 times a day, every day).

There are two behaviors that we track related to establishing consistency. The first is the latency between the start of esophageal insufflation and production of esophageal sound. Based on data from Berlin (1963), Damste (1958), and Diedrich and Youngstrom (1966), the goal is to limit the latency to 0.5 sec or less. Most often, latency decreases with extended practice as the client simply gets the feel for how air is loaded into the esophagus and how it is returned. Second, we pay attention to the degree of physical effort apparent in the esophageal voice production. The goal is for voicing to be as effortless as possible. There are a number of indications of increased effort such as: stoma noise (turbulent airflow through the stoma during voicing), visual distracters (e.g., head bobbing, facial grimacing, eye squinting, etc.), strained voice quality, and intermittent aphonia. Means of addressing these behaviors are addressed subsequently.

*Indirect Therapy Approach.* Our first approach to training reliable esophageal phonation on demand is very similar to the indirect method described by Duguay (1999). We take on the role described by Duguay (1999): set up the opportunity for clients to show you the behavior, make careful observations so you know what they are doing, cheer them on when they are successful, identify key behaviors as needed, and give limited instruction to reinforce the behaviors. First, the SLP can ask whether any sounds have been made spontaneously. If so, we ask for a demonstration. Many will report that they have made some intermittent sounds. If the client can provide a demonstration, the SLP's job is to watch and listen carefully. The SLP must figure out how they are getting air into the esophagus. Are they injecting air into the esophagus? If so, are they using the lips or the tongue or the cheeks? Are they inhalers? Do they use a consonant to insufflate the esophagus? We also look for any difficulties in getting air in or out of the esophagus. Do they struggle? Are there unusual body movements? What does the voice sound like?

There are a few likely scenarios to emerge from this casual solicitation of esophageal voice. Scenario number 1 is the ideal outcome. Some patients can already produce esophageal voice with some consistency and without exceptional effort. In this case, the SLP can simply solicit multiple repetitions of the behavior. Based on careful observations, the SLP can take a more active role in giving the patient stimuli to produce so that the patient does not get distracted by having to generate his or her own sounds. For example, if the patient is an "inhaler," a variety of vowels or vowel initiated syllables can be requested. If he or she is a consonant press injector, the clinician can ask for production of consonant-vowel (CV) stimuli beginning with a pressure consonant. The goal is two-fold: (1) to allow additional opportunities to observe the client, and (2) to provide the client with extended practice of the target behavior so that consistency increases. In general we do not ask the patient to self-analyze at this point, opting for success in execution of the behavior. The insight and analysis will follow shortly.

A second likely scenario when using the indirect therapy approach is that the individual produces esophageal voice, but inconsistently, perhaps 20% to 50% of the time. If there is no evidence of significant struggle, the approach may be the same as described for scenario 1. With more time and more repetitions of the behavior at which they have been successful, the consistency in the behavior is likely to increase. If, however, there is notable effort or struggle, the SLP must make some decisions. Practicing bad habits is not helpful. A semi-direct or direct intervention (described below) may be warranted to find a less effortful means of producing voice. Alternatively, some clients only need to have the behavior identified and the briefest of instruction given to limit its occurrence. If that is sufficient, the SLP can consider him- or herself lucky and resume practicing stimuli on which the client is most successful. If the effort behaviors are more entrenched, a shift to direct instructions regarding esophageal voice production and elimination of the distracters is likely to be needed.

A third scenario that may arise when using the indirect approach is that the client produces little, if any, esophageal voice. The SLP must try to figure out whether the client is demonstrating either of the primary subcomponents: insufflating the esophagus and getting air out. One option is to move straight to semi-direct or direct instruction. Alternatively, the SLP may want to make further observations, still using a nondirective approach. For example, the SLP might engage the patient in a nonstructured interaction with the patient using "mouthed" speech. One indication of air entering the esophagus would be audible "klunking," or a brief noise associated with air entering the esophagus (Diedrich & Youngstrom, 1966). Another is a report from the client of feeling bloated, signaling that the air enters the esophagus, but proceeds to the stomach. Inadvertent belching or occasional bursts of esophageal voice also indicate that air can be returned. If any or all of these behaviors are observed, the SLP can begin to reinforce them when they occur ("Did you hear that? That means air went into your esophagus! Next time you hear it (or feel it), try to say a word as quickly as you can."). In our experience, some clients have "aha!" type experiences wherein a behavior is pointed out to them, they hear it or feel it, and then they can get it under increasing control with little clinician input. We do not count on it, by any means, but we also do not assume that all patients need detailed instruction to show us the behavior.

Regardless of the scenario that might occur, once the individual is able to consistently produce esophageal voice (approaching or at 100% success), it is important to have the clients recognize how they created the sound. The SLP should explain the component behaviors observed, pointing out if they are "inhaling," injecting, or using a consonant to load the esophagus. The client should practice the esophageal voice now with this insight. Prior to this, the patient was merely asked to show the behavior, not dissect it. The SLP and patient can be content with that until some degree of consistency in the behavior is established. Subsequently though, patient insight is important so that he or she can begin to control and manipulate the actions as therapy progresses toward increasing duration and other aspects of the sound production.

*Semi-direct Therapy Approach.* The indirect approach to soliciting esophageal voice and establishing consistency does not work for everyone. A second therapeutic approach involves clinician modeling of the intended behavior (described by Duguay [1999] as a "semi direct method"). Duguay (1999), Salmon (1971), and Shanks (J. C. Shanks, personal communication, July 18, 2003) suggest that the clinician provide a visual and auditory model for the patient to imitate. The model incorporates a variety of esophageal insufflation techniques: inhalation, injection via tongue pressing, injection via lip pressing, and injection from various pressure consonants. The steps below are a variant from Duguay (1999):

1. sniff with the mouth open and say /a/ (inhalation technique)
2. sniff with the mouth open while simultaneously jutting the jaw up and out, saying /a/ (inhalation technique with a head posture change)
3. press the lips together forcefully and say /a/ (injection via lip press)
4. press the tongue tip to the alveolar ridge forcefully and say /a/ (injection via tongue press)
5. say /pa/ with strong plosion on /p/ (injection via bilabial consonant)
6. say /ta/ with strong plosion on /t/ (injection via lingua-alveolar consonant)
7. say /ka/ with strong plosion on /k/ (injection via velar consonant)

The order of the models can be varied and different vowels and consonants might be attempted. Two clinician-client interactions utilizing variants of the above steps for soliciting esophageal sound are depicted on the CD (see Chapter 8: Video: Indirect Instruction). Mid- or low tongue position vowels are preferred early on (Graham, 2005; Hyman, 1994). Voiceless rather than voiced stop consonants are a common first choice for the consonant assist technique because of their higher intraoral pressure (Diedrich, 1999; Moolenaar-Bijl, 1953). Other voiceless obstruents such as s, sh, ch or s-blends, would be reasonable to try as well.

The sequence in this imitation mode is as follows: the SLP demonstrates one of the steps, the patient imitates, the SLP demonstrates the next step, the patient imitates, and so on throughout the full set of steps. The client's job is to pay careful attention and try to replicate the model exactly. The clinician's job is to provide accurate models and carefully observe the client's imitation. The goal is to identify which method facilitates esophageal insufflation and voice production. Many repetitions of the full set of steps are needed. It is an opportunistic approach with the intent of putting the client in favorable situations likely to result in esophageal insufflation. The client's best insufflation technique is identified in the process and the SLP can then develop stimulus materials that take advantage of that facilitative technique. Once the useful technique is identified, the goal reverts to increasing consistency of the behavior. Ideally, the clinician can produce esophageal voice with each method being modeled, but it is not essential as long as he or she can provide an accurate visual model and an acceptable "fake" esophageal voice (i.e., glottal fry).

*Direct Therapy Approach.* In the event that the less direct approaches are unsuccessful, the clinician must be prepared to give more specific direction on getting first sounds. The SLP should be ready to instruct across all of the insufflation methods. Superior ES speakers are likely to use more than one esophageal loading technique, so it is reasonable to attempt training all of them.

Teaching the inhalation method involves clinician modeling of the behavior and specific instructions.

Various instructions have been offered and each should be tried with the client, as needed. Recall that the inhalation method requires an open vocal tract (oral and/or nasal), a fairly relaxed PE segment, and creation of even more negative pressure than usual within the esophagus. The most common instructions are as follows (Diedrich, 1999; Salmon, 1971):

1. leave the mouth open and tongue down (or, alternately, the mouth can be closed if the nasal cavity and velopharyngeal port are patent)
2. "sniff" (or, alternately, "gasp in surprise," "inhale quickly until the lungs are half full," "yawn quickly," "suck air in")
3. move the jaw/head forward and upward simultaneously with the sniff
4. open the mouth and say /a/ by squeezing the stomach and exhaling

Some clients will indicate that they cannot sniff through their nose (or yawn with their mouth, etc.). This is true following laryngectomy. The goal, however, is to get a quick pulmonary inhalation that creates a sudden drop in esophageal pressure. An alternate set of instructions described by Duguay (1999) requires the patient to exhale deeply, cover the stoma partially with a hand or finger, open the mouth, and inhale quickly (a video of this stoma coverage technique is included in the CD segment, Inhalation Method). A slow pace and relaxed approach is necessary so that PE segment tension is not unduly increased. If there is success at insufflating the esophagus, the goal reverts to establishing consistency of the behavior on the simplest stimulus for the inhalation technique, a vowel.

For injection techniques, air under pressure in the oral cavity and pharynx is forced through the PE segment into the esophagus. For the consonant press method, the patient is asked to produce voiceless stops, fricatives, or /s/ blends in isolation so that the SLP can listen for the sound(s) on which the greatest oral plosion or frication occurs. A stronger burst or fricative noise suggests higher intraoral air pressure. Once a best consonant (or set of consonants) is identified, the SLP constructs a series of CV stimuli for use in therapy. The client produces the CVs with a strong burst on the consonant. Clients are asked to feel the compression of the air in the mouth as they practice with a stop consonant stimulus (Salmon, 1971). Other instructions such as "articulate the sound carefully" or "press with the lips/tongue as you say it" may help elevate the intraoral pressure. Fricatives or /s/ blends might be better for some speakers as these are of high pressure and also long duration, allowing additional time for air to be pressed into the esophagus. Again, once ES voice is produced, the goal reverts to establishing consistency before moving on to more complex stimuli.

The glossopharyngeal press can be accomplished in a variety of ways (Diedrich & Youngstrom, 1966). One set of instructions to try would be as follows:

1. put your tongue up on your palate like you are going to say the /t/ sound
2. press your tongue against your palate, pushing the air that is in your mouth back
3. when you feel the air go down, quickly open your mouth and say /a/.

The lips can be open or closed for the above. Some have used instructions describing tongue tip elevation against the alveolar ridge and mid-tongue contact with the posterior hard palate to trap a bolus of air against the palate (Graham, 2005; Salmon, 1971). The client is then instructed to rock the tongue backward and forward in a pumping action to propel the air bolus into the throat. A different approach involves pressing the lips together ("like you are going to say /p/") while also squeezing the cheeks in; the tongue remains inactive on the floor of the mouth. Once sound is produced, the client practices the behavior until sound is consistently produced on the vowel.

***Increasing Phonation Duration.*** Up to this point, the patient and the clinician should be relatively pleased even with short bursts of esophageal sound (<0.5 sec) as long as it can be produced on demand. However, greater duration is needed to develop useable esophageal speech. Targets of 2–3 seconds of sustained phonation or 5–9 syllables per esophageal air charge have been suggested (Diedrich & Youngstrom, 1966; Duguay, 1999). There is no substitute that we know of to increase duration other than significant practice following a hierarchy of stimuli that pushes the client to ever longer productions.

Increased phonatory duration can be realized by loading more air into the esophagus, better controlling esophageal air release, limiting the escape of esophageal air into the stomach, or some combination of these. It is not always clear which parameter needs to be addressed and it is not always obvious what changes the client implements to increase the duration. However, we try to be systematic in our observations and experimentation with the patient. We spend time working on loading more air into the esophagus. Usually we do this by simply talking the client through the goal. Imagery can be useful, encouraging the client to envision a larger air bolus in the mouth, or more air being sucked into the throat as he or she sniffs. This must be done with care as an increase in general tension of the head and neck might ensue, negatively affecting generation of esophageal voice. An instruction to increase loudness has also proven useful for some individuals although an increase in tension is possible with this as well.

Controlling the release of esophageal air during ES voicing can be attempted by instructing the client to "stretch" the vowel longer and longer. Most clients seem to respond well to feedback documenting the actual duration that they achieve. There are many software programs that allow display of an audio signal and measurement of its duration. A stop watch or wall clock with a second hand can give similar data to use as feedback and encouragement.

The hierarchy of stimuli utilized in this training is not unlike that from other areas in the field of communication disorders. Complexity of the stimuli increases from isolated phonemes, to CV or VC construction, to multisyllabic words and phrases, to more complex speech. There are important considerations within each hierarchy level. For the individual using the inhalation or the glossopharyngeal press, practice begins with vowels. The client can be pushed to extend the duration of the vowel through repeated practice. It is not unusual to also work simultaneously on VC or CV syllables using a liquid, glide, or perhaps a nasal. The hierarchy progresses to bi- and trisyllabic words and phrases loaded predominantly (or exclusively) with vowels and sonorants. The intent is to avoid high pressure consonants that the client might use to load the esophagus at the start or in the middle of the production. In this manner, the clinician and the patient can focus on the inhalation or the press technique, respectively.

For the consonant injector, the hierarchy begins with CV stimuli initiated with a voiceless stop consonant, fricative, affricate, or /s/ blend. For most consonant injectors we simultaneously work on syllable repetitions such as /pa pa pa pa/ to practice rapid reloading off of the consonant. As the speaker becomes proficient at using the voiceless obstruents to load the esophagus, the voiced counterparts are added to the CV stimuli. From there on out, we increase the number of syllables requested, but continue to load the stimuli with high pressure consonants (e.g., "pig pen," "tic-tac," etc.).

**Developing Usable Esophageal Speech.** As patients increase the duration and number of syllables per air charge, they may well begin using ES in some situations outside of therapy. Although some may disagree, we usually request that individuals learning ES do significant practice at home regarding consistency and duration of voicing, but refrain from using their esophageal voice in communicative exchanges outside of therapy until the SLP gives permission. The concern is that individuals may get into bad voicing habits if they try to use ES before they have the fundamentals of its production firmly in place. However, when they can produce voice on demand without exceptional effort and they can produce 4-5 syllables on an air charge, we ask them to start using ES in at least some situations that are more controlled (e.g., limited background noise, limited stress, etc.). In order to make ES more usable, though, therapy must continue with a focus on a number of other parameters including articulation, loudness, pitch and pitch variation, speaking rate, and voice quality.

*Articulation.* There is a strong correlation between articulatory accuracy and overall intelligibility of ES (Anderson, 1950; Shames, Font, & Matthews, 1963). A general increase in articulatory precision is encouraged, although care is needed to avoid unnatural movements of the articulators that might draw undue attention. Stronger burst releases and increased frication noise (more intense and longer) are encouraged to provide clearer acoustic cues to the listener. A more general pattern of precise speech can have other articulatory benefits (Ferguson, 2004; Krause & Braida, 2004) including slower rate and fewer instances of omitting or slighting consonants in the final position, which should prove beneficial in maximizing intelligibility (Hyman, 1994).

There are specific articulation issues that arise with ES that may require attention. First, individuals using predominantly consonant injections must be monitored to ensure that there are no perceptible intrusions of pressure consonants in unwanted locations. These people may produce a pressure consonant to load air into the esophagus even though what they want to say is not initiated with a pressure consonant (e.g., "It is mine" is produced as "*P*it is mine"). One option is to wean them off of the consonant injection. Alternatively, it is sometimes possible to minimize the plosion of the injection consonant so that the burst is less perceptible to a listener (in essence this is moving them towards a press maneuver). An example of an ES speaker who has intrusive consonants is included on the CD (see Chapter 8: Video: Distracters).

A second common error is that listeners may misperceive voiceless sounds as voiced (Hyman, 1955; Sacco, Mann, & Schultz, 1967). In connected speech, linguistic context often is sufficient to carry the meaning. However, it may be necessary to specifically maximize voicing distinctions with some individuals. Differentially increasing the burst/frication intensity for voiceless phonemes relative to their voiced cognate has been suggested (Christensen & Dwyer, 1990; Connor, Hamlet, & Joyce, 1985). In this approach, the individual is taught to "push harder" or create a stronger "burst/noise" on the voiceless consonant. Minimal word pair drills can be used for this work. Others have suggested training an increase in duration of the vowel that follows a voiced consonant (Sacco et al., 1967).

The nasals /m/, /n/, and /ng/ may be perceived as /p/, /d/, and /g/ in many esophageal speakers (Duguay, 1999). Struben and van Gelder (1958) and Diedrich and Youngstrom (1966) suggested that ES speakers may not release air nasally on nasal consonants in an attempt to conserve the limited air available to them during speech production. Again, linguistic context may be sufficient to carry the meaning. However, if the issue is of concern, Graham (1997) has suggested using contrastive stress drills pitting plosives against their nasal counterparts as one means of establishing more nasal resonance. Duguay (1999) indicated that practicing humming may sensitize the ES user to the issue and help resolve the denasalization.

Difficulty producing the glottal aspirate /h/ is also a common problem. The listener perceives the /h/ as omitted (e.g., "heart" becomes "art"). In attempting an /h/, airflow through the PE segment to create frication is likely to also set the PE tissue into vibration, changing the /h/ into a vowel. One approach is to train prolongation of the vowel that follows the /h/ (Duguay, 1999). This may work because production of a word such as "hit" takes longer than "it." Shanks (1994) has suggested using a lingua-alveolar fricative (similar to the German "ich") as a substitute that listeners are likely to interpret as /h/ in the context of running speech.

***Loudness.*** Reduced loudness is a pervasive problem in ES. Shanks (J. C. Shanks, personal communication, July 18, 2003) asks individuals using ES to reconcile themselves to this fact, at least for the first year or two while focusing on optimizing other aspects of speech. This may be satisfactory for some. Others, however, may have a strong need for a louder voice. This is a challenge: there is a limited amount of air available for voicing and increasing loudness may increase tension within the speech system, deleteriously affecting PE segment vibration. Haroldson (1999) has suggested that experimentation with varying levels of effort while being ever mindful of creating too much PE segment tension may result in identification of an optimal effort level for intensity increases. Salmon (2005) indicated that digital pressure on the PE segment might serve to increase loudness for some individuals as well. Other alternatives such as amplification or situational use of an AL can also be considered.

***Pitch and Pitch Variation.*** While some individuals are able to push their mean speaking fundamental frequency upward on a regular basis, many cannot. Again, experimentation with speaking effort level might be considered. Subtle head position changes might also change the PE segment dynamics so that pitch (and perhaps loudness and quality) is altered. Perhaps more tenable is training transient changes in pitch so that the voice is not monotone and appropriate intonation is conveyed. Excellent esophageal speakers often have a fairly large pitch range in connected speech (Shipp, 1967; Snidecor & Curry, 1959). Extended practice with singing, repetition of interrogative sentences, or production of highly inflected multisyllabic words or phrase can serve to maximize a speaker's pitch varying capabilities.

***Speaking Rate.*** ES speakers are slower speakers than laryngeal speakers (Snidecor, 1968). Occasionally we have to work with an ES speaker to slow him or her down to increase articulatory precision. More often, however, we are trying to achieve a rate that more closely approximates normal while still preserving acceptable articulation. The increased time needed for insufflating the esophagus and returning air for voicing creates longer pauses in ES speech. Additionally, the smaller volume of air available for ES results in the need for more frequent pauses to reload the esophagus. Consequently achieving more efficient air insufflation and air return are both primary means of increasing speaking rate. One option is to teach the consonant injection technique to be used in combination with either of the other insufflation methods. With consonant injection, fewer pauses are needed as the speaker capitalizes on pressure consonants in running speech to reload the esophagus.

***Voice Quality.*** Esophageal voice is aberrant relative to laryngeal speech. The low fundamental frequency often gives a perception of glottal fry. Others may have varying degrees of hoarseness because of the propensity of the PE segment to vibrate aperiodically. With extended practice, some individuals may be able to increase the fundamental frequency enough to get out of glottal fry. Others may strike a balance regarding the degree of effort or muscular tension in the neck that promotes more periodic vibration and subsequently less hoarseness. In general, we reserve work on improving voice quality in ES until the end. Exceptions to this are situations in which the voice is very breathy, strained, or "wet-gurgly." A breathy voice suggests a hypotonic PE segment. Digital pressure on the neck at the level of the PE segment can often improve the breathy ES voice dramatically. Changes in head position may also prove beneficial (e.g., turning the head up or down or to the left or right). A strained voice or one with intermittent aphonia suggests hypertonicity or spasm of the PE segment. There are various treatment options including general attempts at head/neck relaxation, surgical interventions (myotomy, neurectomy), and injection of botulinum toxin (see Chapter 9). A wet-sounding voice is indicative of saliva or food/liquid pooling on or near the PE segment. For some this occurs mainly during and after meals. Strategies to clear the pharynx of residual food such as multiple swallows, effortful swallows, or altered head positions can be tried.

**Distracters in Esophageal Speech Production.** Some of the more commonly occurring distracters during ES are depicted on the CD (see Chapter 8: Video: Distracters). The specific behaviors shown are clunking, stoma blast, extra mouth movements, double pumping—or pressing twice to load the esophagus, and intrusive consonant production. An additional segment is included in this clip demonstrating pharyngeal speech. This is an unwanted behavior characterized by use of the hypopharynx, not the esophagus, as the air reservoir for speech. The base of the tongue and the pharyngeal walls approximate to serve as the pharyngeal sound source. The voice quality, duration, and control are generally not sufficient to be considered an attractive alaryngeal speech option.

Distracters during ES can be broadly cast into two categories: unwanted noises and visual distractions. "Klunking" refers to a sound made when air is injected into the esophagus. The first step in minimizing this sound is to draw the speaker's attention to it. This can be done in many ways: audio recording and playback of speech, feeling the neck to sense when air charging and klunking occur, a stethoscope on the neck to amplify the klunk, etc. For some speakers, simply asking them to inject with less force may reduce the distracting noise. For others, shifting to the inhalation method may be possible (klunking happens predominantly with injectors).

Stoma noise is also a common distracter in ES that must be addressed. Less forceful pulmonary exhalation should be targeted. The first step is to test the speaker's hearing—reduced hearing acuity can limit the ability to recognize when stoma blast occurs (Kahane & Irwin, 1975). Placing a stethoscope near the stoma can help highlight occurrences of stoma noise for the patient. With the client watching in a mirror, a tissue or feather near the stoma can serve to detect expiratory airflow. With either of these types of feedback, the client can begin to monitor when stoma noise is occurring and then manipulate the force of the exhalation.

A distracting behavior that may occur for those using the consonant press injection is often referred to as "intrusive consonant production." This refers to the situation wherein a given speaker utilizes a particular consonant on a regular basis to load the esophagus with air. During connected speech, this individual will produce the consonant of choice (i.e., the one that helps put air into the esophagus) at inappropriate times when the esophagus needs to be reloaded. For example, if a speaker is only able to use a bilabial sound to insufflate the esophagus, he or she would produce the bilabial whenever air needed to be reloaded, even when a bilabial sound is not called for (e.g., he may say, "/b/+My name is (pause to reload air) /b/+Tim" for "My name is Tim" if he is loading air before "my" and "Tim").

There are also a number of visible behaviors that can detract from ES. These include head bobbing or flexion during insufflation, extensive upward thrust of the jaw or head during inhalation attempts, facial grimacing, lip pursing, lip smacking, multiple oral movements associated with injection attempts, eye rolling, and poor eye contact, among others. Many of these are indicative of inefficient or effortful loading of the esophagus. Often times, the behaviors can be extinguished by identifying them for the client using verbal feedback from the SLP, working in front of a mirror, or through videotape review. The client can then begin to eliminate the distracters, using the feedback in a manner similar to reducing secondary behaviors associated with stuttering (Duguay, 1999).

## Artificial Larynx Speech

### Relevance in the Context of Western Medicine

Unlike ES, there appears to be little doubt that communication using an artificial larynx, in particular an electrolarynx (EL), remains a popular choice for many individuals following total laryngectomy. Several studies have reported that 40% or more of laryngectomized individuals utilize an EL (Carr, Schmidbauer, Majaess, & Smith, 2000; Hillman et al., 1998; Salmon, 2005). For some individuals, AL use may be confined to the immediate postoperative period as an early means of communication or, in the long term, serve only as a backup to TE or ES speech (Ward et al., 2003). For a large pro-

portion of the population though, AL remains the primary means of communication (Hillman et al., 1998; Salmon, 2005).

The reasons for this relatively high rate of AL use are likely to be related to several factors. AL training is the only one of the three primary alaryngeal speech modes that can begin within the first few days after the laryngectomy surgery, usually on approximately the 2nd-4th postoperative day. The ability to reestablish verbal communication in this early time period cannot be underemphasized. After surgery the patient has the option of mouthing or writing notes. To be able to quickly use the device and say, "I love you" or "I'm fine," to his or her significant other is very powerful. While writing, gesturing, and mouthing speech can be useful, reacquiring verbal communication while still in the hospital can serve very functional purposes (e.g., communicating needs to nurses, etc.) and also can help lift the spirits of the patient and the loved ones.

In addition to being trainable early in the postsurgical time period, the training is relatively straightforward. Most individuals can be taught to have usable AL speech with appropriate SLP instruction and diligent practice. Although success at using an AL is not guaranteed for all those who attempt it, most appear capable of learning it, unless there are premorbid cognitive deficits present.

As indicated in Tables 8-1, 8-2, and 8-3, there are advantages and disadvantages to AL use, just as there are with the other alaryngeal speech options. Some of the advantages are particularly strong and may be a primary reason for drawing clients to AL use. In addition to the ability to train AL use early on, the intensity of speech is generally greater than that of ES as well as TE speech in some cases and may be perceived better in the presence of competing noise (Clark & Stemple, 1982). Other advantages of significance include independence from the SLP once functional AL speech is attained (as is the case with ES), limited cost beyond the initial purchase of the device and SLP training, relatively short therapy process (although continual refinements can be attempted), and a speaking rate that can be manipulated fairly easily. These advantages may be enough for many speakers to choose AL speech in spite of some of the drawbacks such as the use of a hand during talking (most use a handheld device), mechanical quality to the voice, and restrictions in intonation and pitch variability.

Even if the AL is not chosen as the primary method of communication following the laryngectomy, it is attractive as a secondary communication option because of the ease of use and training. In the survey by Salmon (2005), 40% of TE and 40% of ES speakers reported using an EL as their backup mode of communication. Duguay (1985) reported the need for an AL to be trained and used, even if only as a backup system to ES or TE speech. He described being in three separate motor vehicle accidents with laryngectomized individuals, who were superior ES speakers, who were unable to speak due to the effect that stress and anxiety had on their method of speech. The same could be true if a TE speaker was suddenly thrown into a traumatic situation, creating excess tension in the PE segment tissue. Additionally, many centers around the world encourage training of proficient EL usage when TE speech is a person's primary mode of communication in order to allow communication to occur even when TE valve/prosthesis problems arise or when TE speech production is uncomfortable, as may be the case during or following radiation therapy (Ward et al., 2003).

## Artificial Larynx Speech Rehabilitation Processes and Techniques

### Preoperative Discussion

As noted above in the preoperative counseling regarding ES speech, we advocate giving patients and their loved ones an overview of all three alaryngeal speech methods. We describe the AL use in basic terms and might demonstrate its use if the patient or family request. Again, we do not do extensive demonstrations or descriptions unless their questioning prompts it. We do inform them that they will not have a voice when they come out of the surgery and that mouthing speech, writing notes, and gesturing are possible with EL training to be initiated a few days after the surgery.

### Various Types of Artificial Larynges

Lerman (1991) gives an excellent historical account of the AL and how they have evolved (as do Keith, Shanks, and Doyle, 2005, and Salmon, 1999). Although

there are some exciting possibilities for future developments in EL devices (see Meltzner et al., 2005), the devices currently in use by patients are in many respects relatively unchanged compared to devices available 20–25 years ago, with a few exceptions. Typically devices are grouped either by the manner in which the vibratory source is powered (pneumatically or electronically) and/or the method of delivering the vibratory sound into the vocal tract (intraorally or through neck tissue). Two devices, which do not fit easily into the usual classifications, are the JusTalk (JustMed, Inc.) and the Ultra-Voice Plus II (Ultra-Voice Ltd.). The JusTalk device generates a tone through a speaker placed at the corner of the mouth (not through a tube into the mouth as with traditional intraoral devices) while the other introduces sound from a speaker embedded within an interdental appliance. These and the other main types of devices will be described in more detail in the subsequent section.

**Pneumatic Devices.** The lungs power a pneumatic device. Devices typically consist of a steel or soft rubber cover which fits over the stoma, a pipe leading to and away from a cylindrical chamber which houses a stretched rubber membrane held in position by a rubber band, and a plastic or rubber tube that is inserted into the mouth. Air from the lungs travels into the metal housing, forcing the rubber membrane within the device to vibrate. This sound is then transmitted through the tube into the oral cavity where it can be shaped into speech. An example of a pneumatic device is shown in Figure 8–2. A video sample of a person using a pneumatic device is on the CD (see Chapter 8: Video. Pneumatic Artificial Larynx).

Pneumatic devices in use today are intraoral in nature (i.e., all require a tube entering from the corner of the mouth to deliver sound into the oral cavity). Pneumatic devices typically offer the most natural sound of all of the AL devices. Pitch can be varied by adjusting the width and tension of the vibrating membrane or by increasing breath pressure during voicing. Manipulating the force of exhalation can also alter loudness. Pneumatic devices are generally less expensive than electronic artificial larynges. This is a consideration when trying to select a device, perhaps even more so when choosing a device as a backup communication option rather than as the primary mode (see discus-

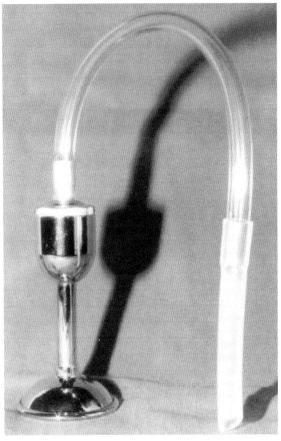

**A.**

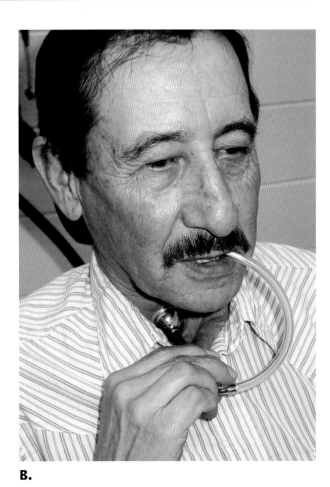

**B.**

**Figure 8–2.** Example of (**A.**) the Tokyo Artificial Larynx (Photo courtesy of Limco Solutions) and (**B.**) the pneumatic device in use.

sion in Chapter 15 regarding the popularity of less expensive pneumatic devices in non-Western health settings such as China).

**Electronic Devices.** Electronic devices are battery powered and can be broadly classified as neck-type or intraoral. Figure 8–3 shows a drawing of the use of a neck-type EL device. Figure 8–4 depicts a sampling of various neck-type ELs (some with oral adaptors also depicted). For the neck-type EL, a button is depressed to turn the device on and released to turn it off. When activated, a small piston at the head of the device moves up and down against a plastic plate creating a vibration. Holding the head of the device to the

neck, the mechanically generated sound is transmitted through the tissue setting air within the vocal tract into vibration. This sound can then be utilized for speech sound production via movements and shaping of the articulators. In addition to the neck, alternative sites for placing the device against the skin are under the chin or on the cheek. A small sampling of typical neck-type EL users is depicted on the CD (see Chapter 8: Video: Neck-Type EL Users).

Electronic neck devices typically have separate buttons for pitch and loudness manipulations. In some cases these control buttons are readily accessible in the outer surface of the device itself and can be adjusted with a thumb or finger. In certain devices,

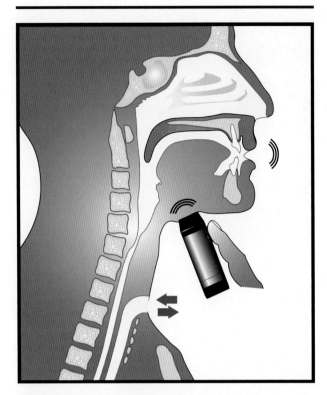

**Figure 8–3.** Schematic of using a neck-type EL.

pitch and loudness control knobs are located more internally within the EL housing itself. In this case, setting and changing pitch and loudness can be more cumbersome as the outer sleeve of the device or the end cap must be removed. In other devices, pitch can be increased or decreased depending on the extent to which a button or lever is depressed.

Some ELs are constructed to be solely intraoral in nature (e.g., Cooper Rand, see Figure 8–5). In these devices vibration is generated in a manner similar to the method described above but there is a small tube coming from the sound generator that can be placed inside the mouth to deliver the vibration directly to the oral cavity. Again a small on-off switch is manipulated to activate and deactivate the voice. Many of the neck-type ELs can be converted to operate as an intraoral EL by placing an adaptor over the head of the device. A tube coming off of the adaptor can be inserted in the mouth to deliver sound into the oral cavity. Use of intraoral ELs is depicted on the CD (see Chapter 8: Video: Intraoral EL Users).

There are two other devices that are variants of intraoral ELs. The first is an interdental device called the UltraVoice Plus II (UltraVoice Ltd.; there are earlier versions of this device as well) (see Figure 8–6). This intraoral device is a denture or retainer that houses a loudspeaker that projects a voice tone into the oral cavity. Also imbedded in the denture or retainer is a radio circuit that receives a signal from a computerized control unit worn on the speaker's belt or carried in the hand. When a switch on the control unit is activated (with a finger or with a hands-free switch), a signal is sent to the radio circuit in the denture, which drives the loudspeaker. Another newer EL called the JusTalk (JustMed, Inc.) (see Figure 8–7) introduces a voice signal into the oral cavity from a small head mounted speaker positioned on or very near the lips. Also on the head mount is a microphone that detects the speech. The microphone signal is routed to a digital signal processing unit that can be held in the hand or clipped to a belt or pocket. This unit reportedly enhances and then plays the modified signal through a speaker. Video samples of individuals using each of these units are included on the CD (see Chapter 8: Video: Other EL Devices). Both of these devices have attempted to address one of the primary limitations of most ELs, namely that one hand is occupied during EL speech.

Another recent attempt to offer a hands-free EL has become commercially available from Griffin Laboratories. A holder for the TruTone™ or SolaTone is strapped to the chest. The EL is placed in the holder, which can be adjusted to position the head of the EL against the neck. By tipping the chin down (or raising the shoulder/chest up) a prominence on the holder depresses the pressure-sensitive on-off switch of the TruTone. A video sample of a client using the TruTone hands-free holder is included on the CD (see Chapter 8: Video: Other EL Devices). Note that the TruTone user is still able to take advantage of the variable pitch control to produce intonation contours.

### Selection of an Instrument

It is important for patients to be introduced to a variety of instruments before they decide which one to purchase. Unfortunately, this exposure to multiple devices prior to purchase may not happen in many cases. Ideally, SLPs will have a stockpile of ALs for the purpose of loaning out a device so that patients can

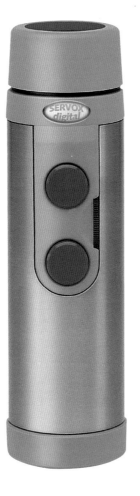
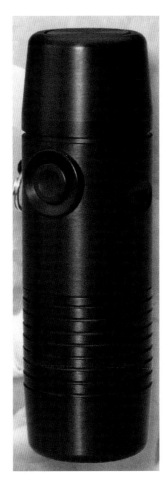
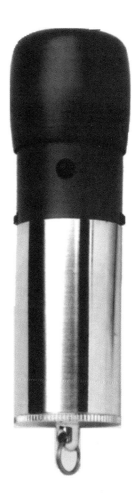

**Figure 8–4.** Examples of different models of neck-type EL devices. From left to right, the Servox Digital (photo courtesy of Servox AG, www.servoxdigital.com), the TruTone (photo courtesy of Griffin Laboratories, Inc.), and the Romet (photo courtesy of Romet, Inc.).

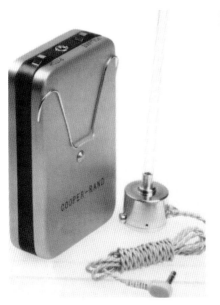
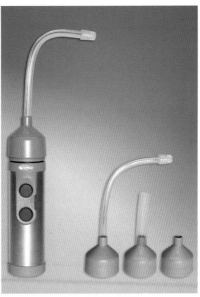
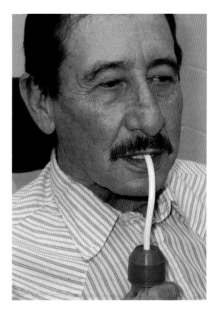

**Figure 8–5.** Intraoral EL options. From left to right, the Cooper-Rand intraoral device (photo courtesy of Luminaud, Inc.), the Servox Digital neck-type EL with intraoral adaptors (photo courtesy of Servox AG, www.servoxdigital.com), and a patient using a Servox with intraoral adaptor.

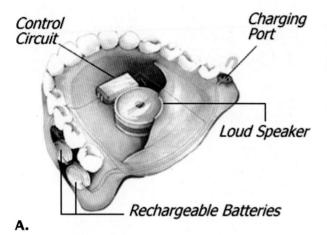

A.

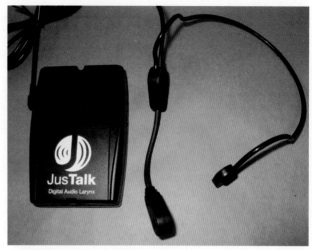

**Figure 8–7.** JusTalk EL device. (Photo courtesy of JustMed, Inc.)

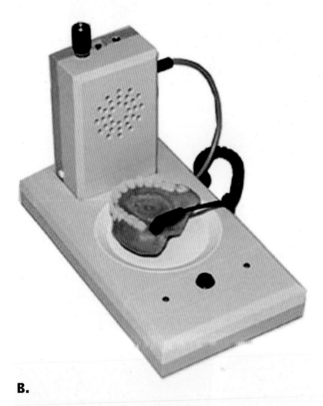

B.

**Figure 8–6.** UltraVoice Plus II generates a tone from a speaker embedded in an interdental appliance. (Photos courtesy of UltraVoice Ltd., www.ultravoice.com.)

experiment to find the one that works best for them. Salmon (1999) stated that before one can appropriately select which device is best for an individual patient, the clinician must first determine the best placement on the neck or cheek (or inside the mouth if using an intraoral device), activate the AL, and listen to the quality of the tone produced. Not all necks are alike and not all patient and spouse preferences are the same. Other features to consider include: size and location of on-off control switches and how they compare to the patient's finger size and dexterity; ease of pitch and loudness controls; type of power supply for the EL (nickel metal hydrite batteries, 9V batteries, rechargeable AA battery, etc.); durability; overall size of the device; cost; and whether the AL is being used as a primary mode of communication or a backup to TE or ES. Other patient related factors that might impact which specific device is selected include their overall health, strength, cognitive abilities, hearing, and vision. Family members' concerns and preferences also can inform and shape the decision that is made.

Clinicians need to give as much information as possible to their patients during this selection process so that an informed decision can be made. Lewin (2004) stated that the method of alaryngeal speech production for a patient should be selected on the basis of the individual's needs, personality, physical capabilities, level of independent functioning, family support, and motivation. Patients who have had a stroke, for example, postlaryngectomy, may find they are no longer able to use the AL in the manner they used it previously. Because of physical or cognitive changes, they may need to alter how they use the device or perhaps even seek out a different device that better suits their current condition.

The individual features of each instrument need to be paired with the needs of the patients or their significant others. For example, if a patient or the spouse is hearing impaired, certain devices (e.g., Cooper-Rand, Luminaud, Inc.) that have greater ability to increase intensity may be preferred. If the patient was a pipe-smoker, he/she might prefer an intraoral AL, such as the Cooper-Rand (Luminaud, Inc.), because it mimics to some extent pipe-smoking. For other individuals, it may be important to produce a very quiet voice at times, prompting consideration of other devices with readily accessible loudness control or possibly the UltraVoice Plus II (UltraVoice Ltd.), which has a "whisper" mode. Still others might place heavy importance on intonation abilities and so devices with a single pressure-sensitive button that manipulates pitch (e.g., TruTone) may be preferred. A petite woman might prefer a small EL such as the Romet (Romet, Inc.).

### Postoperative Training in the Use of an Artificial Larynx

Graham (1997) identified five target behaviors in AL training: placement, on-off control, articulation, appro-

priate rate and phrasing, and attention to nonverbal behaviors. Although each of these target behaviors is relevant for both pneumatic and EL devices, the following discussions will be focused on EL training. Most professionals focus on some variation of these five behaviors, after the initial device is selected (Lerman, 1991; Duguay, 1983; Hyman, 1994; Salmon, 1999).

**Placement.** Accurate and consistent placement of the EL is the first step in the rehabilitation process after selecting a device. Proper placement is necessary before other EL speech production parameters can be addressed. Usually, the EL device is held against the neck, although underneath the chin or on the cheek are also possibilities (use of an intraoral tube/device is discussed separately later) (see Figure 8–8). With patients who have had more extended laryngectomy surgery, or who have had extensive radiation, it may be challenging to find the best placement and alternate locations may have to be sought (e.g., higher or lower or more posterior than is typical). The intent is to identify the location on the neck or face that allows the best sound transmission into the vocal tract. This spot is often referred to as the "sweet spot" (Salmon, 1999).

As a first step to locating the sweet spot, the clinician should ask permission to feel the neck, when trying to determine which device and which placement

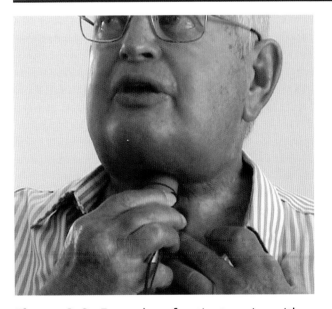
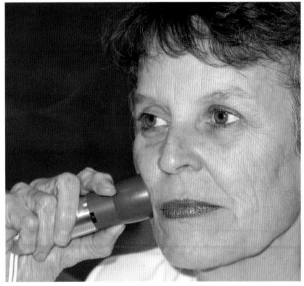

**Figure 8–8.** Examples of patients using either neck or cheek EL placement.

site might work best for the patient, as it might be tender or painful in the early postoperative period. With permission, the SLP palpates the sides of the neck and under the chin in search of soft, pliable surface tissue. In addition to tissue compliancy, the clinician has to consider the individual patient and his/her needs. For example, Lerman (1991) poses the issue of the patient with a hearing loss. He reported better placement on the neck opposite the hearing aide, due to the interference with the hearing aid from the noise produced by the speech aid. In the early stages postsurgery and during radiotherapy the optimal position for the EL may also vary, as parts of the neck and face may be tender, swollen, or too painful to be optimal for communication. Once the optimal section of tissue on the neck/cheek has been identified, the SLP assists the patient to place the device firmly and flush against the tissue, while activating the EL. Typically in initial sessions, having the patient count or recite something meaningless will assist in concentrating on the primary goal, which is finding the best spot that gives good resonance. The clinician's and the patient's ears serve as the primary judge in helping to locate the best spot or spots. Having the patient listen to the tonal quality while positioning the device in several different places will assist the patient to fully understand that all tissue placements are not the same and simply pressing the device against the neck anywhere will not necessarily give him/her the best sound.

Once the best site is identified, the "sweet spot" can be marked with tape or with a marker. The patient can then practice moving the device away from and then back onto the "sweet spot." Often times gaining feedback from a significant other is an important aspect of this part of the training process. The family members need to know that there is a difference in how the device can and should sound, which will help them in their acceptance of their loved ones' new voice. Stressing the importance of hitting the target location every time is essential to optimal use of the EL. Attempts at identifying the sweet spot and practice hitting this location are included on the CD (see Chapter 8: Video: EL Placement).

For some patients, radiation fibrosis or scarring of the neck and/or cheek tissue prevent good conduction of the vibratory tone, and instead lead to distracting mechanical buzzing that hinders intelligibility. In these instances, intraoral EL devices should be considered.

Placement for the intraoral tubing, however, also has to be carefully considered and evaluated. The oral tube poses its own problems in terms of possibly interfering with articulatory movements of the tongue and lips. Salmon (1999) reported that a standard placement of an intraoral tube is approximately 1.5 to 2 inches into the corner of the mouth, resting on the upper lateral surface of the tongue. Deem and Miller (2000) stated the tubing should be angled upward toward the hard palate, but with the tongue not occluding the tip of the tube. Pneumatic devices involve an additional placement consideration beyond where the tip of the oral tube rests. For a pneumatic device, such as the Tokyo Artificial Larynx (Limco Solutions) or the ToneAir II Pneumatic (Communicative Medical, Inc.) speech aids, correct positioning of the metal or plastic stoma cup must be achieved to capture the pulmonary air. This includes firm and complete coverage around the stoma site so that there is not excess air escape between the stoma cup and neck tissue. For the JusTalk device (JustMed, Inc.), proper placement of the microphone/headset is critical for its success. Correct placement for all forms of EL communication is paramount to intelligible speech.

**On-Off Timing.** For electronic AL users, they must learn how to operate the on-off switch in a manner that promotes good speech. For the pneumatic device they must learn how to initiate and halt the pulmonary air supply that powers the vibration of the membrane or reed. A basic rule to assist patients to achieve this coordination is to instruct them to ensure the device is on when their articulators are moving. Alternatively, when a person is simply thinking of an idea or pausing in a sentence, the device should be deactivated. If the on-off skill is not mastered, EL speech can be distracting to the listener, leaving him/her unable to focus adequately on the intended message. Training of this skill is essential and may be one of the main reasons listeners are turned off to the EL initially. Graham (1997) states that the speech pathologist should use the speech aid to demonstrate the errors to the laryngectomized patient, so the patient can begin the process of monitoring his or her own speech patterns. When teaching on-off timing, demonstration of how the inappropriate communication is perceived is important. Often patients do not realize they are speaking in a choppy, distracting manner, by constantly turning the device on and off with each syllable. Turning the device on and off prematurely can also affect the meaning of what is intended in sentences where there are overlapping phonemes or juncture considerations, such as in the phrase: I /am/ Mable vs. I'm /able. The use of pausing or the on-off timing technique will make a difference in communicating what is intended in such cases. Demonstration and practice of appropriate phrasing, timing, and pausing can be facilitated initially with structured reading passages, which contain notation about where and when pauses and device activation/deactivation should occur. Working in front of a mirror to help get the EL in position before the lips start to move is often helpful.

**Articulation.** As for all forms of alaryngeal speech, articulation needs to be addressed in the rehabilitation process. The key characteristics of articulatory production during AL speech have been described by a number of authors (e.g., Cady, 1981; Goldstein & Rothman, 1976; Isshiki & Tanabe, 1972; Weiss & Basili, 1985). In summarizing this research, Salmon (1999) reported that, in general, nasals and glides are perceived as accurate. However, common articulatory concerns include: voiced/voiceless confusions, difficulty producing frication, omission or weak production of consonants in medial and/or final positions, and inability to produce a perceptually distinct /h/. As with ES, many (but not all) of the common articulatory problems in AL speech relate to the need to generate higher intraoral air pressures for production of distinct stop bursts and fricative noise. Shanks (J. C. Shanks, personal communication, July 18, 2003) has described a variety of therapy tasks that can be used to train increased intraoral air pressure including activities such as: blowing out a match, making a kissing sound, spitting seeds, blowing bubbles. These activities can be useful to have them feel what high intraoral pressure might feel like and to help demonstrate for patients that they can produce higher oral pressures. However, once the patient has grasped the concept, we move quickly into speech stimuli.

Before proceeding with articulatory training, it is assumed that the patient has mastered the basics of AL use, namely accurate placement and on-off control of the device. It is often helpful to do auditory training on any of the tasks described below. This would entail demonstration of the intended behavior by the clinician, identifying the important perceptual feature that is being targeted, and having patients serve as the judge for the clinician's demonstrations (and then ultimately their own productions) with the clinician helping to shape their listening skills and judgment over time. Spouses and other family members can also be used as monitors within and outside of therapy if the clinician properly trains them and if the dynamics within the family are conducive to such feedback.

Misperception of voiceless consonants as voiced is perhaps the most commonly encountered articulatory error. The AL device is designed to generate a voice signal whenever it is activated and transient "devoicing" for a voiceless consonant can be difficult. In this case, then, the voice signal continues during stop gaps and frication noise, causing the listener to perceive the consonant as voiced. Some excellent EL speakers learn to turn their device off briefly when producing a voiceless consonant. Others may be able to do very slight adjustments in the amount of pressure with which the device is pressed to the neck (usually more pressure to "dampen" the EL voice signal) during voiceless consonants. However, both of these approaches require a very rapid motor movement of the fingers/hand to be carried out in coordination with speech movements. This skill may not be easily acquired, or even possible, for many speakers. In other cases, training speakers to differentiate cognates based on the strength of the burst or frication noise is more tenable. Voiceless consonants are typically produced with higher intraoral air pressure and stronger burst/frication intensity. Most speakers can be trained to "push harder" or produce a strong burst on voiceless stop consonants and fricatives through drill work with minimal word pairs. The clinician and the patients' ears are generally sufficient to serve as the judge for producing stronger versus weaker bursts, although one could also use instrumentation (small oral catheter and pressure transducer with visual display of oral pressure) or other types of feedback (e.g., tissue/feather held in front of the lips to help visualize strength of a burst release). Poorer speakers do not pay enough attention to these details, along with omitting plosives and fricatives. The CD includes samples of patients working on generating stronger bursts and fricative noises (see Chapter 8: Video: Generating Strong Bursts and Frication) and doing voiced-voiceless word pairs (see Chapter 8: Video: Voiced-Voiceless Contrasts).

Fricatives in general usually have to be specifically targeted in therapy because they are difficult for the AL user to produce. In the nonlaryngectomized speaker, an oral air stream through a point of constriction is generated from pulmonary airflow. In the laryngectomized speaker, the lower airway is diverted out the stoma precluding use of a pulmonary air stream to create frication. Therefore, a new method must be trained for generating an oral air stream. Fortunately, most users can be trained to compress air within the oral cavity and then move the articulators quickly to create a small flow of air through a point of constriction. Usually, the clinician can simply model the production of this fricative burst on a voiceless fricative in isolation (the clinician must hold the breath and create the air flow as the laryngectomee patient does—solely with the oral articulators). The instructions usually center on pressing with the articulators more forcefully and moving them sharply to create a small burst of noise. This initial training is best done without the device in place so that the clinician and patient are able to hear when the fricative noise is generated. Once the patient is able to produce the fricative noise on sounds in isolation, a typical hierarchy of stimuli can be constructed wherein complexity of the sample is gradually increased (greater length, varying place of fricative production, varying position of the fricative from syllable initiating to final positions, etc.). At some point, there can be significant overlap between the work on fricative production and the voiced/voiceless distinction goal. The patient can be trained to produce more or less intense frication for voiceless and voiced fricatives.

During EL speech initial consonants are generally perceived more accurately than those in final position (Cady, 1981; Isshiki & Tanabe, 1972; although see Weiss & Basili, 1981, who reported the opposite). In nonlaryngectomized speakers, final consonants are often slighted (i.e., produced with less pressure and reduced intensity), but intelligibility is not impacted. It is not surprising then that the laryngectomized speaker might retain this same pattern of speech production, but unfortunately there are enough other issues with EL speech that the slighting of final consonants is not well tolerated by listeners and so intelligibility may suffer. EL users must be trained to not slight medial and final consonants. Sometimes asking patients to adopt a "clear" speech pattern (e.g., "Pretend your listener is hard of hearing or is having trouble understanding you.") is sufficient to get more precise inclusion of consonants in all positions of words. However, sometimes more specific training is required. This often involves drill work, using high pressure consonants (stops, fricatives, and affricates) that are embedded in medial and final word positions. The instruction is to produce the word with all consonants clearly included, using perceptual judgments as the criterion. Again, the stimuli can be increased in complexity from single words to short phrases, sentences, and eventually conversation. As with the other articulatory training work, this is best done initially without using the EL so that the ears can better hear the bursts and frication, although at some point the EL must be included. The timing of this varies between patients, but we try to start it soon after the patient appears to have grasped the concept of not slighting the sound (usually that means somewhere within the first session and on single words or short phrases).

The /h/ sound is problematic for EL users, just as it is for those who use ES. Again, the issue is an inability to generate a voiceless fricative air stream at the most posterior and inferior aspects of the altered vocal tract. Some EL users are able to transiently turn off the device when an /h/ is intended to help mark the sound (similar to what some can do to mark voiceless sounds in general), although this is not common in our experience. More typically, we let context help carry the meaning. However, one could also use a pharyngeal fricative to mark the /h/ in a manner similar to what was described for ES above.

Articulation when using an intraoral device deserves specific comment. Placing a tube between the lips and into the oral cavity obviously introduces the possibility that articulatory movements could be impeded or disrupted. Great care must be taken by the speech pathologist and patient to identify the best tube placement. While one might find a "sweet spot" for tube tip placement near the alveolar ridge or in the mid-portion of the oral cavity, the trade-off in terms of articulatory disturbance may be unacceptable. Striking a balance between obtaining the best oral resonance while still allowing the most clear articulatory behavior is imperative. When using an intraoral AL, the speaker must address all of the same issues as noted above for neck-type ELs.

**Pitch, Loudness, Rate, and Stress.** In order to maximize naturalness in EL communication, pitch, loudness, rate, and stress patterning features each may need to be directly addressed during therapy. Speaking pitch can be set and adjusted on some ELs by manually turning a small dial or via digital programming with a computer (e.g., Servox Digital, Servox AG). In these cases, the pitch is set and the device generates a relatively constant fundamental frequency whenever the device is activated. Some devices have two separate buttons that can be preset to specific pitches. Switching between the two pitch buttons during running speech can be done to generate transient increases or decreases in pitch to mark stressed syllables and generate intonation contours. The therapist should help patients learn how to manipulate the EL pitch control feature of their device and to identify the best pitch(es) to preset. Other devices have a variable pitch control switch (e.g., TruTone, Griffin Laboratories) that alters the pitch depending on the extent to which the switch is depressed or moved. Using multisyllabic words or phrases and an instruction to produce a specific pitch intonation contour, the patient can work on controlling the variable pitch button so that the most natural sounding pitch changes are produced. Besides presetting the device or learning how to use the variable control switch, an EL user may be able to change the pitch of the voice in other ways. For example, it has been suggested that an individual can tighten the neck muscles or move the instrument either higher or lower than the "sweet spot" to change pitch to help mark stress or create appropriate intonation contours (Salmon, 1999). Samples of patients attempting pitch changes for intonation purposes are on the CD (see Chapter 8: Video: Intonation with an EL).

Loudness of EL speech is often a relative strength compared to ES and TE speech. ELs usually have volume control knobs that can be adjusted to meet the needs of a particular situation (assuming batteries are fully charged). If anything, clinicians often note that EL users tend to leave their device set with the loudness level too high. Consequently, for many patients, direct training is needed in relation to setting loudness levels and monitoring/adjusting these for different commu-

nicative settings. As with ES and TE speech, manipulations of mouth opening can also be used to alter loudness (i.e., opening the mouth may increase loudness; more closed mouth speech is usually softer). Others have reported that they can alter the amount of pressure that they use in sealing the EL device against the skin. By increasing the pressure against the skin, the vibration from the EL device can be dampened to decrease speech loudness.

Appropriate rate and stress patterning are needed to optimize EL speech. In general, a slightly slower overall rate of speech is usually targeted in therapy. A slower rate presumably allows the speaker time to make more precise (and perhaps longer) articulatory contacts while also allowing the listener more processing time. Care should be given, however, to avoid an excessively slow rate because it could deleteriously affect the naturalness of the EL speech.

A decreased ability to mark word stress is possible in EL speech. Nonlaryngectomized individuals mark stress via pitch, loudness, and durational changes. EL users may be restricted in their ability to finely manipulate these parameters, particularly pitch and loudness, and so they may sound monotone. However, with practice many EL speakers can become proficient in placing emphasis and stress. Certainly, EL users can be taught to pause briefly just prior to a word that they would like to emphasize. Additionally, they should be able to learn to increase the duration of a vowel within a stressed syllable. Contrastive drills in which shifting the syllable stress shifts linguistic meaning (e.g., "*pro*duce" [vegetables and fruit] vs. "pro*duce*" [to make]; "*add*ress" [street] vs. "ad*dress*" [speak to]) can be useful for practicing stress placement. Samples of patients practicing word stress are included on the CD (see Chapter 8: Video: Word Stress with an EL).

Additional therapeutic tasks that can help maximize intonation, stress, and rate issues are singing, reading poems, or other potentially rhythmic and highly stressed passages or role playing as they try to convey particular emotions (e.g., sadness, surprise, anger, etc.). In these types of tasks, an EL user is likely to manipulate several production parameters simultaneously (pitch, loudness, pausing, duration). Often, there is fairly limited direct "teaching" that has to be done. Rather, the clinician's role may be to carefully observe, give verbal reinforcement or feedback of perceptually accurate/good productions, and provide sufficient practice time and materials that allow the skill to develop. With practice the laryngectomized individual can begin to feel a sense of control over the communication process.

**Distractions and Other Considerations.** Graham (1997) refers to distractions as nonverbal behaviors that need to be eliminated, such as facial grimacing while you are trying to talk. Looking uncomfortable during AL use can be a distracter in itself. When people are speaking, they should look as though they want to speak to their listener. Holding their arm in an awkward position while using the AL can also be distracting. A comfortable, natural posture with the shoulder down and the elbow close to the body pointing downward is encouraged. Likewise, unusual head positioning (chin up, head turned, etc.) during AL use can be visually distracting to the listener. The use of a mirror while practicing will assist the new user to see how others view him/her when voicing. The patient must also learn to keep the device on only when wanting to communicate, being careful to not make extraneous noises or buzzes when the device is not in place on the sweet spot. Often, a well meaning clinician does not want to hurt the patient's feelings and does not point out these distractions, but in the long run, the overall communication can be negatively impacted. These are all issues that need to be discussed, so as not to distract from the communication process.

Some thought should also be given to which hand is used to hold the AL. Although the natural inclination of the patient will be to use the dominant hand, we usually discourage this. Using the nondominant hand allows the individual to speak while simultaneously writing or doing other activities with the dominant hand. Sometimes, however, the location of the sweet spot causes us to rethink our usual position. Most often we discourage individuals from crossing the right to the left or vice versa in order to hit their sweet spot unless they can do it very unobtrusively.

Device functionality and issues with battery life are now factors the AL users have to consider as integral to their day-to-day communication. All patients should be taught to carry extra batteries in a protective case at all times. They should be aware of issues relating to their battery life, such as the fact that carrying batteries in your pocket with lose change or keys can sap the batteries' energy, or worse yet, generate heat or fire.

Other issues which need to be discussed include the use of AL devices in a variety of contexts. The most important of these may be the use of the telephone. The ability to use a telephone can be important in gaining independence and socialization for some patients (Salmon, 1990). Telephones have built-in microphones and typically can be used quite well by many AL users. However it is important that the patient is instructed to hold the receiver of the phone up and away from the mouth, instead of down by the head of the instrument; otherwise the sound of the instrument will drown out speech. The use of other ancillary devices, such as an FM microphone in conjunction with the speakers in your car, can also be useful in certain situations (e.g., conversing during car rides, ordering food at a drive-up window, conducting banking through drive-through services, etc.).

# Conclusion

Clinicians must be prepared to educate laryngectomy patients about all three of the primary modes of alaryngeal speech. In this chapter, information regarding ES and AL speech is reviewed. For each of these two modes of communication, information is offered regarding its relevance within the context of Western medicine. The bulk of the chapter then focuses on the rehabilitation process itself. Use of an AL is a skill that all or nearly all laryngectomy patients are likely to need, either as a primary or a secondary mode of communication. In contrast, the number of individuals who use ES is likely to diminish in the upcoming years given advances in the other forms of alaryngeal speech and an ever-decreasing number of SLPs who are familiar with and capable of training ES. However, there are individuals for whom ES may be the best communication option and SLPs must be prepared to take on the necessary training. Additionally, Doyle and Eadie (2005) have raised the interesting suggestion that perhaps the more aggressive use of Botox and surgical myotomy for TE speech rehabilitation could benefit individuals attempting to learn ES. If this ultimately is shown to be the case, ES could reemerge as a more prominent option in the future.

## Vendor List and Contact Details

Communicative Medical, Inc.
P.O. Box 65174
Vancouver, BC 98665
CANADA
www.communicativemedical.com

Cooper-Rand Artificial Larynx
Luminaud, Inc.
8688 Tyler Blvd
Mentor, Ohio 44060
www.luminaud.com
info@luminaud.com

H.E.L.P. Help Employ Laryngectomized Persons:
Video Tape Series
The National Clearing House of Rehabilitation
Training Materials
816 W. 6ᵗʰ Street
Oklahoma State University
Stillwater, Oklahoma 74078-0435

JusTalk Artificial Larynx
JustMed, Inc.
14780 SW Osprey Drive, Suite 260
Beaverton, Oregon 97007
www.justmedinc.com
joel@JustMedInc.com

Lauder Enterprises, Inc.
11115 Whisper Hollow
San Antonio, Texas 78230-3609
www.voicestore.com
info@voicestore.com

Romet Artificial Larynx
Romet, Inc.
9501 W. Sahara Ave. #1023
Las Vegas, Nevada 89117
800-979-0119 or 702-233-3975

Servox Eco, Servox Artificial Larynx
Servox AG
Biberweg 24-26
D-53842 Troisdorf
Cologne, Germany
www.servox.de
info@servox.de

Tokyo Artificial Larynx
Mark Welch
Limco Solutions
4736 North 13th Street
Omaha, Nebraska 68110-1426
402-980-3420
www.limcosolutions.com

TruTone Artificial Larynx
Griffin Laboratories, Inc.
27636 Ynez Road, Suite L 7199
Temecula, California 92591
www.griffinlab.com

UltraVoice Plus II
UltraVoice Ltd.
3612 Chapel Road
Newtown Square, Pennsylvania 19073
www.ultravoice.com

## References

Ainsworth, W. A., & Singh, W. (1992). Perceptual comparison of neoglottal, oesophageal and normal speech. *Folia Phoniatrica, 44*, 297–307.

Anderson, J. O. (1950). *A descriptive study of elements of esophageal speech.* Unpublished doctoral dissertation, Ohio State University, Columbus.

Atkinson, M., Kramer, P., Wyman, S. M., & Inglefinger, F. J. (1957). The dynamics of swallowing: I. Normal pharyngeal mechanism. *Journal of Clinical Investigation, 36*, 581–588.

Bates, G. J., McFeeter, L., & Coman, W. (1990). Pharyngolaryngectomy and voice restoration. *Laryngoscope, 100*, 1025–1026.

Beamer, M. W. (1954). *A qualitative study of the personality adjustment of laryngectomized subjects.* Unpublished master's thesis, Texas State College for Women, Denton, TX.

Bennett, S., & Weinberg, B. (1973). Acceptability ratings of normal, esophageal, and artificial larynx speech. *Journal of Speech and Hearing Research, 16*, 608–615.

Berlin, C. I. (1963). Clinical measurement of esophageal speech: I: Methodology and curves of skill acquisition *Journal of Speech and Hearing Disorders, 28*, 42–51.

Berlin, C. I. (1964). Hearing loss, palatal function and other factors in post-laryngectomy rehabilitation. *Journal of Chronic Disease, 17*, 677–684.

Bertino, G., Bellomo, A., Miani, C., Ferrero, F., & Staffieri, A. (1996). Spectrographic differences between tracheal-esophageal and esophageal voice. *Folia Phoniatrica, 48*, 255-261.

Blom, E. D., Singer, M. I., & Hamaker, R. C. (1985). An improved esophageal insufflation test. *Archives of Otolaryngology, 111*, 211-212.

Blom, E. D., Singer, M. I., & Hamaker, R. C. (1986). A prospective study of tracheoesophageal speech. *Archives of Otolaryngology-Head & Neck Surgery, 112*, 440-447.

Blood, G. W. (1981). The interactions of amplitude and phonetic quality in esophageal speech. *Journal of Speech and Hearing Research, 24*, 308-312.

Brown, D. H., Hilgers, F. J. M., Irish, J. C., & Balm, A. J. M. (2003). Postlaryngectomy voice rehabilitation: State of the art at the millennium. *World Journal of Surgery, 27*, 824-831.

Cady, B. (1981). *Phonemic intelligibility in artificial larynx speech.* Unpublished doctoral dissertation, University of Kansas, Lawrence.

Carpenter, M. A. (1999). Treatment decisions in alaryngeal speech. In S. J. Salmon (Ed.), *Alaryngeal speech rehabilitation* (2nd ed., pp. 55-77). Austin, TX: Pro-Ed.

Carr, M. M., Schmidbauer, J. A., Majaess, L., & Smith, R.L. (2000). Communication after laryngectomy: An assessment of quality of life. *Otolaryngology-Head & Neck Surgery, 122*, 440-447.

Cheesman, A., Knight, J., McIvor, J., & Perry, A. (1986). Tracheoesophageal "puncture speech": An assessment technique for failed oesophageal speakers. *The Journal of Laryngology and Otology, 100*, 191-199.

Christensen, J. M., & Dwyer, P. E. (1990). Improving alaryngeal speech intelligibility. *Journal of Communication Disorders, 23*, 445-451.

Clark, J. G. (1985). Alaryngeal speech intelligibility and the older listener. *Journal of Speech and Hearing Disorders, 50*, 60-65.

Clark, J. G., & Stemple, J. C. (1982). Assessment of three modes of alaryngeal speech with a synthetic sentence identification (SSI) task in varying message-to-competition ratios. *Journal of Speech and Hearing Research, 25*, 333-338.

Connor, H. P., Hamlet, S. L., & Joyce, J. C. (1985). Acoustic and physiologic correlates of the voicing distinction in esophageal speech. *Journal of Speech and Hearing Disorders, 50*, 378-384.

Damste, P. H. (1958). *Oesophageal speech after laryngectomy.* Groningen, The Netherlands: Hoitsema.

Deem, J. F., & Miller, L. (2000). *Manual of voice therapy.* Austin, TX: Pro-Ed.

de Raucourt, D., Rame, J. P., Daliphard, F., Le Pennec, D., Bequignon, A., & Luquet, A. (1998). Voice rehabilitation with a voice prosthesis: Study of 62 patients with 5 years follow-up. *Review of Laryngology, Otology, and Rhinology, 119*, 297-300.

Dey, F. L., & Kirchner, J. A. (1961). The upper esophageal sphincter after laryngectomy. *Laryngoscope, 71*, 99-115.

Diedrich, W. M. (1999). Anatomy and physiology of esophageal speech. In S. J. Salmon (Ed.), *Alaryngeal speech rehabilitation: For clinicians by clinicians* (2nd ed., pp. 1-28). Austin, TX: Pro-Ed.

Diedrich, W., & Youngstrom, K. (1966). *Alaryngeal speech.* Springfield, IL: Thompson.

Doyle, P. C. (1994). *Foundations of voice and speech rehabilitation following laryngeal cancer.* San Diego, CA: Singular.

Doyle, P. C. (2005). Clinical procedures for training use of the electronic artificial larynx. In P. C. Doyle & R. L. Keith (Eds.), *Contemporary considerations in the treatment and rehabilitation of head and neck cancer: Voice, speech, and swallowing* (pp. 545-570). Austin, TX: Pro-Ed.

Doyle, P. C., Danhauer, J. L., & Reed, C. G. (1988). Listener's perceptions of consonants produced by esophageal and tracheoesophageal talkers. *Journal of Speech and Hearing Disorders, 53*, 400-407.

Doyle, P. C., & Eadie, T. L. (2005). Pharyngoesophageal segment function. In P. C. Doyle & R. L. Keith (Eds.), *Contemporary considerations in the treatment and rehabilitation of head and neck cancer: Voice, speech, and swallowing* (pp. 521-543). Austin, TX: Pro-Ed.

Duguay, M. J. (1978). Why not both? In S. J. Salmon & L. P. Goldstein (Eds.), *The artificial larynx handbook* (pp. 3-10). New York: Grune and Stratton.

Duguay, M. J. (1983). Teaching use of an artificial larynx. In W. H. Perkins (Ed.), *Current therapy of communication disorders* (pp. 127-135). New York: Theime-Straton.

Duguay, M. J. (1985). Using Speech Aides. *Seminars in Speech and Language, 7*, 17.

Duguay, M. J. (1999). Esophageal speech training: The initial phase. In S. J. Salmon (Ed.), *Alaryngeal speech rehabilitation: For clinicians by clinicians* (2nd ed., pp. 165-201). Austin, TX: Pro-Ed.

Eadie, T. L., & Doyle, P. C. (2004). Auditory-perceptual scaling and quality of life in tracheoesophageal speakers. *Laryngoscope, 114*, 753-759.

Ferguson, S. H. (2004). Talker differences in clear and conversational speech: Vowel intelligibility for normal hearing listeners. *Journal of the Acoustical Society of America, 116*, 2365-2373.

Frith, C., Buffalo, M. D., & Montague, J. C. (1985). Relationships between esophageal speech proficiency and surgical, biographical and social factors. *Journal of Communication Disorders, 18*, 475–483.

Frowen, J., & Perry, A. (2001). Reasons for success or failure in surgical voice restoration after total laryngectomy: An Australian study. *The Journal of Laryngology and Otology, 115*, 393–399.

Gardner, W. H. (1971). *Laryngectomee speech rehabilitation.* Springfield, IL: Thompson.

Gates, G. A. (1980). Upper esophageal sphincter: Pre and post-laryngectomy—A normative study. *Laryngoscope, 90*, 454–464.

Gates, G. A., Ryan, W., & Lauder, E. (1982). Current status of laryngectomee rehabilitation: IV. Attitudes about laryngectomee rehabilitation should change. *American Journal of Otolaryngology, 3*, 1–7.

Geraghty, J. A., Wenig, B. L., Smith, B. E., & Portugal, L. G. (1996). Long-term follow-up of tracheoesophageal puncture results. *Annals of Otology, Rhinology, and Laryngology, 105*, 501–503.

Gilmore, S. I. (1999). Failure in acquiring esophageal speech. In S. J. Salmon (Ed.), *Alaryngeal speech rehabilitation: For clinicians by clinicians* (2nd ed., pp. 221–268). Austin, TX: Pro-Ed.

Glaze, L. E. (2005). Counseling the laryngectomized patient and family: Considerations before, during, and after treatment. In P. C. Doyle & R. L. Keith (Eds.), *Contemporary considerations in the treatment and rehabilitation of head and neck cancer: Voice, speech, and swallowing* (pp. 353–378). Austin, TX: Pro-Ed.

Goldstein, L. P., & Rothman, H. B. (1976). *Analysis of speech produced with an artificial larynx.* Annual convention of the American Speech and Hearing Association, Houston, TX.

Graham, M. S. (1997). *The clinician's guide to alaryngeal speech therapy.* Boston: Butterworth-Heinemann.

Graham, M. S. (2005). Taking it to the limits: Achieving proficient esophageal speech. In P. C. Doyle & R. L. Keith (Eds.), *Contemporary considerations in the treatment and rehabilitation of head and neck cancer: Voice, Speech, and Swallowing* (pp. 379–430). Austin, TX: Pro-Ed.

Gress, C. D. (2004). Preoperative evaluation for tracheoesophageal voice restoration. *Otolaryngology Clinics of North America, 37*, 519–530.

Haroldson, S. K. (1999). Toward advancing esophageal communication. In S. J. Salmon (Ed.), *Alaryngeal speech rehabilitation: For clinicians by clinicians* (2nd ed., pp. 203–219). Austin, TX: Pro-Ed.

Hillman, R. E., Walsh, M. L., Wolf, G. T., Fisher, S. G., &

Hong, W. K. (1998). Functional outcomes following treatment for advanced laryngeal cancer: Part I—Voice preservation in advanced laryngeal cancer; Part II—Laryngectomy rehabilitation: The state of the art in the VA system. *Annals of Otology, Rhinology, and Laryngology, 107*(5), 1–27.

Hyman, M. (1955). An experimental study of artificial larynx and esophageal speech. *Journal of Speech and Hearing Disorders, 20*, 291–299.

Hyman, M. (1994). Factors influencing the intelligibility of alaryngeal speech. In R. L. Keith & F. L. Darley (Eds.), *Laryngectomee rehabilitation* (3rd ed., pp. 309–321). Austin, TX: Pro-Ed.

Isshiki, N., & Tanabe, M. (1972). Acoustic and aerodynamic study of a superior electrolarynx speaker. *Folia Phoniatrica, 24*, 65–76.

Izdebski, K., Fontanesi, J., Ross, J., & Hetzler, D. (1988). The effects of irradiation on alaryngeal voice of totally laryngectomized patients. *International Journal of Radiation Oncology, Biology, Physics, 14*, 1281–1286.

Kahane, J. C., & Irwin, J. A. (1975). *Comparison of hearing sensitivity and stoma noise in 90 esophageal speakers.* Paper presented at the annual convention of the American Speech Language Hearing Association, Washington, D.C.

Keith, R. L., Ewart, J. C., & Flowers, C. R. (1974). Factors influencing the learning of esophageal speech. *British Journal of Disorders of Communication, 9*, 110–116.

Keith, R. L., Shanks, J. C., & Doyle, P. C. (2005). Historical highlights: Laryngectomy rehabilitation. In P. C. Doyle & R. L. Keith (Eds.), *Contemporary considerations in the treatment and rehabilitation of head and neck cancer: Voice, Speech, and Swallowing* (pp. 17–57). Austin, TX: Pro-Ed.

Koike, M., Kobayashi, N., Hirose, H., & Hara, Y. (2002). Speech rehabilitation after total laryngectomy. *Acta Otolaryngology, Supplement, 547*, 107–112.

Krause, J. C., & Braida, L. D. (2004). Acoustic properties of naturally produced clear speech at normal speaking rates. *Journal of the Acoustical Society of America, 115*, 362–378.

Lerman, J. W. (1991). The artificial larynx. In S. J. Salmon & K. H. Mounts (Eds.), *Alaryngeal speech rehabilitation* (pp. 27–45). Austin, TX: Pro-Ed.

Levitt, M. N., Dedo, H. H., & Ogura, J. H. (1965). The cricopharyngeus muscle: An electromyographic study in the dog. *Laryngoscope, 75*, 122–136.

Lewin, J. S. (2004). Advances in alaryngeal communication and the art of tracheoesophageal voice restoration. *ASHA Leader*, 20–21.

Lewin, J. S. (2005). Problems associated with alaryngeal speech development. In P. C. Doyle & R. L. Keith (Eds.), *Contemporary considerations in the treatment and rehabilitation of head and neck cancer: Voice, speech, and swallowing* (pp. 593-623). Austin, TX: Pro-Ed.

Louden, R. G., Lee, L., & Holcomb, B. J. (1988). Volumes and breathing patterns during speech in healthy and asthmatic subjects. *Journal of Speech and Hearing Research, 31,* 219-227.

Martin, D. E., Hoops, H. R., & Shanks, J. C. (1974). The relationship between esophageal speech proficiency and selected measures of auditory function. *Journal of Speech and Hearing Research, 74,* 80-85.

Max, L., DeBruyn, W., & Steurs, W. (1997). Intelligibility of oesophageal and tracheo-oesophageal speech: Preliminary observations. *European Journal of Disorders of Communication, 32,* 429-440.

McAuliffe, M. J., Ward, E. C., Bassett, L., & Perkins, K. (2000). Functional speech outcomes after laryngectomy and pharyngolaryngectomy. *Archives of Otolaryngology-Head & Neck Surgery, 126,* 705-709.

McIvor, J., Evans, P. F., Perry, A., & Cheesman, A. D. (1990). Radiologic assessment of post laryngectomy speech. *Clinical Radiology, 41,* 312-316.

Mehta, A. R., Sarkar, S., Mehta, S. A., & Bachher, G. K. (1995). The Indian experience with immediate tracheoesophageal puncture for voice restoration. *European Archives of Otorhinolaryngology, 252,* 209-214.

Meltzner, G., Hillman, R. E., Heaton, J. T., Houston, K. M., Kobler, J., & Qi, Y. (2005). Electrolaryngeal speech: The state of the art and future directions for development. In P. C. Doyle & R. L. Keith (Eds.), *Contemporary considerations in the treatment and rehabilitation of head and neck cancer: Voice, speech, and swallowing* (pp. 571-590). Austin, TX: Pro-Ed.

Merwin, G. E., Goldstein, L. P., & Rothman, H. B. (1985). A comparison of speech using artificial larynx and tracheoesophageal puncture with valve in the same speakers. *Laryngoscope, 95,* 730-773.

Miani, C., Bertino, G., Bellomo, A., & Staffieri, A. (1998). Analysis of qualitative voice and speech quality judgements after total laryngectomy. *Acta Otorhinolaryngologica Italia, 18,* 143-147.

Mjones, A. B., Olofsson, J., Danbolt, C., & Tibbling, L. (1991). Oesophageal speech after laryngectomy: A study of possible influencing factors. *Clinical Otolaryngology and Allied Sciences, 16,* 442-447.

Moolenaar-Bijl, A. (1953). Connection between consonant articulation and the intake of air in esophageal speech. *Folia Phoniatrica, 5,* 212-216.

Pauloski, B. R. (1998). Acoustic and aerodynamic characteristics of tracheoesophageal voice. In E. D. Blom, M. I. Singer, & R. C. Hamaker (Eds.), *Tracheoesophageal voice restoration following total laryngectomy* (pp. 123-141). San Diego, CA: Singular.

Perry, A., & Edels, Y. (1985). Recent advances in the assessment of failed oesophageal speakers. *British Journal of Communication Disorders, 20,* 229-236.

Quer, M., Burgues-Vila, J., & Garcia-Crespillo, P. (1992). Primary tracheoesophageal puncture vs. esophageal speech. *Archives of Otolaryngology-Head & Neck Surgery, 118,* 188-190.

Richardson, J. L. (1981). Surgical and radiological effects upon the development of speech after total laryngectomy. *Annals of Otology, Rhinology, and Laryngology, 90,* 294-297.

Robbins, J., Fisher, H. B., Blom, E. D., & Singer, M. I. (1984). A comparative acoustic study of normal, esophageal, and tracheoesophageal speech production. *Journal of Speech and Hearing Disorders, 49,* 202-210.

Sacco, P. R., Mann, M. B., & Schultz, M. C. (1967). Perceptual confusions among selected phonemes in esophageal speech. *Journal of the Indiana Speech and Hearing Association, 26,* 19-33.

Sako, K., Cardinale, S., Marchetta, F., & Shedd, D. (1974). Speech and vocational rehabilitation of the laryngectomized patient. *Journal of Surgical Oncology, 6,* 197-202.

Salmon, S. J. (1971). Use of imagery in teaching esophageal speech. *California Journal of Communication Disorders, 2,* 17-24.

Salmon, S. J. (1983). Artificial larynx speech: A viable means of alaryngeal communication. In Y. Edles (Ed.), *Laryngectomy: Diagnosis to rehabilitation* (pp. 142-162). Rockville, MD: Aspen.

Salmon, S. J. (1988). Factors predictive of success or failure in acquisition of esophageal speech. *Head and Neck Surgery, 10,* 5105-5109.

Salmon, S. J. (1994). Methods of air intake for esophageal speech and their associated problems. In R. L. Keith & F. L. Darley (Eds.), *Laryngectomee rehabilitation* (3rd ed., pp. 219-234). Austin, TX: Pro-Ed.

Salmon, S. J. (1990). The efficacy of speech-language pathology intervention: Laryngectomy. *Seminars in Speech and Language, 11*(1), 256-272.

Salmon, S. J. (1999). Artificial larynx devices. In S. J. Salmon (Ed.), *Alaryngeal speech rehabilitation: For clinicians by clinicians* (pp. 79-104). Austin, TX: Pro-Ed.

Salmon, S. J. (2005). Commonalities among alaryngeal speech methods. In P. C. Doyle & R. L. Keith (Eds.),

*Contemporary considerations in the treatment and rehabilitation of head and neck cancer: Voice, speech, and swallowing* (pp. 59-74). Austin, TX: Pro-Ed.

Schaefer, S. D., & Johns, D. F. (1982). Attaining functional esophageal speech. *Archives of Otolaryngology, 108,* 647-649.

Shames, G. H., Font, J., & Matthews, J. (1963). Factors related to speech proficiency of the laryngectomized. *Journal of Speech and Hearing Disorders, 28,* 273-287.

Shanks, J. (1994). Developing esophageal communication. In R. L. Keith & F. L. Darley (Eds.), *Laryngectomee rehabilitation* (3rd ed., pp. 205-218). Austin, TX: Pro-Ed.

Shipp, T. (1967). Frequency, duration, and perceptual measures in relation to judgments of alaryngeal speech acceptability. *Journal of Speech and Hearing Research, 10,* 417-427.

Simpson, I. C., Smith, J. C. S., & Gordon, T. (1972). Laryngectomy: The influence of muscle reconstruction on the mechanism of oesophageal voice production. *Journal of Laryngology and Otology, 86,* 961-990.

Singer, M. I., & Blom, E. D. (1980). An endoscopic technique for restoration of voice after laryngectomy. *Annals of Otology, Rhinology, and Laryngology, 89,* 529-533.

Singer, M. I., Blom, E. D., & Hamaker, R. C. (1981). Further experience with voice restoration after total laryngectomy. *Annals of Otology, Rhinology, and Laryngology, 90,* 498-502.

Snidecor, J. C. (1968). *Speech rehabilitation of the laryngectomized.* Springfield, IL: Thomas.

Snidecor, J. C., & Curry, E. T. (1959). Temporal and pitch aspects of superior esophageal speech. *Annals of Otology, Rhinology and Laryngology, 68,* 1-14.

Snidecor, J. C., & Isshiki, N. (1965). Air volume and air flow relationships of six esophageal speakers. *Journal of Speech and Hearing Disorders, 30,* 205-216.

Struben, W. H., & van Gelder, L. (1958). Movements of the superior structures in the laryngectomized patient. *Archives of Otolaryngology, 67,* 655-659.

Tardy-Mitzell, S., Andrews, M. L., & Bowman, S. A. (1985). Acceptability and intelligibility of tracheo-

esophageal speech. *Archives of Otolaryngology, 111,* 213-215.

Trudeau, M. D. (1994). The acoustical variability of tracheoesophageal speech. In R. L. Keith & F. L. Darley (Eds.), *Laryngectomee rehabilitation* (3rd ed., pp. 383-394). Austin, TX: Pro-Ed.

Van As-Brooks, C. J., Hilgers, F. J. M., Koopmans-van Beinum, F. J., & Pols, L. C. W. (2005). Anatomical and functional correlates of voice quality in tracheoesophageal speech. *Journal of Voice, 19,* 360-372.

Van As-Brooks, C. J., Koopmans-van Beinum, F. J., Pols, L. C. W., & Hilgers, F. J. M. (2003). Perceptual evaluation of tracheoesophageal speech by naïve and experienced judges through the use of semantic differential scales. *Journal of Speech-Language-Hearing Research, 46,* 947-959.

Van As, C. J., Op de Coul, B. M. R., van den Hoogen, F. J. A., Koopmans-van Beinum, F. J., & Hilgers, F. J. M. (2001). Quantitative videofluoroscopy. A new evaluation tool for tracheoesophageal voice production. *Archives of Otolaryngology-Head and Neck Surgery, 127,* 161-169.

Van den Berg, J., & Moolenaar-Bijl, A. J. (1959). Cricopharyngeal sphincter, pitch, intensity, and fluency in esophageal speech. *Practical Otorhinolaryngology, 21,* 298-315.

Van den Berg, J., Moolenaar-Bijl, A. J., & Damste, P. H. (1958). Esophageal speech. *Folia Phoniatrica, 10,* 65-84.

Ward, E. C., Koh, S. K., Frisby, J., & Hodge, R. (2003). Differential modes of alaryngeal communication and long-term voice outcomes following pharyngolaryngectomy and laryngectomy. *Folia Phoniatrica et Logopaedica, 55,* 39-49.

Weinberg, B., & Bennett, S. (1972). Selected acoustic characteristics of esophageal speech produced by female laryngectomees. *Journal of Speech and Hearing Research, 15,* 211-216.

Weiss, M. S., & Basili, A. G. (1985). Electrolaryngeal speech produced by laryngectomized subjects: Perceptual characteristics. *Journal of Speech and Hearing Research, 28,* 294-300.

Winans, C. S., Reichbach, E. J., & Waldrop, W. F. (1974). Esophageal determinants of alaryngeal speech. *Archives of Otolaryngology, 99,* 10-14.

# Chapter 9

# PROSTHETIC TRACHEOESOPHAGEAL VOICE RESTORATION FOLLOWING TOTAL LARYNGECTOMY

Corina J. van As-Brooks and Dennis P. Fuller

## Introduction

While the former chapter focused on nonprosthetic forms of voice rehabilitation, the current chapter will focus on voice rehabilitation using a voice prosthesis.

During a total laryngectomy the entire larynx, including the hyoid bone, epiglottis, thyroid cartilage, cricoid cartilage, and the first two or three tracheal rings are removed. After removal of the larynx, the trachea is diverted forward to the neck and sutured into the original skin incision or a separately created skin incision. The inferior pharyngeal constrictors (previously attached to the larynx) and pharyngeal mucosa are closed to reestablish the digestive tract. Figure 9–1 schematically shows the anatomical situation before and after total laryngectomy, and during phonation after total laryngectomy with a voice prosthesis in situ.

In addition to providing preoperative information and postoperative voice and speech training, in most countries the speech-language pathologist (SLP) also plays an important role in fitting and replacing the voice prosthesis and in troubleshooting problems that may occur with the voice prosthesis. Although at times it seems that selecting and fitting the prosthesis is the primary focus of rehabilitation, fitting a voice prosthesis is only a first step. In analogy to the voice and speech training provided to nonprosthetic speakers, the prosthetic speakers also require dedicated rehabilitation of voice and speech beyond simply the insertion of the prosthesis, in order for them to achieve optimal voice quality and speech intelligibility. The current chapter focuses on both the rehabilitation of voice and speech and on the voice prosthesis.

## Historical Review: Tracheoesophageal Speech

Tracheoesophageal speech requires an opening between the trachea and esophagus. This opening enables the patient to speak by closing off the tracheostoma (stoma) and thereby causing the air to divert through the opening between the trachea and the esophagus into the esophagus. Historically, various techniques have been used to establish this opening between the trachea and esophagus. At present, tracheoesophageal voice prostheses are the method of choice.

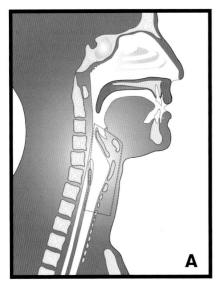 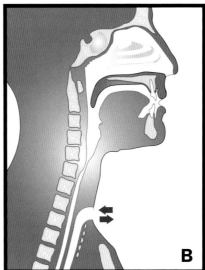 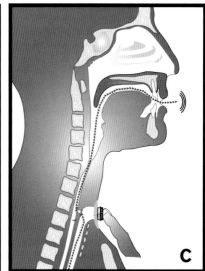

**Figure 9–1.** Schematic drawing of the anatomical situation before total laryngectomy with the red dotted line showing the structures that will be removed during surgery **A.**, of the anatomical situation after total laryngectomy **B.**, and of prosthetic tracheoesophageal speech **C.**

## The First Total Laryngectomy and Artificial Larynx

The Viennese surgeon Billroth is credited for performing the first total laryngectomy secondary to laryngeal carcinoma in 1873. His fellow, Gussenbauer, described the procedure and also described the artificial larynx that was used in this patient (Gussenbauer, 1874). In this early procedure, for reasons of surgical safety, the anterior pharyngeal wall was not closed, leaving the patient with a large, unrepaired defect above the tracheostoma. Already at the time of this first laryngectomy, concerns were expressed about vocal and pulmonary rehabilitation and an artificial larynx was developed for this patient. Specifically, the artificial larynx was connected to the pharyngeal defect and to the tracheostoma, and it contained a metallic reed for voice production and a respirator for pulmonary rehabilitation. The report says that "the patient was able to speak with a clear voice that was loud enough to be heard at the other side of a large hospital room."

This first artificial larynx was based on a design from the Czech physiologist Johann Czermak (Luchsinger & Arnold, 1965) who designed a "sound producing" prosthesis for an 18-year-old female who had suffered "closure of her larynx" and required a tracheotomy. The Czermak design was a tube that was placed over the tracheal stoma upon exhalation which routed the pulmonary air over a metal reed and then through a hollowed rubber tube that was placed in the mouth. Pulmonary airflow through the reed produced the "artificial voice," the user simply articulated, and intelligible speech was created. In 1894 Gluck and Sorensen succeeded in primary closure of the pharyngeal defect, which subsequently ended the need for artificial larynges such as the one described above and enabled the use of esophageal speech (for more on esophageal speech, see Chapter 8).

## Tracheoesophageal Shunt Procedures

Reportedly, the first tracheoesophageal "puncture" was made by a patient himself. Guttman (1932) detailed a laryngectomized patient who used a hot ice pick to create an opening between the trachea and hypopharynx. This enabled the patient to force air through the puncture by closing off the tracheostoma with a finger.

Over the years, a number of surgical tracheoesophageal shunt procedures have been described. Asai (1972) introduced a dermal tube shunt procedure. When successful, the speaker inhaled through the stoma, occluded the stoma with a thumb or finger, and then exhaled. The pulmonary air was consequently routed from the trachea, through the dermal tube, into the esophagus and resulted in esophageal pseudo voice. When completed successfully, this type of tracheoesophageal voice resulted in a length of phonation and vocal prosody that approached that of laryngeal speakers. Similar but surgically unique procedures followed, reported by Montgomery and Toohill (1968), McGrail and Oldfield (1971), Serafini (1972), Amatsu (1980), and Staffieri (1981). Although the voice sound was often good, patients often presented with a high incident of aspiration, dermal tube stenosis, spontaneous dermal tube closure, and/or poor air flow into the esophagus. Over the course of the following decade, fewer of these procedures were completed and at the same time a relatively simple prosthesis was developed that achieved the same physical use and routing of pulmonary air without any of the tracheoesophageal shunt complications.

## Voice Prostheses for Tracheoesophageal Speech

During 1973 Taub and Bergner introduced a surgical procedure with a prosthetic fitting that used pulmonary air to vibrate the new voice source. They circumvented the earlier reported dermal tube difficulties by surgically developing a fistula on the lateral neck just anterior to the external carotid artery. After fistula healing, they connected the tracheostoma to the surgical fistula with a prosthesis that, with increased pulmonary flow and pressure, closed a flutter valve and routed air through the surgical fistula and into the esophagus to produce pulmonary driven esophageal voice. Although some patients reported some complaints about the weight and bulk of the prosthesis, Taub did report a greater than 90% success rate of pulmonary driven esophageal voice production (Taub, 1975).

Singer and Blom (1980) developed an endoscopic procedure with prosthetic fitting that, with continued variations and modifications to both the procedure and the prosthesis, is still considered state of the art

over two and a half decades later. They proposed puncture of the tracheoesophageal wall, dilation of the puncture and fitting with a so-called duckbill silicone voice prosthesis (see Figure 9–2). This seemed an improvement over the Taub and Bergner procedure. The prosthesis was smaller and lighter than previous designs, and the prosthesis puncture was also smaller and located within the trachea, away from the carotid artery. Singer, Blom, and Hamaker (1981) were soon to report a success rate of tracheoesophageal voice production as high as Taub and Bergner with larger numbers of patients and fewer postoperative complications.

## Surgical Techniques and Factors Influencing Voice Production

Not all total laryngectomy procedures are carried out in a similar way. For example, the surgeon will choose a specific type of pharyngeal closure, may or may not choose to create a primary TE puncture, may or may not place a voice prosthesis, may carry out additional procedures that influence the tonicity of the neoglottis, may have to remove more tissue causing the need for reconstruction, may construct the tracheostoma differently, and may attempt to create a flatter peristomal area. All of those techniques may influence voice, speech, swallowing, and the use of devices for rehabilitation. In the following sections each of these additional surgical aspects is discussed.

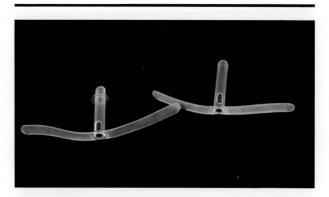

**Figure 9–2.** Photograph of the first Blom-Singer duckbill voice prosthesis initially without esophageal retention collar (right) and later with esophageal retention collar (left).

## Pharyngeal Closure

Usually the pharynx is closed in three layers: mucosa, submucosa, and muscle. Some surgeons prefer a one-layer (mucosa) or two-layer (mucosa and submucosa) closure and leave the muscular layer unclosed or half-closed (see next section for more on this topic).

The pharynx can be closed in a vertical line (I-shape) or in a T-shape; this often depends on the preference of the surgeon and the remaining tissue available for closure. During a T-shape closure, the surgeon starts at one lateral side and sutures the lateral side of the pharynx to the base of tongue until the midline is reached; subsequently, the same is done for the contralateral side. Then, the remaining part of the pharynx is sutured together vertically resulting in a T-shape. During a vertical or I-shaped closure the lateral sides of the pharynx are sutured together in the midline. The occurrence of a pharyngeal pouch is lower when a T-shape closure is used (Davis, Vincent, Shapshay, & Strong, 1982). It is sometimes hypothesized that patients with a T-shape closure have better voice/pitch control and better swallowing due to the connection between the pharynx and base of tongue. See Chapter 10 for aspects related to postlaryngectomy dysphagia.

## Primary or Secondary Tracheoesophageal Puncture (TEP)

The term primary puncture is used when the puncture is created at the time of surgery. The term secondary puncture is used when the procedure is done as a separate procedure any time from weeks to years after the total laryngectomy has been completed.

Blom and Singer's first TE punctures were done as secondary procedures (Singer et al., 1980). Only a few years later, TEP as a primary technique at the time of laryngectomy was introduced (Maves & Lingeman, 1982). Although the TEP was developed at the time of the larynx removal, the placement of the actual voice prosthesis still occurred at a later stage. The advantages of primary TEP are that it eliminates the need for a second surgical procedure (together with accompanying risks and cost) and that the catheter used to maintain the puncture can be used as a feeding tube (Maves et al., 1982). Another advantage is that with pri-

mary TEP the patient will produce voice sooner. Also emotionally it is important for the patient to be able to communicate in the early postoperative period.

Complication rates between primary and secondary puncture procedures have been shown to be no different (Silverman & Black, 1994). Postoperative radiotherapy is not considered a contraindication for primary puncture (Kao, Mohr, Kimmel, Getch, & Silverman, 1994; Silverman et al., 1994). The only contraindication for primary puncture is separation of the tracheoesophageal wall at the puncture site, for example, when the patient undergoes a laryngopharyngoesophagectomy with gastric pull-up (Pou, 2004). In those patients a secondary puncture will have to be carried out after a period of wound healing. Other reasons for secondary puncture are that some patients initially may choose a communication option other than a voice prosthesis and decide at a later date that they now desire this option. In rare situations, a primary TEP fistula may have to be altered or allowed to close, or closes inadvertently due to accidental removal of the prosthesis.

A primary or secondary procedure can be the result of institution tradition/policy, physician choice, clinician choice, and/or patient choice. For most patients, the timing of the creation of the TEP fistula does seem to be more convenient for the patient and all professionals if done at the time of the total laryngectomy.

## Primary or Delayed Placement of the Voice Prosthesis

With the introduction of indwelling voice prostheses, primary insertion of the voice prosthesis was introduced (Manni, Van den Broek, de Groot, & Berends, 1984; Hilgers & Schouwenburg, 1990). Instead of stenting the TEP with a catheter or feeding tube, the prosthesis is placed at the time of surgery. During the surgery, after removal of the larynx but before final closure of the pharyngeal defect the TEP fistula is created and a prosthesis inserted. After a period of healing, the prosthesis can be changed like usual.

Research shows that in general this first indwelling voice prosthesis that is placed at the time of surgery lasts as long and often even longer than average (Op de Coul et al., 2000; Elving, Van Weissenbruch,

Busscher, Van Der Mei, & Albers, 2002). On the contrary, prostheses that are fitted a few (2-6) days postoperatively after secondary puncture (after removal of the catheter) seem to last a shorter duration due to the need for resizing (Leder & Sasaki, 1995). In fact, Leder and Sasaki (1995) report that the most common reason for voice prosthesis resizing after initial fitting is that the prosthesis is protruding too far into the trachea. The first voice prosthesis after initial fitting lasted on average 26 days and the main reason for replacement was the need for resizing: 78% required resizing to two full sizes (8 mm) shorter (Leder et al., 1995). For the indwelling voice prostheses placed at the time of surgery the first prosthesis exchange is usually for leakage through the device and occurs around a median of 135 days (Op de Coul et al., 2000). The reason(s) for this difference between the two methods are not clear. It is sometimes speculated that the presence of a catheter or nasogastric (NG) feeding tube in the fistula may cause irritation with subsequent edema, or angulation of the fistula, while the presence of a voice prosthesis could possibly prevent edema and maintain a stable puncture site. The most important argument for primary TEP with "delayed" fitting of the prosthesis is that the TEP can be used for the NG tube, thus eliminating the need for uncomfortable placement of the NG tube through the nose. However, some surgeons choose to insert the prosthesis at the time of surgery and pass the feeding tube through the lumen of the voice prosthesis.

As with the choice for primary or secondary puncture, whether or not the prosthesis is placed at the time of surgery can be the result of institution tradition/policy, physician choice, clinician choice, and/or patient choice. In any case the SLP should be aware of these differences to provide optimal treatment to the patient. Usage of a prosthesis that is too long or too short may lead to a variety of problems and should therefore be avoided by proper management.

## Surgical Techniques to Influence the Tonicity of the Neoglottis

During the procedure of total laryngectomy there are a variety of surgical techniques that can be employed, which can potentially influence postsurgical voice and swallowing. It is presently well known that the neoglottis consists of the muscles of the upper esophageal sphincter and/or the inferior and middle pharyngeal constrictor muscles. Among other aspects, the tonicity of the neoglottis plays an important role in voice production. The tension in the PE segment may be too high (hypertonicity or spasm) leading to the inability to produce voice, or a strained, squeezed, intermittent voice sound (See CD, Chapter 9: Audio: "Hypertonicity"), or too low (hypotonicity) resulting in voice quality that is soft, weak, breathy, whispery, aphonic, and sometimes intermittently "bubbly" (see CD, Chapter 9: Audio: Hypotonicity).

Singer and Blom (1981) found that 12% of their patients failed to achieve tracheoesophageal voice because of pharyngoesophageal spasm. They successfully carried out a secondary myotomy (cutting the muscle) to prevent the spasm from occurring. In the same study they describe myotomy carried out as a primary intervention immediately during surgery. All patients achieved fluent postoperative voice.

A myotomy may be carried out as a "long" myotomy, including the upper esophageal sphincter and pharyngeal constrictor muscles, or as a "short" myotomy, including the upper esophageal sphincter only (see CD, Chapter 9: Video: Myotomy). Other methods that may be carried out at the time of the laryngectomy to prevent hypertonicity or spasm of the neoglottis are unilateral neurectomy (cutting the nerve) of the pharyngeal plexus (Singer, Blom, & Hamaker, 1986), nonclosure of the pharyngeal constrictor muscles (Olson & Callaway, 1990), and half closure of the pharyngeal constrictor muscles (Deschler, Doherty, Reed, Hayden, & Singer, 2000). Currently, it is common practice to carry out a myotomy, neurectomy, or modified closure to prevent postoperative voice problems due to hypertonicity or spasm (Bayles & Deschler, 2004).

Despite using the preventive measures mentioned above, some patients may still present with pharyngoesophageal spasm. Hoffman et al. (1997) introduced the use of Botox for chemical denervation of the pharyngoesophageal segment to treat pharyngoesophageal spasm. Currently, the use of Botox has replaced secondary myotomy as a treatment for postoperative spasm of the neoglottis (Hamaker & Blom, 2003).

## Pharyngeal Reconstruction

In addition to surgical removal of the larynx, depending on the size and location of the tumor, a part of the pharynx (total laryngectomy with partial pharyngectomy), the entire pharynx (pharyngolaryngectomy), or the entire pharynx and esophagus (laryngopharyngo-esophagectomy) may have to be removed and reconstructed as well. The surgeon has various options available for reconstruction. The tissues that are most often used for reconstruction are a pedicled myocutaneous (muscle and skin) pectoralis major flap, free radial forearm flap, free jejunal graft, lateral or anterolateral thigh flap, and full or tubed gastric pull-up.

The amount of tissue removed and the type of reconstruction may have an impact on postsurgical speech and swallowing (see Chapter 10). In most of the reconstructive cases, the pharyngoesophageal segment that serves as the voice source after standard total laryngectomy may have been resected. The neoglottis will now consist of some part of the reconstructive tissue. Patients who have undergone one of the forms of extensive pharyngeal reconstruction often are not able to use esophageal speech (see also Chapter 8). However, an electrolarynx can be used, and tracheoesophageal speech by means of a voice prosthesis is a viable option for many (Hilgers et al., 1995; Ward, Koh, Frisby, & Hodge, 2003).

In the following sections, the surgical reconstructions that are most often used are described briefly. For a more detailed description of the procedures and the corresponding impact of these reconstructions on swallowing, the reader is referred to Chapter 10.

### Pectoralis Major Flap

The pectoralis major (PM) flap is a myocutaneous flap consisting of muscle and skin of the chest. The flap is pedicled, which means that it remains attached to the feeding vessels under the clavicle and it is rotated into the pharyngeal defect (see Figure 9–3). The PM flap is an important tool for the repair of specific pharyngeal defects after partial or full pharyngectomy and was first introduced in 1981 (Baek, Lawson, & Biller, 1981).

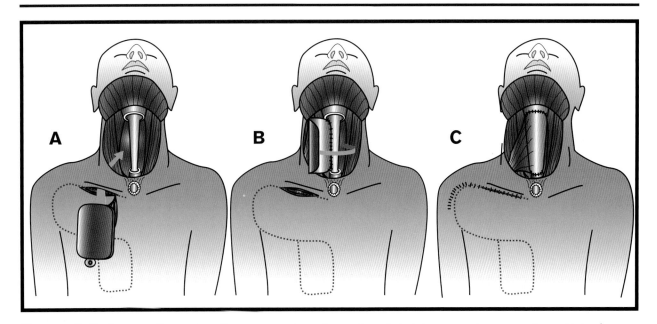

**Figure 9–3.** Pectoralis major flap reconstruction after total laryngectomy and partial pharyngectomy **A.** The pedicled flap is harvested, remains attached to the feeding vessels at the clavicle, and is passed through under the skin to the neck **A.**, sutured in place **B.**, restoring the digestive tract **C.**

Tracheoesophageal voice quality after this type of reconstructive surgery does not differ significantly from voice after standard total laryngectomy for loudness, pitch, and jitter measurement, but perceptual evaluation on 10 parameters has shown that the patients with standard total laryngectomy scored better on all parameters (Deschler, Doherty, Reed, & Singer, 1998).

### Radial Forearm Flap

A radial forearm flap is a free, revascularized fasciocutaneous (fascia and skin) flap of the forearm. This flap is usually tubed and used for reconstruction of circumferential defects of the pharynx after total laryngopharyngectomy (also called pharyngolaryngectomy) (see Figure 9–4) (Harii et al., 1985). With this reconstruction, an acceptable voice can be achieved, but percep-

tual parameters of the voice quality with the radial forearm flap are found to be significantly different from the voice quality after standard total laryngectomy. Both naïve and trained raters found that intelligibility, pitch usage, fluency, communicative effectiveness, and pleasantness were worse in the radial forearm group; the trained raters also rated the radial forearm group worse for loudness usage, wet voice, and extraneous noise while the naïve raters found it to be worse for speaking rate and loudness usage (Deschler, Doherty, Reed, Anthony, & Singer, 1994).

### Jejunal Graft

A jejunal graft is a free revascularized transplant of the jejunum that can be used to reconstruct circumferential defects after total laryngopharyngectomy (see Figure 9-5) (McConnel, Hester, Jr., Nahai, Jurkiewicz,

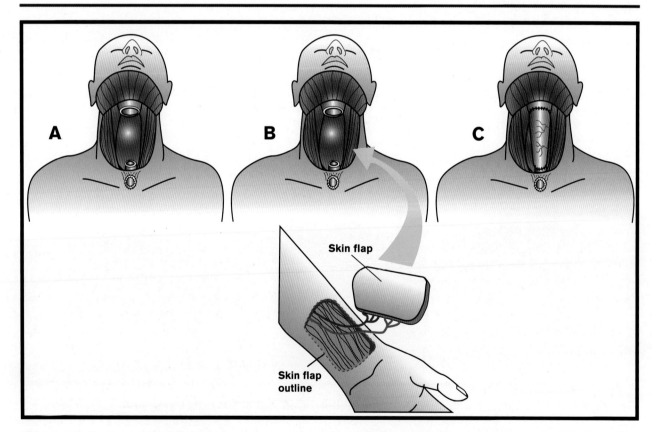

**Figure 9–4.** Free radial forearm reconstruction after total laryngopharyngectomy **A.** The free flap is harvested with attached feeding vessels, a tube is created, and it is transferred to the neck **B.** and sutured in place to restore the digestive tract **C.**

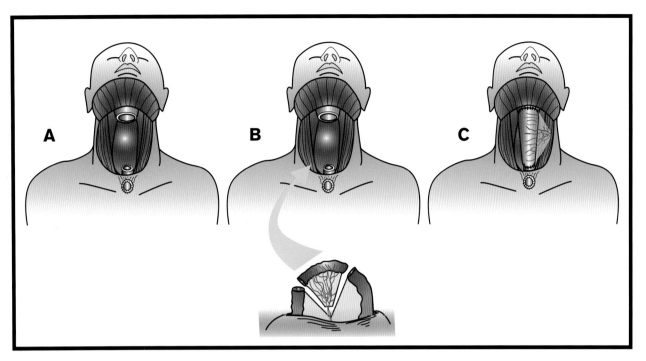

**Figure 9–5.** Jejunal graft reconstruction after total laryngopharyngectomy **A.** The graft is harvested and transferred to the neck **B.** and sutured in place to restore the digestive tract **C.**

& Brown, 1981). After this type of reconstruction, the patient may experience trouble in voice and swallowing due to the peristaltic activity of the graft. The voice is regularly blocked by the autonomous peristalsis, and sounds "wet" due to the continuous production of intestinal secretions (Haughey & Forsen, 1992). In comparison to total laryngectomy speakers, studies have shown that tracheoesophageal speech following jejunal transplant is less intelligible, and of reduced vocal quality; however, patients are satisfied with their voice outcomes and achieve functional speech (McAuliffe, Ward, Bassett, & Perkins, 2000). In spite of the wet-sounding voice quality, patients prefer the use of a voice prosthesis over other forms of communication (Mendelsohn, Morris, & Gallagher, 1993).

### Free Lateral and Anterolateral Thigh Flap

The lateral thigh flap consists of the skin and subcutaneous tissue overlying the lateral thigh. It often supplies a large amount of tissue and can therefore be

used for larger defects of the neopharynx (Hayden & Deschler, 1999). The anterolateral thigh flap is harvested from the anterior part of the lateral thigh and has similar characteristics to the lateral thigh flap. Lewin et al. (2005) showed that in comparison with jejunal graft reconstruction the anterolateral thigh flap resulted in similar complication rates and better speech and swallowing outcomes.

### Gastric Pull-Up

This type of surgery is usually necessary in patients who need a total laryngopharyngoesophagectomy. Either the complete stomach is pulled up to replace the pharynx and esophagus (see Figure 9-6) (Silver, 1976) or the stomach is surgically formed into a tube and then pulled up (Marmuse, Guedon, & Koka, 1994). Hilgers et al. (1995) found that the voice results after tube reconstruction were more often judged to be good than the voice results after full stomach transfer. After the latter the voice more often sounded amphoric, with little strength.

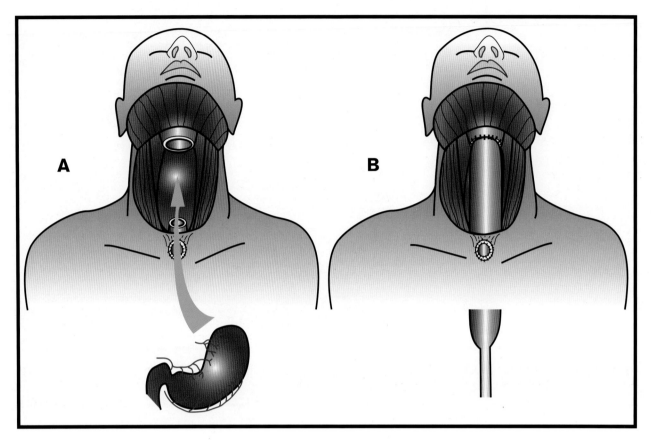

**Figure 9–6.** Gastric pull-up reconstruction after total laryngopharyngoesophagectomy **A.** The stomach is prepared and pulled up into the neck **A.** and sutured to the pharyngeal defect to restore the digestive tract **B.**

## Tracheostoma Construction

Construction of the tracheostoma is an important part of the surgery. Variations in stoma size, shape, and location are the biggest challenges in the restoration of speech and pulmonary function following total laryngectomy and tracheoesophageal puncture (Lewin, 2004).

A stoma that is too large, irregular, or deep (see Figure 9–7) may be difficult to occlude for speech and it may be difficult to apply baseplates or intraluminal attachments for heat and moisture exchangers (HMEs) or hands-free speaking valves. A stoma that is too small may cause difficulty breathing and may cause problems with prosthesis insertion and maintenance.

Although surgical procedures for "stomaplasty" are available to improve the characteristics of the stoma

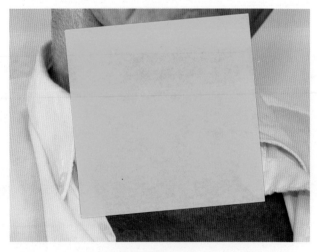

**Figure 9–7.** Photograph of a laryngectomized patient with a deep stoma. (Photo provided as a courtesy of Atos Medical, www.atosmedical.com.)

(Verschuur, Gregor, Hilgers, & Balm, 1996), it is obviously better to avoid these problems in the first place (Verschuur et al., 1996). In general, the stoma will be either created in unity with the surgical incision or separately (see Figure 9-8). It is thought that the latter method causes fewer problems with the stoma configuration and that it eliminates the need for a postoperative laryngectomy tube which is thought by some to cause healing problems of the stoma (Verschuur et al., 1996).

In addition to the creation of the stoma itself, it is often proposed to cut the sternal heads of the sternocleidomastoid muscles (see CD, Chapter 9: Video: Cutting the Sternal Heads). This causes no functional deficits, but results in a flatter peristomal area (see Figure 9-9), which allows for easier application of baseplates or intraluminal devices for HMEs and hands-free speaking valves (Hilgers, 2003).

## Tracheoesophageal Speech

As can be seen in Figure 9-1, tracheoesophageal speech is pulmonary driven. Upon occlusion of the tracheostoma, the exhaled pulmonary air is diverted through the lumen of the voice prosthesis into the esophagus. There, it sets the new voice source, the neoglottis (also referred to as PE segment or pseudoglottis) into vibration. The success rates for tracheoesophageal speech are often higher than those reported for esophageal speech (see also Chapter 8). For tracheoesophageal speech, success rates of up to 90% are reported (Op de Coul et al., 2000).

Of the different forms of alaryngeal communication, tracheoesophageal speech most closely resembles

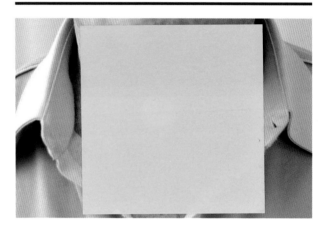

**Figure 9-9.** Photograph of the flat peristomal area of a laryngectomized patient of whom the sternal heads of the sternocleidomastoid muscle were cut during surgery. (Photo provided as a courtesy of Atos Medical, www.atosmedical.com.)

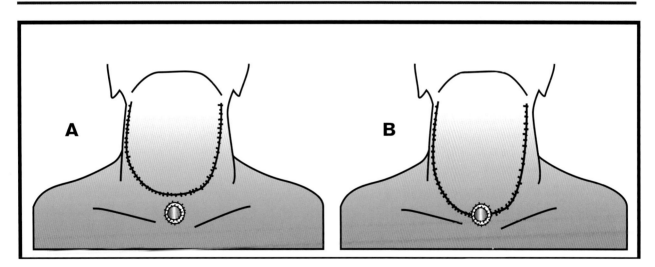

**Figure 9-8.** Illustration of two different methods of stoma construction: separate from the surgical incision **A.** and in unity with the surgical incision **B.**

the mechanism of normal laryngeal speech production. The only difference lies within the voice source. In Table 9–1 the initiator, voice source, resonator, and vocal tract for the different types of alaryngeal communication and normal laryngeal communication are shown.

Due to the differences in nature between the different types of alaryngeal speech, differences in voice and speech can be expected. In general, tracheoesophageal speech is found to be more like normal speech than esophageal speech (Baggs & Pine, 1983; Pindzola & Cain, 1988; Robbins, Fisher, Blom, & Singer, 1984) and is often reported to be superior to esophageal speech (Debruyne, Delaere, Wouters, & Uwents, 1994; Max, Steurs, & De Bruyn, 1996) and electrolarynx speech (Williams & Watson, 1987). However, as stressed in Chapter 8, the superiority of one type of alaryngeal speech over the other is not determined by voice and speech outcome alone. For a more in-depth discussion on this topic and the choice of alaryngeal speech method, we refer the reader to Chapter 8.

Although people tend to discuss tracheoesophageal speech as having certain qualities, it is important to realize that tracheoesophageal voice quality is highly variable between patients. As outlined previously, the anatomy and physiology of the neoglottis plays an important role in tracheoesophageal voice quality (van As-Brooks, Hilgers, Koopmans-van Beinum, & Pols, 2005; van As, Op de Coul, van den Hoogen, Koopmans-van Beinum, & Hilgers, 2001; Van Weissenbruch, Kunne, van Cauwenberghe, Albers, & Sulter, 2000). Perceptually, male and female tracheoesophageal speech appears not to be significantly different from each other (van As, Koopmans-van Beinum, Pols, & Hilgers, 2003).

Female tracheoesophageal speakers often have a low fundamental frequency (115 Hz average), comparable to that of males (109 Hz average) (van As-Brooks, Koopmans-van Beinum, Pols, & Hilgers, 2006). See examples on CD (Chapter 9: Audio: Male Tracheoesophageal Speaker; Audio: Female Tracheoesophageal Speaker). Also both the surgery and any reconstruction can cause alterations in the vocal tract and alterations at the level of the sound source that may result in decreased intelligibility (Doyle, Danhauer, & Reed, 1988; Hammarberg, Lündström, & Nord, 1990; Jongmans, Hilgers, Pols, & van As-Brooks, 2006; Lundstrom & Hammarberg, 2004; Miralles & Cervera, 1995; Searl, Carpenter, & Banta, 2001). Consequently, not all patients have the same voice quality or achieve the same levels of speech intelligibility. In general, patients that have undergone reconstruction of the pharynx in combination with the total laryngectomy have less optimal voice sound (van As et al., 2003). See CD for speech samples (Chapter 9: Audio: "TE Speech Post-Jejunal Reconstruction" 1, 2, and 3).

## Voice Prostheses

Today, a variety of different voice prostheses is available that can be divided into two main categories: nonindwelling voice prostheses that are replaced by the patients themselves and that are regularly removed, cleaned, and reinserted by the patient, and indwelling prostheses that require replacement by a medical professional and remain in situ until a replacement is necessary. Although all the different voice prostheses that

**Table 9–1.** Initiator, Voice Source, Resonator, and Articulator for Each of the Three Types of Alaryngeal Speech, and for Laryngeal Speech

|  | **Electrolarynx** | **Esophageal** | **Tracheoesophageal** | **Laryngeal** |
|---|---|---|---|---|
| Initiator | Battery | Esophageal air reservoir | Pulmonary air | Pulmonary air |
| Voice Source | Vibrating membrane | Neoglottis | Neoglottis | Glottis |
| Resonator | Vocal tract | Vocal tract | Vocal tract | Vocal tract |
| Articulator | Articulatory organs | Articulatory organs | Articulatory organs | Articulatory organs |

are available have their own unique characteristics, the general design of a voice prosthesis is quite consistent (see Figure 9-10).

The prosthesis has retaining flanges at each end. Depending on the type of prosthesis these flanges vary in dimension. Indwelling prostheses typically have larger and more rigid flanges than non-indwelling prostheses to help secure the prosthesis and facilitate long-term placement. The smaller flanges on the non-indwelling prosthesis still help secure the prosthesis, but also facilitate repeated insertion and removal. When the prosthesis is in position, the tracheal flange will be located in the trachea and the esophageal flange will be located in the esophagus. At the time of insertion the tracheal end of the prosthesis has a safety strap attached. In indwelling types of prostheses the safety strap will be removed from the prosthesis after placement. Figure 9-11 shows an indwelling voice prosthesis in situ. In non-indwelling types of prostheses the safety strap (and safety medallion in some models) is retained

to keep the prosthesis secured to the skin of the neck and to assist removal and reinsertion. Figure 9-12 shows a non-indwelling voice prosthesis with safety strap in situ and Figure 9-13 shows a non-indwelling voice prosthesis with safety strap and safety medallion (to prevent aspiration of the prosthesis) in situ.

The term "voice prosthesis" is a paradox as the voice prosthesis does not actually generate sound.

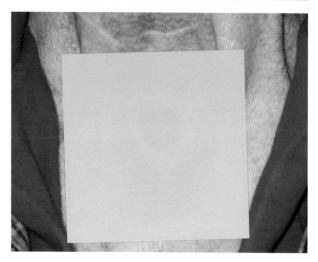

**Figure 9–11.** Photograph of an indwelling (Provox2) voice prosthesis in situ.

**Figure 9–12.** Photograph of a non-indwelling (Blom-Singer) voice prosthesis in situ, with safety strap taped to the skin.

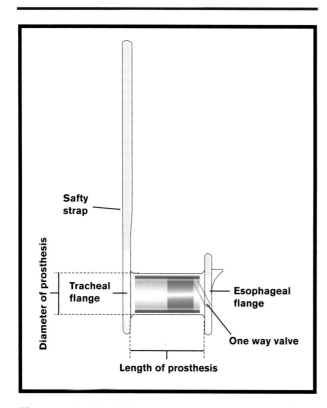

**Figure 9–10.** Schematic representation of the features of a voice prosthesis.

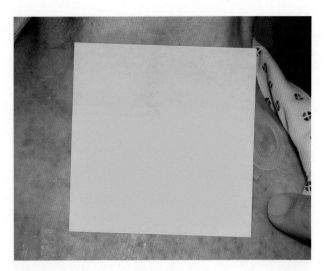

**Figure 9–13.** Photograph of non-indwelling prosthesis with safety strap and safety medallion taped to the neck.

However, its airflow characteristics have some influence on the aerodynamics of voicing and therefore may influence voice quality as well. The aerodynamic characteristics of the voice prosthesis are determined by its design. For example, factors that may influence the airflow resistance (and thus effort to speak and resistance against inadvertent opening at swallowing or inhalation) are the inner diameter of the voice prosthesis, and the design and position of the valve. The voice prosthesis is only partly responsible for effortless esophageal speech; more important factors are the tonicity of the pharyngoesophageal segment and contact between the esophageal end of the voice prosthesis and the posterior esophageal wall (Karschay, Schon, Windrich, Fricke, & Herrmann, 1986). Weinberg and Moon (1986) have shown that the difference in airway resistance that exists among TE puncture prostheses impacts substantially on the actual in vivo process of TE voice production. They conclude that in order to maximize alaryngeal phonatory and speech efficiency, the choice of the appropriate voice prosthesis is important. Some patients may experience an immediate difference in voice and speaking effort when converting to another type of voice prosthesis (Hancock, Houghton, van As-Brooks, & Coman, 2005).

Nowadays, most voice prostheses are placed anterograde through the stoma. The earlier indwelling voice prostheses required retrograde insertion with a guidewire through the mouth and throat (See CD, Chapter 9: Video: Retrograde Insertion). Retrograde insertion is still used for primary placement of the voice prosthesis during surgery (although not through the mouth and throat but through the pharyngeal defect) and for troubleshooting certain problems.

Voice prostheses are available in a variety of lengths. The thickness of the tracheoesophageal wall varies between individuals and therefore the length of the TEP does too. It is important that the length of the prosthesis matches the length of the TEP.

Prostheses also are available in different diameters: 16 French, 17 French, 20 French, or 22.5 French. The larger diameter prostheses typically have lower airflow resistance and therefore require less effort to speak. Non-indwelling types are typically smaller in diameter to facilitate insertion by the patient. Also, the first prosthesis fitted may be of a smaller diameter to avoid substantial dilatation of the still healing tissue after removal of the catheter.

The final key element of the voice prosthesis is the one-way valve. Located near or at the esophageal flange, the one-way air valve enables pulmonary air to pass into the esophagus for sound production and prevents esophageal contents from entering the trachea. In most models of voice prosthesis this valve is a hinged flap, though some prostheses use a different mechanism; the Blom-Singer duckbill voice prosthesis (InHealth Technologies, www.inhealth.com) has an 8 mm long rounded tip with a slit in the middle and the Groningen Ultra Low Resistance voice prosthesis (Medin Instruments, www.medin.nl) has a low profile rounded tip with a semicircular slit along the side.

## Development of Different Types of Voice Prostheses

The original duckbill prosthesis (Singer et al., 1980) was a 16 French diameter, nonflanged device that the patient could remove, clean, and replace him- or herself. Frequent instances of prosthesis extrusion resulted in the addition of an esophageal retention collar (Blom & Hamaker, 1996). Also, in some patients the esophagus was too narrow to accommodate the tip of the duckbill prosthesis causing deformation of the long valve slit at the esophageal side, resulting in leakage or impeded speech airflow (Blom et al., 1996). This problem was addressed by introducing a prosthesis with a shortened tip (Smith, 1986).

After the development of the first voice prosthesis by Singer and Blom in 1980, several other commercial prostheses followed: the Panje Voice Button, a self-retaining, patient managed device (Panje, VanDemark, & McCabe, 1981); the Groningen voice prosthesis, an indwelling device, replaced retrograde by a clinician (Manni et al., 1984); the indwelling Provox voice prosthesis (retrograde insertion) (Hilgers et al., 1990); the Blom-Singer indwelling (Leder & Erskine, 1997); the indwelling Provox2 voice prosthesis (anterograde insertion) (Hilgers et al., 1997); the indwelling VoiceMaster (anterograde insertion) (Eerenstein, Schouwenburg, Van Der Velden, & De Boer, 2001); the Provox ActiValve (special prosthesis with *Candida* resistant valve and valve seat supported by magnets, for early leakage caused by underpressure and/or *Candida*) (Hilgers et al., 2003); the Blom-Singer Advantage (special prosthesis with valve coated with silver oxide for patients with *Candida* problems) (Leder, Acton, Kmiecik, Ganz, & Blom, 2005); and the non-indwelling Provox NID (Hancock et al., 2005).

Features of each of these prostheses can be found in the literature cited above and from the manufacturers. Currently, the Blom-Singer and Provox prostheses are among those that are internationally most widely used. Therefore, in this chapter the discussion will be limited to those prostheses. In Figures 9–14 to 9–18 a range of the indwelling and non-indwelling Blom-Singer and Provox prostheses is shown. It is important

to note that these are single examples only, and that these models also are available in different diameters and lengths for individual patient needs.

## Indwelling versus Non-Indwelling

As mentioned previously, conceptually, the main difference between indwelling and non-indwelling devices is that the non-indwelling device is to be removed and changed by the patient, while an indwelling device is to be removed and refit by a professional. There are other slight differences in the design of the two different types of devices. In general, the indwelling prostheses are sturdier devices that can be cleaned while in place, remain in the fistula for long periods of time, and do not need to be replaced by the patient. The average device life of a low-pressure non-indwelling is between 2 to 3 months (Akbas & Dursun, 2003; Blom, Singer, & Hamaker, 1986; Singer et al., 1980) and the average device lifetime for indwelling types of prostheses is reported to be around 5 months to over 10 months (Aust & McCaffrey, 1997; Laccourreye,

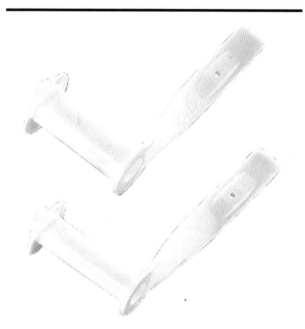

**Figure 9–15.** Photograph of Blom-Singer Low Pressure non-indwelling voice prosthesis. (Photo provided as a courtesy of InHealth Technologies, www.inhealth.com.)

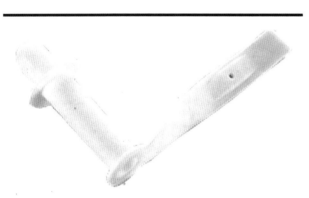

**Figure 9–14.** Photograph of Blom-Singer duckbill voice prosthesis. (Photo provided as a courtesy of InHealth Technologies, www.inhealth.com.)

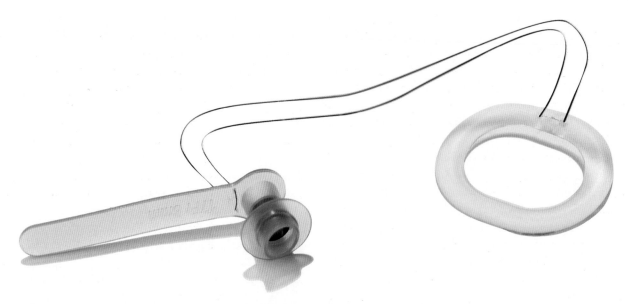

**Figure 9–16.** Photograph of Provox NID non-indwelling voice prosthesis. (Photo provided as a courtesy of Atos Medical, www.atosmedical.com.)

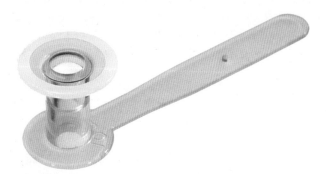

**Figure 9–17.** Photograph of Blom-Singer indwelling voice prosthesis. (Photo provided as a courtesy of InHealth Technologies, www.inhealth.com.)

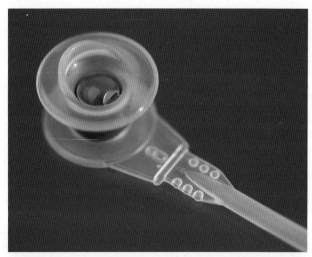

**Figure 9–18.** Photograph of indwelling Provox2 voice prosthesis. (Photo provided as a courtesy of Atos Medical, www.atosmedical.com.)

Menard, Crevier-Buchman, Couloigner, & Brasnu, 1997; Op de Coul et al., 2000).

The non-indwelling prosthesis also needs to be secured to the skin of the neck with a safety strap (and safety medallion) in order to prevent accidental aspiration. However, accidental aspiration of the prosthesis model without a safety medallion can still occur and is reported in about 1.2% to 6.7% of the patients (Andrews, Mickel, Hanson, Monahan, & Ward, 1987; Geraghty, Wenig, Smith, & Portugal, 1996). Other complications commonly associated with non-indwelling prostheses are incorrect insertion methods leading to a false passage or closure of the esophageal side of the tracheoesophageal puncture, and an inability to reinsert resulting in complete closure of the tracheoesophageal puncture (Leder et al., 1997). A common frustration experienced by non-indwelling voice prosthesis users is the need to periodically change the prosthesis (Leder et al., 1997).

Whether the patient is to use an indwelling or a non-indwelling device can be a decision made by the patient or the professional. A non-indwelling prosthesis can only be successful when the patient is able to take excellent care of the prosthesis and will recognize potential problems in time to see the clinician for evaluation. If not, an indwelling device should be inserted.

Patients with poor vision, poor dexterity, poor cognitive ability, high anxiety about self-care, and/or problems of uncontrolled bleeding (anticoagulation treatment) are not considered to be good candidates for a non-indwelling device. Patients with tissue issues or poor condition due to other treatments may not be able to tolerate the frequent changes of a non-indwelling device. Patient selection criteria for an indwelling device are less strict. Almost all patients will be suitable to use an indwelling device, except if they had severe cognitive deficits, severe tissue problems, or very poor pulmonary function.

A patient using a non-indwelling device may be more independent from the clinician because of the ability to self-exchange the prosthesis. However, also non-indwelling users should be routinely checked by their clinician and may need to come in for troubleshooting. For patients who live some distance from their professional care givers or who wish to travel, the use of a non-indwelling prosthesis may be more convenient.

For some patients control of *Candida* may determine the need to select a non-indwelling voice prosthesis. *Candida* are a yeastlike imperfect fungi that are normally present on the skin and in the mucous membranes of the mouth, intestinal tract, and urinary tract (Myers, 2006). The esophageal end of the prosthesis is exposed to this intestinal pool of *Candida*. The buildup of *Candida* can destroy the integrity of the prosthesis, particularly valve function. The non-indwelling prosthesis allows for daily or more frequent removal and cleaning of the prosthesis. Consequently, the patient or the professional caregiver may decide to place a non-indwelling prosthesis to control the effect of the fungus on the esophageal side of the prosthesis. The frequent cleaning and treatment with antifungal agents may extend the life of the non-indwelling prosthesis to a level the patient was unable to achieve with the indwelling device.

A non-indwelling device is also less costly than the indwelling devices. Some would add though that they are also less durable and hence it is not sure whether a less costly device would also imply that it is indeed more cost-effective. This needs to be determined on an individual basis for each patient with device selection influenced by factors such as the financial limits of the patient, hospital regulations, or insurance coverage.

Although there are recognized differences between devices and possible selection criteria for determining which type would suit patients the best, this does not mean that he/she can not try the alternative. Clinicians should encourage patients to select the style that most appropriately fits their means and quality of life. Some patients may alternate back and forth over a period of time before a decision is confirmed.

## Special Purpose Voice Prostheses

In addition to the "normal" types of voice prosthesis, some additional commercial products as well as individual special modifications are available to assist patients with particular issues. For example, a voice prosthesis with a larger esophageal flange can be helpful to solve leakage around the prosthesis in enlarged fistulas (Blom-Singer Large Esophageal Flange, InHealth Technologies, www.inhealth.com). Alternatively, some clinicians choose to glue custom made silicone washers to the esophageal or tracheal flange of the prosthesis to solve this problem.

A voice prosthesis in which the valve mechanism is made out of *Candida* resistant fluoroplastic and closure of the valve is supported by magnets (at three different strengths) (Provox Activalve, Atos Medical AB, www.atosmedical.com; see Figure 9–19) is available for patients with excessive *Candida* growth and/or for patients who generate negative esophageal pressures during swallowing or inhalation. While patients with *Candida* problems only would in general use the Light version, patients with underpressure problems may be helped with a stronger version (Strong, or XtraStrong magnet strength). Device life in patients who experienced extremely short device lives (average 30 days) improved on average 14-fold when using this device (Hilgers et al., 2003).

A voice prosthesis in which the valve of the prosthesis is coated with silver oxide (Advantage, InHealth

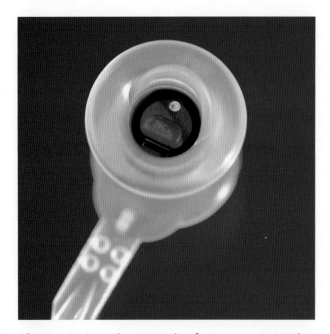

**Figure 9–19.** Photograph of a Provox ActiValve voice prosthesis with a valve and valve seat made out of *Candida* resistant fluoroplastic that is supported by magnets to increase resistance. (Photo provided as a courtesy of Atos Medical, www.atosmedical.com.)

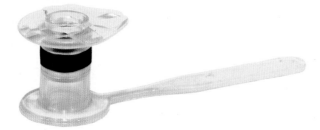

**Figure 9–20.** Photograph of a Blom-Singer Advantage indwelling voice prosthesis with a valve coated with silver oxide to protect the valve against *Candida*. (Photo provided as a courtesy of InHealth Technologies, www.inhealth.com.)

Technologies, www.inhealth.com; see Figure 9–20) may resist *Candida* for a longer period of time. In patients with device failure after an average of 41 days, device life was on average extended by 77 days, in patients with device failures after an average of 86 days and 149 days, device life was extended by an average of 82 and 12 days respectively (Leder et al., 2005).

# Tracheoesophageal Voice Rehabilitation

Tracheoesophageal voice rehabilitation involves patient selection, preoperative counseling, fitting a voice prosthesis, teaching the patient how to speak, and troubleshooting problems that may arise. In the following sections each of these aspects is covered.

## Patient Selection

Tracheoesophageal speech requires acquisition of new self-care tasks and issues. It is recommended that, with few exceptions, all tracheoesophageal speech candidates considered for primary puncture must be physically able and emotionally willing to perform the self-care issues that using TE speech requires. This includes willingness to perform the daily hygiene tasks to keep the prosthesis working, periodically checking for leakage around or through the prosthesis, and returning for professional care when it is time to change the prosthesis (indwelling) or changing and cleaning the device on a regular basis (non-indwelling). If these issues are not clear or resolved before the surgery, then the clinician may choose to make the TEP a secondary procedure to ensure that the patient truly wants this procedure as a communication option and is willing to perform those tasks to be a successful prosthesis user.

The clinician should keep in mind that patients who may initially not have been good candidates for prosthetic voice rehabilitation or for a specific type of prosthesis may be at a later stage, or vice versa.

If a secondary puncture is considered, some clinicians may decide to use esophageal insufflation testing as a method to predict postoperative voice quality (Blom, Singer, & Hamaker, 1985). During this test, a catheter is passed through the nose into the esophagus at a level below the neoglottis. The opposite end of the catheter is attached either to a tracheostoma adapter (see Figure 9–21), which allows air to be diverted through the catheter into the esophagus, or to an external air supply which is used to provide small amounts of air into the esophagus. Results of this test are not always predictive of postoperative outcome; factors such as positioning of the tube, patient

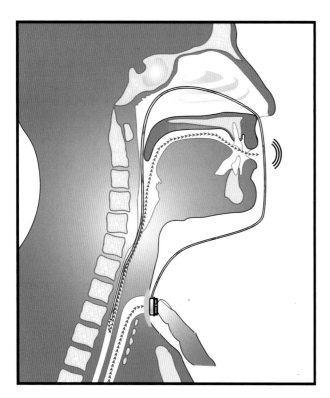

**Figure 9–21.** Schematic drawing of insufflation test using a stoma adapter.

anxiety, and fixation of the stoma adapter may influence the outcome (Gress, 2004).

Some clinicians may choose not to do an insufflation test, rather they inspect the pharynx for stenosis and webs, the tracheostoma for size, and carry out a Modified Barium Swallow to evaluate the PE-segment and then do a secondary puncture. Postoperative problems with hypertonicity or spasm are solved by injecting Botox in the PE-segment or doing a secondary myotomy (Hilgers, 2003).

## Preoperative Visit

It is recommended that the speech-language pathologist meets with the patient prior to the total laryngectomy. The main purpose of this visit is to provide the patient with information about the consequences of a total laryngectomy, such as changes to voice, pulmonary function, olfaction, and swallowing. Anatomical changes should be reviewed using simple drawings,

and postoperative speech options should be demonstrated or shown in a picture or videotape. The amount of detail to be covered during this visit depends on the patient. Some patients may demonstrate a high need for information, while others are coping with other things and are not yet open to more detailed information.

## Prosthesis Measurement, Fitting, Maintenance, and Change

Correctly measuring, fitting, maintaining, and changing the prosthesis is an important process in the ultimate success of tracheoesophageal speech rehabilitation. Active participation of the patient is essential.

### Measurement

Proper length of the prosthesis is critical. As will be demonstrated in the Troubleshooting section, fitting a prosthesis that is either too long or too short will result in problems that can affect both tissue health and vocal output. All commercial companies supply purpose-built measuring devices to facilitate this process. For both main types of measurement process, see CD footage (Chapter 9: Video: "Measurement of TEP Provox," and "Inserting Blom-Singer Indwelling Prosthesis").

The use of the existing prosthesis is another means of measurement that most seasoned clinicians use at the time of prosthesis change. The exterior flange can be grasped with a forceps and gently pulled in an anterior direction. If the space between the tracheal mucosa and the tracheal flange is less than 2 mm the prosthesis can be replaced by a like sized device. If that distance is greater than 2 mm, the prosthesis should be removed and replaced for a shorter device.

Prosthesis measurement and placement are skills that are mastered with hands-on experience. It is recommended that any clinician should seek the assistance of an experienced clinician for mentoring of both measuring and fitting skills.

### Placement of a Non-Indwelling Prosthesis

Fitting or placement of the prosthesis should follow within moments of the completion of the measurement

*Non-Indwelling?*

process. Since a non-indwelling prosthesis is designed for patient manipulation, it is important that the patient be instructed in the resizing and refitting process. Depending on each device used, there are different steps involved in loading and inserting the prosthesis. We refer the readers to the manufacturer instructions of the device they are using for specific details. However the following is an explanation of the general key steps involved.

At the first fitting, if the prosthesis was not placed at the time of surgery, the clinician will dilate the TEP up to the required diameter for insertion of the voice prosthesis. This can be done by using catheters gradually going up in size, or professional dilators developed for this purpose. A dilator is a tapered, curved instrument that has a small diameter at the tip and a larger diameter at the end. The diameter at the end of the dilator should be 2 Fr larger than the diameter of the voice prosthesis to facilitate insertion. Dilators are available in different diameters, corresponding to the prosthesis diameter.

The first prosthesis placements should be done with supervision of the clinician, until the patient has proven to be proficient at it. Before removal of the old prosthesis, the patient should be instructed how to check prosthesis size and prepare the new prosthesis for insertion. Once the old prosthesis has been removed, most patients will need to insert a dilator into the TEP (see CD: Chapter 9: Video: Insertion of Dilator). This ensures that swallowed secretions cannot be aspirated through the open TEP and also ensures that the TEP is sized and ready for insertion of the new prosthesis. The distal end of the loaded prosthesis is then lubricated with a water soluble product. Once this is ready, the dilation tool is removed and the prosthesis gently inserted into the TEP. In some instances a gel cap is used to facilitate insertion (see discussion in Placement of Indwelling Prosthesis section). The inserter is then removed and the position and fit of the prosthesis is checked by gently tugging on the prosthesis in an anterior motion and the prosthesis is rotated. The safety strap (and in some models also the safety medallion) is then taped to the neck above the stoma. To ensure the valve is functioning properly, patients should be encouraged to trial voicing, and also to drink something to check that there is no leakage either around or through the prosthesis. See CD for a demonstration of a non-indwelling prosthesis placement (Chapter 9: Video: "Provox NID Loading" and "Provox NID Placement").

## Placement of an Indwelling Prosthesis

As discussed in the non-indwelling section, there are different equipment and loading procedures for each of the commercial prostheses, and the reader is instructed to the individual manufacturer instructions. However, in general the process of inserting an indwelling prosthesis begins in the same manner as for the non-indwelling device, with removal of the existing device and placement of a dilator in situ in the TEP. Placement of a dilator may not always be necessary; some clinicians prefer to have the new prosthesis prepared for insertion, remove the old one, and immediately place the new one. Sizing may also be required. The preparation of the indwelling device for insertion however differs for the different devices. As previously discussed, flanges of an indwelling device are thicker and larger in diameter and therefore the prosthesis cannot be simply pushed through the TEP. Rather, to aid insertion, the esophageal flange must be folded into either a gel cap or insertion canister. Once this has been achieved, and the prosthesis loaded onto the insertion stick, the dilator is removed and the prosthesis inserted. See CD (Chapter 9: Video: "Provox2 Loading," "Provox2 Placement," and "Inserting Blom-Singer Indwelling Prosthesis") for a demonstration of the different replacements. If a gel cap system was used, the clinician should allow time for it to dissolve and allow the esophageal flange to unfold in the esophagus. Rotating the insertion stick helps to ensure the flanges are fully opened and correctly positioned. The safety strap can then be cut and the insertion stick can be removed. Voicing and swallow trials are also recommended to test the functioning of the prosthesis. See these processes performed at the end of the prosthesis change in the footage "Inserting Blom-Singer Indwelling Prosthesis" (CD, Chapter 9: Video: "Inserting Blom-Singer Indwelling Prosthesis").

## Patient Education

The SLP plays an important role in educating the patient and his or her support family about everything they need to know about the prosthesis, the fistula, and the mechanics of tracheoesophageal voice production. Equally important, the clinician needs to understand the patient's communication demands as well as his or her skills to engage in self-care. Some patients seem eager to learn these new skills while others may try to make these the responsibility of the spouse or other member of the support family. Obviously, the latter individuals may require more concentrated teaching of care and self-observation skills. Time spent at this level will minimize any potential difficulties for both the patient and the family later in the learning and care process.

The educational process should begin the moment the clinician meets the patient and continues through the fitting process until and beyond establishment of functional tracheoesophageal communication. Most critical of the education process is teaching self-care and prosthesis troubleshooting. Key elements of the education process include stoma and tissue inspection and what changes to be alert for, proper fit and maintenance of the voice prosthesis, proper voicing and alertness to voice changes, and prosthesis failure.

One of the first instruction tasks a clinician should undertake with a patient after the initial prosthesis fitting should be how to evaluate the prosthesis and determine when it needs replacement. This is easily done with a swallow of a brightly colored (blue or green) fluid. Instruct the patient to take an average mouthful and hold. Then, swallow while viewing the tracheal end of the prosthesis. It is important to have the patient observe for at least 3 to 5 seconds after completion of the swallow. If the prosthesis has been cleaned and continues to leak with the colored fluid test, it is time to change the prosthesis. It is important to indicate that a leaking prosthesis is not an emergency situation. There are plugs available that can be inserted on a temporary basis to ensure the TEP remains patent and to prevent aspiration, or patients can be instructed to insert their dilation device or a catheter to achieve the same purpose, until they can attend the clinic (see Figure 9–22).

Equally important, the clinician should teach the patient how to clean the prosthesis. Some models can only be cleaned by means of a flushing device, while others can be cleaned by means of a brush and/or flushing device. All prosthesis manuals contain instruc-

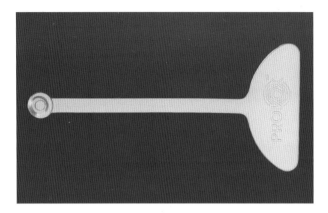

**Figure 9–22.** Photograph of a plug that can be used to temporarily stop leakage through the prosthesis. The small stopper at the left-hand side is inserted in the lumen of the voice prosthesis, while the medallion at the right-hand side is taped to the neck. (Photo provided as a courtesy of Atos Medical, www.atosmedical.com.)

tions how to clean the prosthesis. Flushing requires loading the supplied flushing device with either tap water or saline solution and gently inserting the tip of the flushing device into the lumen of the prosthesis and directing water through the prosthesis by compressing the syringe bulb. Brushing requires gentle insertion of the brush into the lumen of the voice prosthesis, followed by gentle back and forth and twisting motions. In either case, it is important to warn the patients that they should follow the guidelines of the manufacturer, and use only the products and solutions recommended.

It is important to influence the patient to take ownership or responsibility of self-care. Establishing the need to do self-care will not only benefit the patient, but will also benefit all medical and rehabilitation personnel that will be a part of the postoperative process. Conversely, some spouses/partners must be gently persuaded to be less active to allow the patient to learn some independent self-care skills. It may be necessary to remind the patients that if their partners did not assist them with their daily self-care tasks before the surgery, then they should not be doing it now. Only in rare instances of impaired visual or motor skills should an exception be made to this guideline.

## Postoperative Voice and Speech Training

The real reason a TEP with a prosthesis fitting has been done in the first place is to provide a pseudo-voice that allows for verbal communication. However, a TEP does not reduce the need for "post-prosthesis" therapy. Voice production rarely "just happens" but usually requires elements of proper stoma closure, proper pulmonary air pressure/flow, and appropriate muscle tension. While some patients only require a few sessions to be proficient TE speakers, others require many more.

Voice training can only start after wound healing has completed and the surgeon has given approval. In general, this takes about 10 days. In the following sections, the various aspects of postsurgical tracheo-esophageal speech training are addressed.

### The First Session

For many patients (and clinicians) the first session is an emotional moment. The patient may have been worried about the ability to even produce voice, or about the sound of the new voice. The moment of the first sound production is a highly anticipated moment. It is important for the clinician to recognize the importance of this moment and to communicate with the patient about the results. If the patient is unhappy with the sound, then this is the time to explain that our training is aimed at improvement and that the sound of the voice often changes over time.

Before starting, make sure the voice prosthesis is clean. If the patient is wearing an HME, make sure the baseplate has an airtight seal with the skin.

The training usually starts simply by asking the patient to produce a sustained vowel, preceded by an /h/ sound, for example /hay/, /hooooo/, /haaaaa/. Even though laryngectomized patients often are not able to actually produce a real /h/ sound, aiming to start with an /h/ promotes a gentle onset of voicing.

Take the following steps:

- Ask patient to say /haaaa/
- Have thumb/finger ready at level of tracheostoma to occlude
- Observe patient for short prephonatory inspiratory breath
- Occlude stoma so that patient can speak
- Release thumb/finger immediately after sound production stops
- Repeat the procedure with some more sounds and short sentences starting with an /h/ sound

### Training Sequence

The steps described in the previous section can be repeated with the patient occluding the stoma guided by the therapist and then by himself. Some patients will do this easily, while others have a hard time achieving a good seal or good timing of occlusion. In a separate section on stoma occlusion, various aspects related to stoma occlusion will be discussed.

After the initial sustained vowels starting with an /h/, the next steps are words beginning with an /h/ ("hello"), short sentences beginning with an /h/ ("How are you"), short sentences starting with other sounds, longer sentences, longer sentences with pauses (to train phrasing), and just regular conversation.

In most cases, already during the first training session, the patient will be able to speak in short sentences and participate in a short conversation. This usually depends on the ability to achieve good stoma occlusion.

### Basic Aspects to Address

**Stoma Occlusion.** Stoma occlusion may be obtained by thumb or finger directly on the tracheostoma, on top of an HME, or by means of a hands-free speaking valve. In Figure 9–23 different methods of stoma occlusion are shown. Airtight and well-timed stoma occlusion is a very important aspect of tracheoesophageal voice rehabilitation. Problems with stoma occlusion lead to disturbing noises either at the beginning (untimely occlusion), during (incomplete occlusion), and/or at the end (too early release of occlusion) of a sentence (CD: Chapter 9: Audio: Stoma Noise). This draws attention to the handicap and it is distracting and disturbing. Also, less air is available for speech which in turn leads to shorter phonation times and problems with phrasing. Eliminating stoma noise is important, and the use of a stethoscope may be considered for patient feedback; this is especially helpful when the patient is hearing impaired.

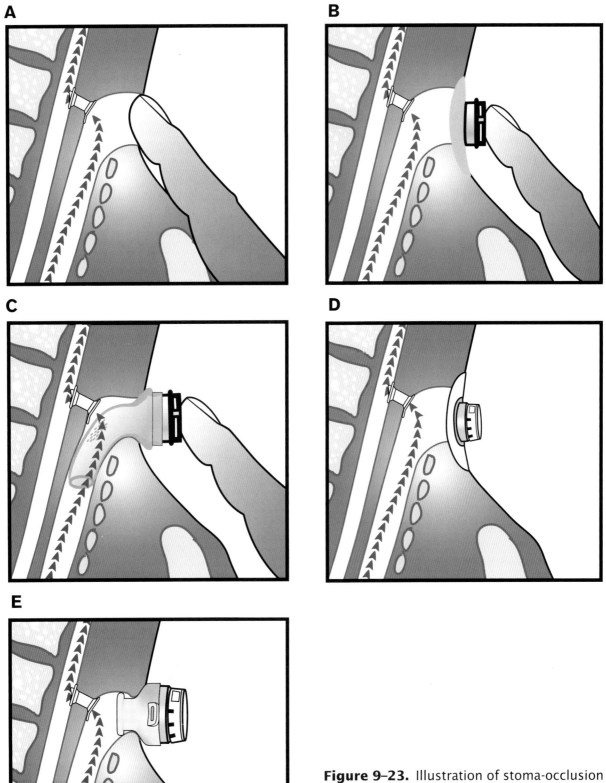

**Figure 9–23.** Illustration of stoma-occlusion by means of a finger **A.**, a finger on top of an HME attached by means of a baseplate **B.**, a finger on top of an HME attached in a laryngectomy tube **C.**, a hands-free speaking device in a baseplate **D.**, and a hands-free speaking device in a stoma button **E.**

When the stoma is occluded with the finger or thumb directly over the stoma, find the finger or thumb that fits the shape of the stoma best and that allows easiest occlusion. See footage on CD of a patient learning finger occlusion, trying both finger and thumb closure (Chapter 9: Video: "Learning Finger Occlusion"). When the stoma is occluded on top of an HME, it is usually not necessary to use the thumb for occlusion. Use the finger that is easiest to use and make sure the occlusion is airtight. When voice rehabilitation commences, some patients will already use an HME while others do not. Starting the patient with a manually closed HME eliminates the need for thumb or finger occlusion on the healing stoma. However, even the HME user should learn how to occlude the stoma with a thumb or finger. This can be done at a later stage when the stoma has healed. Whether direct digital occlusion of the stoma or digital occlusion via an HME is used, the same points should be taken into consideration.

*Finger pressure.* The patient needs to be instructed on how to achieve a stoma seal without too little or too much digital pressure. With too little pressure, the patient may create additional stoma noise and provide hyperfunctional pulmonary support to compensate. With too much digital pressure the patient may functionally compress the neoglottis that would normally vibrate, thus resulting in aphonia.

*Timing.* Timing of occluding the stoma and releasing the finger pressure is important. With occlusion that is too late, the first few words of an utterance get lost, and with occlusion release that occurs too early, the last few words can be lost and instead replaced by stoma noise. The patient needs to learn how to quickly release the finger (without stoma noise), allow air to enter the lungs, and occlude again (without stoma noise) to continue to speak.

*Distractions.* Stoma occlusion should be as inconspicuous as possible. Large movements, an elbow pointing outwards, or an awkward position of the arm draw attention to the handicap. Hold the arm close to the body, do not move the entire arm to achieve stoma occlusion, and instead lift the thumb or finger only.

*Preferred hand.* It is often advised to use the nondominant hand for stoma occlusion; this leaves the dominant hand free for other tasks.

**Posture.** The position of the body and head may influence the voice quality. Body posture influences pulmonary support and head position influences the soft tissues of the neoglottis. In some occasions, alterations in head position may actually be used to achieve changes in voice quality (see CD, Chapter 9: Video: "Head Position and Voice Change"). Some patients have the tendency to use head movements to accentuate aspects of speech. This should be avoided as it is distracting. Instead, teach the patient how to accentuate differently (see Pitch and Loudness Control). Some laryngectomees are tempted to raise the chin in an attempt to create space for stoma occlusion. This is not necessary and should be corrected.

**Pulmonary Support.** The applied pulmonary support to create the airflow through the prosthesis and eventually through the neoglottis is of critical importance. Without instruction, some patients will habitually produce excessive pulmonary support to initiate and continue voice production. Without instruction, they will be the same individuals who will claim that it is impossible to maintain an adhesive seal with an HME or hands-free speaking device. On rare occasions, the clinician may find an individual who has such poor pulmonary support, usually due to poor pulmonary health, that he or she may need instruction to overcome hypofunctional pulmonary support. Very rarely, it is seen that the patient occludes the stoma, but does not exhale to speak.

Another factor related to pulmonary support is the coordination of stoma occlusion and pulmonary support. The patient will have to learn to start/stop pulmonary flow and apply/release finger pressure simultaneously; otherwise stoma noise will occur. Esophageal or electrolarynx speakers who convert to a voice prosthesis or who use both esophageal/electrolarynx speech and tracheoesophageal speech may have more problems with coordination of stoma occlusion and pulmonary support, since they are not coordinated in esophageal and electrolarynx speech.

Instruction and training may be similar to those given to "normal" patients with voice problems and may be focused on controlled "abdominal" breathing rather than "thoracic" breathing. Instruction and training for coordination problems may consist of sustained vowel phonation, starting phonation with an open mouth (to avoid air injection on plosives in esophageal speakers), education, and feedback.

**Muscle Tension.** Some individuals develop a functional habit of squeezing at the level of the neoglottis. The knowledge that the new voice source is located in the neck may cause some laryngectomees to generate extra force in this area when trying to produce voice, while this is actually counterproductive. These individuals may require some instruction to drive the voice with proper pulmonary flow while maintaining a relaxed neoglottis at the same time.

### More Specific Aspects to Address

Once the patient has mastered tracheoesophageal speech using the basic techniques described above, the patient and clinician may choose to improve speech even further by working on voice quality, intonation and inflection, intelligibility, speech rate, fluency, HME use and attachment, and hands-free speaking device and attachment.

**Voice Quality.** Aspects of voice quality that deserve attention during training are the sound of the voice, pitch, and loudness. The sound of the voice is mainly determined by the anatomical and physiological characteristics of the neoglottis. However, also pulmonary support, tension in the neck area, and posture play a role. For example, when the voice is sounding strained, tension in the neck area can be lowered by using proper abdominal pulmonary support. Patients may focus on the neck area too much since that is where the surgery took place and that is where the sound is originated. Removing the focus from the neck area and aiming for relaxation of the neck area and abdominal breath support influence voice quality and makes it less tiring for the patient to speak.

The pitch of the voice mainly depends on the characteristics of the neoglottis. While some patients are able to vary pitch independently from loudness, in most patients the pitch tends to rise when loudness increases. Pitch can be trained by exercising pitch glides and singing.

Loudness is a problem for many laryngectomized patients. It is often not possible to speak very loudly which is a problem in some social circumstances. Trying to speak more loudly takes quite an effort and does not lead to much loudness gain. It may even lead to decreased intelligibility. Therefore, it is important to instruct the patient that in general, but especially in circumstances where increased loudness is desired, it is often better to focus on articulating more precisely, and trying to speak more clearly (see section on Intelligibility). Clearer speech will not only improve intelligibility but also decrease the amount of pressure on the seal of a baseplate used for an HME or hands-free device. Loudness can be trained by crescendo and decrescendo exercises.

Improved pitch and loudness control will help to achieve melodious speech.

**Fluency.** Fluency of speech may be influenced by problems with coordination of stoma occlusion and pulmonary support, phonation time, phrasing, tonicity, and swallowing. Coordination, phrasing, phrase length, pausing at natural places, easy stoma occlusion and release, and maximum phonation time can be the subject of exercises. If it is thought that the tonicity of the neoglottis is a problem, this should be further evaluated (see section on Troubleshooting). In most laryngectomized patients, a swallow disrupts the fluency of speech. Immediately after a swallow it is more difficult to produce voice. The reason is anatomical: the swallow affects the neoglottis and moves food or saliva through the neopharynx and esophagus, the same anatomical structures which are used for speech. The patient should understand this and should be advised to avoid an immediate start of voicing after a swallow.

**Intonation and Inflection.** Not all laryngectomees have the ability to use pitch to produce intonation or contrastive stress. Using loudness and pauses may help. Exercises to improve intonation and inflection may comprise of pitch glides, crescendo, decrescendo, practicing contrastive stress in sentences, practicing the intonation pattern used for asking questions, and singing.

**Intelligibility.** The alterations in the voice source and vocal tract not only influence voice quality, but also intelligibility. Intelligibility of tracheoesophageal speech is not as good as normal speech.

Many laryngectomees will try to speak more loudly in an attempt to be heard or out of habit. In general, the attempt to speak more loudly does not generate a much louder voice sound, it is tiring for the speaker, and it does not improve intelligibility. It is important to teach the laryngectomee to focus on clear speech and good articulation and to keep the loudness at a comfortable level. Practice voiced-voiceless distinction, clear speech, and precise articulation.

Laryngectomized patients who have received radiation in the head and neck area may also experience hypomobility of the jaw (trismus). Among other things, this may affect speech, biting off food, and mastication. This condition can be treated effectively by passive stretching of the jaw musculature and joint by using the Therabite jaw mobilization system (Atos Medical AB, Hörby, Sweden) (Buchbinder, Currivan, Kaplan, & Urken, 1993).

**Speech Rate.** Speech rate is often very personal. It may need some attention in the laryngectomized patient. Speaking too fast will decrease intelligibility while speaking too slowly will decrease the interest of the listener.

**HME and Attachment.** Nowadays many laryngectomized patients use an HME. An HME is a device that warms and humidifies the inhaled air as a replacement of the lost nose functions. It is attached in front of the stoma by means of a baseplate, laryngectomy tube, or laryngectomy button. More information on the research behind these devices and the various available options can be found in Chapters 11 and 12.

Although the primary purpose for using an HME is to improve or maintain pulmonary function, the SLP plays an important role in education and compliance. The HME can be attached to the peristomal area by means of a baseplate or by means of a laryngectomy tube or tracheostoma button (see Chapter 11). The SLP will need to teach the patient how to apply the baseplate and how to maintain a good seal, or how to use the intraluminal attachment. The SLP will also need to teach the patient how to occlude the device properly. The key is often to try a variety of baseplates to find the one that works best and to apply it correctly. The steps to be followed to create a good seal are described in Chapter 11. Another important key issue is the amount of pressure put on the seal during speech. The lower the speaking pressure, the longer the adhesive will generally last.

**Hands-Free Speech and Attachment.** A hands-free speaking valve is a device, usually combined with an HME, that contains a flexible membrane. The membrane does not close at usual exhalation levels, but it does close when the expiratory airflow increases when the patient attempts to speak. Chapter 11 provides more details about these devices. Not all laryngectomees may be able to use a hands-free speaking valve. It depends on factors such as the anatomy of the stoma, speaking pressure, and tonicity of the PE segment. The hands-free device can be attached to the stoma area by means of a baseplate or tracheostoma button (see Figure 9–23D and E). Laryngectomees that are able to use a stoma button (like the Barton-Mayo button or Provox LaryButton, see Chapter 11) are often more successful using a hands-free device (Lewin et al., 2000) compared to patients using a baseplate.

The main problem of hands-free devices is maintaining a good, airtight stoma seal. A large, deep, or irregular stoma may make it more difficult to achieve a good seal. High speaking pressures may put excessive pressure on the seal and hence cause it to loosen quickly (see sections on Voice Quality and Intelligibility for reducing loudness and improving speech clarity). The pressure produced during coughing may also cause problems with the seal. Some hands-free devices have adjustable cough relief valves. It is often advised to adjust these to a setting where they open relatively easily. That way, the pressure on the seal does not become extremely high during coughing. In fact, when the patient would speak (too) loudly, the relief would also open. Hence, this can serve as a feedback mechanism for the patient to control the amount of pressure on the seal while speaking. If the patient desires to occasionally speak more loudly or shout, the cough relief valve can be supported by a finger.

Another aspect of using a hands-free device is selection of the proper speaking membrane, as various resistances are available. The membranes with a lower resistance close more easily for speech, but may also close inadvertently while exhaling with some more force during physical activity. Some hands-free devices come with the option of locking the membrane during physical activities.

Creating a good seal of the baseplate or a good intraluminal attachment of the stoma button is probably the most important factor for success. The SLP plays an important role in, together with the patient, finding an optimal solution. For guidance on obtaining a good seal, see Chapter 11. This is often a process of trial and error and persistence; what may work for one patient may not for the other. Even if the patient would not be able to use the device "full-time" it may still be a valuable device to him or her to use for special occasions.

## Troubleshooting

The following sections discuss the most common problems that experienced clinicians have realized with TEP devices (either indwelling or non-indwelling). The problems can be prosthesis-related, puncture-related, or speech-related. Sometimes it is challenging to diagnose the cause of a problem; sometimes "problems" encountered by patients can be resolved by a word of assurance. Although the following list and discussion of problems may appear to be of considerable length, the reader must be advised that the first listed problem, fluid leaking through the prosthesis, constitutes the problem that the patient and clinician will encounter most often. A regimen of patient education, checking the proper length of the prosthesis at each prosthesis change, routine prosthesis and stoma care, and annual patient follow-up with an otolaryngologist will prevent most difficulties.

### Leakage of Fluid through the Lumen of the Prosthesis

Leaking through the device either of swallowed liquids and saliva (see footage on CD: Chapter 9: Video: "Leak through Prosthesis—Water" and "Leak through Prosthesis—Saliva") may be caused by a number of different problems:

*Potential problem 1*: A colony of *Candida* is blocking the valve door open. The device life of a voice prostheses is often limited because a biofilm (often referred to as *Candida,* a yeast that is present in the biofilm) forms on the esophageal side of the prosthesis, leading to leakage of the valve or increased airflow resistance (Busscher, Free, Van Weissenbruch, Albers, & Van Der Mei, 2000). Biofilms on voice prostheses consist of a large variety of oral and skin microorganisms, including streptococci, staphylococci, and yeasts (Mahieu, van Saene, Rosingh, & Schutte, 1986; Neu et al., 1994). Figure 9–24 shows a voice prosthesis that was removed for leakage through the device because of biofilm formation.

**Figure 9–24.** Photograph of voice prostheses removed for leakage due to *Candida.*

*Resolution*: Flush and/or brush the prosthesis. If the device continues to leak, test with colored fluid. If the prosthesis continues to leak after cleaning and shows signs of leakage with colored fluid, change the prosthesis.

*Potential problem 2*: Dried mucus or food particle blocking the valve door open.

*Resolution*: Flush and/or brush the prosthesis.

*Potential problem 3*: Increased negative pressure developed during the swallowing act or during inhalation. Examples of this are found on the CD (Chapter 9: Video: "Underpressure—Swallow" and "Underpressure—Inhalation"). Excessive negative pressures in the esophagus during swallowing may force the valve of the prosthesis to open during the act of swallowing and subsequent leakage of post-swallow residual through the device may occur. If this problem is suspected the clinician can usually see the valve opening during swallowing or inhalation, and sometimes a clicking sound from the valve can be heard.

*Resolution:* Consider a modified barium swallow (MBS) evaluation to ensure peristaltic movement during the swallow and/or rule out a stenosis or other obstruction. Instruction to reduce the swallowing force may be of benefit as well. If this particular problem persists, the clinician may want to consider placement of a specialized voice prosthesis using magnets

(ActiValve, Atos Medical AB, Hörby, Sweden) to counteract the negative pressure in the esophagus (see section on Special Purpose Voice Prostheses).

*Potential problem 4*: If the patient is using a duckbill prosthesis the slit valve may be pushed open against the posterior esophageal wall.

*Resolution*: Ensure the length of the prosthesis is correct. If the prosthesis is too long, refit with a proper sized prosthesis. Otherwise, use a different type of voice prosthesis.

## Excessive Candida *Growth Leading to Early Valve Failure*

*Potential problem*: Some patients may experience excessive amounts of biofilm/*Candida* formation causing early valve failure (4 to 8 weeks or less).

*Resolution*: Some patients control the fungus growth with topographic and/or systemic fungal control agents. Also, some dietary changes may aid in the control of biofilm formation on the voice prosthesis (Busscher et al., 1998; Free et al., 2003; Schwandt et al., 2004; Free et al., 2000); "flushing" the prosthesis with air may help to prevent biofilm formation as well (Free et al., 2003). Furthermore, a different voice prosthesis may be tried (see discussion in Indwelling versus Non-Indwelling section and section on Special Purpose Voice Prostheses).

## Leakage of Fluid around the Prosthesis

Leakage around the device can be the result of the following problems:

*Potential problem 1*: The prosthesis too long. As a result, the prosthesis has "pistoned" or shifted back and forth, usually during the swallow. This pistoning effect may cause leakage around the prosthesis (see Figure 9–25A). If the current prosthesis can be extended or pulled into the trachea side by more than 2 mm, the patient should be remeasured and fitted with the correct size of prosthesis.

*Resolution*: Remeasure and fit with the proper sized prosthesis.

*Potential problem 2*: Allergies. The length of the fistula may vary due to swelling of the tissue during allergy season; the prosthesis that fit well during allergy season may become too long and piston. On the contrary, as a result of allergies the prosthesis that was fitting well before the allergy season may become too short; this will not lead to leakage around the prosthesis but to other problems covered later.

*Resolution*: Refit with the proper sized prosthesis. This candidate may wear two or three different sized devices during the year.

*Potential problem 3*: TEP enlargement due to tissue problems. If it has been determined that the voice prosthesis is the proper length, but the fistula has dilated to the point that fluid continues to leak around the prosthesis, the patient may have poor tissue tone. The lack of tissue flexibility and elasticity may be the product of prolonged pistoning of a prosthesis that was too long, previous cancer treatments (radiotherapy, chemotherapy), recurrent or metastatic disease, poor functioning thyroid (due to radiotherapy), poor nutrition the way the puncture was created (vertical cut versus punctures), and/or tissue changes due to gastroesophageal reflux.

*Resolution*: All voice prosthesis users should be followed annually by an otolaryngologist. Among other things, it is advised to routinely check the thyroid function and prescribe medication if a problem is diagnosed. Good tissue does not go "bad" without a reason, and leakage around any voice prosthesis that cannot be solved with simple downsizing deserves proper investigation to uncover the cause of the problem. A prosthesis with a larger esophageal flange (see section on Special Purpose Voice Prostheses) may be used to temporarily solve the leakage until the cause has been found and treated, or as a long-term solution when the leakage problem cannot be solved. Other methods that are used to treat an enlarged TEP are purse-string suture, or injections with filling materials like collagen or autologous fat. Ultimately, if the problem cannot be solved, surgical closure of the puncture may be indicated.

*Potential problem 4*: TEP enlargement due to excessive force of air to voice. This type of patient is usually using too much pulmonary support and/or has hypertonicity, spasm, or stenosis of the neoglottis. This can cause excessive dilation of the TEP as the air can be forced around and past the prosthesis. Even more dilation occurs if the patient has an issue with tissue health.

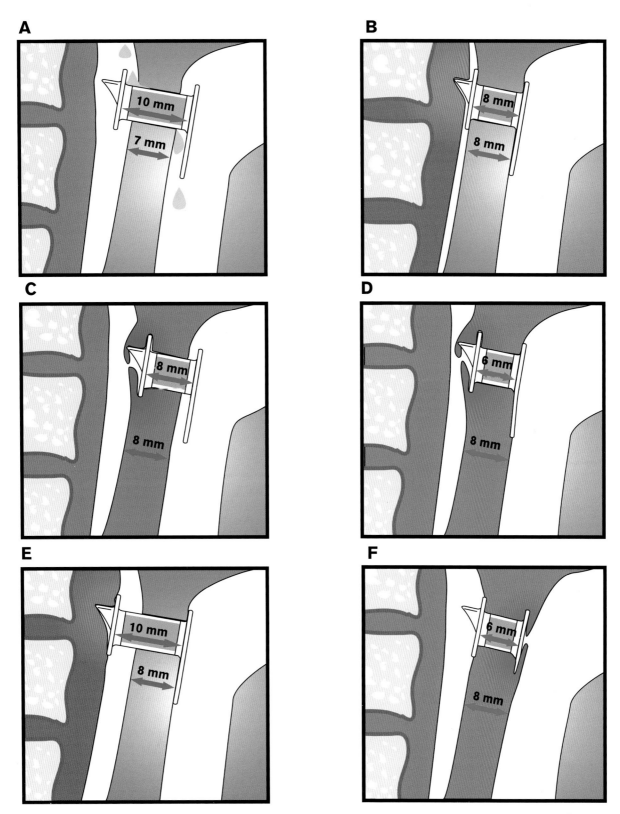

**Figure 9–25.** Illustration of leakage around the prosthesis due to pistoning **A.**, a prosthesis being blocked by the posterior esophageal wall **B.**, a prosthesis embedded in esophageal mucosa after incomplete insertion or partial dislodgement **C.**, a prosthesis embedded in esophageal mucosa because it was too short **D.**, a too-long prosthesis being pushed in the posterior esophageal wall **E.**, and a too-short prosthesis overgrown by tracheal mucosa **F.**

*Resolution*: Instructruct the patient to reduce the amount of pulmonary force to initiate and sustain voice. Suggest an easy onset of voice and encourage voice with minimum amount of pulmonary force. Evaluate for tonicity or stenosis. Treatment for hypertonicity or spasm may be needed (see section on strained/effortful voice production), or esophageal dilatation may be needed to improve swallowing (see also Chapter 10).

## Strained, Tight or Effortful Voice, or No Voice Sound At All

There may be a number of reasons that a patient experiences strained or effortful voice, including:

*Potential problem 1*: The patient may be using an excessive amount of strain and tension thus creating too high tension in the area of the neoglottis.

*Resolution*: Instruction to onset voice with a minimal amount of effort and the only effort should be pulmonary push. Suggest onset of the easiest or quietest voice possible.

*Potential problem 2*: The patient may use too high finger pressure for stoma occlusion. The patient may be physically applying pressure for stoma occlusion that also occludes the esophagus. Alternatively, the patient may be physically applying pressure for stoma occlusion and at the same time push the prosthesis into the posterior wall of the esophagus and preventing voice production; this is more likely to occur when the esophagus is narrow (see Figure 9-25B).

*Resolution*: In either scenario, instruct to seal the stoma with less pressure, in a slightly different direction, or by means of an HME and/or hands-free device.

*Potential problem 3*: The esophageal side of the prosthesis may have become occluded by *Candida*. If this is a patient who was speaking well and gradually loses voice, this cause should be considered.

*Resolution*: Change the prosthesis.

*Potential problem 4*: The esophageal side of the prosthesis has become embedded in the esophageal mucosa. If the patient has had a recent prosthesis change, achieved voice for the first few days, but noticed increased effort was needed to produce voice over time and/or the voice sound changed over time, the distal end of the prosthesis may not have been delivered or pushed completely into the esophagus (see Figure 9-25C). The patient may have also noticed some blood on the brush when cleaning the voice prosthesis. This may also occur if the patient was fitted with a too-short voice prosthesis or the prosthesis has become too short because of swelling or infection of the tissues (see Figure 9-25D).

*Resolution*: Remove the prosthesis, dilate the fistula with a dilator for at least 30 minutes and reinsert the prosthesis, or place a 20 French rubber catheter, and refit the prosthesis 24 hours later. If the remaining opening of the TEP has become too small to introduce the dilator, it may be possible to insert the prosthesis retrograde by means of a guide wire (CD. Chapter 9: Video: "Retrograde Insertion"). In extreme cases, when the patient comes into the clinic with the puncture completely closed at the esophageal side, a secondary puncture is the only solution. Since the consequences of this problem can be quite significant, it is important to instruct the patient to always contact the clinician if a change in voice quality or speaking effort occurs.

*Potential problem 5*: The prosthesis is too long. A prosthesis that is too long may be pushed into the posterior esophageal wall and obstructed for voicing when occluding the stoma (see Figure 9-25E). The prosthesis may have been improperly fitted or the tissue density may have changed.

*Resolution*: Refit with the proper sized prosthesis.

*Potential problem 6*: There is a spasm or hypertonicity of the neoglottis.

*Resolution*: Diagnosis of hypertonicity may involve open tract phonation to rule out a prosthesis-related problem; insufflation testing through the prosthesis to rule out a functional problem (for example the patient exerting too much pressure); manipulation of the neoglottis; videofluoroscopy recording of swallowing and (attempted) phonation; and/or a diagnostic block of the pharyngeal plexus using lidocaine (Hamaker & Cheesman, 1998).

*Resolution*: The first attempt should always be the least invasive one: voice training by an SLP. Training may consist of relaxation of the neck area and use of pulmonary support; speaking with a "forward focus" towards the lips as supposed to focusing on the neck area; low pitch; gentle onset of voice; manipulation of the neoglottis (see Figure 9–26 and CD, Chapter 9: Video: "Manipulation of Neoglottis and Resonance 1–5"); or resonance voice training. Sometimes, a block of the pharyngeal plexus with lidocaine is used therapeutically. Although it works only for a short period of time, for some patients it is enough to just feel exactly how voice should be produced. If all of the above does not help, usually Botox injections or a secondary myotomy will be used.

## Soft, Weak, Breathy Voice

*Potential problem*: Hypotonicity of the neoglottis.

*Resolution*: Check head position; a small adjustment in head position may make a big difference in voice quality (see CD, Chapter 9: Video: "Head Position and Voice Change"). If that does not help, apply digital pressure to the neck with a finger (see CD, Chapter 9: "Digital Pressure Applied to Neck") or use a custommade band around the neck to obtain closure of the neoglottis needed for speech. More recently also surgical options have been explored (Hilgers, van As-Brooks, Polak, & Tan, 2006).

## The Tracheal Flange Seems to Be Angled Forward

*Potential problem*: The prosthesis is too short, cleaned with oil-based agents, or aged. If the prosthesis is over 6 months old, exposure to mucus and *Candida* may have discolored, stiffened, and/or distorted the shape of the exterior flange.

*Resolution*: If the prosthesis is too short, refit with the proper sized prosthesis. If the prosthesis works, is not causing irritation, and there is no risk for parts of the flange to break off, then no direct action is required.

## The Tracheal Flange Is Discolored or Shows Signs of Candida Growth

*Potential problem*: With age, the tracheal flange can become discolored and disfigured due to *Candida* growth, use of oil-based or other nonrecommended cleaning agents, and possibly gastroesophageal reflux. Also, a variety of patient issues may contribute to the discoloration that can be due to pulmonary, digestion, and/or personal hygiene in nature.

*Resolution*: If the prosthesis works, then no action is required.

## Appearance of a Pink or Raised Ring of Tissue around the Fistula

*Potential problem*: A small number of patients will develop a small ring of granulation tissue around the fistula on the tracheal wall. Initially this will appear to have a flat anterior surface, but will usually grow as a complete circle around the fistula (also referred to as *donut*). Over time this may increase in density and thus increase the length of the fistula by extending into the trachea.

*Resolution*: Remeasure the fistula length and place a longer prosthesis if necessary. It should be cautioned that an increase in prosthesis length should only be done once. Eventually, the clinician should refer the patient to the otolaryngologist for removal of the tissue ring. The tissue can usually be removed under local anesthesia in the office and the patient can be refit with a prosthesis immediately.

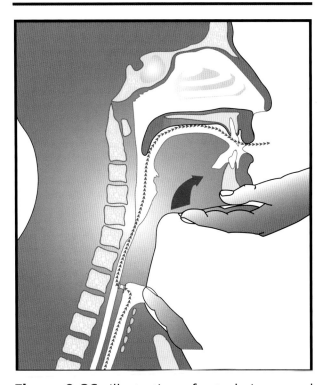

**Figure 9–26.** Illustration of a technique used for manipulation of the neoglottis to overcome hypertonicity.

### TEP Is Situated Too Low or Too High

A number of reasons may lead to a TEP being too low or high, including:

*Potential problem 1*: Some patients experience tissue changes over time. A fistula that may have initially been in the perfect position may shift over time. A fistula that is too high is one where the angle or tract of the TEP delivers the distal end of the prosthesis into the pharynx rather than the esophagus. Insertion and cleaning of the prosthesis may be difficult or impossible.

*Resolution*: Remove the prosthesis, allow fistula to heal or close, and consider for a secondary puncture at a later date. To prevent aspiration of liquid, consider placement of an inflatable, cuffed tracheostomy tube for about a week.

*Potential problem 2*: The fistula tract may migrate or be positioned in line with or below the lower rim of the tracheal stoma.

*Resolution*: If the prosthesis can be removed and reinserted, no action is required. If the clinician or the patient has difficulty changing or cleaning the prosthesis, then closure of the TEP and conduction of a secondary procedure should be considered.

### Prosthesis Is Missing from Fistula

The prosthesis may be missing (or considered missing) from the fistula for two main reasons:

*Potential problem 1*: In the very rare combined conditions of a thin tracheoesophageal party wall and poor tissue flexibility, the prosthesis may be lost from the TEP. More commonly in non-indwelling prostheses, the patients can dislodge the prosthesis with violent coughing or forceful cleaning in situ or may have no idea of when or where the prosthesis went until they have a drink of fluid.

*Resolution*: If the patient recovers the dislodged prosthesis, refit with the proper sized prosthesis (also take note of the previous discussion under Leaking around the Prosthesis about tissue health and care).

If the patient does not know where the prosthesis actually came to rest after being dislodged, stint the fistula with a dilator and/or catheter and send the patient for a chest x-ray to rule out aspiration of the prosthesis into the lungs. If the patient continues to cough, more than likely the prosthesis has been aspirated and is lodged either in the bronchi or lung lobe. As aspiration of the prosthesis is a rare occurrence, it is suggested that a similar prosthesis be described or shown to the radiologist. If the chest x-ray is negative, refit with the proper sized prosthesis. If the chest x-ray is positive, the prosthesis must be removed immediately by a physician because of the risk of airway obstruction or pneumonia.

*Potential problem 2*: In rare occasions, it may seem that the prosthesis is gone, but in fact the tracheal mucosa may have grown over the tracheal side of the prosthesis (Figure 9–25F). This could happen when the prosthesis was too short; it is very rare since this process would be slow and the patient would usually discover the problem before the prosthesis has "disappeared."

*Resolution*: The prosthesis should be removed, the fistula dilated, and the patient should be refitted with a prosthesis of the proper length.

### Prosthesis Turned Sideways in Fistula

*Potential problem*: This is an extremely rare problem. If the patient has been fit with a prosthesis that was one or two sizes too small in length, the distal and tracheal flanges compress the tissue. Within days to weeks, the position of the prosthesis will appear to be rotating either in a lateral (side to side) or vertical (top to bottom) direction. This will be evidenced by acute swelling of the tissue around the tracheal flange and erosion of the posterior flange through the common tracheal-esophageal wall. The patient may present with complaints of aspiration.

*Resolution*: Remove the prosthesis by pulling on the tracheal flange and refit with a longer prosthesis or stint the fistula with a catheter for a period of 24 to 48 hours. When the patient returns, resize and refit with the proper sized prosthesis.

### Infection of the TEP

*Potential problem*: The TEP may be infected, which may lead to swelling of the tissue and problems with the voice prosthesis.

*Resolution*: Refer the patient to an otolaryngologist for evaluation and prescription of antibiotics. If the prosthesis still has the proper fit, it can remain in situ. If the prosthesis seems too short, it should be (temporarily) replaced with a longer prosthesis or with a catheter until the infection has cleared.

## Gastric Filling/Bloating

A number of problems can contribute to the patient experiencing gastric filling or bloating, including:

*Potential problem 1*: Negative pressure in the esophagus during inhalation opens up the valve and allows air to enter the esophagus and stomach. This is more likely to happen during forceful inhalation during physical activities.

*Resolution*: The different prostheses available all have unique features. Changing to a different voice prosthesis may help. Also, prostheses with increased valve resistance are available (see special purpose voice prostheses section).

*Potential problem 2*: The patient may be swallowing with too high pressure; this may be habitual or caused by hypertonicity, spasm, or stenosis of the PE segment.

*Resolution*: Give the patient directions for swallowing with less pressure. Evaluate for problems with the PE segment. Hypertonicity or spasm may have to be treated with Botox or a secondary myotomy (see section on strained, effortful voice); esophageal stenosis may have to be treated with dilatation.

*Potential problem 3*: Air may be forced downwards into the esophagus and stomach during speaking due to hypertonicity or spasm of the PE segment.

*Resolution*: Evaluate the PE segment and treat hypertonicity or spasm when necessary (see section on strained, effortful voice).

## Conclusion

Since its first introduction 25 years ago, prosthetic tracheoesophageal speech has become the most widely used method of alaryngeal communication. The SLP plays an important role in patient education, prosthe-

sis measurement and fitting, postoperative voice and speech training, and troubleshooting. This chapter has aimed to cover all aspects that are important to help the patient achieve optimal tracheoesophageal speech.

## References

Akbas, Y., & Dursun, G. (2003). Voice restoration with low pressure Blom-Singer voice prosthesis after total laryngectomy. *Yonsei Medical Journal, 44*, 615–618.

Amatsu, M. (1980). A one stage surgical technique for postlaryngectomy voice rehabilitation. *Laryngoscope, 90*, 1378–1386.

Andrews, J. C., Mickel, R. A., Hanson, D. G., Monahan, G. P., & Ward, P. H. (1987). Major complications following tracheoesophageal puncture for voice rehabilitation. *Laryngoscope, 97*, 562–567.

Arslan, M., & Serafini, I. (1972). Restoration of laryngeal functions after total laryngectomy. Report on the first 25 cases. *Laryngoscope, 82*, 1349–1360.

Asai, R. (1972). Laryngoplasty after total laryngectomy. *Archives of Otolaryngology, 95*, 114–119.

Aust, M. R., & McCaffrey, T. V. (1997). Early speech results with the Provox prosthesis after laryngectomy. *Archives of Otolaryngology–Head and Neck Surgery, 123*, 966–968.

Baek, S. M., Lawson, W., & Biller, H. F. (1981). Reconstruction of hypopharynx and cervical esophagus with pectoralis major island myocutaneous flap. *Annals of Plastic Surgery, 7*, 18–24.

Baggs, T. W., & Pine, S. J. (1983). Acoustic characteristics: Tracheoesophageal speech. *Journal of Communication Disorders, 16*, 299–307.

Bayles, S. W., & Deschler, D. G. (2004). Operative prevention and management of voice-limiting pharyngoesophageal spasm. *Otolaryngologic Clinics of North America, 37*, 547–558.

Blom, E. D., & Hamaker, R. C. (1996). Tracheoesophageal voice restoration following total laryngectomy. In E. N. Myers & J. Suen (Eds.), *Cancer of the Head and Neck* (pp. 839–852). Philadelphia: WB Saunders.

Blom, E. D., Singer, M. I., & Hamaker, R. C. (1985). An improved esophageal insufflation test. *Archives of Otolaryngology, 111*, 211–212.

Blom, E. D., Singer, M. I., & Hamaker, R. C. (1986). A prospective study of tracheoesophageal speech. *Archives of Otolaryngology–Head and Neck Surgery, 112*, 440–447.

Buchbinder, D., Currivan, R. B., Kaplan, A. J., & Urken, M. L. (1993). Mobilization regimens for the prevention of jaw hypomobility in the radiated patient: A comparison of three techniques. *Journal of Oral and Maxillofacial Surgery, 51,* 863-867.

Busscher, H. J., Bruinsma, G., Van Weissenbruch, R., Leunisse, C., Van Der Mei, H. C., Dijk, F. et al. (1998). The effect of buttermilk consumption on biofilm formation on silicone rubber voice prostheses in an artificial throat. *European Archives of Otorhinolaryngology, 255,* 410-413.

Busscher, H. J., Free, R. H., Van Weissenbruch, R., Albers, F. W., & Van Der Mei, H. C. (2000). Preliminary observations on influence of dairy products on biofilm removal from silicone rubber voice prostheses in vitro. *Journal of Dairy Science, 83,* 641-647.

Davis, R. K., Vincent, M. E., Shapshay, S. M., & Strong, M. S. (1982). The anatomy and complications of "T" versus vertical closure of the hypopharynx after laryngectomy. *Laryngoscope, 92,* 16-22.

Debruyne, F., Delaere, P., Wouters, J., & Uwents, P. (1994). Acoustic analysis of tracheo-oesophageal versus oesophageal speech. *The Journal of Laryngology and Otology, 108,* 325-328.

Deschler, D. G., Doherty, E. T., Reed, C. G., Anthony, J. P., & Singer, M. I. (1994). Tracheoesophageal voice following tubed free radial forearm flap reconstruction of the neopharynx. *The Annals of Otology, Rhinology, and Laryngology, 103,* 929-936.

Deschler, D. G., Doherty, E. T., Reed, C. G., Hayden, R. E., & Singer, M. I. (2000). Prevention of pharyngoesophageal spasm after laryngectomy with a half-muscle closure technique. *The Annals of Otology, Rhinology, and Laryngology, 109,* 514-518.

Deschler, D. G., Doherty, E. T., Reed, C. G., & Singer, M. I. (1998). Quantitative and qualitative analysis of tracheoesophageal voice after pectoralis major flap reconstruction of the neopharynx. *Otolaryngology-Head and Neck Surgery, 118,* 771-776.

Doyle, P. C., Danhauer, J. L., & Reed, C. G. (1988). Listeners' perceptions of consonants produced by esophageal and tracheoesophageal talkers. *Journal of Speech and Hearing Disorders, 53,* 400-407.

Eerenstein, S. E., Schouwenburg, P. F., Van Der Velden, L. A., & De Boer, M. F. (2001). First results of the VoiceMaster prosthesis in three centres in the Netherlands. *Clinical Otolaryngology, 26,* 99-103.

Elving, G. J., Van Weissenbruch, R., Busscher, H. J., Van Der Mei, H. C., & Albers, F. W. (2002). The influence of radiotherapy on the lifetime of silicone rubber voice prostheses in laryngectomized patients. *Laryngoscope, 112,* 1680-1683.

Free, R. H., Van Der Mei, H. C., Dijk, F., Van Weissenbruch, R., Busscher, H. J., & Albers, F. W. (2000). Biofilm formation on voice prostheses: Influence of dairy products in vitro. *Acta Otolaryngologica, 120,* 92-99.

Free, R. H., Van Der Mei, H. C., Elving, G. J., Van Weissenbruch, R., Albers, F. W., & Busscher, H. J. (2003). Influence of the Provox Flush, blowing and imitated coughing on voice prosthetic biofilms in vitro. *Acta Otolaryngologica, 123,* 547-551.

Geraghty, J. A., Wenig, B. L., Smith, B. E., & Portugal, L. G. (1996). Long-term follow-up of tracheoesophageal puncture results. *The Annals of Otology, Rhinology, and Laryngology, 105,* 501-503.

Gress, C. D. (2004). Preoperative evaluation for tracheoesophageal voice restoration. *Otolaryngologic Clinics of North America, 37,* 519-530.

Gussenbauer, C. (1874). Ueber die erste durch Th. Billroth am Menschen ausgefuhrte Kehlkopf-Extirpation und die Anwendung eines künstlichesn Kehlkopfes. *Archives Klinische Chirurgie, 17,* 343-356.

Guttman, M. R. (1932). Rehabilitation of the voice in laryngectomized patients. *Archives of Otolaryngology, 15,* 478-488.

Hamaker, R. C., & Blom, E. D. (2003). Botulinum neurotoxin for pharyngeal constrictor muscle spasm in tracheoesophageal voice restoration. *Laryngoscope, 113,* 1479-1482.

Hamaker, R. C., & Cheesman, A. D. (1998). Surgical management of pharyngeal constrictor muscle hypertonicity. In E. D. Blom, M. I. Singer, & R. C. Hamaker (Eds.), *Tracheoesophageal voice restoration following total laryngectomy* (pp. 33-39). San Diego, CA: Singular.

Hammarberg, B., Lundström, E., & Nord, L. (1990). Consonant intelligibility in esophageal and tracheoesophageal speech. A progress report. *STL-QPR, 7.* Huddinge University Hospital and Karolinska Institute, Stockholm, Sweden.

Hancock, K., Houghton, B., van As-Brooks, C. J., & Coman, W. (2005). First clinical experience with a new non-indwelling voice prosthesis (Provox NID) for voice rehabilitation after total laryngectomy. *Acta Otolaryngologica, 125,* 981-990.

Harii, K., Ebihara, S., Ono, I., Saito, H., Terui, S., & Takato, T. (1985). Pharyngoesophageal reconstruction using a fabricated forearm free flap. *Plastic and Reconstructive Surgery, 75,* 463-476.

Haughey, B. H., & Forsen, J. W. (1992). Free jejunal graft: Effects of longitudinal myotomy. *The Annals of Otology, Rhinology, and Laryngology, 101,* 333-338.

Hayden, R. E., & Deschler, D. G. (1999). Lateral thigh free flap for head and neck reconstruction. *Laryngoscope, 109,* 1490-1494.

Hilgers, F. J. M. (Ed.). (2003). *A practical guide to post-laryngectomy rehabilitation. Including the Provox system* [CD-ROM] (4th ed.). The Netherlands Cancer Institute, Amsterdam, the Netherlands.

Hilgers, F. J. M., Ackerstaff, A. H., Balm, A. J. M., Tan, I. B., Aaronson, N. K., & Persson, J. O. (1997). Development and clinical evaluation of a second-generation voice prosthesis (Provox 2), designed for antero-grade and retrograde insertion. *Acta Otolaryngologica, 117,* 889-896.

Hilgers, F. J. M, Ackerstaff, A. H., Balm, A. J. M, Van den Brekel, M. W., Tan, I. B., & Persson, J.-O. (2003). A new problem-solving indwelling voice prosthesis, eliminating the need for frequent *Candida-* and "underpressure"-related replacements: Provox Acti-Valve. *Acta Otolaryngologica, 123,* 972-979.

Hilgers, F. J. M., Hoorweg, J. J., Kroon, B. N. R., Schaefer, B. S., de Boer, J., & Balm, A. J. M. (1995). Prosthetic voice rehabilitation with the Provox system after extensive pharyngeal resection and reconstruction. In J. Algaba (Ed.), *Surgery and prosthetic voice rehabilitation after total and subtotal laryngectomy. Proceedings of the 6th International Congress on Surgical and Prosthetic Voice Restoration after Total Laryngectomy, San Sebastian, Spain, Sept. 29-Oct. 1, 1995. Excerpta Medica International Congress Series 1112* (pp. 111-120). Amsterdam, Lausanne, New York, Oxford, Shannon, Tokyo: Elsevier.

Hilgers, F. J. M., & Schouwenburg, P. F. (1990). A new low-resistance, self-retaining prosthesis (Provox) for voice rehabilitation after total laryngectomy. *Laryngoscope, 100,* 1202-1207.

Hilgers, F. J. M, van As-Brooks, C. J., Polak, M. F., & Tan, I. B. (2006). Surgical improvement of hypotonicity in tracheoesophageal speech. *Laryngoscope, 116,* 345-348.

Hoffman, H. T., Fischer, H., VanDenmark, D., Peterson, K. L., McCulloch, T. M., Karnell, L. H., et al. (1997). Botulinum neurotoxin injection after total laryngectomy. *Head & Neck, 19,* 92-97.

Jongmans, P., Hilgers, F. J. M., Pols, L. C. W., & van As-Brooks, C. J. (in press). The intelligibility of tracheoesophageal speech with an emphasis on the voiced-voiceless distinction. *Logopedics Phoniatrics and Vocology.*

Kao, W. W., Mohr, R. N., Kimmel, K. A., Getch, C., & Silverman, C. (1994). The outcome and techniques of primary and secondary tracheoesophageal punc-ture. *Archives of Otolaryngology-Head and Neck Surgery, 120*(3), 301-307.

Karschay, P., Schon, F., Windrich, J., Fricke, J., & Herrmann, I. F. (1986). Experiments in surgical voice restoration using valve prostheses. *Acta Otolaryngologica, 101,* 341-347.

Laccourreye, O., Menard, M., Crevier-Buchman, L., Couloigner, V., & Brasnu, D. (1997). In situ lifetime, causes for replacement, and complications of the Provox voice prosthesis. *Laryngoscope, 107,* 527-530.

Leder, S. B., Acton, L. M., Kmiecik, J., Ganz, C., & Blom, E. D. (2005). Voice restoration with the Advantage tracheoesophageal voice prosthesis. *Otolaryngology-Head and Neck Surgery, 133,* 681-684.

Leder, S. B., & Erskine, M. C. (1997). Voice restoration after laryngectomy: Experience with the Blom-Singer extended-wear indwelling tracheoesophageal voice prosthesis. *Head & Neck, 19,* 487-493.

Leder, S. B., & Sasaki, C. T. (1995). Incidence, timing, and importance of tracheoesophageal prosthesis resizing for successful tracheoesophageal speech production. *Laryngoscope, 105,* 827-832.

Lewin, J. S. (2004). Nonsurgical management of the stoma to maximize tracheoesophageal speech. *Otolaryngologic Clinics of North America, 37,* 585-596.

Lewin, J. S., Barringer, D. A., May, A. H., Gillenwater, A. M., Arnold, K. A., Roberts, D. B., et al. (2005). Functional outcomes after circumferential pharyngoesophageal reconstruction. *Laryngoscope, 115,* 1266-1271.

Lewin, J. S., Lemon, J., Bishop-Leone, J. K., Leyk, S., Martin, J. W., & Gillenwater, A. M. (2000). Experience with Barton button and peristomal breathing valve attachments for hands-free tracheoesophageal speech. *Head & Neck, 22,* 142-148.

Lündstrom, E., & Hammarberg, B. (2004). High-speed imaging of the voicing source in laryngectomees during production of voiced-voiceless distinctions for stop consonants. *Logopedics Phoniatrics and Vocology, 29,* 31-40.

Luchsinger, R., & Arnold, G. (1965). *Voice-Speech-Language.* Belmont, CA: Wadsworth.

Mahieu, H. F., van Saene, H. K., Rosingh, H. J., & Schutte, H. K. (1986). *Candida* vegetations on silicone voice prostheses. *Archives of Otolaryngology-Head and Neck Surgery, 112,* 321-325.

Manni, J. J., Van den Broek P., de Groot, M. A., & Berends, E. (1984). Voice rehabilitation after laryngectomy with the Groningen prosthesis. *Journal of Otolaryngology, 13,* 333-336.

Marmuse, J. P., Guedon, C., & Koka, V. N. (1994). Gastric tube transposition for cancer of the hypopharynx and cervical oesophagus. *The Journal of Laryngology and Otology, 108,* 33-37.

Maves, M. D., & Lingeman, R. E. (1982). Primary vocal rehabilitation using the Blom-Singer and Panje voice prostheses. *The Annals of Otology, Rhinology, and Laryngology, 91,* 458-460.

Max, L., Steurs, W., & De Bruyn, W. (1996). Vocal capacities in esophageal and tracheoesophageal speakers. *Laryngoscope, 106,* 93-96.

McAuliffe, M. J., Word, E. C., Bassett, L., & Perkins, K. (2000). Functional speech outcomes after laryngectomy and pharyngectomy. *Archives of Otolaryngology-Head and Neck Surgery, 26*(6), 705-709.

McConnel, F. M., Hester, T. R., Jr., Nahai, F., Jurkiewicz, M. J., & Brown, R. G. (1981). Free jejunal grafts for reconstruction of pharynx and cervical esophagus. *Archives of Otolaryngology, 107,* 476-481.

McGrail, J. S., & Oldfield, D. L. (1971). One-stage operation for vocal rehabilitation at laryngectomy. *Transactions—American Academy of Ophthalmology and Otolaryngology, 75,* 510-512.

Mendelsohn, M., Morris, M., & Gallagher, R. (1993). A comparative study of speech after total laryngectomy and total laryngopharyngectomy. *Archives of Otolaryngology-Head and Neck Surgery, 119,* 508-510.

Miralles, J. L., & Cervera, T. (1995). Voice intelligibility in patients who have undergone laryngectomies. *Journal of Speech and Hearing Research, 38,* 564-571.

Montgomery, W. W., & Toohill, R. J. (1968). Voice rehabilitation after laryngectomy. *Archives of Otolaryngology, 88,* 499-506.

Myers, T. (Ed.). (2006). *Mosby's Dictionary of Medicine, Nursing & Health Professions.* St. Louis, MO: Mosby-Elsevier.

Neu, T. R., Verkerke, G. J., Herrmann, I. F., Schutte, H. K., Van Der Mei, H. C., & Busscher, H. J. (1994). Microflora on explanted silicone rubber voice prostheses: Taxonomy, hydrophobicity and electrophoretic mobility. *The Journal of Applied Bacteriology, 76,* 521-528.

Olson, N. R., & Callaway, E. (1990). Nonclosure of pharyngeal muscle after laryngectomy. *The Annals of Otology, Rhinology, and Laryngology, 99,* 507-508.

Op de Coul, B. M. R., Hilgers, F. J. M., Balm, A. J. M., Tan, I. B., van den Hoogen, F. J. A., & van Tinteren, H. (2000). A decade of postlaryngectomy vocal rehabilitation in 318 patients: A single institution's experience with consistent application of Provox indwelling voice prostheses. *Archives of Otolaryngology-Head and Neck Surgery, 126,* 1320-1328.

Panje, W. R., VanDemark, D., & McCabe, B. F. (1981). Voice button prosthesis rehabilitation of the laryngectomee. Additional notes. *The Annals of Otology, Rhinology, and Laryngology, 90,* 503-505.

Pindzola, R. H., & Cain, B. H. (1988). Acceptability ratings of tracheoesophageal speech. *Laryngoscope, 98,* 394-397.

Pindzola, R. H., & Cain, B. H. (1989). Duration and frequency characteristics of tracheoesophageal speech. *The Annals of Otology, Rhinology, and Laryngology, 98,* 960-964.

Pou, A. M. (2004). Tracheoesophageal voice restoration with total laryngectomy. *Otolaryngologic Clinics of North America, 37,* 531-545.

Robbins, J., Fisher, H. B., Blom, E. C., & Singer, M. I. (1984a). A comparative acoustic study of normal, esophageal, and tracheoesophageal speech production. *Journal of Speech and Hearing Disorders, 49,* 202-210.

Schwandt, L. Q., Van Weissenbruch, R., Stokroos, I., Van Der Mei, H. C., Busscher, H. J., & Albers, F. W. (2004). Prevention of biofilm formation by dairy products and N-acetylcysteine on voice prostheses in an artificial throat. *Acta Otolaryngologica, 124,* 726-731.

Searl, J. P., Carpenter, M. A., & Banta, C. L. (2001). Intelligibility of stops and fricatives in tracheoesophageal speech. *Journal of Communication Disorders, 34,* 305-321.

Serafini, I. (1972). Reconstructive laryngectomy. *Revue de Laryngologie, Otologie, et Rhinologie (Bourdeaux), 93,* 23-38.

Silver, C. E. (1976). Reconstruction after pharyngolaryngectomy-esophagectomy. *American Journal of Surgery, 132,* 428-434.

Silverman, A. H., & Black, M. J. (1994). Efficacy of primary tracheoesophageal puncture in laryngectomy rehabilitation. *Journal of Otolaryngology, 23,* 370-377.

Singer, M. I., & Blom, E. D. (1980). An endoscopic technique for restoration of voice after laryngectomy. *The Annals of Otology, Rhinology, and Laryngology, 89,* 529-533.

Singer, M. I., & Blom, E. D. (1981). Selective myotomy for voice restoration after total laryngectomy. *Archives of Otolaryngology, 107,* 670-673.

Singer, M. I., Blom, E. D., & Hamaker, R. C. (1981). Further experience with voice restoration after total laryngectomy. *The Annals of Otology, Rhinology, and Laryngology, 90,* 498-502.

Singer, M. I., Blom, E. D., & Hamaker, R. C. (1986). Pharyngeal plexus neurectomy for alaryngeal speech rehabilitation. *Laryngoscope, 96,* 50-54.

Smith, B. E. (1986). Aerodynamic characteristics of Blom-Singer low-pressure voice prostheses. *Archives of Otolaryngology–Head and Neck Surgery, 112,* 50–52.

Staffieri, M. (1981). Phonatory neoglottis surgery. *Ear Nose Throat Journal, 60,* 254–258.

Taub, S. (1975). Air bypass voice prosthesis for vocal rehabilitation of laryngectomees. *The Annals of Otology, Rhinology, and Laryngology, 84,* 45–48.

Taub, S., & Bergner, L. H. (1973). Air bypass voice prosthesis for vocal rehabilitation of laryngectomees. *American Journal of Surgery, 125,* 748–756.

Van As, C. J., Koopmans-van Beinum, F. J., Pols, L. C. W., Hilgers, F. J. M. (2003). Perceptual evaluation of tracheoesophageal speech by naïve and experienced judges through the use of semantic differential scales. *Journal of Speech, Language, and Hearing Research, 46,* 947–959.

Van As, C. J., Op de Coul, B. M. R., van den Hoogen, F. J. A., Koopmans van Beinum, F. J., & Hilgers, F. J. M. (2001). Quantitative videofluoroscopy: A new evaluation tool for tracheoesophageal voice production. *Archives of Otolaryngology–Head and Neck Surgery, 127,* 161–169.

Van As-Brooks, C. J., Hilgers, F. J. M., Koopmans-van Beinum, F. J., & Pols, L. C. W. (2005). Anatomical and functional correlates of voice quality in tracheoesophageal speech. *Journal of Voice, 19,* 360–372.

Van As-Brooks, C. J., Koopmans-van Beinum, F. J., Pols, L. C. W., & Hilgers, F. J. M. (2006). Acoustic signal typing for evaluation of voice quality in tracheoesophageal speech. *Journal of Voice 20*(3), 355–368.

Van Weissenbruch, R., Kunne, M., van Cauwenberghe, P. B., Albers, F. W. J., & Sulter, A. M. (2000). Cineradiography of the pharyngoesophageal segment in postlaryngectomy patients. *Annals of Otology Rhinology and Laryngology, 109,* 311–319.

Verschuur, H. P., Gregor, R. T., Hilgers, F. J., & Balm, A. J. (1996). The tracheostoma in relation to prosthetic voice rehabilitation. *Laryngoscope, 106,* 111–115.

Ward, E. C. Koh, S. K., Frisby, J., & Hodge, R. (2003). Differential modes of alaryngeal communication following pharyngolaryngectomy and laryngectomy. *Folia Phoniatrica et Logopaedica, 55,* 39–49.

Weinberg, B., & Moon, J. B. (1986). Impact of tracheoesophageal puncture prosthesis airway resistance on in-vivo phonatory performance. *Journal of Speech and Hearing Disorders, 51,* 88–91.

Williams, S. E., & Watson, J. B. (1987). Speaking proficiency variations according to method of alaryngeal voicing. *Laryngoscope, 97,* 737–739.

# Chapter 10

# SWALLOWING REHABILITATION FOLLOWING TOTAL LARYNGECTOMY

Elizabeth C. Ward, Sophie M. Kerle,
Kelli L. Hancock, and Kylie Perkins

## CHAPTER OUTLINE

## Introduction

Total laryngeal resection and subsequent reconstruction procedures result in significant anatomical and physiological change to the swallowing mechanism. Not only are most of the anatomical structures involved in swallowing actually removed during surgery, but the remaining tissues of the pharynx are repositioned as part of the reconstruction, or in the case of more extensive tumors, partially or totally removed and new tissues are added to close the pharyngeal deficit. As a consequence, the process of swallowing is drastically altered and complications can arise due to the type and extent of surgical reconstruction as well as the effects of adjuvant radiotherapy and alterations to sensory awareness. However, regardless of the enormity of change, most patients regain the ability to eat orally following total laryngeal resection, with over half resuming full normal oral diet in the long term (Ward, Bishop, Frisby, & Stevens, 2002).

It is the aim of the current chapter to detail the changes in swallowing physiology that occur following laryngectomy, outline the potential complications of surgery and postoperative radiotherapy which may impact on swallowing function, and detail the rehabilitation process to facilitate optimal swallowing outcomes for this population.

## Surgical Impact on Swallow Physiology

The impact of surgical removal of the larynx, and in many cases excision of tissues from the base of tongue and pharynx, alters normal swallow physiology. In the following section, the normal swallow and the changes to the normal swallow created by total laryngectomy and pharyngolaryngectomy will be discussed.

### The Normal Swallow

The normal swallow is a complex synergy of biomechanical actions that create the necessary pharyngeal pressures for efficient bolus flow from the mouth to the esophagus. The anterior movement of the larynx creates a short, patent, digestive conduit with mechanical stretching of the upper esophageal sphincter (UES) resulting in its relaxation and the opening of the esophagus. This increases the volume of the digestive tract and creates a negative, suction pressure that will assist in drawing the bolus into the proximal esophagus (Cerenko, McConnel, & Jackson, 1989).

Once the larynx has repositioned, the base of the tongue (in contact with the soft palate) thrusts posteriorly, creating a positive propulsion force behind the bolus tail and clearing the bolus from the oropharynx (Cerenko et al., 1989; McConnel, 1988). A pressure *gradient* therefore exists, between the positive pressure exerted at the oropharynx and the negative suction pressure of the hypopharynx (Cerenko et al., 1989; McConnel, 1988). This pressure gradient is primarily responsible for efficient bolus flow but is assisted by the sequential stripping action of the pharyngeal constrictor muscles once the bolus has passed (McConnel, 1988).

### Total Laryngectomy

For patients who present with advanced laryngeal cancer, a total laryngectomy may be performed. Generally speaking, total laryngectomy removes all of the structures that comprise the anterior wall of the upper digestive tract, including all laryngeal cartilage, the epiglottis, the hyoid bone, and portions of the base of the tongue, along with the strap muscles of the neck (see Figure 10–1). The defect consists of pharyngeal mucosa and constrictor muscle remnants. There are several variations of the type/pattern of closure associated with total laryngectomy. The decision as to the type of closure chosen will be dependant on the surgeon's experience, preference, and institutional guidelines considering variables such as pharyngocutaneous fistula formation and previous radiotherapy. The two most common patterns of closure described in the literature are referred to as T-closure and vertical closure. The surgeon also has the option to close the defect in two or three layers. The usual method of reconstruction of the defect is a three-layer closure. That is, mucosa, submucosal tissue and pharyngeal constrictor muscles are each closed in a separate layer. This method of closure has been associated with high pharyngoesophageal pressures. Alternatively, the two-layer nonmuscular closure technique leaves the pharyngeal

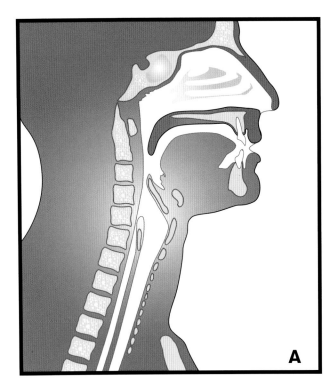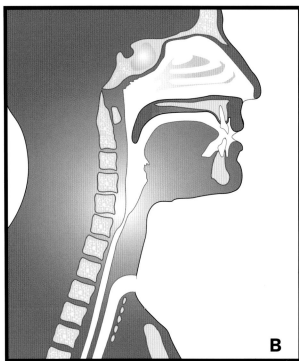

**Figure 10–1.** Schematic representation of the anatomical situation before **A.** and after **B.** total laryngectomy.

muscle open in an attempt to eliminate the complications associated with a three-layer closure. A direct relationship between dysphagia after total laryngectomy and the type/pattern of closure is not clear; however, several authors have reported an association between the presence of features such as pseudo-epiglottis and type of closure and offered possible explanations for their occurrence (see discussion in Logemann, 1998).

Clearly, this removal of key anatomical structures and reorganization of remaining tissues has a dramatic effect on pharyngeal swallowing physiology. Firstly, the absence of the larynx prevents pharyngeal shortening and esophageal opening, as well as the development of the negative component of the pressure gradient. In some cases total laryngectomees may compensate for this by increasing the positive force of lingual propulsion (McConnel, Mendelsohn, & Logemann, 1986). However, in many cases this is not possible due to significant resection of the tongue base (McConnel et al., 1986) and/or iatrogenic hypoglossal nerve palsy (Lewin et al., 2006). The inability to estab-

lish a pressure gradient for swallowing is also often compounded by functional obstructions to bolus flow that result from surgical reconstruction of the neopharynx. Narrowing pharyngeal lumens due to tissue prominence, stricture, and stenosis, as well as pseudo-epiglottis formation, and cricopharyngeal dysfunction (discussed later in the chapter) can often create a high resistance neopharynx, further hindering bolus descent (see CD, Chapter 10; MBS files: "Laryngectomy—Hold-Up Narrow Pharyngeal Lumen and Pseudoepiglottis"). Postoperative radiotherapy is also frequently required and is known to fibrose and subsequently weaken lingual and pharyngeal musculature as well as contribute to late stricture formation.

Changes in esophageal motility following total laryngectomy may also be the cause of dysphagia in this patient population (Choi et al., 2003; Dantas, Aguiar-Ricz, Gielow, Filho, & Mamede, 2005). During total laryngectomy, the cricopharyngeus, the main muscular component of the upper esophageal sphincter (UES) is transected. Postoperatively it exhibits reduced maximum pressure and duration of contraction during swallowing (Choi et al., 2003; Welch, Luckmann, Ricks, Drake, & Gates, 1979). Also, with the removal of the larynx which served as the anterior attachment point, the UES changes shape into a symmetrical ring, altering its contractile ability (Welch et al., 1979). Given that cricopharyngeal contraction normally initiates esophageal peristalsis, changes in its functional capacity could explain the reduction in strength and duration of esophageal contraction in the proximal esophageal body (Choi et al., 2003). Some authors suggest that damage to the nerves during surgery is responsible for such deficits (Choi et al., 2003; Dantas et al., 2005); for example, a simple interruption to the pharyngeal plexus, the motor innervation of the proximal esophagus (Choi et al., 2003). Alternatively, damage to sensory innervation of the esophagus could interrupt the reflexive esophageal accommodation to the bolus (Dantas et al., 2005). In any case, proximal esophageal motility may be affected following laryngectomy but may or may not contribute to dysphagia (Choi et al., 2003). Distal esophageal motility remains unaffected by laryngectomy surgery (Choi et al., 2003).

## Pharyngolaryngectomy

A pharyngolaryngectomy involves more extensive resection than a total laryngectomy, and is used in the management of advanced laryngeal cancers which involve the hypopharynx or cervical esophagus. During pharyngolaryngectomy, the anterior structures of the digestive tract are removed as per total laryngectomy. However, due to the tumor extent, resection typically includes part or all of the lateral and posterior walls of the pharynx from the base of the tongue to the proximal esophagus. The surgical incision may need to be circumferential removing part or the entire pharyngeal wall. Reconstruction of the pharynx requires the use of local or distal reconstructive flaps as insufficient pharyngeal mucosa remains for primary closure following resection. These flaps are used to re-create a swallowing conduit, connecting the base of tongue to the upper esophagus.

Generally speaking, the swallowing characteristics of patients who have undergone pharyngolaryngectomy are similar to those patients who have undergone total laryngectomy, characterized by difficulties establishing the pharyngeal pressures necessary for

efficient swallowing due to the absence of the mechanical function of the larynx in combination with impaired tongue function. Exacerbating these problems, functional obstructions to bolus flow (stricture, stenosis) may be located at either the upper anastomosis of the graft (level of hyoid bone) or the lower anastomosis of the graft (with the upper esophagus) in the pharyngolaryngectomy population (see CD, Chapter 10: MBS files: "Pharyngolaryngectomy—Obstruction at Lower Anastomosis"). Additional swallowing complications for this population may arise as a result of the type of tissues used in the surgical reconstruction. These will be discussed further in the subsequent sections.

### Impact of Reconstruction Type on Swallowing Outcomes

There is controversy in the surgical literature regarding the type of reconstructive flap that engenders the best outcomes for speech and swallowing. Indeed, certain centers tend to favor one technique over another. However, ultimately the surgeon considers many factors and chooses the reconstructive technique according to the individual. As such, the speech language pathologist may be presented with a variety of clinical situations following pharyngolaryngectomy and must be familiar with each of the reconstructive procedures and their impact on swallowing. Free jejunal grafts and gastric transpositions have been the most commonly discussed in the literature and are certainly purported to be the most commonly employed methods for circumferential pharyngoesophageal reconstruction (Sloan, Blackwell, Harris, Genden, & Urken, 2003).

**Visceral Free Flaps.** Visceral free flaps describe the use of visceral organs to reconstruct the pharynx. Both jejunum (small intestine) and all parts of the colon (large intestine) have been used as pharyngeal grafts. These grafts are harvested replete with their vascular and nervous supplies and relocated and reattached to the neck.

**Jejunal Interposition.** Free jejunal transplant is the standard technique for pharyngeal and proximal esophageal tumors (Triboulet, Mariette, Chevalier, & Amrouni, 2001). A free jejunal graft is a piece of jejunum (small intestine), complete with its vascular supply, used to complete the digestive tract. The section of bowel is attached to the upper pharyngeal stump and the lower esophageal stump. Ideally, the interposition is oriented such that peristaltic contractions occur from top to bottom to avoid opposition to bolus transit. The jejunal arteries and veins are anastomosed to recipient vessels in the neck (Sloan et al., 2003) (see Figure 10-2).

The jejunal graft itself frequently causes swallowing difficulties. While the jejunal segment retains some random isoperistaltic movement, the timing of contraction is not always synchronous with the swallow. This can result in delivery of the bolus to a closed graft. In an attempt to overcome this, patients can often present with repetitive lingual pumping (McConnel, Hester, Mendelsohn, & Logemann, 1988). Increased temporal measures of the swallow as well as immediate oral and nasal backflow are also sequelae of this incoordination (McConnel et al., 1988; Walther, 1995). Peristalsis in the graft may also be problematic if it occurs in a distal to proximal direction (reverse peristalsis), also causing oral and/or nasal backflow of the bolus (Ward, et al., 2002). Examples are provided on the CD (Chapter 10: MBS files: "Pharyngolaryngec-

tomy—Graft Occasionally Closed to Bolus" and "Pharyngolaryngectomy—Graft Closed to Bolus").

Activity in the graft however is reported to decrease over time following transplantation. Eventually, jejunal grafts are expected to become inert passages (Sloan et al., 2003). Postoperative radiotherapy is reported to contribute to reducing graft movement (McConnel et al., 1988). This may not always be the case clinically however, with graft movement reported as a late swallowing complication in 8% of pharyngolaryngectomees who present to speech language pathology (Ward et al., 2002). Significant dysphagia can also be associated with a jejunal segment that is longer than required. This redundancy is capable of creating a potential obstruction to bolus passage. Research indicates that strong lingual propulsion and a patent graft are the factors that most contribute to successful swallowing in jejunal reconstructions (Walther, 1995).

***Colonic Interposition.*** Previously, sections of colon were frequently used in a similar reconstructive procedure to the jejunal interposition (Sloan et al., 2003). However, following reports of high incidence of major medical and reconstructive complications as well as an

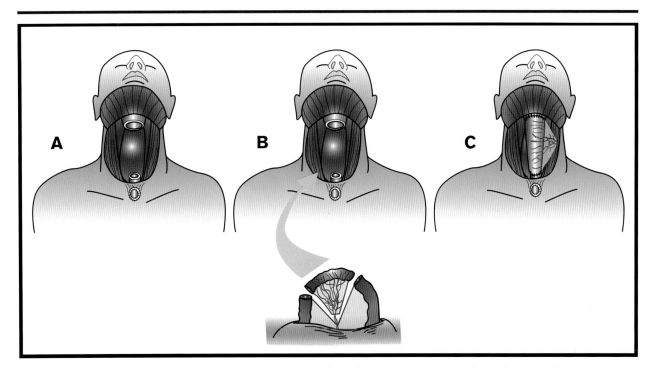

**Figure 10–2.** Schematic representation of jejunal graft reconstruction after pharyngolaryngectomy **A.** The graft is harvested and transferred to the neck **B.** and sutured in place to restore the digestive tract **C.**

overall perioperative mortality of 20%, this technique has become less favored and mainly used exclusively for patients for whom gastric transposition is not possible (e.g., those with previous gastric surgery; Sloan et al., 2003).

Some aspects of the post-colonic interposition swallow have been detailed in the literature. Patients are reported to be capable of tolerating a semisolid diet with normal fluid intake (Moerman, Fahimi, Ceelen, Pattyn, & Vermeersch, 2003). However, they report the need for smaller portions and more frequent meals throughout the day (Moerman et al., 2003). Delayed pharyngeal responses to solids are noted in most patients with repeated swallowing movements and oral residue (Moerman et al., 2003). Often, the colon becomes distended over time (Sloan et al., 2003) and, due to limited or absent colonic peristalsis, bolus transport occurs primarily due to gravity (Moerman et al., 2003). This also results in significant regurgitation (Moerman et al., 2003). Increased neopharyngeal transit times also occur due to stagnation at the anastomotic sites (Moerman et al., 2003). Similarly to cases of jejunal interposition, the propulsion force of the base of the tongue against an open reconstructive tract is the most important factor to guarantee swallowing success (Moerman et al., 2003).

### Ileocolic Free Graft.

The ileocolic free graft is a relatively recent technique used for restoring voice and swallowing following pharyngolaryngectomy with or without partial esophagectomy. In this procedure, a section of colon is used to complete the digestive tract as per colonic interposition. However, the last loop of the ileum containing the ileocecal valve is also included to form the tracheoesophageal party wall, such that the sphincter may provide a shunt for tracheoesophageal speech (Succo, Mioli, Merlino, & Sartoris, 2000). Morbidity rates are reported to be no more excessive than other popular reconstruction techniques such as jejunal interposition and radial forearm flap (Succo et al., 2000).

In a study of eight patients with ileocolic free graft, satisfactory swallowing was achievable between 18 and 38 days following surgery (Succo et al., 2000). There was no evidence of aspiration through the ileocecal valve for any patient on the modified barium swallow. Stenosis and stricture were not reported in this series (Succo et al., 2000). Bolus transit was a problem initially due to asynchronous swallowing and colonic

motility. However, over time, peristalsis was reported to develop some synchronicity, lessening these problems in the long term (Succo et al., 2000).

### Gastric Pull-Up.

Free jejunal transplant is the standard technique for proximal pharyngeal lesions; however, gastric transposition is the technique of choice when the surgical resection must extend below the thoracic inlet (Triboulet et al., 2001). A gastric pull-up involves the elongation of the stomach to pull through the diaphragm and complete the digestive tract (see Figure 10–3). Some surgeons may favor this option, as it requires only a single anastomotic site, unlike the free jejunal graft (Sloan et al., 2003). Medically, the gastric pull-up renders good outcomes. It is associated with fewer complications in relation to respiratory complications, local recurrences, and survival without dysphagia (Mariette et al., 2002).

However, dysphagia has been documented in this patient population. Regurgitation is the most common complaint, with 40% of patients experiencing regurgitation following meals in the immediate postoperative period and as a long-term complication (Cahow & Sasaki, 1994; Dudhat, Mistry, & Fakih, 1999). This symptom may be eased by recommending short frequent meals and upright positioning for an hour following meals (Dudhat et al., 1999).

Triboulet and colleagues (2001) reported that 98.5% of patients achieved swallowing ability with an average time for resumption of oral feeding being 19.7 days postsurgery. Dudhat and colleagues (1999) reported that 83% of their patients were tolerating a soft diet within 15 days. Azurin, Go, and Kirkland (1997) reported that 94% of their patients had good-to-excellent swallowing function with only one patient remaining on a mechanical soft diet. Two patients developed late strictures that were easily managed by dilation (Azurin et al., 1997).

### Fasciocutaneous and Myocutaneous Flaps.

Fasciocutaneous flaps or skin flaps involve the use of sections of skin (with vascular and nervous supply) as a means of reconstruction. In pharyngeal reconstruction, these flaps are often made into a tube with the skin on the inside of the tube forming the watertight walls of the neopharyngeal lumen. Two types of skin flaps are used for pharyngeal reconstruction: anterior/lateral thigh flaps and the radial forearm flap (detailed

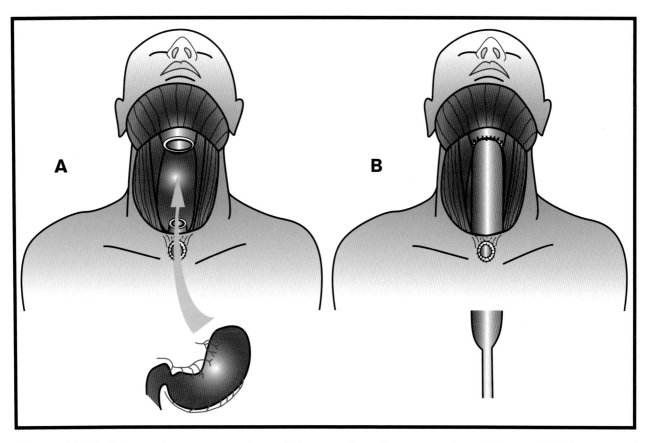

**Figure 10–3.** Schematic representation of the gastric pull-up procedure. The stomach is pepared and pulled up into the neck **A.** and sutured to the pharyngeal defect to restore the digestive tract **B.**

further in this chapter). Fasciocutaneous flaps provide an adynamic, nonmuscular segment which relies on propulsive forces generated from above to drive the bolus through the neopharynx. Increased neopharyngeal transit times result from slowed bolus movement and stasis. Patients are encouraged to alternate liquid and solid bolus types to facilitate bolus transit through an adynamic structure. As is the case with jejunal flaps, swallowing problems may also arise from stricture or stenosis at either the upper or lower anastomoses.

Myocutaneous flaps are similar to fasciocutaneous flaps in that sections of skin are tubed to recreate the pharyngeal lumen. However, a myocutaneous flap also includes some subcutaneous muscle as part of the flap. This allows for additional bulk especially where the defect is large. Two types of myocutaneous flaps are used for circumferential pharyngeal reconstruction: radial forearm flap and pectoralis major flap (detailed further in the subsequent section).

***Anterior/Lateral Thigh Flaps.*** In patients who have sufficiently small amounts of subcutaneous thigh fat (a feature common in many cancer patients due to weight loss), the surgeon may decide to use an anterior or lateral thigh flap to reconstruct the digestive tract (Hayden & Deschler, 1999). This reconstruction involves the use and transposition of skin, subcutaneous tissue, vascular pedicle, and nervous supply from the anterior or lateral thigh. The flap is made into a tube with the skin forming the interior walls of the neopharyngeal lumen. While these flaps are often sensate, swallowing issues can arise due to the lack of movement in the graft to assist bolus transit (Hayden & Deschler, 1999).

The largest case series of pharyngolaryngectomy patients with lateral thigh flaps was 41 patients in 1999 (Hayden & Deschler, 1999). They reported no perioperative deaths, a 12% salivary fistula rate, and successful deglutition achieved in all patients. One incidence of pharyngeal stenosis that required a revision procedure was recorded. The authors also noted a low failure rate that compared favorably with other reconstructions (Hayden & Deschler, 1999). Despite this, the authors stated that this reconstruction technique was not one they routinely employed but one that may provide good functional results in certain situations (Hayden & Deschler, 1999). Recent evidence would support that the anterolateral thigh flap is a viable reconstructive technique for some patients following pharyngolaryngectomy (Hayden & Deschler, 1999; Lewin et al., 2006; Robb et al., 2003; Suominen, Vuola, & Back, 2005).

*Radial Forearm Flap.* The radial forearm flap (see Figure 10–4) has often been used to reconstruct the pharynx as it is thin, relatively hairless, and renders good results with respect to vascular and nervous transposition (Sloan et al., 2003). Similar to thigh flaps,

a section of skin with vascular and nervous supplies is harvested from the medial aspect of the arm to create a sensate tube with the skin forming the inner, watertight lining of the neopharyngeal lumen.

Studies examining the outcomes following radial forearm flap reconstruction have primarily focused on medical outcomes. Little information is available detailing the characteristics of the postoperative swallow. Reports do indicate, however, that this reconstruction technique has demonstrated a good survival rate (100%) in several series (Anthony et al., 1994; Sharpf & Esclamando, 2003), with relatively low morbidity rates with respect to fistula formation (28%), stenosis (36%), and subsequent dilatations (Sharpf & Esclamando, 2003). The median time for the commencement of oral alimentation was 18 days in one study, with only 1 patient of 25 requiring NPO alimentation to maintain the nutritional needs (Sharpf & Esclamando, 2003). Specific reference was also made to the advantages of

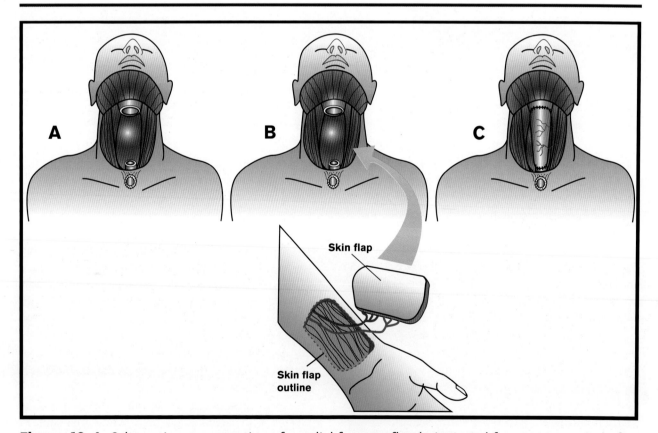

**Figure 10–4.** Schematic representation of a radial forearm flap being used for reconstruction after a total pharyngolaryngectomy **A.** The free flap is harvested with attached feeding vessels, a tube is created, and it is transferred to the neck **B.** and sutured in place to restore the digestive tract **C.**

a passive neopharyngeal conduit as it does not impede bolus transit as much as those with intrinsic peristalsis (i.e., visceral interpositions; Sharpf & Esclamando, 2003). In another study, specific reference was made to the importance of the functional integrity of the tongue base for swallowing. Eighty-eight percent of patients with an intact tongue base were reported to have normal swallowing and to be eating a normal diet (Anthony et al., 1994).

***Pectoralis Major Flap.*** The pectoralis major flap (see Figure 10–5) is a commonly used myocutaneous flap in head and neck reconstruction (Sloan et al., 2003). However, it poses some difficulties for reconstruction of the pharynx and, as such, is less frequently used in contemporary surgical reconstruction of circumferential defects of the pharynx (Reece, 2002). The early technique involved the use of a tubed flap of pectoralis major with maintenance of the local vascular and nervous supply. However, this proved to be too bulky and resulted in less than optimal functional results (Sloan et al., 2003). Modifications of the technique have been described (e.g., Spriano, Pellini, & Roselli, 2002); however, a paucity of data and a lack

of detail in the research literature have led many surgeons to abandon this technique (Reece, 2002).

There are no data available detailing the characteristics of swallowing following pharyngeal reconstruction with the pectoralis major flap. The literature has focused primarily on the medical complications associated with this technique such as graft necrosis, wound dehiscence, fistula formation, infection, and hematoma (Shah, Haribhakti, Loree, & Sutaria, 1990).

## Swallowing Management and Rehabilitation

The management of swallowing dysfunction following laryngectomy is a continuum of care which begins presurgically with counseling, education, and support, progresses through to assessment, troubleshooting, and largely compensatory management during the initial postsurgical and early postdischarge stage, and continues on to involve active rehabilitation and subsequent ongoing monitoring in the long term. At each of these stages, the speech language pathologist must be aware

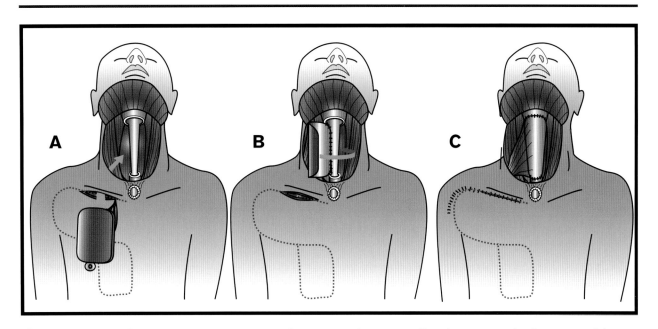

**Figure 10–5.** Schematic representation of a pectoralis major flap being used after a total laryngectomy with partial pharyngectomy **A.** The pedicled flap is harvested, remains attached to the feeding vessels at the clavicle, and is passed through under the skin to the neck **A.**, and sutured in place **B.** to restore the digestive tract **C.**

of the issues which can arise and the appropriate management techniques available to facilitate swallowing and optimize outcomes.

## Presurgical Counseling

Presurgical education and counseling regarding normal swallowing and the anticipated changes following surgery is a critical phase in patient care. In a study of pre- and postsurgical counseling experiences, 92% of laryngectomee respondents considered that the discussion of potential difficulties eating and drinking should be included in both pre- and postoperative counseling for patients undergoing laryngectomy (Ward, Hobson, & Conroy, 2003). Similarly, 86% felt that discussion of changes to taste and smell (see more detailed discussion in Chapter 13) were also important elements of the counseling experience (Ward et al., 2003). A survey conducted by Lennie, Christman, and Jadack (2001) similarly revealed that laryngectomy patients were distressed by the little attention devoted to changes in smell and taste in preoperative counseling. Only 50% of patients in their study reported that they had been made aware of these potential changes. Given that smell is the dominant sense in the identification of flavor, the loss of smell can impact negatively on taste, eating pleasure, and dietary habits (Van Dam et al., 1999). Therefore, as part of holistic management of swallowing and oral intake postsurgery, discussion of both the changes to the swallow and alteration to smell/taste should be addressed with each patient.

Pretreatment swallowing assessment of patients who have previously undergone chemoradiation treatment is particularly warranted. As previously stated, radiotherapy alone or in combination with chemotherapy to the head and neck region often results in fibrosis and scarring of the pharyngeal tissues and structures. Specific changes that can impact on swallowing include reduced range of motion of the tongue base and pharyngeal musculature and structures (Lazarus, Logemann, & Pauloski, 1996). Any existing change in function from prior radiotherapy has the potential to contribute to dysphagia postlaryngectomy. Information gained from the presurgical instrumental swallowing assessment will influence patient counseling regarding possible outcomes postlaryngectomy.

## Swallow Function during Acute Postsurgical/Early Postdischarge Stage

The speech-language pathologist is directly involved in patient care during the acute postsurgery recovery stage and in the early weeks following hospital discharge. During this period, many patients experience swallowing improvement as they undergo healing in the weeks postsurgery, only to later experience some decline in function as they undergo postoperative radiotherapy. In this early stage of care, speech language pathology management is largely comprised of ongoing monitoring of swallowing status, compensatory management of presenting difficulties as healing continues, and providing counseling, education, and support to assist the patient through this initial stage of rehabilitation.

### *Initial Postsurgical Rehabilitation*

The process for early postoperative recovery is similar for total laryngectomy and pharyngolaryngectomy procedures. However, due to the more extensive nature of a pharyngolaryngectomy, initial acute care recovery may take a few days longer (Ward et al., 2002). The following outlines the main stages of care in the initial acute care phase of postoperative management and the role of the speech-language pathologist during this stage of patient management.

**Reestablish Contact.** It is important to reestablish contact with the patient within the first day or two following surgery to reassure the patient, and discuss the process and anticipated timeline for reestablishing communication and addressing the swallowing needs. Much of the information regarding swallowing covered in preoperative counseling will need to be revisited during these sessions. Patients are often unable to retain much of the information provided prior to surgery due to the enormity of the situation and the natural reactions of shock and grief.

**Assessment of Healing and Management of Secretions.** Postsurgery, patients receive nutrition via a nasogastric tube to allow tissues time to heal. In some settings where primary tracheoesophageal puncture (TEP) is performed, the nasogastric tube is inserted via the TEP and functions both as a feeding tube and as a catheter to keep the TEP patent. Within 24 to 48 hours following laryngectomy, patients begin to swallow/manage their saliva. This corresponds with the time at which the pharyngeal mucosa is expected to have sealed in a watertight fashion (Medina & Khafif, 2001).

In some centers, surgeons may request that the healing and swallowing of saliva be formally assessed and monitored early in the postoperative recovery stage. If requested to assess saliva management at this early stage, the clinician should rinse the patient's mouth in either blue dye or institution approved coloring. To ascertain that secretions are not leaking into the surrounding tissue through fistulae or degrading wounds, tracheal suction via the stoma is performed following a period of saliva swallows. If there is evidence of blue dye on suction, then a fistula, inadequate healing, or wound breakdown is suspected. Review by the surgical team is imperative in the case where leaking is detected.

The assessment of secretions may also be requested if it is suspected that secretions are leaking around the TEP feeding tube or catheter into the trachea. To assess this, the clinician should rinse the patient's mouth in blue dye (or approved coloring) and watch closely for evidence around the feeding tube or catheter. Management may involve changing the size of the feeding tube or catheter or inserting a cuffed tracheostomy tube (see Chapter 9 for further information on management of TEP in the early postsurgical stage).

**Evaluate Suitability for Oral Intake.** Most patients following total laryngectomy are assessed for suitability to commence oral intake at approximately 7-10 days postoperatively. Recent reports however suggest that oral intake can be commenced earlier. Studies have found that the early introduction of oral nutrition (within 48 hours) can reduce the trauma associated with tube feeding, minimize the duration of hospital stay, and does not result in fistula formation in total laryngectomy as previously thought (Medina & Khafif, 2001; Saydam, Kalcioglu, & Kizilay, 2002).

For those patients who have undergone reconstruction of the neopharyngeal segment and/or prior nonsurgical treatment, the time postsurgery to safe

reintroduction of oral intake is often extended. Assessment of the stability and integrity of the reconstructed neopharynx can be deferred for up to 6 weeks postsurgery. During this time patients continue to receive enteral nutrition.

The focus of assessment at this point is to determine suitability to initiate oral intake. Given the separation of the respiratory and alimentary tracts following laryngectomy, aspiration is not a concern for these patients. Rather, assessment at this stage determines that adequate healing has occurred, no degraded wounds or fistulae are present, and the patient is suitable to commence oral intake. The presence of any nasal backflow is also monitored for at this stage. Specific institution protocols or surgeon preferences will determine whether a blue dye (or approved coloring) assessment of swallow and/or a radiological examination of swallowing is employed at this initial stage.

***Blue Dye Swallow Assessment.*** A blue dye swallow requires the patient to take sips of blue colored fluid. The patient's skin is monitored for any surface discoloration, hence suggesting wound breakdown/subcutaneous fistulae. If identified, the patient remains nil by mouth and additional healing time will be allowed to see if the fistula will close spontaneously. If they persist, surgical intervention maybe required. The blue dye swallowing assessment is only able to reliably assess for a subcutaneous fistula. The presence of internal tracts/fistulae are only evident using radiological examination and should be used if poor wound healing is an identified patient risk (e.g., postradiotherapy) or in cases where more extensive surgery/reconstruction has occurred.

***Radiological Examination.*** Videofluoroscopic swallowing examinations using a water-soluble contrast agent assesses bolus flow from the oral cavity to the esophagus and the identification of the presence or absence of internal and external fistula. If a fistula is present the examination is ceased, the patient is made nil by mouth, and sufficient time is allowed for further wound healing. If adequate wound healing is determined, the radiological examination may continue following the format of a standard modified barium swallow (MBS) (for MBS procedure details see Chapter 2) providing valuable information regarding the movement and accommodation characteristics of the structures involved in the oral and neopharyngeal stages of swallowing.

**Commence Oral Feeding.** Once it has been established that no leaks are present, and that the patient is adequately healed to avoid the risk of fistula development (as determined by the surgical team), the patient is ready to commence oral feeding. Patients should commence oral intake on a liquid diet to ensure smooth passage through the neopharynx as they become reaccustomed to bolus swallows. This should be gradually upgraded to a soft diet and the patient discharged once he or she is orally consuming a sufficient amount to maintain adequate nutrition without alternative means of feeding or dietary supplementation.

Most patients require dietary modification at discharge. Only 2% of total laryngectomy patients and 0% of pharyngolaryngectomy patients were tolerating a normal diet on discharge from hospital in a study of 55 laryngectomees and 37 pharyngolaryngectomees (Ward et al., 2002). Most total laryngectomy patients were discharged on a soft pureed diet (44%); some were managing soft chewable consistencies (27%); and others were capable of eating soft options of a normal diet (26%) (Ward et al., 2002). Given their longer hospital stays, pharyngolaryngectomy patients tended to be discharged on higher grade diets overall. The majority of pharyngolaryngectomy patients were discharged eating soft chewable consistencies (38%) or soft puree (30%). While some were able to manage softer options of a normal diet (19%), others still required further non-oral feeding (11%) following discharge (Ward et al., 2002).

### Early Postdischarge Swallow Function

Discharge typically occurs at approximately 2 weeks postsurgery for laryngectomy patients and with slightly longer admission sometimes required for pharyngolaryngectomy patients (Ward et al., 2002). Most patients will have follow-up speech language pathology organized for vocal rehabilitation at the time of discharge from acute care. In the early weeks postdischarge, these appointments should also be used to monitor a patient's eating ability and swallowing complaints. For most patients during this period, improvements in swallowing status are noted as postoperative healing continues. Subsequent declines in function, however, may be experienced by some patients while they undergo postoperative radiotherapy, necessitating diet modifications.

**Impact of Radiotherapy.** The majority of patients undergoing laryngectomy will also undergo postoperative radiotherapy. This typically occurs at approximately 4–6 weeks postsurgery and usually comprises a course of 30 treatments over a 6-week period (see Chapter 3 for further discussion). During and immediately following postoperative radiotherapy, patients can experience swallowing change. Depending on the dose, energy level, and amount of tissue irradiated, the side effects of radiotherapy that may cause dysphagia can include edema/swelling of the head and neck tissues, acute and chronic pain, mucosal sensitivity and inflammation, xerostomia (dry mouth), altered or reduced taste, mucosa or bone cell death, and reduced mobility of the tongue lips and jaw impacting on chewing and swallowing (Epstein et al., 1999).

Due to the fluctuating nature of symptoms associated with radiation treatment, speech language pathology intervention for swallowing at this stage is conservative and often supportive in nature. That is, given the potential for change and discomfort, intervention should simply target maximizing the efficiency of the swallowing and minimizing the discomfort associated with oral intake. It is also important to work closely with the dietician to monitor nutrition status.

Mucositis and xerostomia typically occur early in the course of radiation treatment. Mucositis tends to occur 5 to 7 days after initiation of radiation therapy and is treated within the medical framework with palliative pain reduction therapy. In addition, the degree of mucosal inflammation can be controlled to some extent by eliminating secondary causes of inflammation such as alcohol, smoking, coarse or hot foods, alcohol-based mouth rinses, and sodium products that dry the oral tissues (Sloan et al., 2003). Xerostomia is also an early and, for some, a long-term consequence of radiotherapy. Xerostomia tends to occur one week after the initiation of radiation therapy and in some cases causes irreversible salivary gland dysfunction. Reduced saliva production impairs the ability to lubricate and form a cohesive bolus, reduces access to the sense of taste, and increases the friction on the bolus as it is propelled into and through the pharynx, increasing swallowing transit times. Mouth rinses, saliva substitutes, and gustatory stimulants may prove helpful in alleviating some of these symptoms. Generally speaking, patients should be encouraged to increase their water intake, avoid acidic and carbonated drinks, and reduce their sodium intake during radiotherapy (Sloan et al., 2003). Acute and chronic pain is also a common sequelae of radiation therapy. Pain is treated with analgesia provided by the oncological medical team.

### Early Postdischarge Swallowing Intervention.
Dietary modification is the primary compensatory technique employed during the early weeks postsurgery and during radiation therapy. While, generally speaking, smoother foods with a higher fluid content slide more easily through the neopharynx with less propulsion, this is not always the case. In some situations, greater pharyngeal transit times are even observed for thin fluids as presumably they do not have the benefit of weight/cohesion of more viscous liquids or solids to assist their pharyngeal descent.

Various strategies can also be helpful to facilitate bolus transit. Pharyngeal flushing, or taking sips of fluid to "wash down" solid boluses, can be helpful for some patients. Similarly, teaching the patient to perform multiple swallows can facilitate bolus transit. Altering bolus size can also be helpful for some patients, with larger boluses clearing more easily than smaller ones. Altering head position may help bolus transit for some patients with functional obstructions (see CD Chapter 10: MBS files: "Laryngectomy—Using Posterior Head Tilt").

The effortful swallow is a useful compensatory technique that may be taught to patients by the speech language pathologist in the early weeks postsurgery, once healing is complete. The effortful swallow is designed to assist bolus movement through the neopharynx. It functions on the premise that increased tongue base and posterior pharyngeal wall movement will occur if a swallow involves greater physiological effort (Logemann, 1998). Indeed, increased pressure in the oropharynx between the base of the tongue and the posterior pharyngeal wall has been observed during effortful swallows in oral cancer patients (Lazarus, Logemann, Song, Rademaker, & Kahrilas, 2002). This resulted in reduced pharyngeal residue (Lazarus et al., 2002). To elicit an effortful swallow, patients are simply instructed to swallow as hard as possible.

The optimal diet for each individual, and the techniques which best facilitate bolus transit, should be explored under videofluoroscopy. Once the optimal diet level has been ascertained, the patient will require guidance as to specific food and recipe ideas that would be easiest to manage.

### Initial Postsurgery/Early Postdischarge Swallowing Complications

Early swallowing complications may occur in the acute phase of postoperative recovery. A study of a patient cohort group revealed that 27% of total laryngectomees and 65% of pharyngolaryngectomees presented with early swallowing complications (Ward et al., 2002). Early swallowing complications are normally managed with medical intervention or compensatory swallowing strategies.

Predominant early swallowing complications may include:

1. *Edema*: Edema is an inevitable outcome of surgery and postoperative radiotherapy, occurs in all patients, and results in some degree of mild dysphagia. Edema subsides spontaneously within the first few months following surgery, corresponding with the resolution of edema related dysphagia (Gluckman et al., 1985).

2. *Wound degradation/fistulae*: The reported incidence of fistula development following total laryngectomy and pharyngolaryngectomy varies widely in the research literature. Following total laryngectomy, early development of fistulae is reported to occur in between 4% and 75% of cases (Bresson, Rasmussen, & Rasmussen, 1974; Weingard & Spiro, 1983). Following pharyngolaryngectomy, due to the more extensive nature of its reconstruction, the risk of fistula development is significantly greater and reports vary according to the type of reconstructive method used (Medina & Khafif, 2001).

All swallowing should be avoided in the presence of fistulae as the mechanical act of swallowing may exacerbate fistulae formation (Medina & Khafif, 2001). In addition, patients are at risk of aspiration via fistula leaks. Patients should be encouraged to expectorate saliva and commencement of oral intake is contraindicated until the fistulae have been rectified by medical management, be it conservative or surgical.

3. *Functional obstructions to bolus flow*: A number of different factors can create functional obstructions which impair bolus transit and flow through the neopharynx. Of these, the most common types of functional obstruction include stricture/stenosis, pseudoepiglottis, and cricopharyngeal dysfunction.

Surgical stricture may develop in the early phases of recovery but is more commonly a late complication. Stricture may be identified as narrowing or stenosis on radiological examination of the swallow and can manifest clinically as a feeling of the bolus being stuck in the throat or as oral and nasal regurgitation. This occurs at anastomotic sites. Stricture results from the surgical difficulty associated with joining the walls of the pharyngeal stumps (large lumen) with those of the jejunum (smaller lumen). The surgical team performs dilatations for the management of stricture. In some cases, regular dilatations may be necessary. In cases of severe stenosis that does not respond to dilatation, a myotomy may be necessary to release the muscles at distal anastomotic sites in pharyngolaryngectomy patients.

A pseudoepiglottis is a fold of tissue that is a remnant of surgery. It extends from the base of the tongue and protrudes into the neopharyngeal lumen. The etiology of this fold of tissue is not clearly defined in the literature; however, its formation has been related to the nature of closure of the surgical defect (Logemann, 1998). In many cases, the pseudoepiglottis will efface as the bolus passes by, causing little functional obstruction (see CD: Chapter 10: MBS files: "Pseudoepiglottis"). However, in some cases, a pouch is created above the pseudoepiglottis that collects food and liquid. This is clear on a videofluoroscopic study and can clinically manifest as a bad case of halitosis (bad breath). A pseudoepiglottis that creates a pouch requires surgical intervention. In the meantime, the speech language pathologist may instruct the patient in eating soft/liquid consistencies, taking small mouthfuls, washing boluses down with plenty of water, and taking multiple swallows per bolus in an attempt to compensate for the presence of the pouch before surgery (see CD Chapter 10:

MBS files: "Laryngectomy—Pharyngeal Pouch and C4-5 Narrowing" and "Laryngectomy—Hold-Up, Narrow Pharyngeal Lumen, and Pseudoepiglottis").

Alterations to the pharyngeal constrictors in association with increased neopharyngeal pressures may result in formation of a thickening or prominence that appears to arise from the posterior neopharyngeal wall when viewed under videofluoroscopy. The impact of this structure on swallowing should be investigated under videofluoroscopy and treatment should proceed similarly to the treatment procedure outlined for a pseudoepiglottis (see example on CD: Chapter 10: MBS files: "Laryngectomy: Posterior Pharyngeal Wall Prominence").

4. *Oral and nasal backflow*: Nasal backflow is reported as a significant clinical sign of dysphagia during the postoperative recovery period. Nasal backflow occurs in 9% of total laryngectomees and 22% of pharyngolaryngectomees in the first month following surgery (Ward et al., 2002). Few authors have stipulated the physiological underpinnings of nasal backflow at this point in recovery for total laryngectomy patients; however, surgical interruption to the range, strength, and coordination of palatal movement during swallowing is likely. In the case of pharyngolaryngectomy, motor activity in the graft, resulting in uncoordinated delivery of the bolus to a closed graft as well as reverse peristalsis in the graft, is a recognized cause of nasal backflow (McConnell et al., 1988; Ward, Frisby, & O'Connor, 2001). Oral regurgitation is common (40%) in the immediate postoperative phase for those patients who receive gastric transpositions. Patients should be instructed to have small frequent meals, to remain upright for 1 hour following meals, and to sleep with the head elevated (Dudhat et al., 1999). While aspiration is not a concern, regurgitation may cause extreme distress and discomfort for the patient (see example on CD: Chapter 10: MBS files: "Pharyngolaryngectomy—Graft Occasionally Closed to Bolus" and "Pharyngolaryngectomy—Graft Closed to Bolus").

5. *Altered tongue function*: Alterations to tongue mobility and strength can occur due to tissue loss, fibrosis, or denervation. Patients who have undergone total laryngectomy are required to generate greater than normal pressures during the swallow

to achieve effective and efficient bolus transit. Compromised tongue function, particularly in the region of the tongue base, can result in an inability to produce the higher than normal pressures needed for bolus propulsion and clearance through the oral cavity and neopharynx (see CD: Chapter 10: MBS files: "Case Study—Pretreatment"). Concurrent MBS and manometry can provide the ideal assessment of function in this patient group. Specific tests for measuring lingual pressure such as the Iowa Oral Pressure Instrument (IOPI, Blaise Medical Inc.) may also provide valuable information.

## Long-Term Swallowing Function

In the months following surgery and radiotherapy, surgical wounds heal, edema dissipates, and tissues tend to stabilize and adopt their definitive structural and functional characteristics. In addition to this, the patient begins to adjust to the massive lifestyle changes associated with this dramatic surgical procedure (for a discussion of lifestyle changes see Chapter 14). At this point, it is necessary to reassess the patient's swallowing ability, given the high incidence of persistent dysphagia and its reported negative impact on the eating activities, social participation, and level of distress for these patients.

A clinical examination will allow the speech language pathologist to ascertain the diet level patients are tolerating, the specific foods they are avoiding, and any uncomfortable sensations they may be experiencing. Obviously, assessment by palpation in this patient population reveals very little about the swallow as lingual propulsion and graft response are neither externally visible nor palpable. Clinical assessment of the swallow is based primarily on the patient's report of swallowing sensations. Clinically, patients often report symptoms which may include difficulty forming the bolus for dry consistency foods (due to reduced saliva), increased swallowing durations for certain consistencies, increased meal durations, sensations of food "getting stuck," the need to adopt compensatory strategies (multiple swallows, flushing with water, altered bolus sizes), and oral and/or nasal backflow.

Depending on the level of patient and clinician concern, instrumental swallowing assessment may be warranted. Typically a MBS procedure is necessary to define the physiology of the post-laryngeal resection swallow (Ward et al., 2001). The MBS procedure allows the clinician to identify any anatomical features that may contribute to dysphagia. Pseudoepiglottis formation and stricture/stenosis at anastomotic sites will become evident upon barium swallow. It is important to note the presence/absence of any such structures as well as their impact on bolus flow. For example, although present, a pseudoepiglottis may efface for all consistencies and, therefore, have little significance for the presenting dysphagia.

The MBS will also allow the clinician to observe the individual physiology of the swallow. As previously described, dysphagia following laryngeal resection is a function of poor bolus transit subsequent to increased neopharyngeal resistance and reduced lingual propulsion. Physiological features that may be expected in this population include repetitive lingual pumping, delayed pharyngeal response to swallow initiation, reduced area and duration of base of tongue to posterior pharyngeal wall contact, and uncoordinated velopharyngeal closure. For pharyngolaryngectomy patients, additional characteristics may be observed dependent on tissue reconstruction. For example, patients with jejunal reconstruction may present with problems relating to graft motility, including active contractions leading to closure of the graft to bolus delivery or reverse peristalsis.

Given the potential for changes in esophageal motility, the esophageal phase should also be examined by the radiologist on videofluoroscopy. Features of interest at this level would be poor opening of the pharyngoesophageal segment to the bolus, reduced cricopharyngeal contraction, and reduced esophageal motility with poor propagation of peristalsis.

### Long-Term Complications

Although early complications associated with radiotherapy (edema, pain, mucositis, etc.) are no longer impacting on swallowing function at this stage of rehabilitation, the long-term impact of tissue irradiation can impact on swallowing function. Reduced mobility of the oral structures arises as a result of bone and muscle cell death subsequent to radiotherapy. Osteoradionecrosis refers to the death of bony tissue directly resulting from exposure to radiation. Deterioration in muscular activity is thought to be a process of fibrosis (hardening) following damage to capillaries that perfuse muscle fibers in the irradiated region. Being a process, the effects may become symptomatic during the course of radiotherapy or any time thereafter, even years later (Logemann, 1998). Radiation therapy can particularly affect the masticatory muscles and sometimes result in difficulty opening and closing the jaw (trismus). It is recommended that patients commence mouth stretching exercises before, during, and after radiation therapy in an attempt to avoid irreversible trismus (Sloan et al., 2003).

Lingual and pharyngeal muscles are also subject to the effects of radiation and this can dramatically impact upon the efficiency of swallowing. In fact, reduced base of tongue to posterior pharyngeal wall contact is frequently cited as one of the most common dysphagic symptoms following radiation (Lazarus, 1993; Pauloski & Logemann, 2000). Weak lingual and pharyngeal musculature in this patient population tends to result in further increased swallowing transit times and residue as the ability to propel the bolus into and through the high resistance neopharynx is further reduced.

The potential for late stricture formation is also possible as a long-term complication post-surgery/radiotherapy. Stricture formation is the most common late complication following pharyngolaryngectomy, occurring in 20% of patients (Sloan et al., 2003). Management is typically repeated dilatation (McCulloch, Jaffe, & Hoffman, 1997); however, in cases of severe stenosis that do not respond to dilatation, myotomy may be necessary.

The emergence of late swallowing difficulties may also be a symptom of recurrent disease. Assessment by an otolaryngologist is recommended early to exclude any further pathology.

## Post-Early Acute Care Swallowing Rehabilitation

As long as 3 years postoperatively, 58% of total laryngectomy patients and 50% of those with postpharyngolaryngectomy jejunal interpositions are unable to tolerate a full normal diet, avoiding certain foods or requiring consistency modification (Ward et al., 2002). For most of these patients, swallowing function is optimized through the use of the compensatory techniques previously discussed (modifying dietary consistency

and bolus size as well as using techniques such as multiple swallows, flushing with water, and effortful swallows). However, it must be recognized that although a proportion of patients adjust to their altered swallowing capacity, many patients identify elevated levels of disability, handicap, and distress associated with eating (Ward et al., 2002). At this stage of the rehabilitation process, further intervention for the remediation of swallowing is initiated for those patients who express concern regarding residual difficulties and are willing to undergo a period of active rehabilitation.

Although definitive research evidence is yet to be reported, preliminary clinical trials of intensive swallowing rehabilitation of patients following laryngectomy reveal some promise for improving outcomes. In clinical trials being conducted by the lead author of this chapter (Ward and colleagues) intensive swallowing rehabilitation targeting increasing oropharyngeal propulsion force with a view to improving bolus transit through the neopharynx has been found to be beneficial for some patients.

Oropharyngeal propulsion force depends upon the strength of tongue base movement and posterior pharyngeal wall excursion. Consequently, in our clinical setting, the lead author (Ward) uses a therapy regime specifically targeting: (a) bolus propulsion through improving lingual strength, (b) enhancing base of tongue to posterior pharyngeal wall contact, and (c) maximizing effort recruitment for bolus propulsion during swallowing. Each of these will be explained further in the ensuing sections.

**Improving Lingual Strength.** In a single case study of dysphagia following chemotherapy and radiation, Sullivan, Hind, and Robbins (2001) found that a regimen focusing on lingual pressure generation against the hard palate resulted in greater lingual pressure generation during swallowing and nonswallowing tasks. Subsequently, the patient was able to manage a normal diet where previously he required soft foods (Sullivan et al., 2001). Lingual strength training, therefore, may offer some promise for the amelioration of swallowing disorders associated with inadequate lingual propulsion.

Considering the particular swallowing issues of laryngectomy patients, lingual strength training aimed at improving lingual pressure generation during both nonswallow maximal effort tasks and during effortful swallowing may be beneficial for some. Strength training rehabilitation aims to increase the amount of force or tension developed by a muscle or functional muscle group (Clarke, 2003). This occurs with direct exercise over time as the number of motor units recruited during muscular activity increases and the muscle fibers hypertrophy (Clarke, 2003). Such physiological change in response to exercise usually takes between 4 to 6 weeks.

Such training can be conducted using instrumentation such as the IOPI (Blaise Medical Inc.) (see Figure 10–6) to provide the patient with quantifiable feedback of lingual effort during strength training. The Iowa Oral Performance Instrument is a small handheld instrument designed to register tongue pressure against the hard palate. It consists of a pressure sensitive bulb that is placed on the tongue (which can be positioned at tongue tip, blade, or back). The bulb is connected to a manometer that registers the pressure with which the tongue pushes the bulb against the hard palate. However, if the clinician does not have access to an IOPI, comparable outcomes can be achieved using a tongue depressor. Lazarus, Logemann, Huang, and Rademaker (2003) found no significant differences between adults who had performed

lingual strength training with simple tongue depressor exercises and those who had used an IOPI.

**Improving Base of Tongue to Posterior Pharyngeal Wall Contact.** Increased pressure between the base of the tongue and posterior pharyngeal wall, as well as reduced pharyngeal residue, has been observed when the Masako maneuver is employed (Lazarus et al., 2002). Therefore this technique can be beneficial to assist lingual propulsion of the bolus and bolus clearance for patients post laryngectomy. The Masako or tongue hold maneuver involves anchoring the tongue between the teeth and eliciting a strong swallow. The posterior pharyngeal wall movement increases to compensate for the reduced lingual action. As a direct exercise, the Masako maneuver may be used to target permanent augmentation of posterior pharyngeal wall excursion to increase oropharyngeal propulsion. Multiple daily repetitions should be completed of this exercise to facilitate improvement.

**Maximizing Propulsion Effort during Swallows.** Application of the effortful swallow technique can also be beneficial. The effortful swallow technique functions on the premise that increased base of the

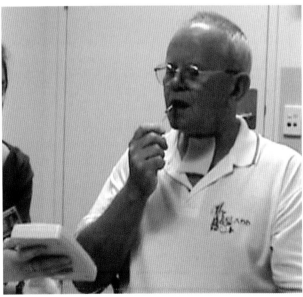
**A.**

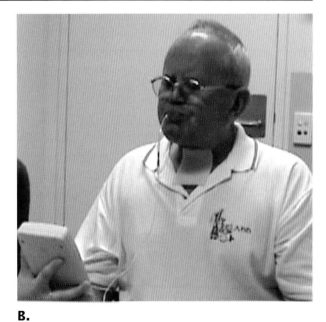
**B.**

**Figure 10–6. A.** Patient placing IOPI bulb in mouth and then **B.** conducting a maximum lingual compression task.

tongue and posterior pharyngeal wall movement will occur if a swallow involves greater physiological effort (Logemann, 1998). This has been confirmed on MBS with the effortful swallow associated with reductions in pharyngeal residue (Lazarus et al., 2002). As such, the effortful swallow, when used as a direct exercise, has the potential to contribute to increased oropharyngeal propulsion twofold.

Although it is recognized that the effortful swallow is seen as a compensatory swallowing technique, when subsequent, effortful swallows are produced by a patient, the effortful swallow also becomes a direct therapeutic exercise. It adheres to the strength training principles of both specificity (being an actual swallowing task) and overload (with greater physiological effort and muscular activity than normal swallowing). Specifically, the patient can complete repetitions of effortful swallows using feedback from either (a) an IOPI in situ, increasing the target effort level of lingual pressure during effortful dry swallows as the weeks progress (60% of maximum lingual pressure in week 1, weeks 2–6 80% of maximum), and/or (b) using surface electromyographic (sEMG) feedback to provide feedback on effort level during both dry and bolus swallows. SEMG is a non-invasive feedback system that employs an electrode on the skin surface to provide visual data regarding the duration and amplitude of muscular activity in the surrounding muscles (Crary &

Groher, 2000). Using a submental placement, patients can receive feedback regarding muscular effort level during effortful swallows (see Figure 10–7). As per the IOPI, systematic increases in target effort can be worked on each session.

**Mode of Delivery.** Intensity and repetition are important elements of behavioral treatment, particularly strength training (Clarke, 2003). In their lingual strength training research Lazarus et al. (2003) had their patients perform five practice sessions per day, 5 days per week for 1 month. Currently optimal intensity levels for treatment have not been established; however, most research suggests three to four sessions a week facilitates change.

Biofeedback is also recognized as beneficial addition to rehabilitation. Both the IOPI and sEMG can be used to provide direct biofeedback on effort level and task performance. The application of biofeedback as an adjunct to therapeutic exercise is an area of rehabilitation that has been relatively well researched. Rehabilitative biofeedback functions on the premise that feedback regarding movement allows modification of subsequent movements. For example, visual or auditory representations of the degree of muscular activity would allow the individual to augment that activity in future movements. During treatment, the instrumentation allows the clinician to provide specific feedback

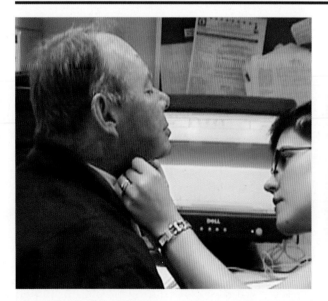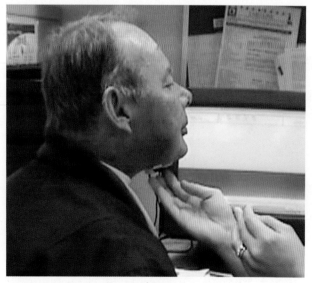

**Figure 10–7.** Clinician positioning the SEMG electrodes in submental position.

of the performance during both nonswallowing (e.g., maximum lingual strength training and Masako maneuver) and swallowing (e.g., IOPI dry swallows, dry and bolus swallows with sEMG) therapy tasks.

Application of a treatment program incorporating the therapeutic techniques just discussed is detailed in the following case study.

**Case Study.** The case study was a 57-year-old male diagnosed with a T1N0 cancer of the right glottis. Initial management involved radiotherapy, 66 Gy in 33 fractions over 47 days. Two months following completion of radiotherapy, a lesion was discovered on the left vocal fold. A total laryngectomy was subsequently performed.

At 6 months following total laryngectomy he self-reported ongoing swallowing difficulties. Although he was tolerating a largely normal diet, he experienced anxiety associated with some foods and avoided eating particularly tough, fibrous, and chewy foods. These foods remained "stuck" and attempts to clear the bolus were uncomfortable and distressing. He was eating three normal size meals per day but was taking, on average, half an hour to consume each meal, longer than it had prior to surgery. Swallowing was effortful and he had to chew more diligently and take smaller mouthfuls. Sometimes he required liquid boluses to flush solids.

Oral motor assessment was within normal limits. Lingual strength was assessed using the IOPI, revealing average maximum pressures of 57 kPa. During normal dry swallows, peak lingual pressure against the hard palate was 9.5 kPa. During effortful dry swallows peak lingual pressure was 15.4 kPa.

Videofluoroscopic examination revealed a prominence or thickening of the posterior pharyngeal wall which was present at rest and during swallowing. This prominence extended from the posterior neopharyngeal wall across the lumen of the neopharynx to the level of the tongue base thereby creating an obstruction to the bolus passage. Liquid swallows were characterized by reduced lingua-velar contact and subsequent premature spilling of the liquid into the neopharynx prior to the pharyngeal response, lingual pumping, and reduced base of tongue to posterior pharyngeal wall contact. This resulted in an uncoordinated, inefficient swallow with residue extending from the base of the tongue to the level of the prominence. A portion of the bolus appeared to pass beyond the prominence;

however, some residue collected above it and was cleared with subsequent swallows. Solid boluses were swallowed with increased effort. Reduced base of tongue to posterior pharyngeal wall contact resulted in a mild increase in pharyngeal transit time, created by numerous attempts to clear material from above the level of the prominence. Most of the residual material eventually cleared with repeated swallows with a thin coating of residue remaining (see CD: Chapter 10: MBS files: "Case Study—Pretreatment").

Therapy involved six weekly therapy sessions with three additional home practice sessions each week. Therapy sessions consisted of sets of direct exercises targeting lingual strength, improved base of tongue and posterior pharyngeal wall movement (Masako maneuver), and bolus propulsion (effortful swallowing). The IOPI was used to provide real-time feedback on lingual function during maximum effort tasks and both normal and effortful dry swallows. SEMG was employed as a means of biofeedback for Masako and effortful swallow exercises.

At reassessment following treatment, the patient was no longer avoiding particular food textures and consistencies and was eating chewy and fibrous foods (particularly steak and salad) with more confidence and minimal concern. He reported that "food was going down more easily" and that effortful swallows (as practiced in therapy) were helpful to propel more difficult consistencies through the neopharynx. Despite these perceived improvements, the need to take small mouthfuls and the duration of mealtime remained unchanged.

There was no change on the clinical oral motor assessment. However, a significant change was observed in lingual pressure generation. Following therapy, maximal lingual pressure increased to 83.7 kPa (from 57k Pa pre-treatment). Peak pressure during normal (39.3 kPa post-, versus 9.5 kPa pre-treatment) and effortful (57.4 kPa post-, versus 15.4 pre-treatment) dry swallows also increased following therapy.

Changes were also noted on videofluoroscopy. Mild premature spilling into the neopharynx persisted post-therapy. However, increased base of tongue to posterior pharyngeal wall contact was noted resulting in a more coordinated, efficient swallow with single swallows observed for most boluses. There was still some evidence of lingual pumping at times. A thin coating of liquid residue also persisted; however, solid boluses were cleared more readily and little residue was observed following solid bolus swallows. Double swallows were sometimes still required to completely clear the neopharynx. Overall, there appeared to be an increase in swallow coordination with reduced time between spilling and the pharyngeal response and a reduction in pharyngeal transit times for most boluses (see CD: Chapter 10: MBS files: "Case Study—Post-Treatment").

The size and location of the prominence had not altered post-therapy. The increased propulsive force generated at the level of the tongue base resulted in an increased ability to drive the bolus past this obstruction. Although this patient presented with relatively specific dietary restrictions, intensive intervention was able to facilitate improved lingual function leading to a physiological change observed on MBS, and a perceived improvement in functional eating ability.

## Conclusion

For the majority of patients, dysphagia is a significant negative consequence of laryngectomy. The physiological basis for the dysphagia can be related to a number of factors, including the removal of the laryngeal structures and altered function of the remaining tissues, the type of surgical reconstruction performed, and for many, the additional negative impact of postsurgical radiotherapy. Consequently, considering the potential multifactorial nature of the swallowing impairment in this population, the application of instrumental assessment of swallow function (i.e., MBS) is critical to accurately identify the causes of the swallowing compromise and ensure appropriate management. Speech pathologists can offer a range of compensatory and rehabilitative strategies which can facilitate improved swallowing in this population. Holistic management should also incorporate rehabilitation of olfaction considering the close relationship between smell, the perception of flavor, appetite, and mealtime satisfaction. Research has shown that total laryngectomy and pharyngolaryngectomy patients with dysphagia experience significantly higher levels of activity limitation and distress than nondysphagic patients (Ward et al., 2002). Therefore, all attempts should be made to optimize swallowing outcomes for this population in order to facilitate improved quality of life.

## References

Anthony, J. P., Singer, M. I., Deschler, D. G., Dougherty, T., Reed, C. G., & Kaplan, M. J. (1994). Long term functional results after pharyngoesophageal reconstruction with the radial forearm free flap. *The American Journal of Surgery*, *168*, 441-445.

Azurin, D. J., Go, L. S., & Kirkland, M. L. (1997). Palliative gastric transposition following pharyngolaryngoesophagectomy. *The American Surgeon*, *63*, 410-413.

Bresson, D., Rasmussen, H., & Rasmussen, P. A. (1974). Pharyngo-cutaneous fistula in totally laryngectomised patients. *Journal of Otolaryngology*, *88*, 835-842.

Cahow, C. E., & Sasaki, C. T. (1994). Gastric pull-up reconstruction for pharyngo-laryngo-esophagectomy. *Archives of Surgery*, *129*, 425-428.

Cerenko, D., McConnel, F. M. S., & Jackson, R. T. (1989). Quantitative assessment of pharyngeal bolus driving forces. *Otolaryngology-Head and Neck Surgery*, *100*(1), 57-63.

Choi, E. C., Hong, W. P., Kim, C. B., Yoon, H. C., Nam, J. I., Son, E. J., et al. (2003). Changes of oesophageal motility after total laryngectomy. *Otolaryngology-Head and Neck Surgery*, *128*(5), 691-699.

Clarke, H. M. (2003). Neuromuscular treatments for speech and swallowing: A tutorial. *American Journal of Speech-Language Pathology*, *12*, 400-415.

Crary, M. A., & Groher, M. E. (2000). Basic concepts of surface electromyographic biofeedback in the treatment of dysphagia: A tutorial. *American Journal of Speech-Language Pathology*, *9*, 116-125.

Dantas, R. O., Aguiar-Ricz, L. N., Gielow, I., Filho, F. V. M., & Mamede, R. C. M. (2005). Proximal oesophageal contractions in laryngectomized patients. *Dysphagia*, *20*, 101-104.

Dudhat, S. B., Mistry, R. C., & Fakih, A. R. (1999). Complications following gastric transposition after total laryngo-pharyngectomy. *European Journal of Surgical Oncology*, *25*, 82-85.

Epstein, J. B., Emerton, S., Kolbinson, D. A., Le, N. D., Phillips, N., Stevenson-Moore, P., et al. (1999). Quality of life and oral function following radiotherapy for head and neck cancer, *Head & Neck*, *21*, 1-11.

Gluckman, J. L., McDonough, J. J., McCafferty, G., J., Black, R. J., Coman, W. B., Cooney, T. C., et al. (1985). Complications associated with free jejunal graft reconstruction of the pharyngoesophagus—A Multi-institutional experience with 52 cases. *Head and Neck Surgery*, *7*, 200-205.

Hayden, R. E., & Deschler, D. G. (1999). Lateral thigh free flap for head and neck reconstruction. *Laryngoscope, 109*(9), 1490-1494.

Lazarus, C. (1993). Effects of radiation therapy and voluntary manoeuvres on swallow functioning in head and neck cancer patients. *Clinics in Communication Disorders, 3*(4), 11-20.

Lazarus, C., Logemann, J. A., Huang, C., & Rademaker, A. W. (2003). Effects of two types of tongue strengthening exercises in young normals. *Folia Phoniatrica et Logopaedica, 55*(4), 199-205.

Lazarus, C., Logemann, J. A., & Pauloski, B. R. (1996). Swallowing disorders in head and neck cancer patients treated with radiotherapy and adjuvant chemotherapy. *Laryngoscope, 106*, 1157-1166.

Lazarus, C. L., Logemann, J. A., Song, C. W., Rademaker, A. W., & Kahrilas, P. J. (2002). Effects of voluntary maneuvers on tongue base function for swallowing. *Folia Phoniatrica et Logopaedia, 54*(4), 171-176.

Lennie, T. A., Christman, S. K., & Jadack, R. A. (2001). Educational needs and altered eating habits following a total laryngectomy. *Oncology Nursing Forum, 28*(4), 667-674.

Logemann, J. A. (1998) *Assessment and Management of Swallowing Disorders.* Austin, TX: Pro-Ed.

Lewin, J. S., Barringer, D. A., May, A. H., Gillenwater, A. M., Arnold, K. A., Roberts, D. B., et al. (2006). Functional outcomes after laryngopharyngectomy with anterolateral thigh flap reconstruction. *Head & Neck, 28*(2), 142-149.

Mariette, C., Fabre, S., Balon, J. M., Patenolre, D., Chevalier, D., & Triboulet, J. P. (2002). Reconstruction after total circular pharyngolaryngectomy: Comparison between gastric interposition and free jejunal flap. *Annals de Chirurgie, 127*(6), 431-438.

McConnel, F. M. S. (1988). Analysis of pressure generation and bolus transit during pharyngeal swallowing. *Laryngoscope, 98*, 71-78.

McConnel, F. M. S., Hester, T. R., Mendelsohn, M. S., & Logemann, J. A. (1988). Manofluorography of deglutition after total laryngopharyngectomy. *Plastic and Reconstructive Surgery, 8*(3), 346-351.

McConnel, F. M. S., Mendelsohn, M. S., & Logemann, J. A. (1986). Examination of swallowing after total laryngectomy using manofluorography. *Head and Neck Surgery, 9*, 3-12.

McCulloch, T. M., Jaffe, D. M., & Hoffman, H. T. (1997). Diseases and operation of head and neck structures affecting swallowing. In A. L. Perlman & K. S. Schulze-Delrieu (Eds.). *Deglutition and its disorders: Anatomy, physiology, clinical diagnosis and management* (pp. 343-381). San Diego, CA: Singular.

Medina, J., & Khafif, A. (2001). Early oral feeding following total laryngectomy. *The Laryngoscope, 111*(3), 368-372.

Moerman, M., Fahimi, H., Ceelen, W., Pattyn, P., & Vermeersch, H. (2003). Functional outcome following colon interposition in total pharyngoesophagectomy with or without laryngectomy. *Dysphagia, 18*, 78-84.

Pauloski, B. R., & Logemann, J. A. (2000). Impact of tongue base and posterior pharyngeal wall biomechanics on pharyngeal clearance in irradiated postsurgical oral and oropharyngeal cancer patients. *Head & Neck, 22*, 120-131.

Reece, G. P. (2002). Pectoralis major myocutaneous flap for hypopharyngeal reconstruction: Discussion. *Plastic and Reconstructive Surgery, 110*, 1414-1416.

Robb, G. L., Lewin, J. S., Deschler, D. G., Haughey, B. H., Brown, D. H., & Langmore, S. E. (2003). Speech and swallowing outcomes in reconstructions of the pharynx and cervical oesophagus. *Head & Neck, 25*, 232-244.

Saydam, L., Kalcioglu, T., & Kizilay, A. (2002). Early oral feeding following total laryngectomy. *American Journal of Otolaryngology, 23*(5), 277-281.

Shah, J. P., Haribhakti, V., Loree, T. R., & Sutaria, P. (1990). Complications of the pectoralis major myocutaneous flap in head and neck reconstruction. *The American Journal of Surgery, 160*, 352-355.

Sharpf, J., & Esclamando, R. M. (2003). Reconstruction with radial forearm flaps after ablative surgery for hypopharyngeal cancer. *Head & Neck, 25*, 261-266.

Sloan, S. H., Blackwell, K. E., Harris, J. R., Genden, E. M., & Urken, M. L. (2003). Reconstruction of major defects in the head and neck following cancer surgery. In E. N. Meyers, J. Y. Suen, J. N. Meyers, & E. Y. N. Hanna (Eds.). *Cancer of the head and neck* (4th ed., pp. 631-670). Philadelphia: Saunders.

Spriano, G., Pellini, R., & Roselli, R. (2002). Pectoralis major myocutaneous flap for hypopharyngeal reconstruction. *Plastic and Reconstructive Surgery, 110*, 1408-1413.

Succo, G., Mioli, P., Merlino, G., & Sartoris, A. (2000). New options for aerodigestive tract replacement after extended pharyngolaryngectomy. *Laryngoscope, 110*, 1750-1755.

Sullivan, P., Hind, J. A., & Robbins, J. (2001). Lingual exercise protocol for head and neck cancer. A case study. *Dysphagia, 16*(2), 154.

Suominen, S., Vuola, J., & Back, L. (2005). Free anterolateral thigh flap in head and neck reconstructions. *Clinical Otolaryngology, 30*, 384-400.

Triboulet, J. P., Mariette, C., Chevalier, D., & Amrouni, H. (2001). Surgical management of carcinoma of the hypopharynx and cervical esophagus. *Archives of Surgery, 136,* 1164–1169.

Van Dam, F. S. A. M., Hilgers, F. J. M., Emsbroek, G., Touw, F. I., van As, C., & de Jong, N. (1999). Deterioration of olfaction and gustation as a consequence of total laryngectomy. *Laryngoscope, 109,* 1150–1155.

Walther, E. K. (1995). Dysphagia after pharyngolaryngeal cancer surgery. Part I: Pathophysiology of postsurgical deglutition. *Dysphagia, 10,* 275–278.

Ward, E. C., Bishop, B., Frisby, J., & Stevens, M. (2002). Swallowing outcomes following laryngectomy and pharyngolaryngectomy. *Archives of Otolaryngology-Head & Neck Surgery, 128,* 181–186.

Ward, E. C., Frisby, J., & O'Connor, D. (2001). Assessment and management of dysphagia following pharyngolaryngectomy with free jejunal interposition: A series of eight case studies. *Journal of Medical Speech Language Pathology, 9*(1), 89–105.

Ward, E. C., Hobson, T. K., & Conroy, A. (2003). Pre and post-operative counselling and information dissemination: Perceptions of patients undergoing laryngeal surgery and their spouses. *Asia Pacific Journal of Speech, Language and Hearing, 8,* 44–68.

Weingard, D. N., & Spiro, R. H. (1983). Complications after laryngectomy. *American Journal of Surgery, 146,* 517–520.

Welch, R. W., Luckmann, K., Ricks, P. M., Drake, S. T., & Gates, G. A. (1979). Manometry of the normal upper oesophageal sphincter and its alteration in laryngectomy. *Journal of Clinical Investigation, 63,* 1036–1041.

# Chapter 11

# STOMA CARE

Elizabeth C. Ward, Lynn M. Acton, and
Ann-Louise Morton

## CHAPTER OUTLINE

## Introduction

Surgical removal of the larynx requires the formation of a tracheostoma (stoma) to reestablish a patent airway. Adjusting to life with a stoma can be overwhelming for many patients, particularly in the first few weeks postsurgery. Consequently, education, training, and emotional support are critical in the early stages to help the patient and the family establish a sound understanding of the physiological changes that have occurred, and the practical skills necessary to manage the stoma. The current chapter is designed to detail for the reader the process of stoma formation and summarize its impact on pulmonary function (this is detailed further in Chapter 12). It also outlines the acute and long-term care issues relating to having a stoma, and provides clinical reasoning regarding the selection and application of various appliances/devices used in stoma protection and management.

## Stoma Formation and Anatomy

The process of forming the tracheostoma is conducted during the total laryngectomy procedure once the laryngeal tissues have been removed and the pharynx has been closed. The actual procedure for stoma formation varies between surgeons. In some institutions, a beveled incision of the trachea is typically performed at the time the larynx is removed. The beveled end of the trachea is then sutured to the anterior neck tissues using interrupted horizontal mattress sutures in a tension-free fashion to form the tracheostoma.

In other institutions, they follow different procedures, preferring to create the tracheostoma separately from the surgical incision (See Figure 11–1). Verschuur, Gregor, Hilgers, and Balm (1996) give a detailed description of what they consider optimal construction of the tracheostoma using this type of approach. Points of consideration raised by these authors include: creating the tracheostoma separately from the surgical incision, the angle of the trachea, complete skin coverage of the tracheal cartilage, and avoiding the use of laryngectomy tubes which may cause irritation and may subsequently lead to stenosis.

Stomas vary between individuals, depending on their own unique anatomy and the surgical procedure (see Figure 11–2). With increasing use of peristomal devices such as heat and moisture exchange (HME) devices and hands-free speaking valves, the need for a peristomal area that accommodates the use of these devices has increased. For this reason, some surgical teams also cut the heads of the sternocleidomastoid

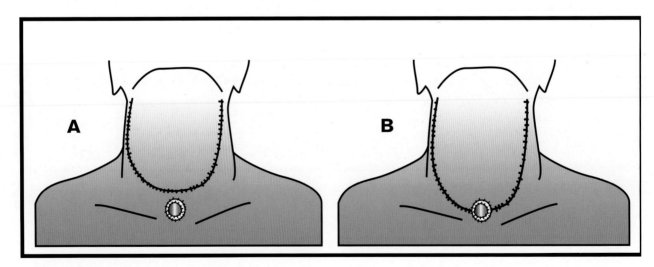

**Figure 11–1.** Schematic drawing of tracheostoma creation separately from the surgical scar **A.** and within the surgical scar **B.**

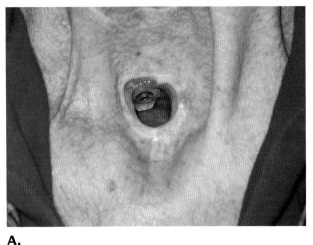

**A.**

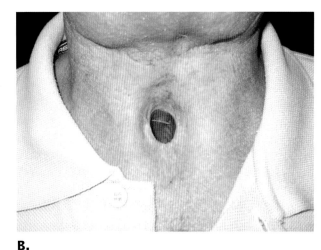

**B.**

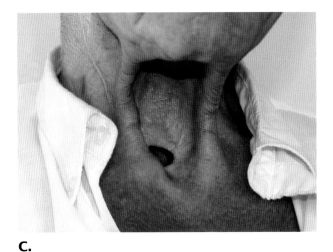

**C.**

**Figure 11-2.** Note individual differences in stoma size and contour of the peristomal area. (Figure 11-2C courtesy of Atos Medical, www.atosmedical.com.)

muscles during surgery. This causes no functional deficits and often leads to a flatter peristomal area (Hilgers, 2003).

Stoma revision may be necessary for laryngectomees who have difficulty maintaining stoma patency. A variety of surgical procedures can be employed, based on the type of problem presented (Verschuur et al., 1996).

## Impact on Pulmonary Function

With the formation of a stoma, a permanent disconnection is created between the upper and lower respiratory tract. Prior to surgery, the upper respiratory tract serves critical functions including the warming, humidification, and filtration of inhaled air. Following surgery, the loss of these functions has a significant impact on pulmonary function (see detailed discussion in Chapter 12).

Maintaining adequate humidification postlaryngectomy is important for respiratory health. The process of humidification increases the moisture content of respiratory secretions, allowing them to remain thin and watery, and enabling them to be cleared easily from the airways. In the absence of natural humidification (i.e., postlaryngectomy), secretions within the respiratory tract can become thick and sticky, and if left uncleared, may accumulate to form a "plug" of mucos, with the potential to block the airway. Consequently, postlaryngectomy, patients need to find alternate means to humidify inhaled air and manage their sputum production and clearance.

Current research evidence supports the use of HME devices which are attached to the stoma to reestablish humidification of inhaled air (Ackerstaff, Hilgers, Aaronson. Balm, & Van Zandwijk, 1993; Hilgers, Aaronson, Ackerstaff, Schouwenburg, & Van Zandwijk, 1991). A variety of different HME systems is available from different manufacturers (see Figure 11-3); some of the systems are interchangeable. The HME device serves to trap moisture within the lower respiratory tract reducing the amount of water loss from the respiratory system and thereby facilitating humidification (see Figure 11-4). Use of an HME device has been demonstrated to decrease sputum production, coughing, and stomal cleaning (Ackerstaff et al., 1993; Hilgers et al., 1991) (see Chapter 12 for a full discussion of research evidence relating to HMEs).

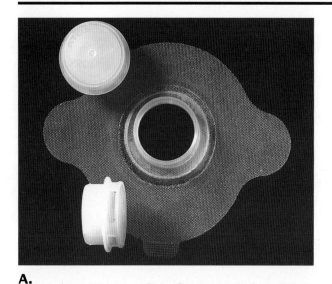

**A.**

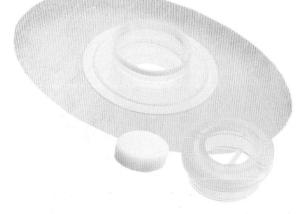

**B.**

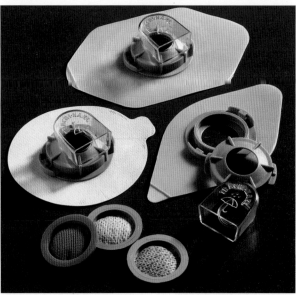

**C.**

**Figure 11–3.** Different types of HME systems: **A.** Provox HME system (Photo courtesy of Atos Medical, www.atosmedical.com). **B.** InHealth Humidifilter system (Photo courtesy of InHealth Technologies, www.inhealth.com). **C.** Kapitex Trachi-Naze system (Photo courtesy of Kapitex Healthcare Limited, www.kapitex.com).

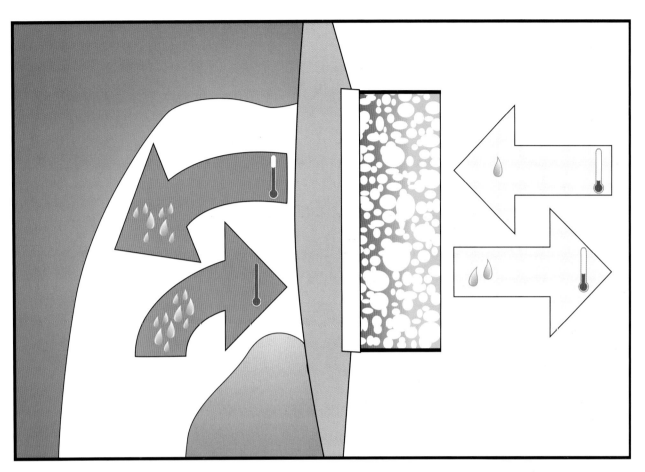

**Figure 11–4.** Schematic drawing of the heat and moisture exchanging function of an HME.

For those patients who do not use HMEs, they need to be advised of other strategies to assist humidification, such as wearing stoma covers or foam pads (which may be moistened to further assist humidification), steaming, and enhancing the level of humidity in the air in their living environment.

The creation of a permanently open stoma also prevents protection of the lower airway from inhaled foreign bodies. Airway protection in this context relates to both the possible inhalation of larger items that may threaten to block the airway and the inability to filter and prevent inhalation of fine, airborne molecules (such as dust and pollens), which can lead to tracheal irritation, allergy, and infection. Laryngectomized patients need to keep their stoma covered at all times to assist airway protection. Although not the primary purpose of the device, clinical anecdotal reports suggest that HMEs can help filter inhaled air to some extent.

Regardless of whether an HME is used, patients are advised to wear some form of stoma cover at all times to protect the lower airway from particle inhalation. Windy weather and dry, dusty environments in particular can place laryngectomees at increased risk of particle inhalation. During seasonal changes when airborne pollens are plentiful, some laryngectomees may need to take extra caution to protect their airway in order to avoid allergic irritation and/or infection. Changes in the amount, consistency, color, or smell of mucus is a possible indication of infection. If this occurs, the laryngectomee should go to the health care professional for a sputum sample and possible course of antibiotics.

## Education Needs of Patient and Caregiver

Prior to surgery, stoma care and the long-term implications of being a "neck-breather" are discussed with the patient. Although differences may exist between settings, patient education and the subsequent acute stoma care training are typically the role of the specialized head and neck nursing staff, with support from other multidisciplinary team members, including the speech-language pathologist and physical therapist. Presurgery, it is important that the patient is prepared about what to expect in the initial days postsurgery, particularly in terms of wounds, drains, and caring for the new stoma.

While presurgical patient preparation is critical to avoid shock and fear in the initial postoperative stage, the majority of patient education regarding stoma care and management is conducted postoperatively, prior to discharge home. The primary objectives of postsurgical education are (a) to teach the patient to maintain an adequate airway at all times, and (b) gain familiarity with the various devices associated with stoma care and maintenance. To achieve these objectives, patients undergo daily training until independence is achieved. Whenever possible, the education process commences within the initial days postsurgery, and practice is repeated daily, with the goal being for the patient to be fully independent in stoma care and use of all equipment associated with the stoma prior to hospital discharge. Training is supported by demonstrations from the nursing staff, written handouts and videos, as well as daily motivation and support from all multidisciplinary team members.

In addition to achieving independence in stoma care and maintenance, it is important that the laryngectomee and the family are aware of how to clear the airway in case of an emergency, and the process of mouth-to-stoma resuscitation prior to discharge home. Most laryngectomy associations/support groups produce materials detailing the process of mouth-to-stoma resuscitation that can be provided to patients. Laryngectomees may wish to carry alert cards in their wallet, or attach notices/stickers to the windshield or dashboard of their vehicles advising of their condition and resuscitation procedures in case of emergency. Figure 11–5 is a display of just some of the materials produced by the Queensland Cancer Fund and Laryngectomee Association of Queensland, Australia.

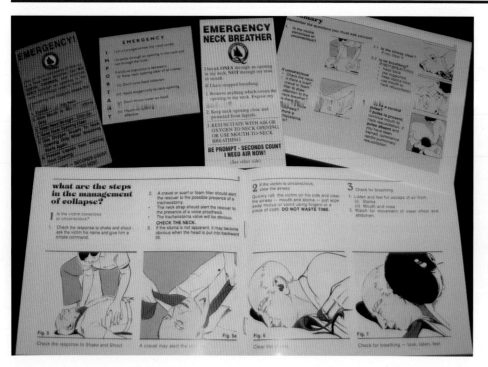

**Figure 11–5.** Examples of various information booklets, flyers, and alert stickers available through support groups and organizations. (Resources photographed with permission from Queensland Cancer Fund and Laryngectomee Association of Queensland.)

## Acute Healing and Stoma Care

Prior to surgery, the patient should be counseled regarding the surgical procedure and what to expect with respect to wound care and healing postsurgery. This typically involves discussion of wound drainage lines, suture care and oral care, enteral feeding tubes (nasogastric tube), and the presence of any airway tubes (tracheostomy tubes, laryngectomy tubes) or devices (HMEs) which may be in situ postsurgery.

To prevent accumulation of fluids within the neck tissues postsurgery, the wound is closed in layers over low-pressure suction drains. In the first 24–72 hours, the amount and consistency of wound drainage is monitored closely by nursing staff to assess for possible postoperative complications with wound healing. If there are no complications, patients can anticipate the removal of these drains by about the 5th day postsurgery.

During the acute stage, the suture lines of the neck and stoma are cleaned regularly, and a thin coating of antibacterial ointment applied, to facilitate healing. The sutures in the neck are typically removed around day 7, while stomal sutures are removed around day 10 in most settings. However, the duration to suture removal may be protracted if the patient has had prior radiotherapy and/or chemotherapy. Oral irrigation and cleaning is typically performed every few hours until the patient recommences an oral diet, at which point cleaning is encouraged after all intake, particularly if surgery has involved sections of the tongue or jaw.

Nasogastric tubes are inserted at the time of surgery, typically prior to pharyngeal closure. The tubing is typically attached to the nose with tape to prevent dislodgement and improve patient comfort. In some centers, and with patients who have undergone a primary tracheoesophageal puncture, the tracheoesophageal puncture (TEP) catheter may be used for immediate postoperative feeding. Other centers avoid this practice to minimize any irritation and distortion of the TEP. Traditionally, the nasogastric tube is removed around day 7–10 when the patient commences an oral diet. Commencement onto an oral diet commonly occurs after a videofluoroscopic assessment to confirm the absence of leaks. In some institutions, however, practice is changing and fluids are being commenced as early as 1 or 2 days postsurgery.

In many institutional settings, on return to the ward/floor from theater/operating room (OR) patients have a high-volume low-pressure cuffed tracheostomy tube (a tube normally used for patients who have undergone a tracheotomy) in situ. This typically remains in situ for approximately 24–48 hours to ensure maintenance of a patent airway. It is then removed and replaced with a laryngectomy tube (also referred to as tracheostoma tube; discussed later in chapter), which is used to keep the stoma patent. The laryngectomy tube typically remains in position for the first 10–14 days. It is then removed, and only used again during postoperative radiotherapy or when the size of the stoma is getting too small. Some settings encourage more long-term use of the laryngectomy tube, eventually taking the patient through a systematic weaning process (to be detailed later in chapter) months after surgery. In other settings, they do not insert either a tracheostomy tube or a laryngectomy tube postsurgery, but rather leave the newly formed stoma unobstructed, and monitor airway patency using clinical observation. In this instance, a laryngectomy tube will only be inserted if there is a noticeable change in the size/shape of the stoma and during any postoperative radiotherapy.

## Early Pulmonary Management

In those settings that insert a tracheostomy tube postsurgery, the patient receives constant humidification through either a T-piece or via a humidification mask placed over the tracheostomy in the first instance. Once the tracheostomy tube is removed and is replaced with a laryngectomy tube (or in cases when no tracheostomy or laryngectomy tube is used), humidification is provided directly to the stoma via a humidification mask or an HME. When humidification is not being provided, stoma covers are worn at all times to help with humidification.

Currently in most settings, HMEs are not typically introduced until postoperative healing is complete. However in some institutions, the use of an HME device may commence as early as the first postoperative day. Preliminary clinical reports of early HME use suggest this can assist in early airway protection and aid retention of substantial humidification, making the need for additional mechanical humidification redundant (see discussion in Chapter 12).

In addition to addressing the issue of humidification, in the early days postsurgery the physical therapist will assist the patient to learn how to clear secretions using a modified cough technique referred to as a "huff." A huff is a modified forced expiratory technique which involves exhaling forcefully from high to mid-lung volumes (Pryor, 1999). The process involves instructing the patient to take in a slow deep breath followed by a quick forceful exhalation. Additional manual assistance may be provided by the physical therapist in the early postoperative period to assist airway clearance (see Figure 11-6).

## Care and Cleaning of Stoma

Within the first week postsurgery, patients are taught how to safely and effectively clean their stoma and any laryngectomy tubes. In the acute recovery phase, cleaning the stoma is typically required multiple times throughout the day. Table 11-1 outlines the stages for cleaning the stoma, and these basic steps are documented on the video footage contained on the CD (see Chapter 11: Video: "Cleaning the Stoma"). Footage such as this can be useful in the early stages of patient education and training.

In addition to cleaning, patients should also be taught to conduct regular stomal inspections. Any dry crusting or mucos plugs that could lead to obstruction of the airway need to be gently removed using blunt forceps/tweezers. Application of skin products such

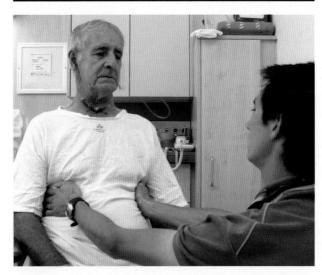

**Figure 11–6.** Physical therapist provides additional manual assistance to facilitate "huff" maneuver for airway clearance.

**Table 11–1.** Steps for Cleaning the Stoma

| Step | Task |
| --- | --- |
| 1. | Wash your hands thoroughly. |
| 2. | Fill a basin with hot, steamy water. |
| 3. | Lean over basin and inhale steam through your stoma for 5–10 minutes. |
| 4. | Have a good cough to help clear accumulated secretions. Leaning forward can help expel secretions more efficiently. |
| 5. | Wet a cloth* in warm water, then wring out thoroughly and clean around stoma. Repeat process until the area is clear of any crusted or dried secretions. You may need to use tweezers to gently remove any dried secretions from around the stoma edge. |
| 6. | Gently dry the area with a clean cloth*. |
| 7. | Place a rim of water soluble lubricant around the edge of stoma to prevent new crusting of mucus†. |

Notes: *Only use a face cloth, towel, or gauze squares—paper towels, tissues, or cotton wool should not be used due to risk of particle inhalation. †Patients undergoing radiotherapy may be advised about suitable creams for use around the stoma site during treatment.

as Vaseline (petroleum jelly) or lanolin may be applied to the skin around the stoma to alleviate irritation/inflammation and prevent the formation of tight scar tissue that may reduce stoma diameter. However, some institutions do not recommend using any products around the stoma that may be harmful when entering the stoma.

## Long-Term Management of the Stoma

On discharge from the hospital, the patient should be independent in stoma care. Over the course of postdischarge rehabilitation and long term adjustment to living with a stoma, the frequency and duration of time involved in stoma care may change due to a number of factors, including postoperative radiotherapy, healing and adjustment to tracheostomal respiration, and external influences such as the weather and the environment in which the laryngectomee lives/works.

## Care and Cleaning of Stoma Postdischarge

Once the patient has returned home, cleaning of the stoma will typically occur up to three to four times daily. As the stoma heals, edema of the head and neck tissues subsides, and the body adjusts to breathing through the stoma, this frequency will usually reduce to one to two times each day. However, frequency of cleaning varies between individuals depending on how much sputum they produce and the extent of crusted mucus formation around their stoma. This can also vary within the individual, depending on weather conditions and the work/home environment (e.g., air conditioned workplace, dusty outdoor environment). If the patient is using an HME device, then the frequency of cleaning is often considerably reduced.

Patients who do not use an HME device may experience "crusting," which is the accumulation of dried secretions around the stoma. If this occurs, inhaling steam for longer durations can assist removal of these dried secretions. Coating the area with water based lubricant, and re-attempting cleaning and removal

5–10 minutes later can also assist. Patients may continue to apply Vaseline (petroleum jelly) or lanolin onto the skin around the stoma to soothe dry and irritated skin, and to assist with the clearance of secretions huffed out of the stoma.

## Impact of Radiotherapy Postsurgery

Regardless of differing clinical procedures relating to the use of laryngectomy tubes postsurgery, most physicians will recommend that laryngectomy tubes are used during postoperative radiation therapy, as the radiation causes the tissues of the neck to swell, and can cause contracture of the stoma. Tissues of the neck and around the stoma can become tight and sore during treatment with skin breakdown as a common side effect. During this time, frequent application of aqueous cream to moisten the skin and maintain skin integrity is required. During radiotherapy, only aqueous creams approved by the radiation staff should be applied to the skin of the head and neck.

While the patient is undergoing radiotherapy he or she may also find that the use of direct steam (such as from a vaporizer) may be painful at this time and may be advised to use more diffuse steam, such as from the shower, to assist humidification. Similarly, silicone skin adhesive and adhesive baseplates or housings for HMEs or hands-free speaking valves should not be used during radiation therapy and for at least 2 weeks after the completion of the irradiation treatment to avoid excessive irritation of the neck tissues and skin breakdown when removing the baseplate. During this time, the HME can be attached directly to the laryngectomy tube.

## Long-Term Humidification

Following discharge from the hospital there are various ways and means to assist humidification, including HME devices and stoma covers that are attached directly to the stoma; inhaled steam (from the shower, an open bowl of hot water, or commercial vaporizers/nebulizers), and appliances such as room humidifiers in the bedroom or family room which can be left on 24 hours a day. For those patients who do not use an HME device, steam humidification at least twice a day is recommended to assist with sputum clearance.

Patients need to be aware of the weather and its impact on their pulmonary function. In particular, dry and windy weather can make sputum thick and sticky, making it difficult to clear. During these periods, it may be necessary to increase periods of humidification (either increasing the duration of HME use, or increased use of steaming). For some patients who are experiencing particular difficulty clearing their sputum, nursing and medical staff may recommend the use of saline lavage. A saline lavage involves squeezing a small dose of saline solution (typically about 2-4 ml, though some settings use 15 ml saline "bullets") into the trachea to moisten the tracheal wall, help elicit a strong cough, and dislodge resistive secretions.

## Stoma Devices

There is a range of equipment and devices associated with caring for, and protecting, the stoma which will be detailed further in the following sections. These include intraluminal equipment such as laryngectomy tubes and tracheostoma buttons, which are used to help maintain the size and shape of the stoma, and devices such as HMEs which facilitate humidification and hands-free speaking valves which, as the name suggests, allow hands free tracheoesophageal speech production. These devices can be used in various combinations with laryngectomy tubes, stoma buttons or peristomal baseplates allowing individuals and their clinicians to choose the system that works best for their individual situation (see examples of different equipment arrangements illustrated in Figure 11-7). There is also an extensive range of brushes, guards, and stoma covers which can assist the person to clean and protect the stoma. We have provided a list of some of the main suppliers of stoma care products at the end of this chapter to assist the readers to locate products which would best suit their patients' needs.

## Laryngectomy Tubes

Laryngectomy tubes (also referred to as cannulas) are used to maintain a patent airway and prevent stoma contracture. Examples of different types of laryngectomy tubes can be seen in Figure 11-8. As mentioned previously, the timing and use of laryngectomy tubes is institution specific. For those settings that use laryngectomy tubes in the early postoperative stage, decannulation procedures vary by physician. Some will remove the laryngectomy tube prior to hospital discharge and only replace it if tracheostoma contracture is noted. Others prefer to have the patient continue to use the tube for longer durations until they are satisfied that stomal stability has been achieved.

To determine if the patient can discontinue use of the tube, some surgeons will trial a systematic "weaning" process. This commences with having the patient remove the tube for 1 hour a day. Once this goal has been achieved and the tube can be easily reinserted each time, the duration of removal is increased by additional 1 hour increments each day. When the laryngectomee is managing to keep the tube out all day (over a period of a few weeks with no decrease in size of the stoma), the patient can go for 24 hour periods without the tube, with only occasional checking that no change in stoma size occurs. For those patients who never achieve stoma patency, long-term use of the tube (either 24 hours a day or just overnight) may be considered instead of surgical revision of the stoma.

### Clinical Reasoning, Selection, and Indications for Laryngectomy Tube Use

There are various types of laryngectomy tubes, with different models varying in length, inner and outer cannula diameter, angle of the tube, the presence/absence of fenestration, how they are secured in position (using neck ties or attached to a baseplate), whether or not they allow attachment of other stoma devices (such as HMEs and hands-free devices), and the type of manufacturing material (metal, silicone, etc.). Determining the optimal tube for each patient depends on many factors, which will be discussed in the following sections. Figure 11-9 shows some laryngectomy tubes of different length and diameter.

**Tube Length.** Laryngectomy tubes are available in different lengths. Selecting the optimal length is dependent on the depth and the shape of each individual stoma/

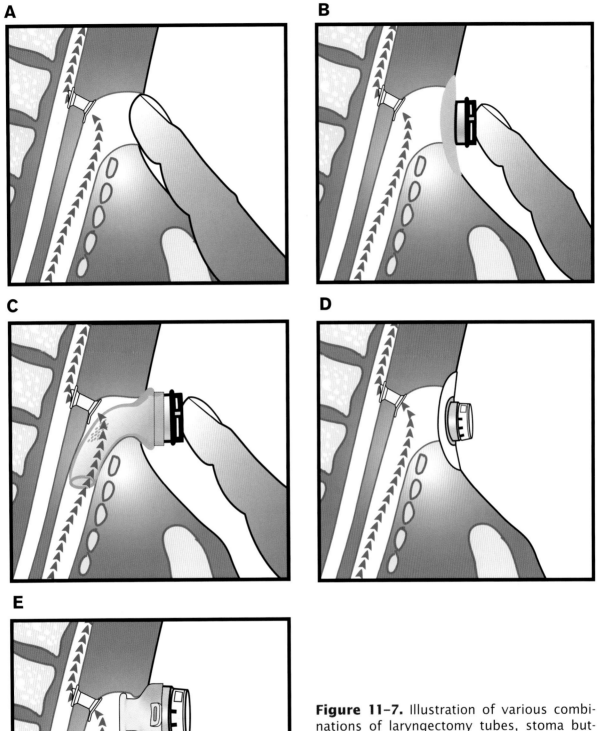

**Figure 11–7.** Illustration of various combinations of laryngectomy tubes, stoma buttons, hands free devices and HMEs and how phonation can be achieved with each combination for a patient using tracheoesophageal speech **A.** No equipment in stoma, **B.** HME attached by means of a base plate, **C.** an HME attached to a laryngectomy tube, **D.** a Hands-free speaking device in a base plate, and **E.** a Hands-free speaking device attached to a stoma button.

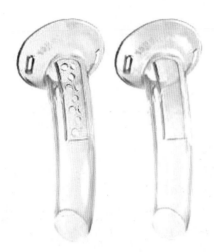

**A.**

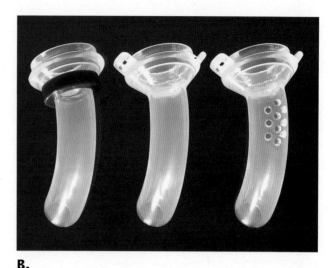

**B.**

**Figure 11–8.** Different types of laryngectomy tubes. **A.** Fenestrated laryngectomy tube for use with neck band (left), nonfenestrated laryngectomy tube for use with neck band (right) (Photo courtesy of InHealth Technologies, www.inhealth.com). **B.** Laryngectomy tubes that enable combination with an HME or hands-free speaking valve. From left to right, laryngectomy tube with blue ring to fit in baseplate, nonfenestrated laryngectomy tube for use with neck band, fenestrated laryngectomy tube for use with neck band. (Photo courtesy of Atos Medical, www.atosmedical.com.)

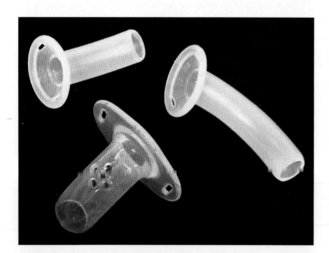

**Figure 11–9.** Laryngectomy tubes with different lengths and diameters.

trachea. Clinical experience would suggest trying a longer tube (e.g., 36 mm) in the first instance, as shorter tubes may tilt forward and dislodge for some patients. Shorter tubes may also rub against the voice

prosthesis causing discomfort or irritation. For some patients, however, the long tubes cause excessive tracheal irritation and in this case, level of comfort with shorter tube lengths should be examined. For most patients, progression to a medium length or shorter tube makes insertion easier and many report greater comfort with the shorter tubes.

### Inner and Outer Dimensions of the Cannula.

Just like other interluminal devices (e.g., tracheostomy tubes) laryngectomy tubes vary in the outer diameter of the cannula in order to achieve optimal fit in different tracheal lumens. The outer dimensions primarily determine selecting the size of the tube, as this is governed by the physical diameter of the patient's airway and stoma. Males typically require larger outer dimensions than females. Equipment is available for determining stoma size to facilitate tube selection.

The inner dimension of the cannula also varies depending on the material the laryngectomy tube is manufactured from (see discussion below). Consideration of the inner diameter of the cannula is particularly important for patients with smaller outer cannula diameters, and/or when optimizing gas exchange is important (e.g., when patient has coexisting respiratory disease). In these cases, the clinician needs to select a cannula with the optimal inner diameter to facilitate maximal respiratory flow.

**Angle of Tube.** Laryngectomy tubes are also manufactured with different angles. The angle of the tube facilitates insertion and removal of the tube with minimal tracheal irritation. Determining which angle of the tube is optimal for any patient is dependent on his or her individual stoma shape and depth, and the observed ease of insertion.

**Fenestration.** While clinicians once used to create manual fenestrations in silicone laryngectomy tubes, there are now both standard and fenestrated commercial models available (see Figures 11-8 and 11-9). Fenestrated tubes are used in those patients who communicate with tracheoesophageal speech. The addition of fenestrations in the posterior wall of the tube allows air to flow through to the voice prosthesis for speech production. However, some patients can still achieve good voice with a short unfenestrated tube in situ, their success is dependent on how the tube is positioned in relation to the voice prosthesis and whether or not it impairs airflow to the prosthesis. In general, nonfenestrated tubes are preferred over fenestrated ones, since the fenestrations could possibly cause granulation tissue to form.

**Method of Securing to Neck.** Most laryngectomy tubes are secured in place using ties or Velcro straps. When conducting routine cleaning of the tubes it is important to replace these ties each time. Other models of laryngectomy tubes have been designed to connect to an adhesive baseplate. The tube can be "clicked" in and out of the baseplate for cleaning. An example of a laryngectomy tube connected to an HME baseplate is shown in Figure 11-10 and can be seen in the footage on the CD (Chapter 11: Video: "Laryngectomy Tube and HME").

**Suitability for Attaching Other Devices.** With the advent of HME devices, some models of laryngectomy tubes have been designed to allow attachment of other devices, such as some models of HMEs and hands-free valves. This is an important factor to consider in

the selection of a laryngectomy tube if early HME use is anticipated with a patient, and to ensure HME use can continue during radiation therapy. An example of this type of system is shown in Figure 11-11 and

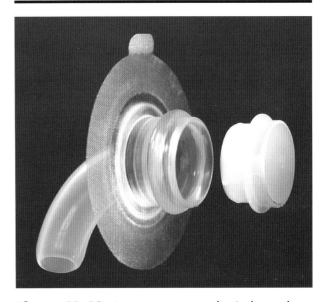

**Figure 11–10.** Laryngectomy tube in baseplate. (Photo courtesy of Atos Medical, www.atos medical.com.)

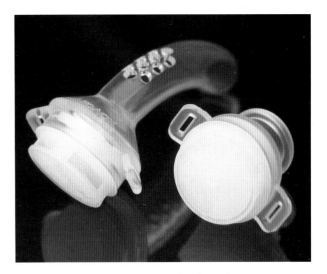

**Figure 11–11.** HME attached to laryngectomy tube (left) and to tracheostoma button (right). (Photo provided as a courtesy of Atos Medical, www.atosmedical.com.)

demonstrated on the CD (Chapter 11: Video: "Laryngectomy Tube and HME").

**Type of Material.** Finally, laryngectomy tubes are manufactured in various materials including PVC, polyurethane, silicone, metal (stainless steel and sterling silver), Teflon, and nylon. Of these, PVC is the most widely used plastic for artificial airways. PVC tubes are designed to avoid reaction; however, they do contain chemicals that may cause allergic or tissue reaction. They are flexible, disposable, and are designed to be adaptable and nontraumatic to the airway. They will soften in heat (as with body temperature) and are porous; therefore, they can retain bacteria. In comparison, polyurethane tubes are flexible at room temperature and become more pliable at body temperature, making them comfortable to wear. They are not as thick as PVC tubes; therefore, the inner diameter of a polyurethane tube will be larger than a PVC tube of the same size outer diameter, leading to increased flexibility and maximum airflow.

Silicone tubes are more "tissue friendly" than PVC tubes. They are durable, flexible, and softer, yielding increased comfort. Silicone is resistant to water absorption which results in a more slippery and less encrusted surface. Silicone tubes retain their shape under various temperature conditions. They also have fewer chemical additives than PVC; therefore, there may be less risk of leaking chemicals into the tracheal tissues. Silicone is also less porous, which results in decreased bacteria adherence to the tube, and they can be sterilized.

Metal laryngectomy tubes are nonreactive when in contact with living tissue but they are rigid and will become cold in low temperatures. Although the sterling silver model of metal laryngectomy tube is more expensive, it is sometimes indicated for patients that have allergic reactions to stainless steel or other PVC/silicone tubes. A metal laryngectomy tube cannot be in place while the patient is receiving radiation treatment. Metal tubes can be sterilized.

Teflon tubes are rigid, remain stable for years, and are very durable. Teflon is a well-tolerated material. The walls of Teflon tubes are particularly thin which results in a higher inner cannula diameter. Nylon tubes are also rigid; however, in contrast to metal and Teflon tubes, they may be degraded by moisture and heat, and may become tissue toxic. The rough surface of these tubes may also be irritating to the tracheal mucosa.

## Cleaning and Maintenance of the Laryngectomy Tube

In the initial stage postsurgery, it is recommended that the laryngectomy tube be removed and cleaned two to three times a day. After discharge, it should be removed at least twice a day for cleaning, once in the morning and once in the evening. Tubes should be cleaned more frequently if increased secretions are noted to ensure airway patency at all times.

The following section details the procedure for care and cleaning of the laryngectomy tube:

1. Wash hands thoroughly prior to handling the laryngectomy tube. The tube should be rinsed with tap water, washed with an antiseptic or soapy water (institution specific), and rinsed again. Special cannula brushes, pipe cleaners, or small bottle brushes may be used to help clean the tubing. See footage on the CD of using both running water and a brush to help remove secretions (Chapter 11: Video: "Cleaning the Laryngectomy Tube"). Stubborn crusting can be removed by soaking the tubing overnight. Within a hospital setting, formal sterilization procedures should follow manufacturers' guidelines for each type of tube.

2. The tube should not be dried with facial tissue as particles of lint may adhere to the tube and be inhaled into the trachea. Allowing the tube to air dry is the preferred method. If the tube needs to be dried manually, a lint-free material should be used.

3. A water soluble lubricant can be used to ease the insertion of the tube. Petroleum-based lubricants should not be used to lubricate the tube as they are not safe for the airway and can damage some tubes (e.g., if using a silicone tube). See CD footage of lubrication and insertion (Chapter 11: Video: "Tracheostoma Tube and HME"). Silicone tubes can be collapsed/folded to ease insertion if the tracheostoma has contracted.

4. If the tube is attached to the neck using ties, then the ties should be replaced each time the tube is cleaned.

## Tracheostoma Buttons

Tracheostoma buttons are shorter than stoma tubes and can also be used to prevent contracture of the tracheal laryngectomy. Figure 11–12 shows some

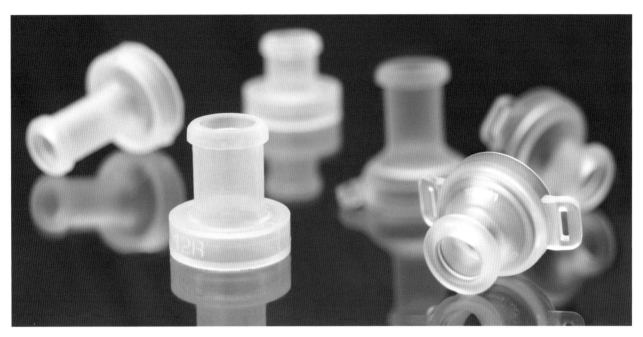

**Figure 11–12.** Different types of stoma buttons that can hold HMEs or hands-free speaking valves. (Photo provided as a courtesy of Atos Medical, www.atosmedical.com.)

examples of stoma buttons that can hold an HME or hands-free device. Figure 11–13 shows some examples of stoma buttons that are used to maintain stoma patency but that do not hold an HME. They do not need to be held in place with tracheostomy tube ties, although for some models it is possible to keep them in place with tracheostomy tube ties if desired. Rather, the fit of a button is airtight within the tracheal lumen so that it is not expelled from the stoma. The button may be taken out at night to allow the stoma to contract slightly, facilitating the airtight seal once reinserted the following day. Gently tugging on the button after insertion and asking the patient to cough forcefully can help check the "fit" of the button. When sizing a patient for a tracheostoma button, the diameter of the button is determined first, followed by the length.

For most clinicians a tracheostoma button is usually trialed if the patient has experienced tracheal irritation and excessive coughing with the longer laryngectomy tube. Some clinicians choose not to use a tracheostoma button prior to trials with a laryngectomy tube, in order to prevent possible stenosis of the lower tracheal airway, which may be associated with the shorter button. For those patients who need to use

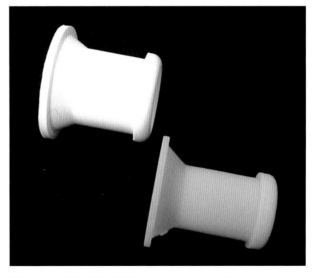

**Figure 11–13.** Different types of stoma buttons that do not hold an external device.

some form of tubing in the long term to maintain stoma patency, many will progress from using a laryngectomy tube to a tracheostoma button in the months post surgery due to the increased comfort and the ease of insertion associated with a button.

Some stoma buttons can also be used to connect with HME or hands-free devices (see Figure 11–11). See footage on the CD of a patient inserting his stoma button and attaching HME device (Chapter 11: Video: "Tracheostoma Button and HME"). The combination of a stoma button with a hands-free device is often more successful than a peristomal baseplate (Lewin, Lemon, Bishop-Leone, Leyk, & Martin, 2000).

As with laryngectomy tubes, there is a range of tracheostoma buttons available commercially. They are manufactured in different sizes, using different materials (e.g., acrylic, Teflon, silicone), and have different designs, with some specifically designed to allow attachment of other devices. For patients using tracheoesophageal speech, a shorter button may not obstruct airflow to the prosthesis; however, in a longer button fenestration of the button is usually required to allow lung air to flow into the voice prosthesis.

### Cleaning the Stoma Button

As per the procedure for cleaning a stoma tube, the laryngectomee should begin by washing the hands, then remove and clean the stoma button with water and allow it to air dry. This should be conducted daily. Sterilization within institutional settings should be performed consistent with the manufacturers' instructions. Application of water-soluble lubrication to the stoma button can assist insertion.

### Peristomal Devices

### Heat and Moisture Exchange (HME) Devices

There is a range of different HME devices available commercially. Regardless of the brand and the individual manufacturing features, HME devices in general serve to humidify and filter inhaled air and increase airway resistance, thereby improving pulmonary physiology by decreasing secretion production and allowing a more thorough and complete expansion of the lungs (see discussion of research evidence supporting HME use in Chapter 12).

The first generation of HMEs were manufactured as one piece that required complete removal if secretions needed to be cleared from the stoma. Second generation products have two component parts: the HME device and the baseplate/housing/adhesive disk (terms vary with different products/manufacturers). There are a number of different HME baseplates available commercially, each designed for a different purpose or need. Currently there are standard baseplates designed for regular skin with standard adhesives, which are less flexible and sticky than other baseplates. There are also models designed for deep and irregular stomas, which are flexible and transparent and have strong adhesive. Other products have been designed for patients with sensitive skin, which are most often used immediately postoperatively or after radiotherapy. Companies also produce baseplates that are combined with double sticking adhesive (foam) disks in varying strengths of adhesive, while others produce baseplates in different sizes (small, large) and different shapes (oval, round) to accommodate various neck shapes. See Figure 11–14 for examples of different types, shapes, sizes, and materials of products currently available. Determining which product best suits each particular patient depends on the ability to achieve an airtight seal between the baseplate and the skin around the stoma.

The HME device itself attaches onto this baseplate. Different manufacturers have created different HME devices; however, the fundamental component of each device is a casing, which attaches to the baseplate and contains a specially treated foam filter. Depending on the manufacturer of the device, this foam filter may be replaceable within the casing, while for other models the whole filter cassette needs to be replaced. Some HMEs are available in different "resistances." Although manufacturers in general recommend to use the "standard" resistance, some patients may benefit from the lower resistance/higher flow devices during physical exercise or when they are experiencing trouble in getting used to the increased breathing resistance with the HME.

HME devices can be used in conjunction with tracheoesophageal speech. Depending on the model and manufacturer, different methods are used to prevent air from being exhaled, and instead, be diverted up through the voice prosthesis. This is typically achieved

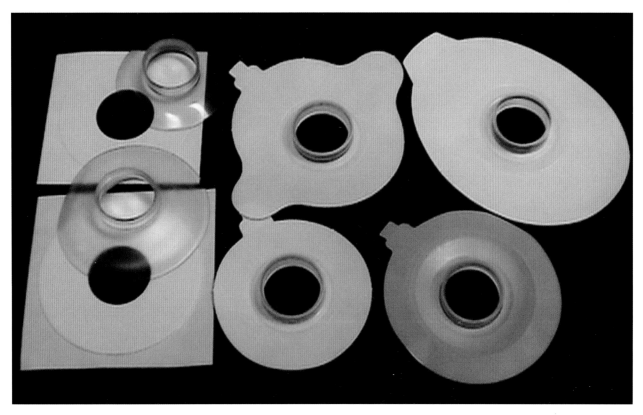

**Figure 11–14.** Range of different types, shapes, and sizes of baseplates.

by pushing down on the top of the HME device with a finger to close it so that speech can be produced (see Figure 11-15).

When laryngectomees first wear an HME, they report it feels "different." They feel increased resistance when they breathe and they may initially notice an increase in secretions. However, their body soon adapts to the HME, and at this point they will notice a significant reduction in secretions. It may take a week to a month for patients who have never used an HME device to become adjusted to the product and to really become comfortable. Many HME manufacturers recognize this and give laryngectomees free sample packs for a trial period. Some companies suggest trying their product for an entire month to fully experience the benefit of wearing an HME. Prior to allowing the laryngectomee to wear the device out of the clinic setting he or she needs to be able to insert/remove the HME and to insert/remove the filter and clean the filter

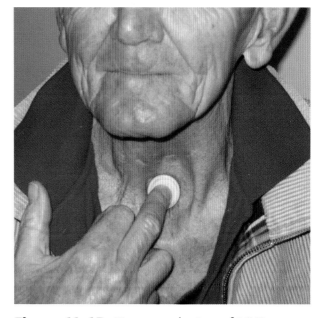

**Figure 11–15.** Finger occlusion of HME.

holder (if using a device with replaceable filters). If the patient uses tracheoesophageal speech, he or she needs to be able to adequately occlude the HME and produce voice. If there are no problems with neck irritation from the adhesive, sleeping with the HME in place is encouraged. This will allow the laryngectomee to receive the benefits of heat and moisture exchange and filtration both day and night.

### Hands-Free Speaking Valves

Hands-free speaking valves eliminate the need for manual occlusion of the tracheostoma in order to produce tracheoesophageal puncture (TEP) speech (see discussion in Chapter 9). During normal respiration, the valve stays in the open position and the laryngectomee inhales and exhales through the tracheostoma. After inhaling through the tracheostoma, when the tracheoesophageal speaker exhales more forcefully to speak, pressure is increased and the airflow pushes the valve closed. This allows the air to be channeled through the voice prosthesis and out of the mouth for speech production without manual occlusion. The valve returns

to its open position when the pressure drops/the airflow is decreased or when the patient inhales. Hands-free valves are not to be used at night when the laryngectomee is sleeping as the valve may become fixed in the closed position, not allowing the valve to open for inhalation.

Similar to HME devices, hands-free systems are comprised of a baseplate or intraluminal attachment, and a hands-free device which fits into this baseplate or intraluminal device (see Figure 11–16). The hands-free valve itself typically consists of casing containing the membrane, which closes off the valve during speech, diverting all air through the prosthesis. The membranes come in different closing resistances to accommodate for different types of speech pattern; for example, a membrane set in a more open position (or low resistance setting) requires increased effort to close for speech, and therefore is best for patients with forceful tracheoesophageal speech. Trial and error is needed to determine the optimal valve sensitivity level (membrane resistance) for patients with different patterns and volumes of tracheoesophageal speech.

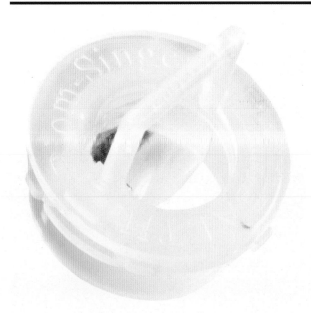

**A.**

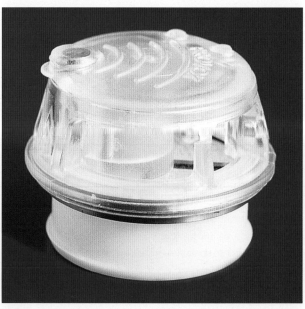

**B.**

**Figure 11–16.** Hands-free devices. **A.** Blom-Singer ATV II (Photo provided as a courtesy of InHealth Technologies, www.inhealth.com.) and **B.** Provox Freehands (Photo provided as a courtesy of Atos Medical, www.atosmedical.com.).

Some hand-free devices also have a cough relief valve, which should open only during coughing and not during loud speech. When talking very loudly, the laryngectomee should talk while pushing a finger on the top of the valve. This will prevent the cough-relief from opening and will support the adhesive seal between the skin and the baseplate. Hands-free valves can also be used with HMEs. For some commercial brands the use of an HME is optional, while for other products, it is an integrated part of the valve.

## Securing HMEs and Hands-Free Devices

In the first speech therapy session, the speech-language pathologist should apply the baseplate to demonstrate the process to the patient. The subsequent session(s) should be devoted to promoting patient independence applying the baseplate. Although the following outlines some guidelines for stoma preparation, it is important to keep in mind that every laryngectomee is different, and so trial and error may be necessary to determine what is best for each individual.

The patient should begin by washing the hands. Then the stoma should be cleaned and cleared of any dried secretions, and the area allowed to dry thoroughly prior to proceeding. Next a skin preparation agent (commercial products such as Skin Prep: Smith & Nephew) can be applied to the skin around the stoma where the baseplate will be secured (this is especially helpful in patients experiencing skin irritation). This is allowed to dry, forming a clear, protective barrier between skin and any tape and/or adhesive. Depending on the model of baseplate being used, the next steps may vary slightly:

- Some baseplates are "all-in-one" with a backing sheet that is removed prior to application. Although it is often not necessary to use extra glue with these baseplates, some patients get better results when a thin layer of silicone glue or liquid adhesive is applied directly to the skin. After applying the glue and waiting the appropriate amount of time to allow for the glue to become "tacky," the backing of the baseplate is removed, and the baseplate is placed over the stoma while gently moving skin away from the stoma. Patients are encouraged to massage the

baseplate onto the skin in order to improve adhesion. Any excess glue should be cleared to prevent it entering the stoma. Once the baseplate is applied, it is suggested that the patient wait about 30 minutes prior to talking hands-free, to allow the glue adequate time to "set." See footage on the CD (Chapter 11: Video: "Preparing Neck and Attaching Baseplate").

- With other systems, there are two components including a double-sided foam or tape disk and a plastic housing, which is attached to the disk. With this system, one side of the protective paper from the double sided foam adhesive disk is removed. The plastic tracheostoma housing is then placed on the exposed side of the adhesive disk, ensuring that both the housing and the adhesive align accurately. The clinician needs to ensure they massage out any air bubbles so that a good seal is maintained. Once this has been achieved, the other side of the adhesive tape is removed and this is attached directly to the patient's prepared skin. See video footage on CD of this type of system (Chapter 11: Video: "Adhesive Disk and Plastic Housing"). For some patients additional application of silicone glue to the patient's skin can also help improve adhesion.

If the patient is using a hands-free speaking valve there are a few things that can help with baseplate adhesion. The most important thing for the patient to do while speaking with a valve is to speak with constant, gentle air pressure. This will put the least amount of stress on the adhesive, thereby increasing the time it stays secured to the neck. Beginning sentences with increased pressure (like a hard glottal attack) should be avoided. Patients should be encouraged to support the device with a finger when speaking loud or shouting, to avoid excessive pressure on the seal. Proper adjustment of the cough relief valve is important as well. It should not open when speaking at a normal level, but should open easily enough to let air escape during a cough.

It is important to keep the prosthesis clean as the more air that goes through the prosthesis, the less air will be in the trachea, potentially breaking down the adhesive seal. Regarding placement of the baseplate, it should be positioned slightly lower than the stoma to aid in the removal of secretions. If patients can keep secretions away from the adhesive, it will help to prolong the duration of the adhesive seal. Any air leaks can be repaired by applying glue to the location of the leak with a cotton-tipped applicator. Once the glue is "tacky" the clinician/patient can use a finger to gently push the baseplate back onto the neck to reestablish the seal. Again, it is best to wait a few minutes before voicing. Footage is available on the CD showing a patient speaking with, and then repairing, an air leak (Chapter 11: Video: "Repairing Seal").

Be aware that adhesive does not stick well to shiny red skin. Ideally you should not be able to visualize where the baseplate was placed. If a large red ring around the stoma is evident, then the baseplate should be left off at least one night to allow the skin to heal. It is also worth investigating other adhesive products to see if the patient is more tolerant of different brands.

Removal of the baseplate is achieved by gently pulling it away from the skin. This is typically easier if the seal has already been degraded. See CD footage (Chapter 11: Video: "Removal"). If there is difficulty removing the baseplate, or for those patients with sensitive skin, there are commercial products available that can be used to help break down the adhesive seal and facilitate easy removal. If using these types of products, it is important that they have been fully washed off the skin before attempting to reattach a new baseplate. Regarding attaching the HME and hands-free devices to the baseplate, this can be achieved by pushing and "clicking" the devices into place. Prior to allowing the laryngectomee to wear the device out of the clinic, he or she needs to be familiar with how to manipulate the different valve settings, and be able to insert and remove the valve; assemble/ disassemble the valve; fix the cough release both in and out of the baseplate; and clean the valve. In no case should the patient wear the hands-free device during the night. It should be replaced with a regular HME.

### Care and Cleaning of HMEs and Hands-Free Devices

HMEs and hands-free devices should be removed and cleaned daily, as valve functioning can be adversely affected by secretions and dried phlegm. In general, soaking in lukewarm water should clean most devices. The device can then be rinsed and allowed to air dry.

Oil-based detergents should not be used, nor should the valve be placed in hot water, boiled, or sterilized as this may result in destruction of the valve. For specific cleaning instructions for each device, the reader is instructed to read the product manual.

## Stoma Care Accessories

In addition to those devices that can be attached to the stoma to facilitate humidification and communication, there is a range of stomal devices which function to protect the airway. These will be discussed in the following sections. As with all other stomal devices, there is a range of airway protection devices available commercially. The current discussion outlines the main types of equipment currently in use. The reader is encouraged to discuss with local distributors current products available for patients.

### Stoma Covers

There is a wide range of different stoma covers available for the laryngectomee. Stoma covers are used to prevent debris from entering the stoma. They also serve to help filter inhaled air, thereby decreasing secretions. Some stoma covers also assist in moisturizing and warming inhaled air. The humidifying function of foam stoma covers (see Figure 11–17) can be enhanced by slightly moistening the foam.

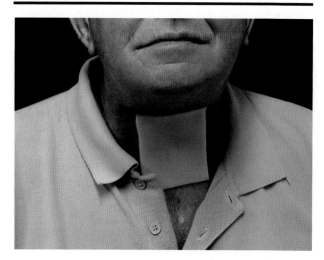

**Figure 11–17.** Patient wearing a foam stoma cover.

The main types of stoma cover are the disposable foam squares secured to the neck with an adhesive strip, or the open weave cloth covers that attach with Velcro around the neck and are able to be washed and reused (see Figure 11-18). Some companies sell fully lined pleated ascots and lace collars that serve to cover the stoma and provide a fashionable alternative. Some patients, particularly female laryngectomees, create their own personalized stoma covers using scarves or beaded necklaces (see Figure 11-19).

### Shower Shields and Guards

Laryngectomees need to be cautious when showering, especially when washing their hair, to avoid aspiration of water into the tracheostoma. Male laryngectomees also need to be vigilant when shaving to prevent aspiration of hair or shaving cream. Shower guards prevent water from entering the stoma during showering. They are not intended for swimming. Shower guards can be made of vinyl, rubber, or nylon. The vinyl shower guards look similar to a bib and they are very lightweight (see Figure 11-20). Other versions of the shower guard have an appearance that is similar to a nose. This design keeps the shower guard elevated off of the tracheostoma. Some laryngectomees report that they feel they can breathe better with this type of

shower guard. All shower guards come with adjustable Velcro straps. Some companies produce shower guards that fit into the HME baseplate (see Figure 11-21).

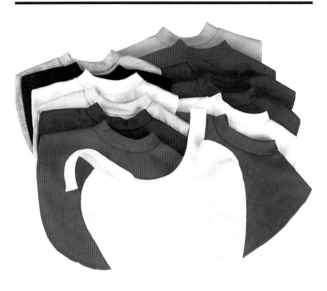

**Figure 11-18.** Cloth stoma covers. (Photo provided as a courtesy of InHealth Technologies, www.inhealth.com.)

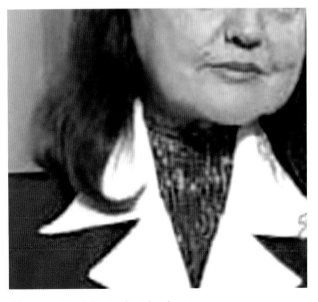
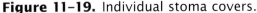

**Figure 11-19.** Individual stoma covers.

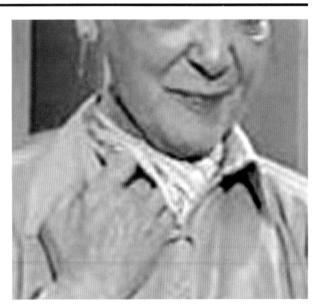

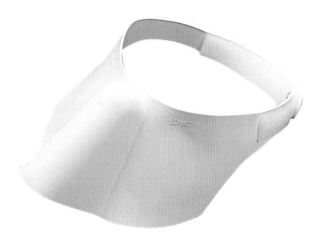

**Figure 11–20.** Shower guard (Photo provided as a courtesy of InHealth Technologies, www.inhealth.com.).

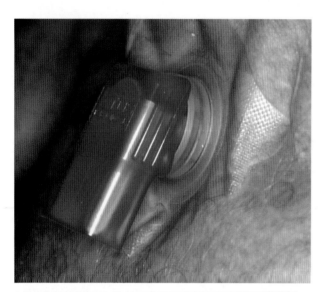

**Figure 11–21.** Shower guard attached to baseplate (Photo provided as a courtesy of Atos Medical, www.atosmedical.com.).

## Conclusion

Adjusting to life with a permanent tracheostoma can be a significant challenge for patients and their families postlaryngectomy. Early and ongoing patient education, hands-on training, and emotional support, are critical to assist the patients and their families adapt to living with, and caring for, their stomas. As demonstrated throughout this chapter stoma management practices vary between institutions; therefore, it is important that the health care professional is aware of the procedures specific to his or her institution. In addition, the range of commercial products available for maintaining, cleaning, humidifying, and protecting the airway is extensive and constantly improving. Clinicians should ensure they remain up to date with the range of products available, and any research evidence supporting their use, in order to optimize stoma care for their patients.

## List of Main Manufacturers of Stoma Care Products

Listed below are some of the main manufacturers of stoma care products and their Web sites. All companies have local distributors that can be contacted.

ATOS Medical AB (Provox products)
E-mail: info@atosmedical.com
www.atosmedical.com

InHealth Technologies (Blom-Singer products)
E-mail: info@inhealth.com
www.inhealth.com

Kapitex Healthcare USA
E-mail: info@kapitex.com
www.kapitex.com

Mallinckrodt Corporate Headquarters (Shiley products)
www.mallinckrodt.com

Smith Medical ASD Inc. (Bivona and Portex products)
www.smiths-medical.com

## References

Ackerstaff, A. H., Hilgers, F. J. M., Aaronson, N. K., Balm, A. J. M., & Van Zandwijk, N. (1993). Improvements in respiratory and psychosocial functioning following total laryngectomy by the use of a heat and moisture exchanger. *Annals of Otology, Rhinology and Laryngology, 102,* 878-883.

Hilgers, F. J. M. (Ed.). (2003). *A practical guide to post-laryngectomy rehabilitation, including the Provox System* (4th ed.) [CD-ROM]. Netherlands Cancer Institute, The Netherlands.

Hilgers, F. J. M., Aaronson, N. K., Ackerstaff, A. H., Schouwenburg, P. F., & Van Zandwijk, N. (1991). The influence of a heat and moisture exchanger (HME) on the respiratory symptoms after total laryngectomy. *Clinical Otolaryngology, 16,* 152-156.

Lewin, J. S., Lemon, J., Bishop-Leone, J. K., Leyk, S., & Martin, J. W. (2000). Experience with Barton button and peristomal breathing valve attachments for handsfree tracheoesophageal speech. *Head & Neck, 22,* 142-148.

Pryor, J. A. (1999). Physiotherapy for airway clearance in adults. *European Respiratory Journal, 14,* 1418-1424.

Verschuur, H. P., Gregor, R. T., Hilgers, F. J. M., & Balm, A. J. M. (1996). The tracheostoma in relation to prosthetic voice rehabilitation. *Laryngoscope, 106,* 111-115.

# Chapter 12

# PULMONARY FUNCTION AND REHABILITATION

Annemieke H. Ackerstaff, J. Karel Zuur, and
Frans J. M. Hilgers

---

## CHAPTER OUTLINE

## Introduction

The anatomical reconstruction associated with a total laryngectomy procedure leads to significant functional changes for the individual. While the full extent of the postoperative issues facing this population will be discussed further in Chapter 14, of perhaps the most significant impact is the loss of the laryngeal structures, requiring a new sound source for voicing and the redirection of the airway through a permanent tracheostoma. Such dramatic alteration to the upper respiratory tract results in a permanent inability to breathe through the upper airways (i.e., nose, mouth), leading to a loss of the warming and humidification functions that once were facilitated by these structures, as well as a detrimental impact on olfaction (discussed in more detail in Chapter 13) (Hilgers & Ackerstaff, 2000). The changes experienced by patients postlaryngectomy, in particular the loss of normal voice and the respiratory symptoms, cause a wide range of additional physical and psychosocial implications for each individual patient (Hilgers, Ackerstaff, Aaronson, Schouwenburg, & van Zandwijk, 1990). This chapter will detail the changes in the respiratory tract postlaryngectomy and its effect on pulmonary function and quality of life, and explore current available treatment options.

## Normal Pulmonary Physiology

Prior to surgery, resting breathing primarily occurs through the nasal airways. During this normal nasal breathing, the passage of the air through the short anterior part of the nasal cavity contributes to the conditioning (heating and humidification) of the inspired air (Keck, Leiacker, Heinrich, Kuhnemann, & Rettinger, 2000). As the temperature of the inspired air increases during its passage through the nasal cavity, it has increased capacity to hold water vapor, increasing the relative humidity (RH) of the air. During normal nasal breathing at rest, a healthy individual with an intact upper airway will alter the ambient air with a temperature of 23°C (71.6°F) and a RH of 30% to a temperature of 32°C (89.6°F) and 99% RH when measured at the level of the trachea (Ingelstedt, 1956).

## Pulmonary Physiology Postlaryngectomy

Complete surgical removal of the larynx leads to a permanent separation of the upper and lower airways (schematically shown in Figure 12–1). (See Chapter 6 for more details regarding the surgical procedure.) Due to this permanent separation, respiration is no longer taking place via the upper respiratory tract, which prohibits normal warming, humidifying, and filtering functions in these patients (Harris & Jonson, 1974; Todisco, Maurizi, Paludetti, Dottorini, & Merante, 1984; Togawa, Konno, & Hoshino, 1980; Torjussen, 1968; Usui, 1979). During rest breathing in laryngectomized individuals, the ambient air of 22°C (71.6°F) and 40% RH is only conditioned to 27–28°C (80.6–82.4°F) and 50% RH at the level of the upper trachea. This is obviously much less than the physiological optimal values of 32°C (89.6°F) and 99% RH mentioned previously for the normal population (Keck, Durr, Leiacker, Rettinger, & Rozsasi, 2005).

The lack of the nasal functions (warming, humidifying, filtering) has unfavorable effects on the lower airways. Those effects are expressed in both the subjective complaints by the patients and objective changes in pulmonary function. Common complaints are irritation of the tracheobronchial mucosa, excessive sputum production, crusting, shortness of breath, and coughing (Hilgers et al., 1990; Pruyn et al., 1986). The respiratory problems, such as coughing, excessive sputum production, and shortness of breath that many laryngectomees suffer from (Hilgers et al., 1990) usually develop and increase during the first 6–12 months postoperatively, and tend to stabilize over the next year (Todisco et al., 1984). Fluctuations in these symptoms may be seen depending on the season, with patients reporting fewer respiratory problems during the summer than during the winter period (Ackerstaff, Hilgers, Aaronson, Balm, & Van Zandwijk, 1993; Hilgers et al., 1990; Natvig, 1984).

In addition to these more overt respiratory changes noted postsurgery, extensive histological changes, such as squamous metaplasia of the respiratory ciliary epithelium, and chronic inflammatory changes of the lamina propria have been observed in the trachea of laryngectomized patients at the level of the carina (Griffith & Friedberg, 1964; Roessler, Grossenbacher, &

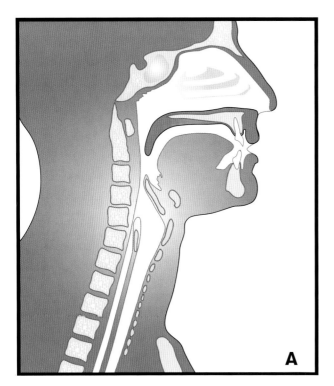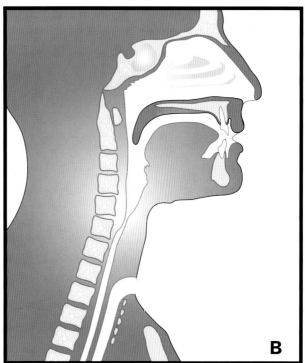

**Figure 12–1.** Schematic illustration of the anatomical situation before **A.** and after **B.** a total laryngectomy leading to a complete separation of the upper and lower airways impairing voicing, respiration, and olfaction.

Walt, 1988). Furthermore, in a small series of patients a progressive bronchial obstruction and bacteriological infection of the tracheobronchial tree during the first postoperative year was observed (Todisco et al., 1984), which eventually causes permanent disturbances in pulmonary function (Ackerstaff, Hilgers, Balm, & Van Zandwijk, 1995b; Hess, Schwenk, Frank, & Loddenkemper, 1999).

Studies that have examined objective pulmonary function postlaryngectomy have documented the significant impact of the surgery on respiratory function (Ackerstaff, Hilgers, Meeuwis, Knegt, & Weenink, 1999a; Hess et al., 1999; Ackerstaff et al., 1995b). A study involving patients who had undergone a laryngectomy procedure 3–24 years prior to participation in the study revealed that long-term pulmonary function is significantly affected (Ackerstaff et al., 1995b). The results of the 58 patients showed that Maximum Vital Capacity (VCmax), Forced Expiratory Volume at 1 second (FEV1), Peak Expiratory Flow (PEF), Maximum Expiratory Flow at 50% (MEF50), and Total Lung capacity

(TLC) were all significantly lower than the predicted values.

In a study specifically designed to measure the extent of the impact of the total laryngectomy on pulmonary function, Ackerstaff, Hilgers, Meeuwis, Knegt, and Weenink (1999b) examined pulmonary function of 16 patients at approximately 3 days before surgery and again at 9 days and 6 months postlaryngectomy. Comparison to predicted respiratory values revealed that prior to surgery, the group had significantly reduced MEF50 and FEV volumes. However, measures of VCmax and TLC were not significantly different from predicted values. Nine days following surgery, significant reductions in VCmax and further declines in FEV measures were observed. Also inspiratory flow measures (Forced Inspiratory Volume at 1 second [FIV1], Peak Inspiratory Volume [PIF], and Maximum Inspiratory Flow at 50% [MIF50]) increased significantly 9 days postsurgery and this increase slightly continued over the next half year postsurgery, while the expiratory flow measured stabilized. No changes were observed across TLC postsurgery.

## Effect of Pulmonary Symptoms on Quality of Life, Voice, and Psychosocial Aspects

Research has revealed significant relationships between the respiratory symptoms experienced postlaryngectomy, the perceived quality of voice, and aspects of daily life such as sleep disturbances, feelings of fatigue and malaise, social contacts, and feelings of anxiety and depression (Ackerstaff, Hilgers, Aaronson, & Balm, 1994; Hilgers et al., 1990). For example, coughing was significantly related to fatigue, whereas sputum production and breathlessness were found to be associated with a much wider range of physical and psychosocial problems, such as voice quality, fatigue, sleeping problems, and depression. With regards to voice quality, there was a significant correlation with fatigue, depression, and social contacts. Table 12–1 shows the significant correlations between the respiratory symptoms, psychosocial aspects, and voice quality reported in the literature (Ackerstaff et al., 1994; Hilgers et al., 1990).

## Assessment of Pulmonary Function Postlaryngectomy

Reliable respiratory assessment is mandatory to ensure accurate assessment of pulmonary function (e.g., prior to and postsurgery), or to monitor the effects of thera-peutic interventions. However for the patients following laryngectomy, standard equipment for measuring pulmonary capacity is no longer applicable, and modifications to the traditional nose/mouthpiece of most spirometric devices is necessary to ensure accurate readings via the permanent tracheostoma. Traditionally, pulmonary function measurements in laryngectomized patients were performed by means of a cuffed trachea cannula (see Figure 12-2), connected to a pulmonary function analyzer (Harris & Jonson, 1974; Todisco et al., 1984). It is not recommended to use

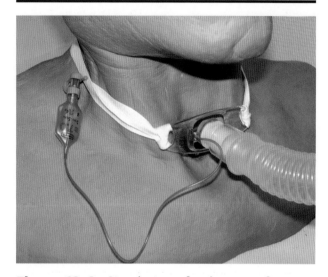

**Figure 12–2.** Simulation of pulmonary function measurement using a cuffed trachea cannula in a life-sized manikin.

**Table 12–1.** Significant Relationships between Respiratory Symptoms (Row 1) and Psychosocial Aspects (Column 1) and Voice Quality (Row 2 and Column 5).

|  | Cough | Sputum | Shortness of Breath | Voice Quality |
|---|---|---|---|---|
| Voice quality |  | <.01 | <.01 |  |
| Fatigue | <.01 | <.001 | <.001 | <.01 |
| Sleeping problems |  | <.05 |  |  |
| Anxiety |  |  | <.001 |  |
| Depression |  | <.01 | <.001 | <.01 |
| Social contacts |  |  |  | <.01 |

Numbers in the cells indicate the p-value for the relationship that was found.

a cuffed cannula. Its insertion is often an unpleasant experience for the patient and may lead to uncomfortable coughing, sometimes lasting for several minutes. Spraying of a local anesthetic does not completely solve this problem, as it often initiates a coughing fit. More importantly, the use of an intratracheal device, such as a cuffed cannula, has a negative influence on the results of forced expiration and inspiration tests, and the cannula decreases the actual diameter of the trachea (Togawa et al., 1980) and thereby increases the airway resistance.

The use of extratracheal devices, such as specially constructed "mouthpieces" has been suggested to avoid this problem (Davidson, Hayward, Pounsford, & Saunders, 1986; Gardner & Meah, 1989; Gregor & Hassman, 1984). Also tracheal masks, manually placed over the stoma, have been used for this reason (Togawa et al., 1980). Ackerstaff et al. (1993) described an easy, comfortable, and reliable pulmonary function assessment that can be achieved by connecting the pulmonary function equipment to an extratracheal adapter that fits into commercially available baseplates used for heat and moisture exchangers (HMEs) (see Figure 12-3). This method more accurately and validly represents the actual lung function of these patients (Ackerstaff, Souren, Van Zandwijk, Balm, & Hilgers, 1993). An

example of the differences in the flow-volume loops between this extratracheal device and a traditional cuffed cannula clearly demonstrates the inadequacy of the latter method (see Figure 12-4). As can be seen in this figure, when measured via the extratracheal

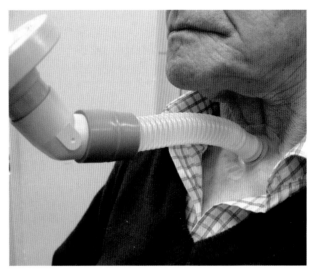

**Figure 12–3.** Example of peristomal attachment of the pulmonary function equipment using a baseplate.

**Figure 12–4.** Flow-volume loops with the dotted line showing the loop obtained with peristomal attachment of the pulmonary function equipment, and the dashed line representing the loop obtained with a cuffed trachea cannula. The solid line shows the normative expiratory loop. *Note.* From "Improvements in the Assessment of Pulmonary Function in Laryngectomized Patients," by A. H. Ackerstaff, T. Souren, N. van Zandwijk, A. J. M. Balm, and F. J. M. Hilgers, 1993, *Laryngoscope, 103,* pp. 1391–1394. Copyright 1993 by Lippincott, Williams and Wilkins. Reprinted with permission.

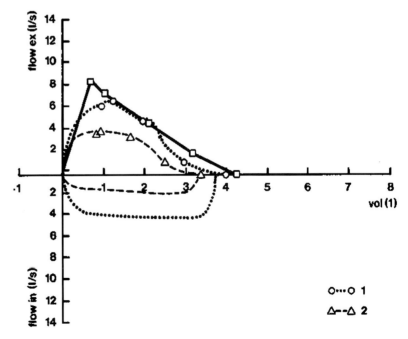

device, the expiratory function in this patient is more or less normal, whereas the trachea cannula method would have suggested a severely disturbed expiratory function. Since there are no predictive values for the inspiratory function it is unclear whether this is normal for this patient, but it is obvious that the method using a peristomal attachment scores "better."

## Heat and Moisture Exchange Devices

Heat and moisture exchange devices (HMEs) have been in clinical use for more than 30 years and are currently the only effective, nonpharmaceutical treatment option for pulmonary symptoms experienced by laryngectomized patients (for an extensive review see Zuur, Muller, de Jongh, van Zandwijk, & Hilgers, 2006). HME devices are attached over the tracheostoma and provide a means for filtering, warming, and humidifying inspired air for the patient postlaryngectomy. There are a number of different types of HMEs available. In Chapter 11, the ones that are most frequently used are described in detail. Figure 12-5 shows an example of an HME.

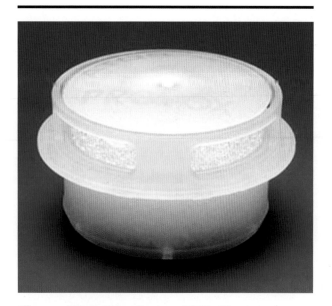

**Figure 12–5.** The Provox HME. (Photo courtesy of Atos Medical, www.atosmedical.com.)

The basic component of an HME is foam, paper, or another substance, which acts as a condensation and absorption surface. In order to enhance the water-retaining capacity, these elements are often impregnated with water-absorbing (hygroscopic) salts like $CaCl_2$, $AlCl_3$, $MgCl_2$, or LiCl (Thomachot, Viviand, Arnaud, Boisson, & Martin, 1998). Some HMEs have been impregnated with a bactericide solution like chlorhexidine in order to control bacterial colonization (Grolman, Blom, Branson, Schouwenburg, & Hamaker, 1997). The principle of heat and moisture exchange in an HME is similar to that of the human airways. During expiration, two phenomena occur: water condensates on the relatively cool HME surface and thermal energy is added to this surface. This limits the loss of heat and moisture into the environment. During inspiration the process is reversed: breathing air passes the warmed and humidified HME surface, leading to evaporation of moisture into, and the direct heating of, the inspired air. During rest breathing in individuals postlaryngectomy, ambient air of 22°C (71.6°F) and 40% RH has been found to be conditioned to 27–28°C/50% RH at the level of the upper trachea without an HME in situ, and to 29-30°C (80.6–82.4°F) and 70% RH using an HME device (Keck, Durr, Leiacker, Rettinger, & Rozsasi, 2005). This corresponds to an increase of approximately 50% of the absolute water content at that specific site. Although this increase is substantial, the intratracheal values obtained during nasal rest breathing in healthy individuals with an intact upper airway of 32°C (89.6°F) and 99% RH (Ingelstedt, 1956) may still not be reached.

Apart from its heat and moisture exchanging capacity, two other physical properties of the HME are also believed to influence respiratory physiology. First, the HME's resistance, in addition to total airway resistance, may reduce dynamic airway compression, thereby improving ventilation and blood oxygenation values (McRae, Young, Hamilton, & Jones, 1996). However, the available evidence in support of this hypothesis is not yet convincing (Zuur et al., 2006). Secondly, the particle filtration capacity of the HME device is frequently referred to by physicians and patients, with anecdotal evidence of a black HME after a day of shopping in the city of London, or a red HME after a tennis match on a gravel court. However, this does not necessarily imply that substantial amounts of particles do not enter the airway. Moreover, due to its large pore size, the HME does not seem to be an efficient barrier for microorganisms. This hypothesis is supported by anesthesiology studies reporting a relatively poor bacterial filtration capacity of simple hygroscopic HMEs (Saravolatz et al., 1986; Shelly, Bethune, & Latimer, 1986; Vanderbroucke-Grauls et al., 1995). Therefore, the significantly decreased incidence of airway infections which has been observed after 6 months use of an HME (Jones et al., 2003), might be attributed to improved humidity values, rather than to sufficient pathogen filtration.

It is also likely that the efficiency of coughing for mucus clearance from the trachea is improved using an HME. By deliberately closing and releasing the valve while coughing, thus imitating the explosive initial "spike" referred to as a supramaximal expiratory flow, which is absent in patients following laryngectomy (Murty, Smith, & Lancaster, 1991), patients experience additional benefit.

## Pulmonary Function Rehabilitation Using HMEs

At the Netherlands Cancer Institute, a series of studies have been carried out that provided both objective and subjective indications that an HME has a positive influence on respiration, phonation, and psychosocial functioning following total laryngectomy (Ackerstaff et al., 1993; Ackerstaff et al., 1995a; Ackerstaff et al., 2003; Hilgers, Aaronson, Ackerstaff, Schouwenburg, & Van Zandwijk, 1991). In the first two studies (Ackerstaff et al., 1993; Hilgers et al., 1991), one with an HME trial period of 6 weeks and one with an HME trial period of 3 months, it could be demonstrated that respiratory problems diminish, resulting in significant reductions in the incidence of coughing, mean daily frequency of sputum production, forced expectoration, and stoma cleaning. In addition, several related physical as well as psychosocial factors were noted to improve. Significant reductions were found in the perception of shortness of breath, feelings of fatigue and malaise, sleep problems, levels of anxiety, and depression. The decrease in sputum production had a positive influence on the quality of voice as reported by the patients (Ackerstaff et al., 1993; Ackerstaff, Hilgers, Balm, & Tan, 1998). Objective measurements by means of pulmonary function tests demonstrated a significant increase of the inspiratory flow measures after using the HME for 3 months (Ackerstaff et al., 1993).

Studies performed in the United States, Spain, and the United Kingdom using similar methodologies have confirmed the above mentioned findings in different cultures and climates (Ackerstaff et al., 2003; Herranz Gonzalez-Botas, Suarez, Garcia Carreira, & Martinez Moran, 2001; Jones et al., 2003). Early application of an HME (i.e., as soon as wounds were healed sufficiently, in general after 2 weeks) cannot prevent respiratory problems completely, but researchers has shown that after 6 months the incidence rates and severity of respiratory problems were significantly lower for the HME users than for those patients who did not use an HME (Ackerstaff et al., 1995a).

Another important issue for the patients following laryngectomy is the loss of approximately 500 ml of water simply by breathing through the stoma in comparison with normal nasal breathing (Toremalm, 1960). By using an HME it is possible to retain 250–300 ml of this excessive water loss in the respiratory system (Toremalm, 1960). This finding alone already might serve to explain much of the decrease in sputum and coughing problems reported because the retained water obviously leads to a lower viscosity and stickiness of the phlegm.

## *Early Introduction of HME Device*

The results of the research projects discussed in the previous section have led to a change in clinical practice at the Netherlands Cancer Institute. HME use is now started on the first postoperative day (see Figure 12-6). An early start has several important advantages, such as early airway protection and unobtrusive stoma coverage, easy adjustment to the airflow resistance of the filter, retention of substantial volumes of water, and thus the redundancy of using the more cumbersome external humidifier. Early familiarization with this medical rehabilitation device for pulmonary rehabilitation enhances compliance and introduces the HME as a self-evident integrated part of postlaryngectomy rehabilitation. Furthermore, this device also enables easier stoma occlusion without interfering with tracheostoma healing.

Also, the use of HMEs in combination with automatic tracheostoma valves (ATVs), such as the Blom-Singer adjustable tracheostoma breathing valve (Van den Hoogen, Meeuwis, Oudes, Janssen, & Manni, 1996;

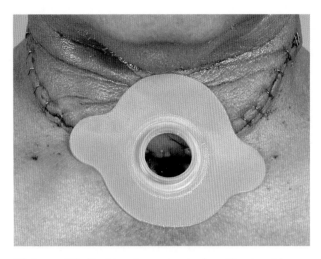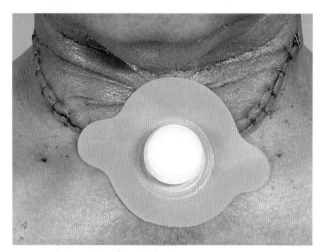

**Figure 12–6.** Newly operated patient with a peristomal, hydrocolloid adhesive; on the right, an HME inserted to protect his airway.

Blom, Singer, & Hamaker, 1982), and the Provox Freehands device (Op de Coul et al., 2005; Hilgers et al., 2003), should be encouraged in this respect. With the Blom-Singer ATV, the HME is optional while the Provox Freehands device was purposely developed in such a way that use of the device without an HME is precluded (Op de Coul et al., 2005; Hilgers et al., 2003). (More information on the different hands-free speaking valves can be found in Chapter 11.)

### HME Use and Compliance

Historically, the early HME devices were not developed with tracheoesophageal speakers in mind. They were initially constructed with the HME and its adhesive baseplate as one single unit, which forced the patient to always remove the entire device for stoma cleaning, and caused adherence problems to the skin. Also, achieving an airtight seal was difficult. Therefore, the compliance rate in the early HME studies was not optimal. Confronted with the choice between adequate pulmonary protection and optimal voicing, patients invariably choose the latter.

Later HME designs have addressed these problems, making the HME device separate to the base adhesive, creating devices that enable easier finger occlusion for those patients using tracheoesophageal speech, and making a variety of adhesives available for different individual needs (see Chapter 11 for more

details). Studies of one particular model of valved HME for easier finger occlusion (see Figure 12–7) showed that with an improved design, and a choice of a variety of adhesives, patient compliance indeed increased (Ackerstaff, et al., 1998; Ackerstaff et al., 2003; Hilgers, Ackerstaff, Balm, & Gregor, 1996; Ackerstaff et al., 2003; Hilgers et al., 1996; Van As, Hilgers, Koopmans-van Beinum, & Ackerstaff, 1998).

In a long-term compliance study of 69 laryngectomy patients, results revealed that 78% of the patients used the device on a daily basis, 6% used it on an irregular basis and 16% did not use it. The reasons for not using the device were mainly disease related (i.e., stoma recurrence, radiotherapy), with only 4 patients reporting they felt uncomfortable using the device. The long-term results were generally quite positive with 94% of the patients reporting an overall considerable benefit, 65% reporting diminished respiratory symptoms, 63% reporting improved digital occlusion, and 55% reporting improved intelligibility (Ackerstaff et al., 1998). A study comparing speech of patients in two conditions, with and without HME use, revealed that although no specific acoustic changes were found, both maximum phonation time and dynamic loudness range were better in the speaking condition using the HME (Van As et al., 1998).

The clinician plays an important role in educating the patient about the effect and use of the HME. Counseling of the patient to improve understanding of the

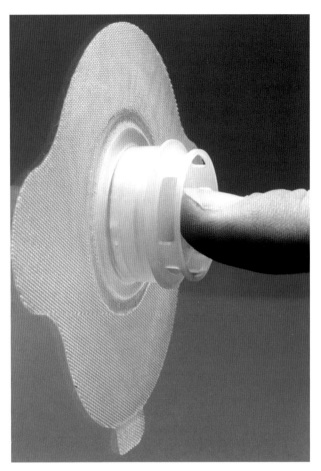

**Figure 12–7.** Valved HME easing airtight finger occlusion. The push-button opens automatically after release of the finger pressure because of a built-in spring. (Photo courtesy of Atos Medical, www.atosmedical.com.)

physiological effects and the practical aspects of these medical devices is of importance to ensure optimal compliance. In our experience, complaints regarding skin irritation (reported in approximately 9% of patients) can sometimes be resolved by alternating between the various types of adhesives. Problems with airway resistance, typically mentioned by about 37% of the patients (especially by the ones who have been laryngectomized already for a long period of time), can be handled by using the HME in the beginning only during nighttime and gradually expanding the use to daytime as well (Ackerstaff et al., 1998), or by starting its use with an HME with lower airflow resistance.

Other problems that may arise include pain during the removal of the adhesive, reports of the adhesive coming loose due to coughing, or that adhesion (mostly due to a deeply situated and/or irregular tracheostoma) in general is inadequate (Hilgers et al., 1996). The period of time that the adhesive adheres well to the skin may vary from less than 1 day to 4 days or longer (Hilgers et al., 1996). Helping the patient to achieve an airtight seal and choosing the optimal adhesive type and shape, stimulating the patient to use the device, and, as already stated before, advising the patient during the first period of use in overcoming the increased resistance and explaining the initial increase of sputum production are all important factors in the rehabilitation program (see Chapter 11 for more details and practical advice).

## Medical Management of Pulmonary Function Postlaryngectomy

In addition to the application of HMEs to normalize (in part) the individual's pulmonary physiology, around 40% of individuals postlaryngectomy may benefit from further medical treatment for their pulmonary symptoms (Hess et al., 1999). A recent guideline of the American Thoracic Society and European Respiration Society considers post-bronchodilator FEV1/VC and FEV1 (% predicted) as the most important parameters in the diagnosis and follow-up of chronic obstructive pulmonary disease (COPD) (Celli & MacNee, 2004). A positive effect of bronchodilator medication on the pulmonary function values is seen in some laryngectomized patients (Ackerstaff et al., 1995b). However, regular treatment with bronchodilators or anti-inflammatory medications is only infrequently provided in this patient population.

Currently, the optimal mode of administering the inhalation medication via the tracheostoma of the laryngectomized individual is not known. For example, metered dose inhalers regularly used in nonlaryngectomees deliver the aerosol particles in such a size and flow that oropharyngeal deposition is limited, which probably limits their effectiveness for direct tracheal inhalation in laryngectomees. The use of a spacer might overcome this problem to some extent (see Figure 12–8)

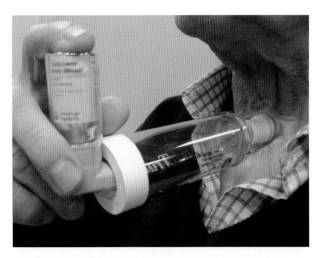

**Figure 12–8.** A small type spacer (AeroTrach, Trudell Medical International, Canada), which is easy to carry in a small sponge-bag most patients use for their stoma care equipment.

(Ackerstaff et al., 1995b; Nakhla, 1997; Webber & Brown, 1984). Further research into the role of medical treatment on the pulmonary complaints of the laryngectomized individual is clearly warranted in view of the aforementioned and frequently encountered impaired pulmonary function and the negative effects of these problems on quality of life.

## Conclusion

Pulmonary function and rehabilitation are key issues in the treatment and after care of laryngectomized individuals. In fact, research has shown that patients rate their pulmonary problems as more problematic than the loss of the normal voice, while medical professionals judged this to be the opposite (Mohide, Archibald, Tew, Young, & Haines, 1992). Moreover, the wealth of evidence of the positive effects of HMEs, not only on pulmonary function but also on psychosocial aspects and voice quality, should be enough reason in this time and age of evidence-based medicine to offer these medical devices to all laryngectomized individuals.

All currently available HMEs provide meaningful airway protection and pulmonary rehabilitation, and thus should be an integral part of any comprehensive postlaryngectomy rehabilitation program. Ongoing research should clarify whether the efficiency of the presently available HMEs can be further improved. Based on the available research in this area and our experience, we can conclude that pulmonary rehabilitation deserves the special attention of those professionals who provide service to individuals following laryngectomy. To ensure a better quality of life, the pulmonary rehabilitation should be, from the start, an integral part of the rehabilitation program. As one of our patients stated, "If you can replace the voice with an artificial voice prosthesis, it makes sense to replace the nose with an artificial moistening and heating device."

## References

Ackerstaff, A. H., Fuller, D., Irvin, M., MacCracken, E., Gaziano, J., & Stachowiak, L. (2003). Multi-center study assessing effects of heat and moisture exchanger use on respiratory symptoms and voice quality in laryngectomized individuals. *Otolaryngology-Head and Neck Surgery, 129*, 705–712.

Ackerstaff, A. H., Hilgers, F. J. M., Aaronson, N. K., & Balm, A. J. M. (1994). Communication, functional disorders and lifestyle changes after total laryngectomy. *Clinical Otolaryngology, 19*, 295–300.

Ackerstaff, A. H., Hilgers, F. J. M., Aaronson, N. K., Balm, A. J. M., & Van Zandwijk, N. (1993). Improvements in respiratory and psychosocial functioning following total laryngectomy by the use of a heat and moisture exchanger. *Annals of Otology, Rhinology and Laryngology, 102*, 878–883.

Ackerstaff, A. H., Hilgers, F. J. M., Aaronson, N. K., de Boer, M. F., Meeuwis, C. A., Knegt, P. P. M., et al. (1995a). Heat and moisture exchangers as a treatment option in the post-operative rehabilitation of laryngectomized patients. *Clinical Otolaryngology, 20*, 504–509.

Ackerstaff, A. H., Hilgers, F. J. M., Balm, A. J. M., & Tan, I. B. (1998). Long term compliance of laryngectomized patients with a specialized pulmonary rehabilitation device, Provox Stomafilter. *Laryngoscope, 108*, 257–260.

Ackerstaff, A. H., Hilgers, F. J. M., Balm, A. J. M., & Van Zandwijk, N. (1995b). Long-term pulmonary function after total laryngectomy. *Clinical Otolaryngology, 20*, 547–551.

Ackerstaff, A. H., Hilgers, F. J., Meeuwis, C. A., Knegt, P. P., & Weenink, C. (1999a). Pulmonary function pre-

and post-total laryngectomy. *Clinical Otolaryngology and Allied Sciences, 24,* 491–494.

Ackerstaff, A. H., Hilgers, F. J., Meeuwis, C. A., Knegt, P. P., & Weenink, C. (1999b). Pulmonary function pre- and post-total laryngectomy. *Clinical Otolaryngology and Allied Sciences, 24,* 491–494.

Ackerstaff, A. H., Souren, T., Van Zandwijk, N., Balm, A. J. M., & Hilgers, F. J. M. (1993). Improvements in the assessment of pulmonary function in laryngectomized patients. *Laryngoscope, 103,* 1391–1394.

Blom, E. D., Singer, M. I., & Hamaker, R. C. (1982). Tracheostoma valve for postlaryngectomy voice rehabilitation. *Annals of Otology, Rhinology, and Laryngology, 91,* 576–578.

Celli, B. R., & MacNee, W. (2004). Standards for the diagnosis and treatment of patients with COPD: A summary of the ATS/ERS position paper. *European Respiratory Journal, 23,* 932–946.

Davidson, R. N., Hayward, L., Pounsford, J. C., & Saunders, K. B. (1986). Lung function and within-breath changes in resistance in patients who have had a laryngectomy. *Quarterly Journal of Medicine, 60,* 753–762.

Gardner, W. N., & Meah, M. S. (1989). Respiration during exercise in conscious laryngectomized humans. *Journal of Applied Physiology, 66,* 2071–2078.

Gregor, R. T., & Hassman, E. (1984). Respiratory function in postlaryngectomy patients related to stomal size. *Acta Otolaryngology, 97,* 177–183.

Griffith, T. E., & Friedberg, S. A. (1964). Histologic changes in the trachea following total laryngectomy. *Annals of Otology, 73,* 883–892.

Grolman, W., Blom, E. D., Branson, R. D., Schouwenburg, P. F., & Hamaker, R. C. (1997). An efficiency comparison of four heat and moisture exchangers used in the laryngectomized patient. *Laryngoscope, 107,* 814–820.

Harris, S., & Jonson, B. (1974). Lung function before and after laryngectomy. *Acta Otolaryngology (Stockholm), 78,* 287–294.

Herranz Gonzalez-Botas, J., Suarez, T., Garcia Carreira, B., & Martinez Moran, A. (2001). Experiencia con el uso del HME-Provox Stomafilter en pacientes laringuectomizados (Experience with the HME-Provox Stomafilter in laryngectomized patients). *Acta Otorrinolaringológica Española, 2001,* 221–225.

Hess, M. M., Schwenk, R. A., Frank, W., & Loddenkemper, R. (1999). Pulmonary function after total laryngectomy. *Laryngoscope, 109,* 988–994.

Hilgers, F. J. M., Aaronson, N. K., Ackerstaff, A. H., Schouwenburg, P. F., & Van Zandwijk, N. (1991). The influence of a heat and moisture exchanger (HME) on the respiratory symptoms after total laryngectomy. *Clinical Otolaryngology, 16,* 152–156.

Hilgers, F. J. M., & Ackerstaff, A. H. (2000). Comprehensive rehabilitation after total laryngectomy is more than voice alone. *Folia phoniatrica et logopaedica, 52,* 65–73.

Hilgers, F. J. M., Ackerstaff, A. H., Aaronson, N. K., Schouwenburg, P. F., & Van Zandwijk, N. (1990). Physical and psychosocial consequences of total laryngectomy. *Clinical Otolaryngology, 15,* 421–425.

Hilgers, F. J. M., Ackerstaff, A. H., Balm, A. J. M., & Gregor, R. T. (1996). A new heat and moisture exchanger with speech valve (Provox® Stomafilter). *Clinical Otolaryngology, 21,* 414–418.

Hilgers, F. J. M., Ackerstaff, A. H., Van As, C. J., Balm, A. J. M., Van den Brekel, M. W. M., & Tan, I. B. (2003). Development and clinical assessment of a Heat and Moisture Exchanger with a multi-magnet automatic tracheostoma valve (Provox FreeHands HME) for vocal and pulmonary rehabilitation after total laryngectomy. *Acta Otolaryngology (Stockholm), 123,* 91–99.

Ingelstedt, S. (1956). Studies on the conditioning of air in the respiratory tract. *Acta Otolaryngology, 56,* 1–80.

Jones, A. S., Young, P. E., Hanafi, Z. B., Makura, Z. G., Fenton, J. E., & Hughes, J. P. (2003). A study of the effect of a resistive heat moisture exchanger (Trachinaze) on pulmonary function and blood gas tensions in patients who have undergone a laryngectomy: A randomized control trial of 50 patients studied over a 6-month period. *Head & Neck, 25,* 361–367.

Keck, T., Durr, J., Leiacker, R., Rettinger, G., & Rozsasi, A. (2005). Tracheal climate in laryngectomees after use of a heat and moisture exchanger. *Laryngoscope, 115,* 534–537.

Keck, T., Leiacker, R., Heinrich, A., Kuhnemann, S., & Rettinger, G. (2000). Humidity and temperature profile in the nasal cavity. *Rhinology, 38,* 167–171.

McRae, D., Young, P., Hamilton, J., & Jones, A. (1996). Raising airway resistance in laryngectomees increases tissue oxygen saturation. *Clinical Otolaryngology, 21,* 366–368.

Mohide, E. A., Archibald, S. D., Tew, M., Young, J. E., & Haines, T. (1992). Postlaryngectomy quality-of-life dimensions identified by patients and health care professionals. *American Journal of Surgery, 164,* 619–622.

Murty, G. E., Smith, M. C. F., & Lancaster, P. (1991). Cough intensity in the laryngectomee. *Clinical Otolaryngology, 16,* 25–28.

Nakhla, V. (1997). A homemade modification of a spacer device for delivery of bronchodilator or steroid therapy in patients with tracheostomies. *Journal of Laryngology and Otology, 111*, 363-365.

Natvig, K. (1984). Influence of different climates on the peak expiratory flow in laryngectomees. *Journal of Laryngology and Otology, 98*, 53-58.

Op de Coul, B. M. R., Ackerstaff, A. H., van As-Brooks C. J., Van den Hoogen, F. J. A., Meeuwis, C. A., Manni, J. J., et al. (2005). Compliance, quality of life and quantitative voice quality aspects of hands-free speech. *Acta Otolaryngology (Stockholm), 125*, 629-637.

Pruyn, J. F. A., de Jong, P. C., Bosman, L. J., van Poppel, J. W. M. J., van den Borne, H. W., Ryckman, R. M., et al. (1986). Psychosocial aspects of head and neck cancer—A review of the literature. *Clinical Otolaryngology, 11*, 469-474.

Roessler, F., Grossenbacher, R., & Walt, H. (1988). Die tracheobronciale Schleimhautbeschaffenheit bei Patienten mit Langzeit-Tracheostoma. *Laryngology, Rhinology, Otology, 67*, 66-71.

Saravolatz, L. D., Pohlod, D. J., Conway, W., Haberaecker, W., Markowitz, N. P., & Popovich, J., Jr. (1986). Lack of bacterial aerosols associated with heat and moisture exchangers. *American Review of Respiratory Disease, 134*, 214-216.

Shelly, M., Bethune, D. W., & Latimer, R. D. (1986). A comparison of five heat and moisture exchangers. *Anaesthesia, 41*, 527-532.

Thomachot, L., Viviand, X., Arnaud, S., Boisson, C., & Martin, C. D. (1998). Comparing two heat and moisture exchangers, one hydrophobic and one hygroscopic, on humidifying efficacy and the rate of nosocomial pneumonia. *Chest, 114*, 1383-1389.

Todisco, T., Maurizi, M., Paludetti, G., Dottorini, M., & Merante, F. (1984). Laryngeal cancer: Long-term follow-up of respiratory functions after laryngectomy. *Respiration, 45*, 303-315.

Togawa, K., Konno, A., & Hoshino, T. (1980). A physiologic study on respiratory handicap of the laryngectomized. *Archives of Otorhinolaryngology, 223*, 69-79.

Toremalm, N. G. (1960). Heat and moisture exchange for post-tracheotomy care. *Acta Otolaryngology (Stockholm), 52*, 1-12.

Torjussen, W. (1968). Airway obstructions in laryngectomized patients. *Acta Otolaryngology, 66*, 161-170.

Usui, N. (1979). Ventilatory function in laryngectomized patients. *Auris Nasis Larynx, 6*, 87-96.

Van As, C. J., Hilgers, F. J. M., Koopmans-van Beinum, F. J., & Ackerstaff, A. H. (1998). The influence of stoma occlusion on aspects of tracheoesophageal voice. *Acta Otolaryngology (Stockholm), 118*, 732-738.

Van den Hoogen, F. J. A., Meeuwis, C., Oudes, M. J., Janssen, P., & Manni, J. J. (1996). The Blom-Singer tracheostoma valve as a valuable addition in the rehabilitation of the laryngectomized patient. *European Archives of Otorhinolaryngology, 253*, 126-129.

Vanderbroucke-Grauls, C. M., Teeuw, K. B., Ballemans, K., Lavooij, C., Cornelisse, P. B., & Verhoef, J. (1995). Bacterial and viral removal efficiency, heat and moisture exchange properties of four filtration devices. *Journal of Hospital Infection, 29*, 45-56.

Webber, P. A., & Brown, A. R. (1984). The use of a conical spacer after laryngectomy. *British Medical Journal (Clinical Research Edition), 288*, 1537.

Zuur, J. K., Muller, S. H., de Jongh, F. H., van Zandwijk, N., & Hilgers, F. J. (2006). The physiological rationale of heat and moisture exchangers in post-laryngectomy pulmonary rehabilitation: A review. *European Archives of Otorhinolaryngology 263(1), 1-8*

# Chapter 13

# REHABILITATION OF OLFACTION AND TASTE FOLLOWING TOTAL LARYNGECTOMY

Corina J. van As-Brooks, Caterina A. Finizia, and Elizabeth C. Ward

---

## CHAPTER OUTLINE

# Introduction

Our sense of smell is important. For instance, it helps us detect danger or spoiled food, and it allows us to enjoy food and our favorite perfume. Nevertheless, the loss of the sense of smell as a consequence of total laryngectomy and more importantly its rehabilitation have historically not received as much attention as the more obvious consequences, such as changes in voice, swallowing, and pulmonary function. Similarly the loss of taste, as a function of cancer treatment (surgery and/or radiotherapy), has received little attention during rehabilitation. The current chapter focuses on the changes in the sense of smell and the sense of taste as a result of total laryngectomy and gives a framework for rehabilitation.

# Normal Sense of Smell

Despite the early proposals in the late 1960s and 1970s of primary and accessory olfactory areas (Henkin & Hoye, 1966; Henkin, Hoye, Ketcham, & Gould, 1968), today it is accepted that qualitative sensations of smell are detected by olfactory cells localized in a particular area of nasal epithelium (referred to as the olfactory epithelium) and conveyed by the olfactory nerve (cranial nerve 1) (Doty & Cometto-Muniz, 2003). In addition to this primary receptor pathway, odorant molecules from pungent odors (such as ammonia) may also stimulate the free nerve endings of cranial nerves, particularly those of the trigeminal nerve (cranial nerve V), located in the lining of the oral and nasal cavity (Doty & Cometto-Muniz, 2003). This chemo-sensation is perceived as irritation, tickling, burning, warming, cooling, and stinging (Doty & Cometto-Muniz, 2003).

The olfactory epithelium is an area of about 1cm², located within each nasal vault at the roof of the nasal cavity, at the adjacent superior part of the nasal septum, and at the superior nasal conchae. The olfactory epithelium is comprised of 100 million olfactory receptor cells interspersed among membrane supporting cells (Heald & Schiffman, 1997). These olfactory receptor cells are bipolar neurons. The mucosal ends of the receptor cells contain cilia that project into the mucous layer of the olfactory mucosa (Ding & Dahl, 2003), which is kept moist by secretions from Bowman's glands.

On arrival at the olfactory mucosa, odorants dissolve in the mucus and their substrates bind with chemoreceptors on the cilia (Sherwood, 2001). From there, the olfactory information is passed to thin nerve fibers (*fila olfactoria*) at the cranial side of the olfactory epithelium. The fila olfactoria join and pass through openings in the *lamina cribrosa* of the ethmoid bone. There, they together form the olfactory bulb. The olfactory bulb is the beginning of the olfactory nerve (cranial nerve 1: CN1), situated under the cerebrum and against the frontal lobe. In Figure 13–1 a detailed drawing of the olfactory epithelium is shown and in Figure 13–2 a more general drawing of the olfactory system is shown.

Two olfactory pathways diverge from the olfactory bulb (Heald & Schiffman, 1997). The first synapses in the medial olfactory area located superior and anterior to the hypothalamus (Heald & Schiffman, 1997). This pathway is a reflex arc mediating such conditioned reactions as licking the lips and salivating in response to a smell stimulus (Heald & Schiffman, 1997). The second pathway leads to the lateral olfactory area in the prepiriform and piriform cortex as well as the cortical portion of the amygdaloid nuclei. This lateral olfactory area is the cerebral location responsible for the conscious perception and analysis of smells. Its complex circuitry also accommodates learned responses to foods including enjoyment and distaste (Heald & Schiffman, 1997).

The sense of smell is described as a chemical sense. Normal sense of smell is referred to by the term normosmia, while hyposmia refers to reduced olfactory acuity, and anosmia is an absence of olfactory acuity. The normal sense of smell occurs upon breathing in through the nose or sniffing. This is known as *orthonasal olfaction*. The orthonasal airflow carries the odor molecules that are present in the surrounding air to the olfactory epithelium. Olfaction may also occur as a result of air entering the nasal cavity posteriorly when breathing out through the nose, chewing, or swallowing. This is known as *retronasal olfaction*. Retronasal olfaction plays an important role in the perception of taste. Therefore, odor molecules may reach the olfactory epithelium either through the anterior nasal entrance (inspiratory breath, orthonasal olfaction), or through the posterior nasal entrance (expiratory breath/chewing/swallowing, retronasal olfaction). Each process will be explained further below.

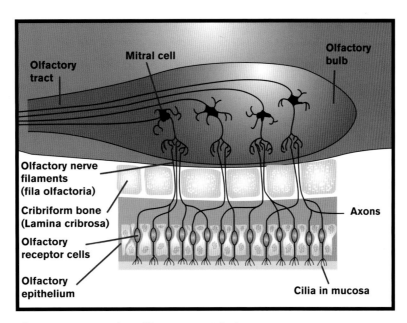

**Figure 13–1.** The olfactory epithelium.

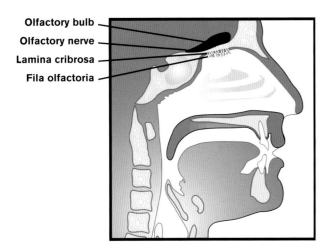

**Figure 13–2.** The different anatomical parts of the olfactory system.

ate turbulent airflow, mixing the incoming air and allowing the delivery of odorants to the epithelium (Frye, 2003). The action of sniffing enhances this delivery system, by increasing the volume flow rate of inspired air and augmenting the deposition of particles in the nose as well as the proportion of particles transported to the olfactory region (Becquemin, Swift, Bouchikhi, Roy, & Teillac, 1991). Indeed, the literature documents positive correlations between volume flow rate of inspired air and several olfactory parameters, including estimation of odor intensity (Rehn, 1978), percentage of odors correctly identified (Schwartz, Mozell, Youngentob, Leopold, & Sheehe, 1987), as well as magnitude of olfactory evoked potentials (Kobal & Hummel, 1991). Adequate delivery of odorants to the olfactory epithelium by nasal airflow, therefore, is crucial for achieving orthonasal olfaction.

## Orthonasal Airflow

During quiet breathing, nasal airflow is primarily shunted along the medial nasal septum at the level of the inferior and medial turbinates (Frye, 2003). Only 15% of the inspired air passes near the olfactory epithelium (Frye, 2003). The turbinates, however, cre-

## Retronasal Airflow

Retronasal olfaction is achieved when odorants diffuse from the oral cavity, through the posterior nasal entrance, and up to the olfactory epithelium (Burdach, Kroeze, & Koster, 1984). Turbulent air created during mouth movements associated with chewing and swallowing can increase the intensity of retronasal odor perception (Burdach & Doty, 1987). Chewing to enhance retronasal olfaction is analogous to sniffing to augment orthonasal olfaction (Burdach & Doty, 1987). This retronasal pathway is also an important form of olfactory stimulation, particularly for identifying the flavors of food in the mouth (Mozell, Smith, Smith, Sullivan, & Swender, 1969).

## Normal Sense of Taste

Similar to the sense of smell, the sense of taste (gustation) is also described as a chemical sense. Impaired taste is referred to as hypogeusia and ageusia refers to the complete inability to taste. The sensation of taste occurs when tastant molecules are released from foods, dissolve in saliva, and bind with taste receptor cells in the taste buds. Soluble carrier proteins in the saliva assist in the transportation of taste stimulants to the taste receptors.

Although it was once thought humans could identify four basic tastes (salty, sour, sweet, and bitter) it is now recognized by many that there is a fifth taste called umami, which refers to savory flavors such as monosodium glutamate (MSG). Different combinations of these five primary tastes are responsible for the thousands of different taste sensations humans are capable of perceiving (Sherwood, 2001). Ten thousand taste buds line the superior tongue surface with additional taste buds found on the soft palate, pharynx, larynx, epiglottis, uvula, and upper esophagus (Sherwood, 2001). While each taste bud responds to varying degrees to all of the primary tastes, it is generally preferentially responsive to one of the tastes (Sherwood, 2001).

Each taste bud contains approximately 50 receptor cells arranged around a central pore (Sherwood, 2001). Tastant solutions must enter the taste pore to stimulate the taste receptor cells. Microvilli on the receptor cells extend into the taste pore and serve as the binding surface for taste stimulation (Heald & Schiffman, 1997). The complex stimulation patterns are transmitted to the central nervous system via several pathways depending upon the location of the stimulated taste bud. Afferent pathways from taste buds include the chorda tympani of the facial nerve (ante-

rior tongue), the lingual branch of the glossopharyngeal nerve (posterior tongue and oral cavity), and the vagus nerve (epiglottis, larynx, and upper esophagus). These cranial nerves synapse in the solitary tract in the medulla, then project into the thalamus and on to the cortical taste area in the parietal cortex (Heald & Schiffman, 1997).

## The Interplay of Olfaction and Taste

During eating, the faculties of smell and taste, in combination with texture and temperature information, contribute to the sensory pool of information pertaining to the food that determines flavor perception. Of the contributing senses (smell, taste, texture, and temperature), smell and taste participate the most significantly in flavor perception. More specifically, of the two senses, smell information has been observed to take precedence over taste information in flavor identification, as experimental deprivation of smell results in an inability to identify a food flavor (e.g., chocolate) (Mozell et al., 1969) yet retained ability to identify the gustatory component of the flavor (e.g., chocolate is sweet). Impaired olfaction therefore, impairs flavor perception to a greater degree than impaired taste (Mozell et al., 1969). Indeed it is thought that 75% of flavor perception is derived from odor (Mann, 2002).

## The Significance of Olfaction and Taste

The loss of the sense of smell (which is most often accompanied by the loss of the sense of taste) has a substantial effect on various aspects of daily life. Miwa et al. (2001) studied the impact of olfactory impairment on quality of life and found that patients with olfactory loss reported on average 4.7 daily activities to be affected. The most cited impairments in this group of patients with olfactory loss were the inability to detect spoiled food (75%), gas leaks (61%), or smoke (50%), as well as problems with eating (53%) and cooking (49%). Overall, only 50% of the subjects in the olfactory loss group were satisfied with life. Similarly, Blomqvist, Bramerson, Stjarne, and Nordin (2004) studied the consequences of olfactory loss in hyposmic and anosmic patients and found that risks associated with the loss, interference with daily routine and deterioration of well-being, were common. Physical health, financial security, profession, partnership, friendship, emotional stability, and leisure were also negatively affected.

It is olfaction that allows the human experience, recognition and enjoyment of a variety of food flavors. Enjoyment of food flavors is determined by classical conditioning, as olfactory templates become associated with pleasant and unpleasant experiences derived from food. The nutritional implications of impaired olfaction, therefore, are serious. When flavor identification, and thus enjoyment, is no longer possible, a person is less likely to be exposed to pleasant experiences, resulting in reduced oral consumption. Certainly, this has been observed in the elderly population, with reduced smell and taste abilities reported to be linked to both diminished food enjoyment and food intake (Asai, 2004).

Although the role of taste in forming food preferences and contributing to nutritional intake appears less predominant than that of olfaction, it serves an equally important role in influencing oral intake. Taste is known to primarily perform biological functions, such as protecting the body from external toxins. Specifically, humans are biologically engineered to dislike bitter tastes, as many poisons in the environment tend to be bitter. The sense of taste is also thought to contribute to some degree to the physiological regulation of nutrients. For example, the palatability of salty foods may be increased in situations of salt deprivation. This is thought to occur as the reserve level of any given nutrient in the body (e.g., sodium) is inherently linked to a gustatory correlate (e.g., salty taste) (Richter, 1942). In this way, gustation also plays an important role in regulating nutrition.

Combined, the senses of smell and taste are known to be important in stimulating physiological events that have profound effects on the nutritional uptake of food (Mattes, 1997). The odor, taste, sight, and thought of foods are known to stimulate a series of physiological events (cephalic phase responses) that result in increased bioavailability of the body's digestive medi-

ators in preparation for food intake (Mattes, 1997). These include saliva, gastric acid, and gastrin as well as pancreatic hormones and enzymes. Increased saliva is necessary for mastication, swallowing, and carbohydrate digestion. It is also thought to influence gastric emptying and nutritional uptake in the small intestine (Lebenthal, 1987). The senses of smell and taste specifically are responsible for producing approximately one third of the total gastric acid secreted during eating (Feldman & Richardson, 1986) as well as significantly increasing the release of gut peptides (Mattes, 1997). These responses play a role in stomach emptying, nutrient absorption, and registering satiety (Mattes, 1997). Indeed, decreased taste and smell abilities have been associated with early satiety and reduced food intake in the elderly population (Asai, 2004).

Cephalic phase responses are also known to play regulatory roles in digestion. The combination of sensory input and cognition associated with the presence of food result in increased body temperature and decreased cardiac output (Mattes, 1997). Decreasing cardiac output is thought to be an anticipatory regulation of the increased cardiac output associated with the eventual digestion of the food. This is crucial given that the distribution of nutrient uptake is dependent upon blood flow (Mattes, 1997). Preingestion smell and taste, therefore, are important not only in invoking a desire to eat, but also for the physiological augmentation of nutritional processes.

In addition to issues relating to oral intake, olfaction plays an important role in personal hygiene, eroticism, and sex. Observing your own body odor is very important within a social context. The inability to do so may lead to excessive use of perfume or excessive bathing or cleaning (Van Toller & Dodd, 1987). Perception of unique personal odors is important in forming and maintaining a social network (Vroon, van Amerongen, & de Vries, 1994). It is also known that perception of certain odors can cause changes in someone's mood (Van Toller & Dodd, 1987). A certain smell can bring back memories from long ago, because of the link between the sense of smell and memory (Mozell, 1971; Laing & Willcox, 1983; Laing & Francis, 1989).

Those parts of the brain that are involved in olfaction are also linked to parts of the brain that deal with the endocrine system that regulate eroticism and sex. Furthermore, olfaction is linked to parts of the brain that play a role in the expression of emotions, swelling of sexual organs, and orgasm (Vroon et al., 1994). Odors influence sexual appetite and activity, and it has been reported that anosmic people often have less sexual interest (Van Toller & Dodd, 1987; Tennen, Affleck, & Mendola, 1991).

## Factors That Influence Olfaction and Taste

Olfactory performance is influenced by many factors, such as head injury, nasal polyps, endocrine conditions, toxins, allergies, and even the common cold. Similarly multiple factors influence taste. It is, however, beyond the scope of this chapter to discuss all possible factors that may influence the sense of smell and taste. Rather this section will be limited to the discussion of some factors that influence the sense of smell and/or taste that are relevant in the laryngectomee population, such as age, smoking, cancer, and its surgical/nonsurgical treatment.

Research has shown that olfactory performance decreases with age and is generally worse in men (Doty, Shaman, Kimmelman, & Dann, 1984; Hoffman, Ishii, & MacTurk, 1998; Larsson, Finkel, & Pedersen, 2000; Hummel, Konnerth, Rosenheim, & Kobal, 2001). Murphy et al. (2002) investigated prevalence of olfactory impairment in 2491 older adults, aged 53 to 97 years, and found adverse effects of age and male gender on odor identification. Specifically, they found an overall prevalence of olfactory dysfunction of 24.5% in their elderly population. Brämerson, Johansson, Ek, Nordin, and Bende (2004) studied olfactory acuity by means of the Scandinavian Odor Identification Test (SOIT) in 1387 volunteers of 20 years and older. The overall prevalence of olfactory impairment was 19.1% (13.3% hyposmia—reduced olfactory acuity, 5.8% anosmia—no olfactory acuity). In the subgroup of individuals 53 years and older, prevalence was found to be 32.9% (Bramerson et al., 2004). Overall the results of this large cohort study confirmed a significant relationship between impaired olfaction and age, male gender, and nasal polyps.

Patients with malignant disease have also been shown to exhibit significantly lower olfactory acuity than noncancer patients, possibly due to the exposure

to cytostatic drugs (chemotherapy) or radiation (Landis, Konnerth, & Hummel, 2004). Irradiation has been reported to have a slight and transient effect on olfactory function, while chemotherapy has been shown to alter chemosensory functions (Doty, Bartoshuk, & Snow, 1991; Ho, Kwong, Wei, & Sham, 2002). There is currently controversy whether or not tobacco smoking affects the sense of smell, with research in this area still being inconclusive. While some studies have shown adverse effects on odor detection and perceived odor intensity of certain odorous substances (Joyner, 1964; Kittel, 1970; Hubert, Fabsitz, Feinleib, & Brown, 1980; Ahlstrom, Berglund, Berglund, Engen, & Lindvall, 1987; Berglund & Nordin, 1992; Weinstock, Wright, & Smith, 1993), as well as odor identification (Frye, Schwartz, & Doty, 1990), others have found no effect (Pangborn, Trabue, & Barylko-Pikielna, 1967; Venstrom & Amoore, 1968; Martin & Pangborn, 1970).

Loss of taste occurs when there is either a disturbance in the saliva or to the taste receptor cells in the taste buds. Similar to olfaction, the sense of taste diminishes with age (Schiffman, 1997), with bitter taste most affected (Frank, Hettinger, & Mott, 1992). Gender may also play a role. Generally speaking, women exhibit greater taste sensitivity in comparison to men (Gromysz-Kalkowska, Wojcik, Szubartowska, & Unkiewicz-Winiarczyk, 2002). As with olfaction, changes in taste sensation and taste sensitivity have been associated with chemotherapy (Wickham et al., 1999; Epstein et al., 2002; Berteretche et al., 2004; Ravasco, 2005; Wilson & Rees, 2005) and radiotherapy to the head and neck area (Harrison et al., 1997; Trotti et al., 1998; Huang, Wilkie, Schubert, & Ting, 2000; Logemann et al., 2001; Zheng, Inokuchi, Yamamoto, & Komiyama, 2002; Ravasco, 2005). Cigarette smoking does influence taste sensitivity, though only to a small extent (Gromysz-Kalkowska et al., 2002).

## Olfaction Following Total Laryngectomy

Hyposmia or reduced olfactory acuity is a common complaint following complete surgical removal of the larynx (Trotti et al., 1998; Lennie, Christman, & Jadack, 2001). The prevalence of hyposmia in this patient population has been reported to range between 68% (Van

Dam et al., 1999) and 100% (Welge-Luessen, Kobal, & Wolfensberger, 2000), according to the method of assessment employed by the investigators. Given that the postlaryngectomy nasal and oral cavities are no longer contiguous with the lower respiratory system, and breathing occurs through a permanent tracheostoma in the anterior neck, significant reduction in nasal airflow is a natural corollary of this altered postlaryngectomy anatomy (see Figure 13-3). Intuitively, therefore, it would be expected that reduced odorant transport to the olfactory epithelium (reduced orthonasal airflow) would be the key contributor to hyposmia following laryngectomy. Researchers concur that olfactory acuity is a function of nasal airflow, and that reduction in nasal airflow may certainly be defined as the key contributing factor to impaired olfaction following laryngectomy (Moore-Gillon, 1985; Tatchell, Lerman, & Watt, 1985; Schwartz et al., 1987; Tatchell, Lerman, & Watt, 1989; Doty & Cometto-Muniz, 2003). When nasal airflow resembling natural breathing and sniffing is reestablished using puffs of air from squeeze bottles (Moore-Gillon, 1985) or prosthetic devices that reconnect the nose and the lungs (Schwartz et al., 1987; Tatchell et al., 1985; Tatchell et al., 1989), improvements in olfactory acuity are evident.

Research has also revealed that olfactory epithelial damage is present in patients following total laryngeal surgery. A recent study which conducted histological examination of the olfactory epithelium of 10 laryngectomy patients and 10 control patients revealed that although there were similarities between the two groups, there was evidence of epithelial degeneration in the laryngectomy group (Miani et al., 2003). The authors concluded that it is the combination of the loss of nasal airflow and degenerative phenomena of the neuroepithelium which contribute to the olfactory deficits in patients following total laryngectomy.

Given the role of smell in the identification of food flavors and its subsequent contribution to nutrition, it is likely that olfactory impairment following laryngectomy would produce changes in the hunger, appetite, dietary habits, and nutritional status of laryngectomy patients. Several studies have suggested that changes in taste and smell are indeed correlated with anorexia, decreased nutrient intake, and malnutrition in cancer patients (DeWys & Walters, 1975; Nitenberg & Raynard, 2000). This is an area that has been well researched due to the clinical importance of maintaining nutrition in this patient population, particularly for those patients with ongoing oncological treatment regimens. The physical ramifications of poor nutrition in the cancer patient have been demonstrated to include impaired wound healing, impaired immune responses, impaired musculoskeletal performance, and generalized fatigue (Larsson, Akerlind, Permerth, & Hornqvist, 1995). Poor nutrition may also be associated with a poor response to therapy, tumor extension, and metastases (Nitenberg & Raynard, 2000). These factors may additionally impact on survival by reducing a patient's ability to withstand the side effects of treatment and therefore to tolerate the treatment per se (Daly & Torosian, 1993). The literature suggests that these issues translate directly into increased morbidity and mortality in those cancer patients with poor nutrition (Daly & Torosian, 1993).

Despite the gravity of poor nutrition in cancer patients and its obvious interaction with smell ability, the impact of hyposmia on eating behaviors and quality of life postlaryngectomy is sparsely documented in the literature and is frequently overlooked in preoperative

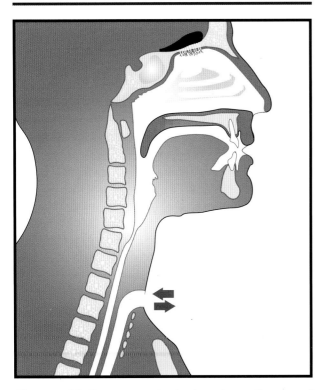

**Figure 13–3.** Anatomical situation after total laryngectomy.

counseling (Van Dam et al., 1999; Lennie et al., 2001). To date, only two studies have investigated the impact of deteriorated olfaction on eating behaviors and quality of life in laryngectomy patients. Van Dam and colleagues (1999) objectively assessed the olfaction of 63 laryngectomized patients and divided them into groups of "smellers" and "nonsmellers." Sixty eight percent of the patients were "nonsmellers" and reported reduced taste and appetite as well as changes in dietary habits and an inability to enjoy food subsequent to changes in the faculty of taste. Of particular clinical importance was the reported 50% of patients who were given no information regarding potential postoperative changes in smell and taste acuity during the preoperative counseling period. Following their operation, 91% of the patients reported that they were not given rehabilitative instruction in how to compensate for any changes in smell and taste (Van Dam et al., 1999).

Lennie and colleagues (2001) issued a "Food Eating Experiences and Diet Questionnaire" to 34 people involved in an Internet based laryngectomy support group. This questionnaire compared pre- and postlaryngectomy eating behaviors by patient report. Eighty nine percent of those surveyed reported reductions in postoperative olfaction and 63% reported less effective taste following laryngectomy. Twenty nine percent of patients reported decreases in both the intensity of hunger sensations and the amount of food consumed per day and 42% of patients reported a decrease in their overall enjoyment of eating. Additionally, these patients reported that little to no attention was given to changes in smell or taste during preoperative counseling. When asked what type of information they wish they had been told, the patients reported that recommendations to cope with loss of smell and taste needed the most additional attention (Lennie et al., 2001).

## Assessment of Olfaction

The patients' self-reported medical history and symptoms provide important information for the diagnosis of olfactory impairment (Nordin, Bramerson, Murphy, & Bende, 2003). To complement this, the clinician can create simple rating scales to help quantify the severity of function/dysfunction using simple 5-, 7-, or 10-point scales with criteria ranging from very poor, to very good, sense of smell. There are also standard questionnaires available to examine olfaction function. Examples of those types of questionnaires are the Questionnaire Olfaction Taste and Appetite, also called AHSP (Appetite, Hunger, and Sensory Perception questionnaire) (de Jong, Mulder, de Graaf, & van Staveren, 1999; Mathey, 2001), the Multi-Clinic Smell and Taste Questionnaire (Nordin et al., 2003), or the Chemosensory Questionnaire (Goldberg, Shea, Deems, & Doty, 2005).

In addition to rating scales and questionnaires, there are a variety of assessments of olfaction commercially available, which have been developed for different clinical purposes and different cultural regions. The different tests mostly discriminate between anosmia, hyposmia, and normosmia. Because each test has its own merits in terms of facility of administration, cost, and reproducibility of results, no globally accepted gold standard exists. Unfortunately, as different tests have been used all over the world, comparison of clinical or research data can be difficult. Study results suggest that data on subjects with diagnoses of anosmia or normosmia are more reliable than data on subjects with different levels of hyposmia (Tsukatani, Reiter, Miwa, & Costanzo, 2005).

Doty, Smith, McKeown, and Raj (1994) compared different olfactory tests (e.g., odor detection, discrimination, identification, and memory) and found that the tests cover different aspects of olfaction, only covering overall olfactory performance when used in combination. For example some tests are combined tests; e.g., "Sniffin Sticks" includes tests for odor threshold, odor discrimination, and odor identification, while the Connecticut Chemosensory Clinical Research Center (CCCRC) test (Cain & Rabin, 1989) includes an odor threshold test and an odor identification test. Some of the different types of tests of olfaction available include:

■ Odor Detection Tests. These assess the person's ability to detect an odor when multiple trials are presented with only one of the trials actually having an odor. An example of an odor detection test is contained as part of the Sniffin Sticks system. In this test there are sets of three sticks of which only one has an odor.

■ Odor Identification Tests. Odor identification tests typically involve presenting an odor to the patient to identify (e.g., orange, smoke). Examples of such assessments include the University of Pennsylvania Smell Identification Test (UPSIT) (Doty et al., 1984), the Cross Cultural Smell Identification Test (CC-SIT) (Doty, Marcus, & Lee, 1996), "Sniffin Sticks" (Hummel, Sekinger, Wolf, Pauli, & Kobal, 1997), the Scandinavian Odor Identification Test (SOIT) (Hummel et al., 1997; Nordin, Bramerson, Liden, & Bende, 1998), the European Test of Olfaction Capabilities (ETOC) (Thomas-Danguin et al., 2003), the T&T Olfactometer (Takagi, 1989), Smell Diskettes (ZGT) (Briner & Simmen, 1999), the Yes-No odor identification test (Corwin, 1989), and the CCCRC odor identification test (Cain & Rabin, 1989).

■ Olfactory Sensitivity Tests (odor detection and recognition thresholds). These assessments involve presenting an odor of varying intensity levels and determining at what point the odor is detected. The Single Ascending Series Butanol Odor Detection Threshold Test (Cain & Rabin, 1989), the Phenyl Ethyl Alcohol Single Staircase Odor Detection Threshold Test (Deems & Doty, 1987), the Single Series Phenyl Ethyl Methyl Ethyl Carbinol (PEMEC) odor detection threshold test (Amoore & Ollman, 1983), the CCCRC threshold test (Cain, Gent, Goodspeed, & Leonard, 1988), and "Sniffin Sticks" (Hummel et al., 1997), are all examples of odor sensitivity tests.

■ Odor Discrimination Tests. In this type of assessment, the person is presented with sets of odors of which all will have the same odor except one, which is different. The person has to identify the one that is different. Examples of this type of assessment tool include the Odor Discrimination Test (Smith, Doty, Burlingame, & McKeown, 1993), and "Sniffin Sticks" (Hummel et al., 1997).

■ Odor Memory Tests. An odor memory test involves presenting a particular odor to the patient, and then, following time delays, having the patient identify that odor from a selection of distracter odors. An example is the Odor Recognition Memory Test (Mair et al., 1986).

■ Tests of Suprathreshold Scaling of Odor Intensity and Pleasantness Perception. In this type of assessment the person must reference or judge odor intensity. An example is the Suprathreshold Amyl Acetate Odor Intensity and Odor Pleasantness rating test (Doty, 1975).

Of these, the more widely used tests currently include the CCCRC test (Connecticut Chemosensorial Clinical Research Center), the University of Pennsylvania Smell Identification Test (UPSIT), the T&T Olfactometer, and the "Sniffin Sticks" assessment battery.

## Rehabilitation of Olfaction Following Total Laryngectomy

Rehabilitation of olfaction is not currently an area of clinical focus in laryngectomy rehabilitation. In fact, only 9% of laryngectomy patients report any postsurgical instruction in the area of smell and taste rehabilitation (Lennie et al., 2001). However, there are both prosthetic devices and behavioral treatment methods available to assist in reestablishing olfaction postlaryngectomy.

### Prosthetic Devices

Clinical attention to impaired olfaction has seen the development of several prosthetic devices. These include the "nipple tube" (Bosone, 1984), the oral tracheal breathing tube (Knudson & Williams, 1989), and the larynx bypass (Schwartz et al., 1987; Tatchell et al., 1985). Essentially, these instruments all act to bypass the larynx and reestablish the airway between the tracheobronchial tree and the nose. With each device, a tube is passed between the sealed stoma and the oropharynx such that inspiration draws air in through the nose, restoring orthonasal olfaction. Examples of patients using different types of laryngeal bypasses are demonstrated in Figures 13–4 and 13–5. The reader is also referred to the video segment on the CD (Chapter 13: Video: "Laryngeal Bypass") to see a patient using a bypass to reestablish nasal airflow.

Research has testified to the efficacy of these devices in restoring olfaction to laryngectomized patients (Schwartz et al., 1987; Tatchell et al., 1985). For example, one study of 25 laryngectomy patients

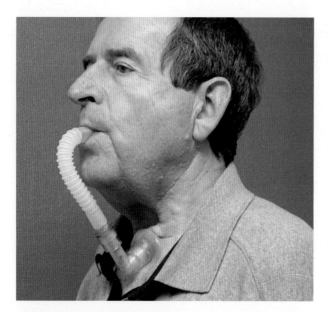

**Figure 13–4.** Photo of a patient using a larynx bypass attached to an HME baseplate. (Photo courtesy of Jan Persson.)

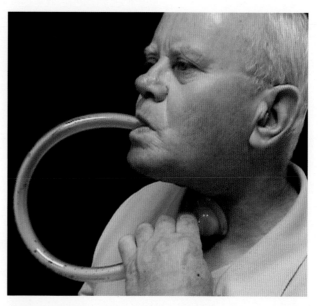

**Figure 13–5.** Photo of a patient using a laryngeal bypass system connected to the stoma using a nipple from a baby's bottle.

using the larynx bypass revealed no significant differences in smell detection thresholds and smell identification accuracy between the laryngectomees and the controls (Tatchell et al., 1985). The functional application of such devices however, remains questionable. The apparatuses themselves are conspicuous and intrusive. It is unlikely their use would extend beyond the laboratory and this limitation was not addressed in the aforementioned articles. As such, it is expected that these olfactory aids would have little impact on olfactory ability in everyday situations. Despite their limitations, they do provide a viable option in clinical practice to assess the olfactory function of laryngectomees.

## Nasal Airflow Inducing Maneuver

Although it is recognized that the loss of respiratory airflow through the upper airways impairs olfaction postlaryngectomy, there are patients who unintentionally compensate for the loss of the sense of smell (Moore-Gillon, 1985; Schwartz et al., 1987; Van Dam et al., 1999). In those patients who were able to smell postsurgery, Van Dam et al. (1999) observed more active use of muscles in the face and neck compared

to the patients who were not able to smell. These observations led to the development of the Nasal Airflow Inducing Maneuver (NAIM), a maneuver that induces orthonasal airflow.

The NAIM is described by Hilgers et al. (2000) and is also referred to as the "polite yawning technique." The "polite yawn" aims to establish a negative pressure in the oral cavity and oropharynx that naturally draws air in through the nose. Negative pressure is attained through increasing the volume of the oral cavity and oropharynx, by tightly sealing the lips and simultaneously lowering the jaw, floor of mouth, tongue, base of tongue, and soft palate in a "polite yawn." By making a movement that is similar to yawning with the lips politely closed, the oral cavity is enlarged and the vacuum that is created causes air to flow into the nose: orthonasal airflow. This airflow carries the odor molecules to the olfactory epithelium and thereby restores the orthonasal airflow and thus the sense of smell. The key points of instruction include:

1. Move the lower jaw and floor of mouth downward in a rapid but relaxed movement
2. Move the tongue downward simultaneously, starting from the palate

3. Keep the lips closed
4. Repeat this movement a few times to allow the air to reach the olfactory epithelium

Figures 13-6A and 13-6B are a schematic representation of how this movement should be carried out, while Figure 13-7 shows a patient at rest and demonstrating the maneuver. While performing the technique it is important not to breathe in too heavily simultaneously with performing the movement. Many laryngectomees initially do breathe in during the movement simply because they are used to inhaling or sniffing when trying to smell. It is not necessary at all and may cause dizziness. Video footage is available on the CD of a patient learning to do the technique (Chapter 13: Video: "Learning NAIM").

Once they have established the technique, some laryngectomees are able to refine the technique using smaller yet as effective movements, making the maneuver less visible and thus more comfortable to use in public. To achieve this goal, it is advised to start with the (easier) regular polite yawning at first. Then teach the patients to use an isolated pumping movement of the back of the tongue and the floor of the mouth and eliminate the downward movement of the jaw (see Figure 13-8A and B). This closely resembles the breathing pattern of frogs (See DVD: Chapter 13: Video: "Frog Breathing"). Many patients also find that small, fast repetitions of the technique (like a series of small rapid sniffs) also helps to optimize nasal airflow yet minimize the obtrusiveness of the technique.

The key points for training the more refined movement include:

1. Keep the lips closed
2. Start in a position where the tongue is held against the palate
3. Stabilize the tip of the tongue against the front teeth or alveolar ridge
4. Move the back of the tongue downwards in a pumping motion
5. Repeat the movement in quick rapid succession

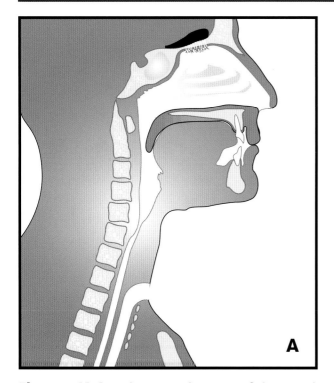 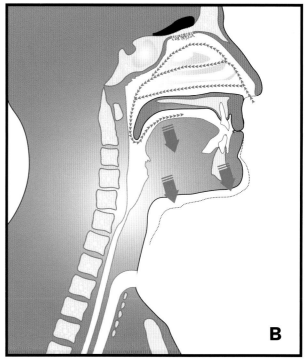

**Figures 13-6.** Schematic drawing of the Nasal Airflow Inducing Maneuver. Position at rest **A.** and orthonasal airflow induced by enlargement of the oral cavity by lowering the tongue, floor of mouth, and mandible **B.**

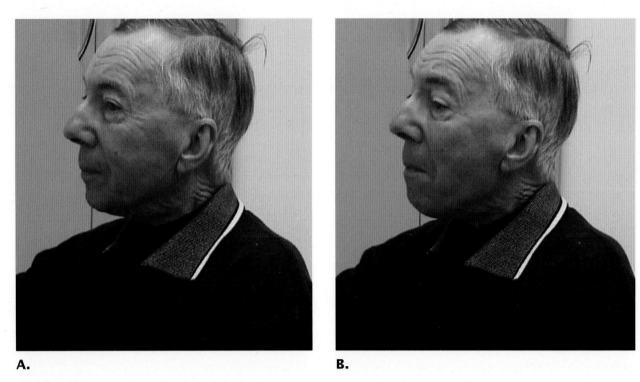

**Figure 13–7.** Patient demonstrating Nasal Airflow Inducing Maneuver at rest **A.** and with jaw lowered **B.**

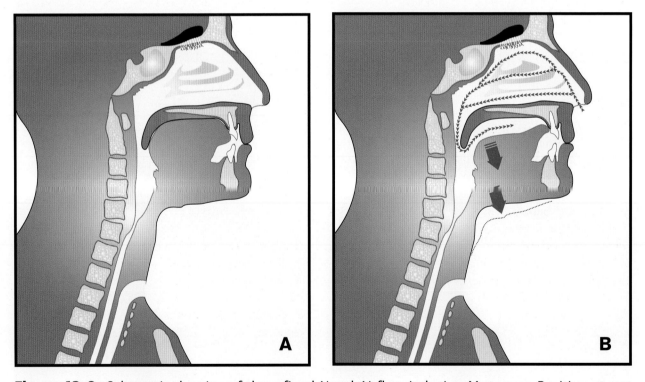

**Figure 13–8.** Schematic drawing of the refined Nasal Airflow Inducing Maneuver. Position at rest **A.** and orthonasal airflow induced by enlargement of the oral cavity by lowering the tongue and floor of mouth only (mandible remains in rest position) **B.**

## Patient Suitability for NAIM Training

Ideally, it is best to determine patient suitability for NAIM training during the presurgery assessment and counseling sessions. In the preoperative session, the loss of olfaction and the possibility of rehabilitation should be discussed. During this visit it is important to find out how good the patient's current sense of smell is by using any of the assessment techniques outlined previously. At this point, those patients who are determined to be anosmic for other reasons can be identified and deemed unsuitable for rehabilitation.

Although early postoperative intervention may be the most beneficial for the patient, studies have shown that patients who have had their total laryngectomy many years prior can still regain their sense of smell using this technique (Hilgers et al., 2000; Risberg-Berlin, Ylitalo, & Finizia, 2006). If the patient has already undergone laryngeal surgery, determining patient suitability for NAIM training can be determined by either anecdotal reports of occasional smell perception postsurgery (such as when near pungent odors such as petrol) or by direct assessment using a laryngeal bypass. Although the laryngeal bypass reestablishes orthonasal airflow, for some patients, particularly those long-term postsurgery, a laryngeal bypass assessment may be unsuccessful. Risberg-Berlin et al. (2006) showed that one cannot rely on the use of a larynx bypass to predict whether a patient is anosmic. Two of the five patients who were not able to smell with the larynx bypass were able to smell with the NAIM technique, and were categorized as smellers after the study. Thus, the results from a laryngeal bypass may give an indication but cannot predict with certainty whether a patient would benefit from olfactory rehabilitation. In addition, some patients who are many years postsurgery may be unable to use the laryngeal bypass, as the tissues of the nasopharynx may be obstructing nasal airflow. For some patients, encouraging them to relax and think about sniffing when inhaling can help reflexively stimulate improved opening of the nasopharynx and establish airflow.

There are some factors, however, that may influence the patient's ability to make the movements associated with the NAIM. Radiation induced fibrosis leading to stiffness in the neck or jaw or hypomobility of the jaw (trismus) may limit the jaw mobility or mouth opening needed for the movement. In this case, concentrating on teaching the smaller base of tongue action right from the start may help. For these patients, additional intervention using a passive jaw mobilization device (Therabite, Atos Medical, Hörby, Sweden) may be beneficial to improve jaw movements for all functions, including smelling.

Some patients may also have difficulty closing the lips due to uni- or bilateral weakness in the lower lip after radical neck dissection (mandibular branch of facial nerve may be affected). Additional lip training or immediate use of the smaller movement may help. Patients with partial or total glossectomy have been found to be able to regain olfaction with the technique even though they cannot carry out the tongue movement in an optimal way. The large movement, using the downward movement of the jaw, is optimal in those cases.

## Treatment Delivery

Except for the first training session, which may take 20 to 30 minutes to establish the technique, subsequent training sessions typically take only 10–15 minutes. Therefore, for early postoperative patients, NAIM training can easily be incorporated as a part of the normal postsurgical training sessions for voice and swallow rehabilitation. For patients who remain hospitalized because of complications with wound healing, rehabilitation of olfaction can be started early while awaiting healing. In patients who had their surgery some time ago, the training can start at any given point in time.

The ultimate goal of olfaction rehabilitation should be the complete restoration of the ability to smell. This can only be achieved by active intervention during which not only proper use of the technique is accomplished, but also proper use of the technique in daily life. The therapist can give the patient suggestions on how to incorporate the technique in daily life and accomplish "automatic" use of the movement. An example of the stages of NAIM training is outlined as follows:

During the first therapy session:

- test olfaction (see section Assessment of Olfaction)
- explain and demonstrate the movement

- ask the patient to imitate
- give feedback to optimize movement
- use a water manometer to check result
- present odors to practice (for example coffee, peppermint, rose, vanilla); do not use the olfaction test for this purpose
- explain that the movement always has to be carried out in order to be able to smell
- explain the importance of frequent (automatic) use of the technique in order to reach a sense of smell as close to "normal" as possible
- propose a training schedule to practice at home with the water manometer and various odors

Then subsequent sessions would involve:

- Ask the patient to demonstrate the movement without the manometer and with the manometer.
- Give further advice based on the observations.
- Present various common odors of different intensity levels to practice (e.g., coffee, sauces, favorite perfumes). Do not use the olfaction test for this purpose. Typically begin with trials of more intense odors and as the patient masters the technique more subtle odors can be introduced, all the while encouraging automatic use of the technique. See footage on the CD of a patient during therapy completing a functional odor identification task during therapy. (Chapter 13. Video. Function odor identification).

During the final session:

- End the therapy sessions when the goal of treatment has been reached (this may differ from patient to patient and for instance may depend on their motivation and the importance of the sense of smell in their daily lives).
- Test olfaction again for treatment evaluation.
- Make a follow-up appointment for long-term outcome evaluation.

**Treatment Intensity.** Currently, researchers are investigating the frequency and duration of NAIM

training and its impact on patient outcomes. In the original research that reported the technique, Hilgers et al. (2000) showed that quite a high percentage of the participating laryngectomees (89%) were able to learn to use the technique in one therapy session. With no further direct intervention, an evaluation after 6 weeks showed that 46% of the laryngectomees that could not smell had mastered the technique and now were able to smell again (Hilgers et al., 2000). Long-term evaluation, however, showed that not all laryngectomees were able to carry out the maneuver correctly (Hilgers et al., 2002). Based on these findings, in later manuals for olfaction training (In Dutch: Polak, Van As, Van Dam, & Hilgers, 2002; In English: Polak, Van As, Van Dam, & Hilgers, 2004) the use of biofeedback techniques, such as using a water manometer, and more intensive training were suggested as possible ways to improve long-term results.

A number of researchers are currently investigating this issue of improving the long-term outcomes of NAIM training. Recently a Swedish prospective intervention study trained 24 laryngectomized patients in the NAIM technique using a more intensive rehabilitation program, consisting of three intervention sessions within a 6-week period (Risberg-Berlin et al., 2006) and with use of a water manometer for biofeedback. Before treatment, 25% of the patients could smell within the normal range (n = 6), 17% of the patients had hyposmia (n = 4), and 58% had anosmia (n = 14). Using the NAIM technique, a success rate of 50% was found in anosmic patients after one session, and as much as 72% of the patients with impaired olfaction showed improvement after three sessions. Follow-up at 6 and 12 months post-treatment revealed that after 6 months the percentage of "smellers" was still similar to that following the intervention period; however, by 12 months an even higher percentage of patients had become smellers. These results demonstrate the importance of long-term follow-up for these patients, giving them the possibility to repeat training in the technique and use it more adequately (Risberg-Berlin et al., 2006).

The third author of this chapter (Ward) and colleagues are currently conducting a randomized NAIM treatment trial, with patients either receiving (a) a single NAIM training session and a water manometer for home practice, or (b) 6 × 15 minute sessions of NAIM training over a 6-week period (one session/week) incorporating the water manometer, functional odor identification activities, as well as home practice. This intensive or nonintensive training was delivered concurrently with dysphagia rehabilitation sessions. Preliminary analysis of the first 20 patients (10 per group) revealed that, although some patients in the nonintensive group became successful smellers, by 8 weeks following initial training a significantly greater proportion of patients in the intensive group had become successful smellers. Long-term data are still being collected. As there was no difference in the performance of both groups on the initial olfaction assessment, the authors consider that these preliminary data support that more intensive training can help optimize olfaction outcomes.

**Use of Biofeedback.** As mentioned previously, biofeedback can help facilitate NAIM training. A water manometer is a particularly useful tool for providing feedback on the success of the maneuver. In particular it shows both the clinician and the laryngectomee whether the movement is carried out correctly, and it can be used as a training instrument to further improve and stabilize the technique. Figure 13-9 demonstrates a patient at rest and then completing the NAIM maneuver. As you can see the water in the manometer is drawn up with the negative pressure of nasal inhala-

tion. If you find you have a patient who moves the water in the opposite direction, he or she is not completing the maneuver correctly and is closing the oral cavity rather than opening it. The patient needs to be reinstructed in the technique, starting with the jaw closed and tongue to the roof of the mouth, and *then* lowered to create negative nasal airflow.

With feedback from the manometer, the patient can work on improving the technique and on transferring from the larger movement to a smaller or more efficient movement. Figure 13-10 shows examples of different water manometers that can be used for patient feedback. Such devices are not currently available commercially. Polak et al. (2002, 2004) give a good description of a simple water manometer that a patient can make out of a tube, foam rubber, a piece of cardboard, and some tape. Obviously, care should be taken that any device is constructed well and cannot potentially inflict harm.

Some points of consideration when using the water manometer:

■ Always close off one nostril while holding the nasal button of the water manometer against the other nostril (explain to the patient that this is only required when practicing with the manometer and is not

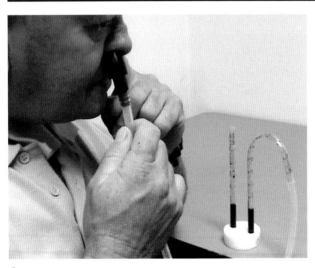 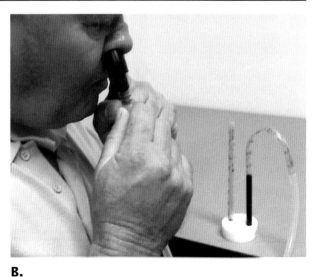

**A.**        **B.**

**Figure 13–9.** Patient using the manometer for biofeedback. Note the movement of the fluid in the manometer from rest **A.** to the lowered jaw movement **B.** creating negative nasal airflow.

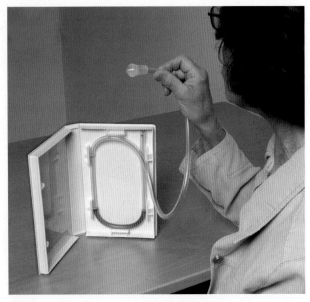

**A.**

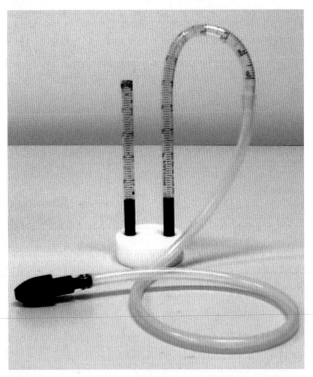

**B.**

**Figure 13–10.** Examples of water manometers. Photo **A.** is an example of a system that can be made by the patients themselves (Photo courtesy of Jan Persson.), while photo **B.** is an example of the equipment used by Polak et al. (2002, 2004) and Ward and colleagues.

necessary when carrying out the technique in daily life).

■ One nostril may be more open than the other and this may vary throughout the day; always try both nostrils for the best result.

■ Patients should be encouraged to move the water in the manometer using the NAIM technique only. In some patients, stomal inhalation will cause the water to move towards the nose as desired due to negative pressures created in the thorax and esophagus. It is also a habit to want to inhale when "sniffing." Once the patient has initially mastered the technique, inhalation during the maneuver can be gradually eliminated. Repeated inhalations during therapy can induce dizziness.

In addition to using the water manometer, both Risberg-Berlin et al. (2006) and Ward and colleagues have found that videotaping the training sessions and using the tapes as a feedback tool is helpful in teaching the technique.

**Individual versus Group Treatment.** Although group treatment leaves less room for individual attention, and the speed, ease, and ability to master the technique varies from person to person, training of this technique can be a nice group activity for patient meetings. As with individual patient sessions, it remains important to train intensively. Therefore it is suggested to briefly pay attention to the technique in a few subsequent meetings.

## Sense of Taste Following Total Laryngectomy

The sense of taste is also impacted following total laryngectomy. In a study by Ackerstaff, Hilgers, Aaronson, & Balm (1994), 15% of the laryngectomized patients reported a decreased sense of taste. Although this proportion is significantly lower than the 52% of laryngectomized patients that reported a decreased sense of smell, it is a problem that should not be neglected. Finizia, Hammerlid, Westin, and Lindström (1998) found similar results, with 50% of their laryngectomized patients reporting "much" or "very much" trouble with their sense of smell, whereas 21% reported "much" or "very much" trouble with their sense of taste.

## Assessment of Taste

As for assessments of olfactory acuity, psychosocial techniques are used to determine sensory intensity, sensory thresholds, quality identification, and quality discrimination. Clinically, basic rating scales can be used to quantify the level and extent of taste perception. There are also standardized questionnaires with questions relating to taste (as well as olfaction), such as the AHSP (de Jong et al., 1999; Mathey, 2001), the Multi-Clinic Smell and Taste Questionnaire (Nordin et al., 2003), or the Chemosensory Questionnaire (Goldberg et al., 2005).

The two main parameters of taste which are evaluated include intensity processing (both threshold detection and intensity ratings) and quality processing (identifying the quality of the sample). Taste intensity and quality are evaluated using whole mouth taste tests, in which the patient has to identify and evaluate different concentrations of taste solutions which are placed in their mouth; and spatial taste tests, in which cotton swabs are used to deliver tastes to particular parts of the mouth and/or throat. Further details of these assessments, and related clinical issues regarding taste assessment, can be found in Frank, Hettinger, Barry, Gent, and Doty (2003).

## Rehabilitation of Taste Following Total Laryngectomy

Following radiation and surgical damage, there is no therapy currently available to restore taste. Although there are medications available that may alleviate some degree of the taste distortion or burning mouth sensation that may be experienced by some following radiotherapy, only time will reveal whether or not regeneration of the nerve cells will occur and to what extent taste will be restored (Mann, 2002).

However, although little can be done to restore taste sensation, there are ways to help optimize residual taste function and also to optimize flavor perception. This can be achieved by instructing patients to use intensive chewing and back and forth movements of the food in the mouth in order to optimize gustation and retronasal olfaction (Hilgers & Ackerstaff, 2000). Increased chewing results in an increased release of odorant molecules from the food, increased saliva production to dissolve tastants, and maximal exposure of foods to the taste buds, while the induction of turbulent airflow in the oral cavity enhances retronasal olfaction (Frye, 2003; Hilgers & Ackerstaff, 2000). In addition, chewing with the lips closed is thought to result in transient increases in the closed oral cavity volume. This generates transient negative oral pressures, inducing nasal airflow and thus also encouraging orthonasal olfaction (Frye, 2003; Hilgers & Ackerstaff, 2000).

Thus, advising the laryngectomee to chew well and use the tongue actively to move the bolus around in the mouth may help optimize residual taste perception, and encourage retronasal and some degree of orthonasal olfaction. Considering that flavor perception is an integration of taste, smell, temperature, and texture, altering the texture or temperature of foods may further enhance the sensory experience of oral intake and stimulate enhanced flavor perception. Other patients may benefit from chemical enhancement of foods (flavor enhanced). At a psychological level, the presentation of food in an attractive and appetizing way, considering temperature, texture, and color, can encourage oral intake and enhance the pleasure of eating (Van Toller, 1999).

## Conclusion

Although deficits of taste and smell are recognized as negative consequences of head and neck cancer and surgical removal of the larynx, little attention has been paid to their rehabilitation postsurgery. The current chapter has provided the reader with a framework for the assessment and rehabilitation of both smell and taste. Considering that the strategies available for optimizing both olfaction and taste are simple and easy to implement within the process of postsurgical intervention, it is hoped that more clinicians will address these issues within the context of holistic rehabilitation for the patient following laryngectomy.

## Acknowledgements

Rianne Polak, Frans Hilgers, and Frits van Dam from the Netherlands Cancer Institute (Amsterdam, the Netherlands) have worked intensively together with the first author of this chapter on investigating and developing the NAIM. The authors would also like to acknowledge the contributions of Sophie Kerle from the University of Queensland to the current chapter.

## References

Ackerstaff, A. H., Hilgers, F. J., Aaronson, N. K., & Balm, A. J. (1994). Communication, functional disorders and lifestyle changes after total laryngectomy. *Clinical Otolaryngology and Allied Sciences, 19*, 295-300.

Ahlstrom, R., Berglund, B., Berglund, U., Engen, T., & Lindvall, T. (1987). A comparison of odor perception in smokers, nonsmokers, and passive smokers. *American Journal of Otolaryngology, 8*, 1-6.

Amoore, J. E., & Ollman, B. G. (1983). Practical test kits for quantitatively evaluating the sense of smell. *Rhinology, 21*, 49-54.

Asai, J. L. (2004). Nutrition and the geriatric rehabilitation patient: Challenges and solutions. *Topics in Geriatric Rehabilitation, 20*, 34-45.

Becquemin, M. H., Swift, D. L., Bouchikhi, A., Roy, M., & Teillac, A. (1991). Particle deposition and resistance in the noses of adults and children. *The European Respiratory Journal, 4*, 694-702.

Berglund, B., & Nordin, S. (1992). Detectability and perceived intensity for formaldehyde in smokers and non-smokers. *Chemical Senses, 17*, 291-306.

Berteretche, M. V., Dalix, A. M., d'Ornano, A. M., Bellisle, F., Khayat, D., & Faurion, A. (2004). Decreased taste sensitivity in cancer patients under chemotherapy. *Supportive Care in Cancer, 12*, 571-576.

Blomqvist, E. H., Bramerson, A., Stjarne, P., & Nordin, S. (2004). Consequences of olfactory loss and adopted coping strategies. *Rhinology, 42*, 189-194.

Bosone, Z. T. (1984). The nipple tube: A simple device for olfaction and nose blowing after laryngectomy. *Journal of Speech and Hearing Disorders, 49*, 106-107.

Bramerson, A., Johansson, L., Ek, L., Nordin, S., & Bende, M. (2004). Prevalence of olfactory dysfunction: The Skovde population-based study. *Laryngoscope, 114*, 733-737.

Briner, H. R., & Simmen, D. (1999). Smell diskettes as screening test of olfaction. *Rhinology, 37*, 145-148.

Burdach, K. J., & Doty, R. L. (1987). The effects of mouth movements, swallowing, and spitting on retronasal odor perception. *Physiology & Behavior, 41*, 353-356.

Burdach, K. J., Kroeze, J. H., & Koster, E. P. (1984). Nasal, retronasal, and gustatory perception: An experimental comparison. *Perception and Psychophysics, 36*, 205-208.

Cain, W. S., Gent, J. F., Goodspeed, R. B., & Leonard, G. (1988). Evaluation of olfactory dysfunction in the Connecticut Chemosensory Clinical Research Center. *Laryngoscope, 98*, 83-88.

Cain, W. S., & Rabin, M. D. (1989). Comparability of two tests of olfactory functioning. *Chemical Senses, 14*, 479-485.

Corwin, J. (1989). Olfactory identification in hemodialysis: Acute and chronic effects on discrimination and response bias. *Neuropsychologia, 27*, 513-522.

Daly, J. M., & Torosian, M. H. (1993). Nutritional support. In V. T. DeVita & S. R. S. A. Hellman (Eds.), *Cancer: Principles and practice of oncology* (4th ed., pp. 2480-2501). Philadelphia: Lippincott.

de Jong, N., Mulder, I., de Graaf, C., & van Staveren, W. A. (1999). Impaired sensory functioning in elders: The relation with its potential determinants and nutritional intake. *The Journals of Gerontology. Series A. Biological Sciences and Medical Sciences, 54*, B324-B331.

Deems, D. A., & Doty, R. L. (1987). Age-related changes in the phenyl ethyl alcohol odor detection threshold. *Transactions—Pennsylvania Academy of Ophthalmology and Otolaryngology, 39*, 646-650.

DeWys, W. D., & Walters, K. (1975). Abnormalities of taste sensation in cancer patients. *Cancer, 36*, 1888-1896.

Ding, X., & Dahl, A. R. (2003). Olfactory mucosa: Composition, enzymatic localization and metabolism. In R. L. Doty (Ed.), *Handbook of olfaction and gustation.* (2nd ed., pp. 51-74.), New York: Marcel Dekker.

Doty, R. L. (1975). An examination of relationships between the pleasantness, intensity and concentration of 10 odorous stimuli. *Perception and Psychophysics, 17*, 492-496.

Doty, R. L., Bartoshuk, L. M., & Snow, J. B. J. (1991). Causes of olfactory and gustatory diseases. In T. V. Getchell, R. L. Doty, L. M. Bartoshuk, & J. B. J. Snow (Eds.), *Smell and taste in health and disease* (pp. 449-462). New York: Raven.

Doty, R. L., & Cometto-Muniz, J. E. (2003). Trigeminal chemosensation. In R. L. Doty (Ed.), *Handbook of olfaction and gustation* (2nd ed., pp. 981-1000), New York: Marcel Dekker..

Doty, R. L., Marcus, A., & Lee, W. W. (1996). Development of the 12-item Cross-Cultural Smell Identification Test (CC-SIT). *Laryngoscope, 106*, 353-356.

Doty, R. L., Shaman, P., Applebaum, S. L., Giberson, R., Siksorski, L., & Rosenberg, L. (1984). Smell identification ability: Changes with age. *Science, 226*, 1441-1443.

Doty, R. L., Shaman, P., Kimmelman, C. P., & Dann, M. S. (1984). University of Pennsylvania Smell Identification Test: A rapid quantitative olfactory function test for the clinic. *Laryngoscope, 94*, 176-178.

Doty, R. L., Smith, R., McKeown, D. A., & Raj, J. (1994). Tests of human olfactory function: Principal components analysis suggests that most measure a common source of variance. *Perception and Psychophysics, 56*, 701-707.

Epstein, J. B., Phillips, N., Parry, J., Epstein, M. S., Nevill, T., & Stevenson-Moore, P. (2002). Quality of life, taste, olfactory and oral function following high-dose chemotherapy and allogeneic hematopoietic cell transplantation. *Bone Marrow Transplantation, 30*, 785-792.

Feldman, M., & Richardson, C. T. (1986). Total 24-hour gastric acid secretion in patients with duodenal ulcer. Comparison with normal subjects and effects of cimetidine and parietal cell vagotomy. *Gastroenterology, 90*, 540-544.

Finizia, C., Hammerlid, E., Westin, T., & Lindström, J. (1998). Quality of life and voice in patients with laryngeal carcinoma: A post treatment comparison of laryngectomy (salvage surgery) versus radiotherapy. *Laryngoscope, 108*, 1566-1573.

Frank, M. E., Hettinger, T. P., Barry, M. A., Gent, J. F., & Doty, R. L. (2003). Contemporary measurement of human gustatory function. In R. L. Doty (Ed.), *Handbook of olfaction and gustation* (2nd ed., pp. 783-804), New York: Marcel Dekker.

Frank, M. E., Hettinger, T. P., & Mott, A. E. (1992). The sense of taste: Neurobiology, aging, and medication effects. *Critical Reviews in Oral Biology and Medicine, 3*, 371-393.

Frye, R. (2003). Nasal patency and the aerodynamics of nasal airflow: Measurement by rhinomanometry and acoustic rhinometry, and the influence of pharmacological agents. In R. L. Doty (Ed.), *Handbook of olfaction and gustation* (2nd ed., pp. 439-460), New York: Marcel Dekker.

Frye, R. E., Schwartz, B. S., & Doty, R. L. (1990). Dose-related effects of cigarette smoking on olfactory function. *The Journal of the American Medical Association, 263*, 1233-1236.

Goldberg, A. N., Shea, J. A., Deems, D. A., & Doty, R. L. (2005). A ChemoSensory questionnaire for patients treated for cancer of the head and neck. *Laryngoscope, 115*, 2077-2086.

Gromysz-Kalkowska, K., Wojcik, K., Szubartowska, E., & Unkiewicz-Winiarczyk, A. (2002). Taste perception of cigarette smokers. *Annales Universitatis Mariae Curie Sklodowska [Medicine], 57*, 143-154.

Harrison, L. B., Zelefsky, M. J., Pfister, D. G., Carper, E., Raben, A., Kraus, D. H., et al. (1997). Detailed quality of life assessment in patients treated with primary radiotherapy for squamous cell cancer of the base of the tongue. *Head & Neck, 19*, 169-175.

Heald, A. E., & Schiffman, S. S. (1997). Taste and smell. Neglected senses that contribute to the malnutrition of AIDS. *North Carolina Medical Journal, 58*, 100-104.

Henkin, R. I., & Hoye, R. C. (1966). Hyposmia secondary to excision of the olfactory epithelium. The definition of primary and accessory areas of olfaction. *Life Sciences, 5*, 331-341.

Henkin, R. I., Hoye, R. C., Ketcham, A. S., & Gould, W. J. (1968). Hyposmia following laryngectomy. *Lancet, 2*, 479-481.

Hilgers, F. J., & Ackerstaff, A. H. (2000). Comprehensive rehabilitation after total laryngectomy is more than voice alone. *Folia Phoniatrica et Logopaedica, 52*, 65-73.

Hilgers, F. J., Jansen, H. A., Van As, C. J., Polak, M. F., Muller, M. J., & Van Dam, F. S. (2002). Long-term results of olfaction rehabilitation using the nasal airflow-inducing ("polite yawning") maneuver after total laryngectomy. *Archives of Otolaryngology-Head and Neck Surgery, 128*, 648-654.

Hilgers, F. J., Van Dam, F. S., Keyzers, S., Koster, M. N., Van As, C. J., & Muller, M. J. (2000). Rehabilitation of olfaction after laryngectomy by means of a nasal airflow-inducing maneuver: The "polite yawning" technique. *Archives of Otolaryngology—Head and Neck Surgery, 126*, 726-732.

Ho, W. K., Kwong, D. L., Wei, W. I., & Sham, J. S. (2002). Change in olfaction after radiotherapy for nasopharyngeal cancer—A prospective study. *American Journal of Otolaryngology, 23*, 209-214.

Hoffman, H. J., Ishii, E. K., & MacTurk, R. H. (1998). Age-related changes in the prevalence of smell/taste problems among the United States adult population.

Results of the 1994 disability supplement to the National Health Interview Survey (NHIS). *Annals of the New York Academy of Sciences, 855,* 716-722.

Huang, H. Y., Wilkie, D. J., Schubert, M. M., & Ting, L. L. (2000). Symptom profile of nasopharyngeal cancer patients during radiation therapy. *Cancer Practice, 8,* 274-281.

Hubert, H. B., Fabsitz, R. R., Feinleib, M., & Brown, K. S. (1980). Olfactory sensitivity in humans: Genetic versus environmental control. *Science, 208,* 607-609.

Hummel, T., Konnerth, C. G., Rosenheim, K., & Kobal, G. (2001). Screening of olfactory function with a four-minute odor identification test: Reliability, normative data, and investigations in patients with olfactory loss. *Annals of Otology, Rhinology, and Laryngology, 110,* 976-981.

Hummel, T., Sekinger, B., Wolf, S. R., Pauli, E., & Kobal, G. (1997). "Sniffin' sticks": Olfactory performance assessed by the combined testing of odor identification, odor discrimination and olfactory threshold. *Chemical Senses, 22,* 39-52.

Joyner, R. E. (1964). Effect of cigarette smoking on olfactory acuity. *Archives of Otolaryngology, 80,* 576-579.

Kittel, G. (1970). [Possibilities of olfactometry. Fatigue measurements in smokers]. *Zeitschrift für Laryngologie, Rhinologie, Otologie und ihre Grenzgebiete, 49,* 376-386.

Knudson, R. C., & Williams, E. O. (1989). Olfaction through oral tracheal breathing tube. *The Journal of Prosthetic Dentistry, 61,* 471-472.

Kobal, G., & Hummel, T. (1991). Human electro-olfactograms and brain responses to olfactory stimulation. In D. G. Laing, R. L. Doty, & W. Breipohl (Eds.), *The human sense of smell* (pp. 135-150). Berlin: Springer-Verlag.

Laing, D. G., & Francis, G. W. (1989). The capacity of humans to identify odors in mixtures. *Physiology and Behavior, 46,* 809-814.

Laing, D. G., & Willcox, M. E. (1983). Perception of components in binary odour mixtures. *Chemical Senses, 17,* 249-264.

Landis, B. N., Konnerth, C. G., & Hummel, T. (2004). A study on the frequency of olfactory dysfunction. *Laryngoscope, 114,* 1764-1769.

Larsson, J., Akerlind, I., Permerth, J., & Hornqvist, J. O. (1995). Impact of nutritional state on quality of life in surgical patients. *Nutrition, 11,* 217-220.

Larsson, M., Finkel, D., & Pedersen, N. L. (2000). Odor identification: Influences of age, gender, cognition, and personality. *The Journal of Gerontology. Series B, Psychological Sciences and Social Sciences, 55,* 304-310.

Lebenthal, E. (1987). Role of salivary amylase in gastric and intestinal digestion of starch. *Digestive Diseases and Sciences, 32,* 1155-1157.

Lennie, T. A., Christman, S. K., & Jadack, R. A. (2001). Educational needs and altered eating habits following a total laryngectomy. *Oncology Nursing Forum, 28,* 667-674.

Logemann, J. A., Smith, C. H., Pauloski, B. R., Rademaker, A. W., Lazarus, C. L., Colangelo, L. A., et al. (2001). Effects of xerostomia on perception and performance of swallow function. *Head & Neck, 23,* 317-321.

Mair, R. G., Doty, R. L., Kelly, K. M., Wilson, C. S., Langlais, P. J., McEntee, W. J., et al. (1986). Multimodal sensory discrimination deficits in Korsakoff's psychosis. *Neuropsychologia, 24,* 831-839.

Mann, N. M. (2002). Management of smell and taste problems. *Cleveland Clinic Journal of Medicine, 69,* 329-336.

Martin, S., & Pangborn, R. M. (1970). A note on responses to ethyl alcohol before and after smoking. *Perception and Psychophysics, 8,* 169-170.

Mathey, M. F. (2001). Assessing appetite in Dutch elderly with the Appetite, Hunger and Sensory Perception (AHSP) questionnaire. *Journal of Nutrition, Health and Aging, 5,* 22-28.

Mattes, R. D. (1997). Physiologic responses to sensory stimulation by food: Nutritional implications. *Journal of the American Dietetic Association, 97,* 406-413.

Miani, C., Ortolani, F., Bracale, A. M., Petrelli, L., Staffieri, A., & Marchini, M. (2003). Olfactory mucosa histological findings in laryngectomees. *European Archives of Otorhinolaryngology, 260,* 529-535.

Miwa, T., Furukawa, M., Tsukatani, T., Costanzo, R. M., DiNardo, L. J., & Reiter, E. R. (2001). Impact of olfactory impairment on quality of life and disability. *Archives of Otolaryngology-Head and Neck Surgery, 127,* 497-503.

Moore-Gillon, V. (1985). The nose after laryngectomy. *Journal of the Royal Society of Medicine, 78,* 435-439.

Mozell, M. M. (1971). *The chemical senses II.* New York: Holt, Rinehart and Winston.

Mozell, M. M., Smith, B. P., Smith, P. E., Sullivan, R. L., Jr., & Swender, P. (1969). Nasal chemoreception in flavor identification. *Archives of Otolaryngology, 90,* 367-373.

Murphy, C., Schubert, C. R., Cruickshanks, K. J., Klein, B. E., Klein, R., & Nondahl, D. M. (2002). Prevalence of olfactory impairment in older adults. *The Jour-

*nal of the American Medical Association, 288,* 2307-2312.

Nitenberg, G., & Raynard, B. (2000). Nutritional support of the cancer patient: Issues and dilemmas. *Critical Reviews in Oncology/Hematology, 34,* 137-168.

Nordin, S., Bramerson, A., Liden, E., & Bende, M. (1998). The Scandinavian Odor-Identification Test: Development, reliability, validity and normative data. *Acta Otolaryngologica, 118,* 226-234.

Nordin, S., Bramerson, A., Murphy, C., & Bende, M. (2003). A Scandinavian adaptation of the Multi-Clinic Smell and Taste Questionnaire: Evaluation of questions about olfaction. *Acta Otolaryngologica, 123,* 536-542.

Pangborn, R. M., Trabue, I. M., & Barylko-Pikielna, N. (1967). Taste, odor, and tactile discrimination before and after smoking. *Perception and Psychophysics, 2,* 529-532.

Polak, M. F., Van As, C. J., Van Dam, F. S., & Hilgers, F. J. (2004). *Olfaction regained, using the polite yawning technique* [CD-ROM]. Amsterdam: the Netherlands Cancer Institute.

Polak, M. F., Van As, C. J., Van Dam, F. S. A. M., & Hilgers, F. J. M. (2002). *Reukrevalidatie voor gelaryngectomeerden. Handleiding voor logopedisten.* Lisse: Swets & Zeitlinger.

Ravasco, P. (2005). Aspects of taste and compliance in patients with cancer. *European Journal of Oncology Nursing, 9,* Supplement 2, S84-S91.

Rehn, T. (1978). Perceived odor intensity as a function of air flow through the nose. *Sensory Processes, 2,* 198-205.

Richter, C. P. (1942). Total self regulatory functions in animals and human beings. *Harvey Lecture Series, 38,* 68-103.

Risberg-Berlin, B., Ylitalo, R., & Finizia, C. (2006). Screening and rehabilitation of olfaction after total laryngectomy in Swedish patients: Results from an intervention study using the Nasal Airflow-Inducing Maneuver. *Archives of Otolaryngology-Head and Neck Surgery, 132,* 301-306.

Schiffman, S. S. (1997). Taste and smell losses in normal aging and disease. *The Journal of the American Medical Association, 278,* 1357-1362.

Schwartz, D. N., Mozell, M. M., Youngentob, S. L., Leopold, D. L., & Sheehe, P. R. (1987). Improvement of olfaction in laryngectomized patients with the larynx bypass. *Laryngoscope, 97,* 1280-1286.

Sherwood, L. (2001). *Human physiology: From cells to systems.* (4th ed.). Pacific Grove, California, USA: Brooks Cole Publishing Co.

Smith, R. S., Doty, R. L., Burlingame, G. K., & McKeown, D. A. (1993). Smell and taste function in the visually impaired. *Perception and Psychophysics, 54,* 649-655.

Takagi, S. F. (1989). *Human olfaction.* Tokyo: University of Tokyo Press.

Tatchell, R. H., Lerman, J. W., & Watt, J. (1985). Olfactory ability as a function of nasal air flow volume in laryngectomees. *American Journal of Otolaryngology, 6,* 426-432.

Tatchell, R. H., Lerman, J. W., & Watt, J. (1989). Speech acceptability and olfaction in laryngectomees. *Journal of Communication Disorders, 22,* 35-47.

Tennen, H., Affleck, G., & Mendola, R. (1991). *Coping with smell and taste disorders.* New York: Raven Press.

Thomas-Danguin, T., Rouby, C., Sicard, G., Vigouroux, M., Farget, V., Johanson, A., et al. (2003). Development of the ETOC: A European test of olfactory capabilities. *Rhinology, 41,* 142-151.

Trotti, A., Johnson, D. J., Gwede, C., Casey, L., Sauder, B., Cantor, A., et al. (1998). Development of a head and neck companion module for the quality of life-radiation therapy instrument (QOL-RTI). *International Journal of Radiation Oncology, Biology, Physics, 42,* 257-261.

Tsukatani, T., Reiter, E. R., Miwa, T., & Costanzo, R. M. (2005). Comparison of diagnostic findings using different olfactory test methods. *Laryngoscope, 115,* 1114-1117.

Van Dam, F. S., Hilgers, F. J., Emsbroek, G., Touw, F. I., Van As, C. J., & de Jong, N. (1999). Deterioration of olfaction and gustation as a consequence of total laryngectomy. *Laryngoscope, 109,* 1150-1155.

Van Toller, S. (1999). Assessing the impact of anosmia: Review of a questionnaire's findings. *Chemical Senses, 24,* 705-712.

Van Toller, S., & Dodd, G. H. (1987). Presbyosmia and olfactory compensation for the elderly. *The British Journal of Clinical Practice, 41,* 725-728.

Venstrom, D., & Amoore, J. E. (1968). Olfactory threshold in relation to age, sex or smoking. *Journal of Food Sciences, 33,* 264-265.

Vroon, P., van Amerongen, A., & de Vries, H. (1994). *Verborgen verleider: Psychologie van de reuk.* Baarn, the Netherlands: Ambo.

Weinstock, R. S., Wright, H. N., & Smith, D. U. (1993). Olfactory dysfunction in diabetes mellitus. *Physiology & Behavior, 53,* 17-21.

Welge-Luessen, A., Kobal, G., & Wolfensberger, M. (2000). Assessing olfactory function in laryngectomees using the Sniffin' Sticks test battery and chemosensory evoked potentials. *Laryngoscope, 110*, 303–307.

Wickham, R. S., Rehwaldt, M., Kefer, C., Shott, S., Abbas, K., Glynn-Tucker, E., et al. (1999). Taste changes experienced by patients receiving chemotherapy. *Oncology Nursing Forum, 26*, 697–706.

Wilson, J., & Rees, J. S. (2005). The dental treatment needs and oral side effects of patients undergoing outpatient cancer chemotherapy. *The European Journal of Prosthodontics and Restorative Dentistry, 13*, 129–134.

Zheng, W. K., Inokuchi, A., Yamamoto, T., & Komiyama, S. (2002). Taste dysfunction in irradiated patients with head and neck cancer. *Fukuoka Igaku Zasshi, 93*, 64–76.

# Chapter 14

# PATIENT SUPPORT AND MULTIDISCIPLINARY MANAGEMENT

Nadine R. Manison and Elizabeth C. Ward

## CHAPTER OUTLINE

# Introduction

The importance of multidisciplinary care for patients with head and neck (H&N) cancer has been highlighted numerous times in the previous chapters of this textbook. Many patients with H&N cancer, regardless of the treatment approach they receive, will require long-term specialist support from a variety of health care professionals, particularly speech-language pathologists (SLPs), nurses, dietitians, and managing medical staff. This service is most efficiently delivered in an integrated, multidisciplinary framework that fosters ongoing communication between team members. Within the present chapter, the multidisciplinary approach to cancer care and the role of the multidisciplinary team members will be outlined along with important principles for counseling and patient support. The final section of the chapter will discuss the management issues associated with some special populations, including patients undergoing total laryngectomy, pediatric patients with H&N cancer, and those patients requiring palliative care. These populations in particular have extensive challenges to face and the provision of high quality and coordinated multidisciplinary management and counseling is pivotal to their care.

# The Multidisciplinary Approach

The cancer framework within Australia, and many other countries, has a strong emphasis on a multidisciplinary approach to cancer care to ensure that services are effective and efficient and fulfill the needs of patients, their families, and other caregivers. In addition to optimizing coordination of standard treatment options, the multidisciplinary approach also helps ensure patients have access to the latest clinical trials and protocols, if applicable.

Although internationally it is accepted that multidisciplinary care is integral to optimal patient management, slight variance exists between health facilities regarding exactly how services are arranged and coordinated. Within many countries, the assessment and management of H&N cancer has become increasingly concentrated in specialist cancer care centers. This allows patients to receive services from teams with the most experience. In some settings, clinical criteria regarding levels of experience are being adopted to ensure ongoing standards. An example of such criteria is the United Kingdom NICE (National Institute for Health and Clinical Excellence, 2004) recommendation for clinicians to manage a minimum of approximately 100 patients per year in order to maintain clinical expertise in the treatment of H&N cancers.

In addition to recognizing the need for skilled team members, many cancer services operate under patient management frameworks based around dedicated cancer types (e.g., H&N, colorectal, breast, lung) to further enhance the quality of care. These frameworks are developed from current best practice, including clinical guidelines, care pathways, consensus statements, and research that exists to support optimal care at critical points. An example of this type of approach is currently being implemented within Victoria, Australia. The Cancer Services Framework has been developed which divides the state of Victoria into eight regions (three metropolitan and five rural) where hospitals, primary, and community centers work together to provide integrated care for the communities they service. Each of these Integrated Cancer Services (ICS) ensures the care provided will be multidisciplinary and well coordinated. The clinical treatment and care is then delivered in streams in each of these ICSs, with each stream focusing on a particular cancer (e.g., H&N, colorectal, breast, lung). Such structure affords patients consistent care across the state, so that all cancer patients will have the benefit of experienced multidisciplinary, multimodality coordinated care in the assessment of their disease, the planning and provision of treatment, and follow-up services.

## Stages of Multidisciplinary Care

The multidisciplinary management of patients with H&N cancer is ongoing from the point of initial diagnosis, and continues for as long as needed. Within each stage of the continuum of care—pretreatment, during treatment, and post-treatment—different members of the multidisciplinary team are needed to address the issues facing the patient. In order to help the patient navigate his or her way through the maze of investigations, appointments, and services on offer, the multidisciplinary team will typically include an individual (usually a specialized nurse with experience in the cancer area) who has responsibility for coordinating the patient's transit through assessment, treatment, and follow-up. This coordinator is also responsible for ensuring that the patient is well informed and for advocating that the patient's own decisions and requirements are respected.

## Pretreatment Planning and Support

Multidisciplinary treatment will usually commence at the planning phase of treatment. Many health services/ hospitals will have a dedicated multidisciplinary H&N oncology meeting that is used to discuss new patients presenting with H&N cancer. At these meetings initial case history information (including past medical history, initial symptoms of disease development, recent biopsy/medical interventions) is presented by the referring surgeons/physician and review of any radiological imaging by the radiologist. Patients are often required to attend the clinic that day so that the multidisciplinary team can examine them and their tumor site.

The pretreatment meeting has become increasingly important as a setting in which all health care professionals can meet to develop the treatment plan appropriate for the patient's psychological and functional needs. The meeting alerts all team members to relevant issues that may influence rehabilitation planning, which also begins at this initial meeting. Attendance at these multidisciplinary team meetings provides team members the opportunity to express their opinions through open discussion, and in some cases debate, leading to a team consensus for optimal patient treatment. At the end of this consultative meeting, a team representative returns to the patient to convey the recommendations and make future appointments/ referrals as required. The plan is documented in the patient's medical history, and letters summarizing the discussion and recommended treatment plan are sent to referring surgeons and/or physicians to ensure communication of information between the treating facility and the community.

The treatment planning phase allows the patient and family to be presented with a choice of treatment options available and to be involved in decision making. At this stage patients may require considerable support and counseling as they take in the diagnosis

and the treatment planned for them. Key members of the multidisciplinary team including the medical staff, the SLP, and the social worker are most likely to spend the greatest amount of time with the patient providing the support, education, and counseling at this point. This ensures the patients have a sound understanding of what is happening to them and the treatment planned for them. On the accompanying CD there is a video segment of a patient describing her initial reactions, and her experience with the team approach in this early stage of care (Chapter 14: Video: "Shock and Adjustment").

## Multidisciplinary Care during Treatment

Once the multidisciplinary team has determined the treatment approach, patient care is delivered by the appropriate specialist clinicians. The approaches used during the acute phase may differ slightly between different hospitals and centers. Although many centers do not have weekly multidisciplinary team meetings, all staff working on the acute wards will be aware of patient progress and status. Clinicians working on the wards communicate easily and frequently ensuring all team members are updated with information from each other throughout the day and across the week. This tends to happen effectively in an ad hoc manner. In some hospitals formal weekly team meetings or discharge planning meetings provide additional forums and opportunity for the team members to communicate.

## Ongoing Multidisciplinary Care

The patient with H&N cancer often presents with complex home care needs at the completion of treatment. Both surgical and nonsurgical management can often be debilitating, with many patients experiencing persistent side effects such as difficulty chewing, swallowing, and speaking, discomfort associated with damaged and sore skin/tissues, and psychological/psychosocial distress associated with postsurgical esthetic and vocational/ lifestyle changes. Both patients and caregivers usually require support to make the adjustments required to live with the effects of H&N cancer. On the CD there are two patients describing the significant adjustments for them and their families on coming home from the hospital (Chapter 14: Video: "Coming Home").

When treatment is completed, patients continue to require input from specialist clinicians such as the social worker and SLP. Now that the person is being managed as an outpatient, the responsibility to ensure good communication between team members requires increased effort. Not all clinicians may be involved (in comparison to the acute phase where virtually all members are involved); therefore, there is less informal discussion in the corridors and sometimes increased time is required to source the colleague needed.

## Limitations of the Multidisciplinary Approach

Although the multidisciplinary model of care is advantageous in many ways, there are also some recognized disadvantages. These may include:

- Only brief consultation time possible with each discipline in early diagnosis/treatment planning stages.
- Patients often experience long waits due to clinic organization and coordination between appointments.
- Appointment times and dates are often inflexible.
- The atmosphere can be intimidating for some patients.
- Such multidisciplinary teams are unlikely to exist in rural centers; therefore, some patients are faced with large distances to travel to specialist centers.

Many of these disadvantages may be overcome by increasing resources. Having additional rooms available and surplus of personnel can help alleviate delays and scheduling problems. In addition, having a good clinical nurse manager in charge of the coordinated care of the patient can help to alleviate much of the pressure regarding scheduling of appointments and timing of visits to professionals. A good nurse manager can also help alleviate patient fears and concerns by keeping the patient well informed throughout the care and ensuring appropriate referrals to additional support services, such as social work and psychology, are provided as needed. The issues of distance to centers will always be a problem for many patients, particularly in countries such as Australia where almost a third of the population live in more rural and remote areas of the country. However it is possible that advances in telehealth networks and the provision of health care via Internet based telerehabilitation services may offer some solutions to this problem in the future.

## The Multidisciplinary Team

Multidisciplinary teams are central to the cancer service. Patients diagnosed with H&N malignancy face extensive and radical treatment with numerous negative physiological, functional, social, and psychological consequences. Thus, specialized teams of professionals are required to coordinate, plan, and manage the complex management of H&N cancer. The multidisciplinary team requires a spirit of cooperation and mutual respect from each member to facilitate activity and energy that results in the best possible patient care. Certain conditions can help facilitate effective multidisciplinary teams and collaboration including:

- Respected team leader with strong leadership and facilitation skills to enable full participation of all disciplines
- Preparation and dissemination of all relevant materials and information in advance of meetings and key decisions
- Inclusion of all disciplines in discussions, and mutual respect between participants leading to productive group dynamics
- Staff awareness of the personal benefits of multidisciplinary collaboration, including ongoing education, enhanced peer respect, and the benefits of supported management decisions
- Regular case discussions highlighting collaboration and enhanced outcome
- Timely communication of outcomes of case discussions to the patient, other team members, and referring practitioner
- Supporting infrastructure; this can range from the availability of general facilities, such as meeting rooms, to resource allocation, such as the formation of special multidisciplinary oncology teams within a health

setting, or departmental allocation of time for attending team meetings within a clinician's caseload

The multidisciplinary team generally consists of specialist physicians, dentist, surgeons, and allied health staff to achieve necessary tumor control and maximum functional outcome after treatment. Although the multidisciplinary team members may vary slightly depending upon the availability of particular staff, the role of team leader is usually held by the otolaryngologist or radiation oncologist. Regular attendees at the initial multidisciplinary meetings include otolaryngologists, plastic reconstructive surgeons, maxillofacial surgeons, radiation oncologists, radiologists, SLP, and dietitian. The multidisciplinary team involved during treatment may include other allied health members as appropriate. Many multidisciplinary teams need to access input from a dentist, social worker, pathologist, and psychologist/psychiatrist/counselor when required, as they are not regular attendees at multidisciplinary team meetings in many centers. The ideal multidisciplinary team to manage H&N cancer would consist of the following broad spectrum of health care professionals. In the following sections each of these professions and their roles will be detailed.

## Otolaryngologist

The otolaryngologist, also referred to as an ear, nose, and throat (ENT) surgeon, specializes in the diagnosis and management of disorders of the H&N, specifically the face, ear, nose, throat, sinuses, neck, and skull base. They are responsible for resection of cancers of the oral cavity, pharynx, or larynx. These surgeons remove the tumor and if possible close the defect primarily with sutures. However, if the defect is too large then the resecting surgeon will hand over to the plastic reconstructive surgeon to close the defect. The otolaryngologist also completes combined craniofacial resections and neck dissections.

Due to their recognized expertise in head and neck management, general practitioners (local medical officers) and other medical staff usually refer patients who present with problems directly to an otolaryngologist. The otolaryngologist is frequently the first specialist the patient has seen. They will complete initial

examinations and usually coordinate appropriate radiological imaging and biopsy procedures to confirm a diagnosis of H&N cancer before presenting the patient to the multidisciplinary team treatment planning meeting. They also work closely with the plastic and reconstructive surgeons, the maxillofacial surgeons, and radiation oncologists.

The otolaryngologist will be the primary treating specialist if the patient is treated with surgery +/− postoperative radiotherapy/chemotherapy. If surgery is required, then he or she will be involved in the patients' management across the continuum of care. The patient will then be reviewed at regular intervals postoperatively, with the frequency of reviews reducing over time. Follow-up with the otolaryngologist is essential to check for tumor recurrence or new tumors. Most patients will be monitored for about 5 years, although the duration does vary depending upon individual factors.

## Plastic and Reconstructive Surgeon

Plastic and reconstructive surgeons provide a wide range of reconstructive and cosmetic surgery services for patients who present with cancer of the H&N. Plastic and reconstructive surgeons have specialized skills in reconstructive microsurgery, craniofacial surgery, and esthetic plastic surgery. They work closely with the otolaryngologist and maxillofacial surgeons. These surgeons are responsible for closure of surgical defects once the tumor is removed, using local or regional pedicled flaps or microvascular free tissue transfer (free flaps) as appropriate to achieve optimal reconstruction.

Like the otolaryngologist, these surgeons may have patients referred to them directly and will often present patients for discussion and treatment planning at the multidisciplinary planning meeting. If patients undergo surgery then they will be involved across the continuum of care. The plastic and reconstructive surgeon may require additional specialized radiological imaging and assessments at the planning phase of treatment to determine the most suitable reconstructive option for an individual (i.e., require leg angiograms to accurately assess viability of vessels for fibular free flaps, or orthopantomography [OPG] scans to assess the mandible for accurate planning of deep circumflex iliac artery [DCIA] free flaps).

Plastic and reconstructive surgeons will also follow the patient closely during the initial months post-surgery, to ensure the flap or tissue used for reconstruction has healed well and functions as designed. Similarly, they monitor recovery and function of the donor tissue sites. Once all the postoperative care is provided, the plastic and reconstructive surgeons may not actively conduct ongoing monitoring; rather, they will continue liaison with the otolaryngologist who has principal responsibility for monitoring the patient in the long term.

## Oral and Maxillofacial Surgeon

Oral and maxillofacial (OMF) surgeons are dental specialists who treat diseases, conditions, defects, injuries, and aesthetics of the mouth, teeth, jaw, and face. The OMF surgeon plays an important role in a vast range of clinical conditions, such as problem wisdom teeth, facial pain, misaligned jaws, or patients suffering facial injuries following trauma. However, they are also particularly skilled in reconstructive and dental implant surgery. The role of the OMF surgeon is often significant in the management of complications associated with H&N cancer treatments including osteoradionecrosis, dental problems, and temporomandibular joint (TMJ) dysfunction. The OMF surgeon works closely with the otolaryngologist and plastic reconstructive surgeons.

Similarly to the otolaryngologist and plastic and reconstructive surgeon, the OMF surgeon often presents patients for discussion at the multidisciplinary planning meeting. If the patient is planned for surgery, OMF surgeons are usually involved; however, input often varies depending upon the size of the tumor and planned procedure. For large H&N cancers, the OMF surgeon is usually responsible for removal of teeth and bone to provide access to the cancer, which is then removed by the otolaryngologist. For smaller H&N cancers, the OMF surgeon may complete the removal of the cancer in addition to management of the teeth and mandible.

At the planning treatment meeting, the OMF surgeon will ensure patients who are planned for radiotherapy have their teeth assessed and arrange their removal, if required, prior to commencement of radiotherapy (see discussions in Chapter 3 regarding radiotherapy and dental management). In some organizations the OMF surgeon may complete this work while others may refer the patient to the dentist/prosthodontist. The OMF surgeon may also complete follow-up surgery after completion of radiotherapy and recovery to facilitate dental reconstruction. The OMF surgeon usually manages the H&N cancer patient at regular intervals and for varied lengths of time depending upon a number of factors, including which other surgical specialists are involved in the patient's care.

## Radiation Oncologist

Radiation oncologists specialize in the treatment of H&N cancer using radiation and chemotherapy treatment regimens. In some health services, patients may be referred to specialist radiation units/centers for opinions and diagnosis of H&N cancer. In these situations, the radiation oncologist usually coordinates appropriate assessments by surgical colleagues and arranges required radiological imaging before presenting the patient to the multidisciplinary planning meeting for discussion. Radiation oncologists advise if the cancer may be best treated with radiotherapy or chemotherapy or a combination of both. They also advise at what time point the radiation or chemotherapy should be delivered, i.e., preoperatively, postoperatively, or as a stand-alone treatment modality. If the patient is not planned for surgery, then the radiation oncologist will be the primary specialist managing the patient, and will monitor and manage the care during the course of the treatment and on an ongoing basis. If the patient is treated with surgery and receives either pre- or postoperative radiotherapy or chemotherapy, then the radiation oncologist usually monitors the patient during the course of the daily/weekly treatment regimen and for some time post-completion of treatment. However the surgeon provides ongoing care and monitoring. Many radiation units are involved in research and thus the patients may be monitored indirectly via participation in research projects investigating new treatments.

## Radiologist

Radiologists have experience in the subspecialty of diagnostic radiology, which is devoted to the imaging diagnosis of disorders of skin, mucosal surfaces, and deep anatomic structures of the head, face, and neck. They provide reports of the CT and MRI scans, as well as any other imaging techniques conducted to accurately assess H&N cancer. The radiologist is usually involved in the multidisciplinary treatment planning meeting and is able to assist the surgeons with planning for surgery by providing detailed information about the structures and tissues the tumor is invading.

The radiologist is not usually involved in direct management of the H&N cancer patient. Once a treatment option is determined at the multidisciplinary treatment planning meeting, the radiologist may be required again post-treatment to provide opinion regarding most suitable radiological imaging if a recurrence or new cancer is suspected. Repeat radiological imaging and opinion may be required in the months or several years post-treatment or not at all.

## Head and Neck Nurse Coordinator/Clinical Nurse Specialist

Cancer management and rehabilitation is best delivered by a multidisciplinary team; however, communication between the team members, the patient, and family is essential. This communication can be maximized by a patient care coordinator who is knowledgeable in H&N cancer management and its rehabilitation principles. Many multidisciplinary teams will have either a H&N nurse coordinator (also called clinical nurse specialist) or a highly experienced nurse within the team. They usually have many years of experience working with patients with H&N cancer and demonstrate a sound understanding of the treatment options for management of this patient group. This nurse plays a significant role during all stages of the patient's care.

As discussed earlier, the patient with H&N cancer usually attends a multidisciplinary treatment planning meeting at a hospital with expertise in H&N cancer treatment. The H&N nurse coordinator schedules the patients to attend these meetings and is often the first person the patient will meet. The nurse will often complete all required paperwork with the patients, escort them to the meeting, and complete additional paperwork and source any additional case history information as required.

Once a treatment plan has been established, the nurse will coordinate any appointments and examinations that the patient requires before commencement of treatment (i.e., CT/MRI scans, blood tests, preadmission clinic appointment for preoperative assessment). The nurse will then be one of the team of professionals who help educate and prepare the patients for the treatment they are about to undergo, whether this is radiotherapy, chemotherapy, or surgery. The nurse informs the patient about the potential side effects of nonsurgical treatments (radiotherapy and chemotherapy) and/or the day-to-day care that will be required immediately after surgery and during the recovery phase in the hospital (i.e., tracheostomy and suctioning, enteral nutrition, pain relief). He or she will also briefly discuss the self-care practices that the patient will learn and need to be able to complete on a long-term basis following surgery (i.e., cleaning a stoma after laryngectomy). The nurse may also address general hygiene issues, particularly for laryngectomees who lose the sense of smell.

The H&N nurse coordinator often does not work on the H&N ward on a daily basis but often visits patients during their treatment (particularly as inpatients) to provide ongoing support and care. The ward nursing staff along with the nurse coordinator or clinical nurse specialist supports the patients through the most difficult postsurgical phase. For those patients who need to use alternative communication options (i.e., communication boards, electronic communication devices, or artificial larynges) the nurses are often able to help encourage the patient to use these devices by taking some additional time to spend to listen and be supportive. The nurse coordinator or clinical nurse specialist remains a key contact for the H&N cancer patients when they return for outpatient reviews following completion of treatment. These nurses usually attend the outpatient clinics and so are able to provide ongoing advice and support about issues such as wound management, general hygiene, and care.

## Dietitian

Impaired nutritional status in the H&N cancer population has been a well documented problem (Mathog, 1991). Maintenance of proper/adequate nutrition is critical to the healing process and success of rehabilitation and recovery following surgery and/or radiotherapy for H&N cancer. The majority of cancer patients will present with nutritional deficiencies due to tumor burden and associated symptoms. Dysphagia, odynophagia, anorexia, and significant weight loss are all common symptoms. A patient with these symptoms may present as cachectic and malnourished. Additionally, chronic high alcohol consumption accompanied by liver damage impairs metabolism, placing the already compromised patient at greater risk of delayed or poor wound healing. Malnutrition may also contribute to reduced tolerance of prescribed treatment regimens.

When possible, the dietitian should be involved with H&N cancer patients from the pretreatment phase. Referring the patient to the dietitian at this phase of treatment allows completion of baseline nutritional assessment, including a detailed nutritional history, anthropometric measurements, and evaluation of laboratory chemistry (Clarke, 1998). In many H&N cancer units the SLP will frequently meet patients prior to commencement of treatment. Informal conversation and questioning will quickly indicate if a referral to the dietitian is required. If patients report a significant loss of weight or a difficulty managing particular food and/or fluids (suggesting the presence of dysphagia and/or odynophagia), then input from the dietitian is crucial. Patients may already be modifying oral intake to make eating/drinking easier. However, by doing so, they may not be meeting their daily nutritional requirements. Involvement of the dietitian can result in the education of patients to ensure that they introduce new food items to meet daily nutritional requirements. In cases of more severe nutritional compromise, the dietitian may suggest commencement of enteral nutrition and even pretreatment hospital admission to maximize the patient's nutritional status before treatment begins.

Nutritional management is critical during treatment regimens, both surgical and radiotherapy (see discussions in Chapter 3). Most of the patients treated surgically will be unable to eat or drink orally for a short period of time postoperatively. During this time the "nil oral" status is used to facilitate wound healing and to allow for resolution of edema. Enteral nutrition is the feeding method of choice at this time. Nasogastric feeding is used as a short-term feeding option. However, those patients who will require long-term

nutritional support are more likely to have enteral nutrition via percutaneous endoscopic gastrostomy (PEG). The dietitian is responsible for recommending appropriate enteral nutrition regimens to meet individual patient requirements.

Once medical staff are satisfied with wound healing, the SLP will assess swallowing function and may commence placing the patient on oral intake. At this point, the dietitian collaborates with the SLP, adjusting the enteral nutrition based upon the oral intake abilities of the patient. The dietitian may prescribe ongoing supplementary enteral nutrition while the patient gradually increases oral intake (as most patients commence some type of modified diet and/or fluids initially). Similarly, H&N cancer patients receiving radiotherapy or combined chemo and radiotherapy treatment also require close monitoring by the dietitian. Patients treated with radiotherapy regimens frequently develop associated symptoms, such as mucositis, xerostomia, trismus, loss of appetite, and pain secondary to tissue/skin damage, that impair their ability to swallow and maintain adequate oral nutrition. In these cases, the dietitian may recommend commencement of enteral nutrition for those who had not required enteral nutrition prior to treatment. Enteral nutrition instigated during treatment may be used as a supplement to some oral intake. However, as treatment progresses (i.e., towards end of treatment regimen), and the ability to tolerate oral intake is further reduced, enteral nutrition may become the primary method of nutrition.

Those patients who will require long-term (postdischarge) use of enteral nutrition (i.e., PEG), will be educated by the dietitian regarding the type and frequency of feeding. Patients returning home on enteral nutrition programs are reviewed at regular intervals to ensure their weight remains stable and nutritional needs continue to be met. For some patients, the completion of treatment will result in a gradual return of swallowing function and an ability to recommence oral intake. The dietitian and SLP must collaborate closely during this period. The dietitian will modify enteral nutrition feeding regimens to help facilitate a return to oral intake (i.e., patient cannot be "full" of enteral nutrition, such that they have no appetite for oral intake). At any stage in the continuum of care, a patient who is not compliant with the completion of enteral nutrition may present a challenge for the dietitian.

## Speech-Language Pathologist (SLP)

SLPs are responsible for the assessment and management of speech, swallowing, and voice function across the continuum of care. Their role is to minimize the impact of the chosen treatment option on communication and swallowing and maximize the functional ability of patients with H&N cancer post-treatment. This can involve the use of a range of compensatory and rehabilitative strategies as well as alternative options (e.g., alaryngeal speech, modified techniques for assisting olfaction) which may be introduced pre-, during, and/or following treatment depending on the patient and the presenting situation.

Pretreatment, the SLP is involved in discussions at the multidisciplinary team meeting. It is important in these meetings that the SLP provides advice about speech and swallowing outcomes in relation to the specific treatments being discussed. The information provided in this forum may direct which treatment method is used (i.e., functional speech and swallowing outcomes of all treatment options are considered). It is also important that SLPs be present so that they have a full understanding of the treatment modality proposed for each patient. This way they can appropriately plan for anticipated outcomes and gauge the extent of clinical involvement that will be required during and post-treatment for each patient.

The SLP meets with the patient before treatment to provide information and counseling about the treatment option planned and its potential impact upon communication and swallowing. It is useful to have a spouse or family members present during this education and counseling session so that they too understand the planned treatment and expected recovery course. The level of information presented will relate to the needs of individual patients. It is important at the end of the pretreatment education session that the patient has been provided with information about the expected speech and swallowing outcomes post-treatment and an approximate time frame for the rehabilitation and intervention to follow (see Chapters 5, 7, and 9 for detailed discussion of presurgical patient counseling, patterns of rehabilitation, and anticipated outcomes for various types of H&N cancer).

If surgery is the treatment option, then the SLP must advise the patient of the expected changes to speech and swallowing as a result of the surgery. In particular, it is important to focus on both the early and late changes anticipated during postsurgical recovery. The early impact of surgery on both communication and swallowing needs to be fully explained to the patient and the caregivers. The patient must be educated about the alternative communication options (i.e., electronic communication devices, whiteboards, pen/paper, yes/no head nods, and gesture) that will be used during this early postsurgical stage. Patients should also be counseled and prepared for any potential changes to their speech production that will occur on account of surgery, and the management plan and prognosis they can expect with postsurgical speech treatment. Regarding oral intake, it is important to discuss with the patient the need to remain nil by mouth after surgery to allow healing, and the potential anticipated timeline until they can recommence some oral intake (modified diet and /or modified fluids). As with communication, it is important the patients understand the anticipated changes they can expect to their swallow function, the timeline for recovery, and the potential prognosis following rehabilitation. Being prepared for these changes, and the associated issues such as the presence of a tracheostomy, postsurgical edema etc., will help alleviate anxiety and distress in the initial postoperative period.

If radiation treatment is being initiated, the SLP advises the patient about the likely effects of radiation treatment that relate to speech and swallowing, such as the impact of xerostomia and mucositis upon swallowing and the potential need for diet and fluid modification to ensure aspiration risk is minimized. SLPs should also advise the patient that the radiation staff will closely monitor pain and the damage to the mucosa and will provide appropriate pain relief. In addition, the possible need for enteral nutrition (i.e., NG tube or PEG) should be discussed.

Postsurgery, the SLP should initiate contact with the surgical patient within the first day or two of surgery to reinforce the postoperative recovery and intervention plan, particularly in relation to communication and swallowing. At this early stage, the patient may not be ready to use a communication device; however, it is important to reassure the patient that a device is available at the bedside as soon as he or she is ready. The simplest device such as a whiteboard or communication picture board is usually the favored option in the early postsurgical days when the patient is sleep deprived and often has significant swelling and pain and thus sleeps/rests for most of the time. For patients who undergo total laryngeal surgery, during this initial postsurgical period the SLP will also commence some education and basic training regarding their new form of verbal communication, i.e., artificial larynx. The SLP usually includes family members, caregivers, and/or friends during this early education period so that they understand the communication options and are able to support the patient. Knowledge about how communication devices work enables the SLP to empower others to facilitate communication with the patient. Nursing staff are particularly useful during this stage, providing patient support and encouragement regarding the patient's new form of communication.

The SLP is responsible for assessing swallowing function once the surgeons have advised the wounds are sufficiently healed. At this point, patients are often commenced on modified diets and/or fluids. SLPs must work with the dietitian regarding commencement of oral intake, particularly if enteral nutrition is also being used. They will also provide patients with oromotor exercises to attempt to increase range of motion and strength of movements to benefit both communication and swallowing. The specific exercises that patients will require will depend upon the nature of the surgery they have undergone. Exercise programs are usually tailored to individual patient needs and abilities, and should not be commenced before the suture lines are sufficiently healed.

For most patients, the SLP will provide ongoing intervention postdischarge from hospital. Patients often require a review of their swallowing and speech function as gradual improvements in swallowing occur and some patients are able to recommence oral intake and/or wean off enteral nutrition completely. The SLP must work closely with the dietitian during this period.

## Social Worker

Living with cancer and the treatment required can be a difficult challenge, and often entails a great deal of stress. The patient with H&N cancer may experience many emotions during the diagnosis and treatment course, some of which may include anxiety, fear, anger, depression, worry, uncertainty, and apprehension. Dealing with fear and the emotional impact of facing a serious disease is a large challenge in itself; however, patients with H&N cancer also have enormous adjustments to make to their daily schedules to accommodate their treatment and often long-term new self-care tasks (i.e., stoma care).

In many H&N units the social worker is the primary provider of psychological services to patients undergoing treatment and their families and caregivers. Social work services are designed to assist individuals, families, groups, and wider community members through counseling, stress management, care planning, case management, system navigation, education, and advocacy (Association of Social Workers, 2006). Social workers provide a range of services directly for patients and their families including counseling, support, education, and resource identification. Their scope of practice involves provision of assessment, treatment, and evaluation services within a therapeutic relationship developed between the social worker and patient.

Where possible the social worker will be present at the initial multidisciplinary meeting to initiate contact with the patient and/or the family/caregiver. Many patients have little suspicion of a likely diagnosis because of the rarity of H&N cancer in comparison to other more widely publicized cancers, such as breast and lung cancer. This lack of awareness about head and neck cancer, and the significant issues associated with its treatment, compound with the additional issues associated with a diagnosis of "cancer." At this stage considerable support for the patient and the family is required. Examples of patients and their spouses explaining their reaction to their diagnosis of cancer can be found in the CD segment "First Reactions" (Chapter 14: Video: "First Reactions").

At the pretreatment phase, the social worker recognizes the supportive care needs of patients and personal risk factors that may highlight need for particular supports; i.e., does person live alone, is he or she a caregiver for partner/spouse? There is also a need to recognize if the patient may require support to cease smoking or may need support to reduce alcohol consumption. These risk factors can be picked up early in pretreatment assessments and discussions. Patients should be referred to the social worker at this point, to begin the process of providing support within and outside the treatment setting.

The patient may also require supportive counseling after being informed of the diagnosis and treatment planned, and during the period while waiting for assessment/biopsy results. At this early stage, the patient and family may be anxious and fearful of the unknown ahead. The social worker can connect persons diagnosed with cancer and their families with essential community, state, and international resources where appropriate. Social workers are also advocates of increasing awareness of the social, emotional, educational, and spiritual needs of patients with cancer and their families.

Social work services are designed to help patients and their families feel more in control. Intervention is focused on helping people cope with the medical, emotional, and social problems they encounter at different points of the cancer experience. Postoperative altered appearance can be devastating for the H&N cancer patient. Laryngectomees (see section later in chapter) typically feel that nothing can prepare them for the altered anatomical and physiological changes that significantly alter their body image. Preparation for these appearance and lifestyle changes may require intensive support and counseling. Family and caregivers may also need support as they learn to accept and adjust to these changes in order to support the patient. These issues and others are discussed by patients in the CD segments "Biggest Worry" (Chapter 14: Video: "Biggest Worry") and "Family Emotions" (Chapter 14: Video: "Family Emotions") as they describe their greatest concerns on finding out they had laryngeal cancer and the response of their family members.

Anecdotal information suggests that patients with H&N cancer are often isolated after treatments and some rarely venture outside. Many have needed to cease employment, temporarily or even permanently for some. While these patients usually attend their regular medical appointments at outpatient clinics, they are often socially isolated. This social isolation can be grossly underestimated during earlier phases of treatment. Thus, ongoing follow-up and access to a social worker is also an important part of the rehabilitation process. Access to the social worker during these outpatient clinic appointments is highly desirable. This allows even brief face-to-face contact to reassess the patient's coping strategies and current psychological status. At this point, the social worker may provide the patient with an appointment time to provide further support and counseling as the patient begins the journey of returning to normal life. Discussion about return to life after cancer treatment may require several sessions and ongoing social work support. The patient may need encouragement to reengage with social networks and local communities. The social worker may be able to direct the patient to local, national, and international support groups. They may also explore further the changes in self and altered relationships.

The above intervention is frequently not possible in many H&N units where access to the social worker is less than required. In these cases the social worker may be called upon to provide other service delivery models to monitor the social, emotional, and psychological well-being of these patients who have recently completed long and challenging treatment regimens. The social worker can provide services over the phone to patients and families, offering an alternative and additional support service once the patient is discharged from treatment. At this point many patients are often reluctant to return to the hospital more than absolutely necessary, after having spent considerable time undergoing treatment (which is frequently multimodality); thus phone contact may provide a more appropriate form of service delivery.

## Psychologist

There is a strong body of evidence that psychological distress is common in patients with H&N cancer and that psychology has a role in reducing that stress (Hutton & Williams, 2001). The psychological problems associated with H&N cancer and its treatment are serious and pervasive, often impacting detrimentally on the patient's quality of life, yet minimal attention is sometimes given to this domain of care. While social workers will monitor the patient's ability to manage these emotions and challenges, at any point during the treatment process they, or another member of the multidisciplinary team, may suggest referral to a psychologist. Seeking assistance from the psychologist may facilitate further exploration of successful methods of coping with emotions. Clinical psychology services usually provide individual counseling and treatment for difficulties and stress associated with a diagnosis of cancer and the disease treatment. Patients with H&N cancer often interact with a number of health care workers during and immediately after their treatment; however, many clinicians are only able to offer general support. Referral to the psychologist enables the patient to receive care from clinicians with expertise in psychological issues.

Where psychology services are available before the commencement of treatment a screening for psychological distress may be completed. There is no body part more exposed to the world than a person's head and neck, and thus any threat to this renders the person vulnerable. The psychologist can begin to explore issues such as altered body image and life role changes. From this, the psychologist can provide valuable input into the multidisciplinary team discussion when treatment plans are being made (surgery and/or radiotherapy).

The self-image and confidence of patients who survive H&N cancer treatment is challenged through the effects of the disease and its treatment on physical appearance and everyday functions such as eating and speaking. Changes to recreational and sexual functioning are also common problems faced by this population. The realization of these impairments is far greater during and particularly following completion of treatment, thus rendering the assistance of the psychologist essential. The psychologist assists the patient to cope and adjust to the new status.

Anxiety about hospital appointments, loss of interest or pleasure in activities, and dislike of altered roles are also common among patients. Literature supports the notion that depression is not uncommon in H&N cancer patients with levels of distress found to be greater in younger patients (Hutton & Williams, 2001). It has been documented that anxiety and depression (psychological distress) are also higher in those patients whose cancer was diagnosed relatively recently. This evidence suggests that H&N cancer patients should receive psychological support early after diagnosis and in the early treatment phase.

## Physiotherapist

Physiotherapy involves the use of exercises to help improve joint movement, reduce pain, and to reduce swelling following H&N surgery. Physiotherapists (also referred to as physical therapists) conduct a wide range of assessment and provide management and intervention throughout the patient's care. The aim of physiotherapists working with patients with H&N cancer is to minimize the effects that the disease or its treatment has on the patient. Physiotherapy also aims to improve quality of life, by maximizing functional ability and independence and providing relief from distressing symptoms. The physiotherapists may complete some or all of the following interventions when managing patients with H&N cancer:

- Respiratory care: management of dyspnea, removal of secretions, nebulization, and oxygen management (This is performed by a Respiratory Therapist in the United States.)
- Education of patient in care of limb/body areas postsurgery, in conservational or adaptive strategies, in appropriate handling strategies
- Positioning and movement
- Education of family/caregiver regarding handling strategies
- Exercise therapy to improve flexibility, strength, and function

The physiotherapist is usually involved in pretreatment assessment on an "as needs" basis. Patients who present with limited fitness and severe airways disease may be seen for pretreatment assessment regarding exercise tolerance, management of secretions, and chest condition. The physiotherapist may prescribe an individual exercise program to help prepare the patient for surgery, or if required, may provide advice regarding strategies to assist secretion clearance and airway maintenance. Some services may have preoperative education information that is given to the patient with H&N cancer at pretreatment assessment that outlines the role of the physiotherapist postsurgery.

During and post-treatment, the physiotherapist plays an important role in managing chest status. Physiotherapy management of pulmonary/respiratory function can reduce complications of treatments and therefore contribute to reducing length of stay in the hospital. Respiratory problems in patients with H&N cancer are often related to underlying chronic obstructive pulmonary disease (COPD); mechanical, sensory, or motor problems of the upper airway caused by the primary malignancy; or therapies directed towards treatment of the cancer (e.g., surgery, radiotherapy)

(Mathog et al., 1991). Aspiration and COPD have been found to be major causes of morbidity and mortality in patients with H&N cancer.

Physiotherapists maximize respiratory function by improving ventilation and aiding the removal of secretions. They will usually see the patient from the initial day postsurgery to complete baseline assessments, including observation of temperature, oxygen saturation, antibiotic usage, and risk factors for postoperative respiratory complications. This initial assessment will also include supported coughing and guidelines to improve breathing efficiency and assist sputum clearance. The physiotherapist will then devise a daily treatment plan that is then carried out by the nursing staff throughout the day.

When working with patients who undergo partial laryngeal surgery, necessitating tracheostomy surgery, the physiotherapist is usually involved in multidisciplinary tracheostomy management, in particular joint cuff deflation assessments with the SLP. During cuff deflation assessments, the physiotherapist will monitor the patients' respiratory function (i.e., oxygen requirements, respiratory rate) and their ability to cough and expectorate sputum and observe the type and amount of sputum produced. The physiotherapist is particularly involved with patients who undergo total laryngectomy. These patients have significant changes to pulmonary function as a consequence of surgery (see Chapter 12) and require assistance and training in how to produce the modified cough maneuver using forced exhalations or "huffs" to assist sputum clearance (discussed previously in Chapter 11).

For patients who undergo more extensive reconstructive surgery, the physiotherapist will guide commencement of certain activities such as the patient's first attempt to sit on the edge of the bed or stand. They will assess the patient's safety to ambulate setting guidelines for distance ambulated and frequency, and work with the reconstructive unit regarding mobilization when muscle flaps have been necessary to achieve surgical reconstruction (e.g., fibular free flaps). Patients who have had radical neck dissections with sacrifice of the spinal accessory nerve will usually benefit from the intervention provided by a physiotherapist. If appropriate exercises are not provided, drooping of the shoulder on the affected surgical side frequently results in limited range of movement. Patients may also complain of pain associated with the

shoulder movement and this may be reduced or managed more effectively with education and instruction by the physiotherapist.

For patients undergoing chemotherapy and/or radiotherapy, exercises during the course of treatment can improve their strength, decrease fatigue, and help maintain physical well-being while receiving treatment. During these treatments the physiotherapist can design exercise programs that cater to the individual needs of each patient. The physiotherapist will work with individuals to optimize their physical function. Patients undergoing chemotherapy and/or radiotherapy may find the mobility of the head and neck region alters as the course of treatment progresses with some patients complaining of "stiffening" in the neck and shoulder region. The physiotherapist will advise on appropriate neck and shoulder exercises to maintain the greatest range of movement possible while minimizing pain and discomfort.

In the long term, the physiotherapist will provide ongoing or new intervention strategies to manage the deficits of the neck and shoulder associated with some of the H&N procedures. Some patients may also require a longer term rehabilitation exercise program if they have required muscle flaps for reconstruction of the surgical defects associated with removal of the tumor mass. For the occasional patient who is discharged home with a tracheostomy tube in situ, the physiotherapist may also provide ongoing monitoring of chest status and sputum clearance.

## Occupational Therapist

The occupational therapist addresses a wide range of functions based upon the prognostic information available, such as type of treatment planned and lifestyle demands. With this knowledge in mind, the occupational therapist plans interventions based on physical, functional, and psychological assessments. Occupational therapists assist patients by educating patients and their families regarding the changes in motion, strength, flexibility, balance, and/or endurance that result from surgery or radiotherapy treatment. They will educate patients in how to use adaptive equipment and compensatory techniques to increase their independence during their daily routines. They also teach patients how to complete basic daily activities such as bathing, dressing, and moving around their environment.

Similar to the physiotherapist the occupational therapist is usually involved in pretreatment assessment of patients with H&N cancer on an "as needs" basis. The occupational therapist may be contacted to assess the patient's current level of independence in areas of self-care, home management, work, or vocational pursuits. At this pretreatment assessment the occupational therapist also aims to assist the patient and family/caregivers to anticipate immediate and future activity demands and challenges as a result of the treatment planned. Evaluation prior to treatment is useful to help the patient establish realistic goals and assist in the development of a supportive therapeutic relationship. The occupational therapist may prescribe adaptive equipment and compensatory techniques to maximize function and improve safety prior to treatment. Some facilities may have preoperative education information that is given to patients with H&N cancer at pretreatment assessment that outlines the role of the occupational therapist postsurgery.

Patients with H&N cancer who are treated with chemotherapy and/or radiotherapy often experience fatigue during the course of their treatment, as well as other symptoms such as generalized muscle weakness and loss of muscle mass. These side effects of treatment may result in limited activity levels and make basic self-care functions more difficult. During the course of treatment the occupational therapist can advise of strategies to modify daily activities, stressing the importance of safety and hygiene. Occupational therapy during this time is focused on energy conservation and work simplification. The occupational therapist usually provides advice and education to prevent overexertion and fatigue that may aggravate an already reduced activity and independence level.

Radiation treatment regimens may result in a "stiffening" of head, neck, and shoulder movements. To prevent restricted range of movement the occupational therapist can provide appropriate exercises. The occupational therapist and physiotherapist often work closely to ensure the exercises provided by each are complementary. During radiation treatment blistering of skin and other tissue reactions are common. The occupational therapist is able to provide education to the patient about protecting irradiated tissue and pre-cautions to reduce trauma; i.e., grooming and hygiene routines require modification to protect the treated skin.

Patients with H&N cancer who undergo surgery will benefit from early intervention from the occupational therapist to assist understanding the altered physical state and resulting deficits associated with their surgery, and any functional impact upon basic daily activities. The occupational therapist will provide the patient with strategies to maximize independence without compromising wound healing and recovery from surgery, and provide specialized exercise regimens for patients who undergo muscle flaps and skin grafts.

When considered appropriate the occupational therapist will suggest assistive devices that can be used to aid self-care independence. Occupational therapy intervention goals also focus on maintaining range of movement, mobility, and independence while simultaneously avoiding the complications associated with bed rest. In some facilities the occupational therapist is available to advise on diversional activities that may be helpful in assisting the patient to adjust to the current level of functioning induced by the treatment being completed. It is important to note that some patients may have difficulty accepting the need to modify self-care regimens or use assistive devices/equipment.

Helping the patient to return to familiar, independent activities is an important goal of recovery for the occupational therapist. Some patients will require ongoing modification of food and/or fluids after the return home. The occupational therapist is involved with menu planning, shopping skills, and assessment of kitchen skills to ensure the patient is able to prepare the required modified diet appropriately (i.e., use blender, store food/fluid appropriately). Patients who have undergone surgery that involved muscle flaps and/or skin grafts will also benefit from outpatient follow-up by an occupational therapist. These patients are usually scheduled for a routine appointment to monitor the donor site limb to ensure maximum function returns with gradual recovery. A tailored exercise regimen is usually developed for individual patients to increase the range of movement and strength in the donor site limb. Patients treated with chemotherapy and/or radiotherapy or surgery that did not involve a muscle flap or skin graft are usually seen for outpatient follow-up as needed. The occupational therapist often relies on the other multidisciplinary team members to refer patients for review if required; this is usually via outpatient clinics.

## Dentist/Maxillofacial Prosthodontist

Patients who require radiation therapy should be referred to a dentist for pretreatment dental evaluation and prophylactic dental care. Radiation treatment has the potential to result in the development of xerostomia, dental caries, and osteoradionecrosis (see discussions in Chapter 3); therefore, dental examinations must be completed before radiation treatment is initiated. The dentist will often also prescribe an appropriate oral hygiene and dental care protocol, or may refer the patient to an oral hygienist for oral care during and after radiation treatment. Dental caries left untreated can worsen rapidly after completion of radiotherapy treatment. Therefore, dental extractions are often recommended pre-radiation treatment. Extractions after radiation treatment may place the patient at a greater risk for developing serious infection, which may lead to erosion of part of the mandible (osteoradionecrosis).

Similarly, patients with H&N cancer who are being treated surgically may be appropriate for preoperative assessment by the dentist for pretreatment planning for any prosthetic intervention post-treatment (e.g., intraoral prosthesis—see discussion in Chapter 5). This is particularly crucial for patients undergoing surgery involving the palate and/or maxilla. For dental prostheses to remain stable and in the correct position they must be anchored securely. Therefore, it is essential that the dentist preserves critical teeth that may be required for anchoring and stabilizing the prosthesis postoperatively or postradiation. The dentist/prosthodontist will ensure that dental extractions pretreatment do not overlook the need to save selected teeth to facilitate intraoral prosthetic intervention. They also specialize in designing and placing dental implants used in the rehabilitation of complicated intraoral and facial defects.

## Facial Prosthetics

Cosmetic deformity is a key issue for patients with H&N cancer. Those patients who undergo surgery of the nose, ear, or orbit present with particular issues.

The advances over the past 30 years have made it possible to fit the patient with temporary prosthetic units almost immediately after surgery, with a more permanent prosthesis available within a couple of months. The prosthetics clinician is able to make prostheses that are tailor made and dependent upon the location of the tumor and the climate the person lives in. Prostheses are often made from polyvinyl chlorides and other silicone rubbers that sometimes require replacement as frequently as 3 to 8 months (due to material shrinkage, discoloration, and breakdown).

In some centers, the facial prosthetics clinician will attend the multidisciplinary planning meeting to meet with the patient before surgery and discuss the potential defect with the surgeon and patient. The clinician will be able to advise surgeons of structures that would be beneficial to preserve (where possible) to maximize attachment of the prosthesis. The patient may need to return for another assessment prior to surgery so the clinician is able to begin working on the prosthesis that will be required postoperatively.

The patient may require several appointments with the prosthetics clinician postoperatively to modify and adjust the prosthesis to achieve the best cosmetic outcome possible. Patients tend to adjust well to their prostheses. Adjustment is facilitated by a return to normal activities and familiar environments (i.e., where the patient can feel comfortable to use the prosthesis).

## Counseling, Information Dissemination, and Support

Both diagnosis and management of H&N cancer can have wide-ranging implications for the patient. Consequently, counseling and patient education are critical components in the rehabilitation process. Patient counseling is a complex communication task, and incompetence in this area can inevitably have a distressing impact on the patient and families (Fallowfield, 1993). Good communication and increased satisfaction of patients with their health care providers is associated with increased compliance and better emotional adjustment. By understanding what is important to patients, health care professionals can help to modify the care environment to enhance patient satisfaction and quality of care (Gourdji, McVey, & Loiselle, 2003).

During counseling, patients should be treated as unique individuals, with their personal priorities central to the process. Clinicians should consider the patients' social circumstances and other psychosocial factors, and use this to tailor the counseling situation. Knowledge of patient preferences with regards to their information needs, and being responsive to these preferences, can help to increase patient satisfaction (Parker et al., 2001; Ptacek & Ptacek, 2001). Sensitivity to spousal needs is also central to providing good patient support (Gates, Ryan, & Lauder, 1982; Ward, Hobson, & Conroy, 2003). Recent research reported that only 58% of spouses felt they had received enough presurgical information and 38% would have liked more information prior to their partners' laryngectomy surgery (Ward et al., 2003). Considering that spousal support is a significant element in rehabilitation, such findings suggest the need for more attention to this aspect of support services.

Rutten, Arora, Bakos, Aziz, and Rowland (2005) provided a systematic review of research on the information needs and sources of information of cancer patients along the continuum of care (diagnosis, during treatment, and post-treatment), and found that the information needs of patients change throughout the continuum. Indeed, patients generally do not want information about everything all the time, but prefer specific information about particular aspects of their condition and its treatment at each different stage of the continuum (Leydon, et al., 2000; Ward et al., 2003). During diagnosis and treatment, information about the stage of disease, treatment options, and side effects of treatment is needed (Rutten et al., 2005). Particularly in the pretreatment phase, studies have found that patients want information on the sequelae of surgery/ treatment, and not just the procedure itself (Edwards, 1998). Table 14–1 outlines some of the key topics that should be discussed pretreatment. The patient should be encouraged to ask questions and engage in discussion with the clinician about concerns and fears. This can help establish the amount of information required by each individual and can be more beneficial than supplying copious amounts of information before surgery (Renner, 1995). On the accompanying CD, this point is emphasized by a patient who describes her own experiences regarding asking questions, seeking out information, and requesting repetition of information (Chapter 14: Video: "Asking Questions").

Post-treatment, patients view the information pertaining to recovery as being more relevant (Rutten et al., 2005). At this stage, providing patients with information regarding the interventions/strategies available to help them adjust to the long-term changes associated with their cancer and its treatment become the focus of discussion. Table 14–2 outlines some of the issues that should be discussed post-treatment.

Apart from the different type of information needed to assist patients at each stage of their care, the quantity of information provided is also an important consideration. In striving to provide comprehensive information, it is important to note that not all patients desire a lot of information all of the time (Leydon et al., 2000). Therefore, regulating the quantity of information received at each stage is important. The manner in which the information is delivered is another factor to consider. Repetition of the same piece of information during diagnosis or the pretreatment stage has been shown to be highly desirable (Newell, Ziegler, Stafford, & Lewin, 2004). Particularly in the initial stages of diagnosis, patients report experiencing shock, numbness, and anxiety, and the inability to absorb the information provided to them (Newell et al., 2004; Ward et al., 2003). Therefore it is important to check that the patient has understood what has been discussed and revise and summarize key information to help recollection (Fallowfield, 1993; Ptacek & Ptacek, 2001).

The modality in which the information is provided (verbal, written, visual) is also an important consideration. Due to the initial shock and impact of diagnosis, it is important that the provision of written/ printed information accompany all verbal discussions. This information can provide a valuable permanent reference for patients and their families. Clinicians should remain conscious of the literacy levels of their patients when supplying written information. Including diagrams (e.g., in the care of surgical patients) with the written materials can also be of great assistance to the patient. Similarly, providing patients with access to visual education materials, such as documentaries or informational videos, can be extremely beneficial. If time allows, the ability for the clinician to watch these videos with the patient and answer additional questions can be extremely helpful. Having copies of the videos available for loan can also assist in the educa-

**Table 14–1.** Key Topics for Discussion Pretreatment

| Topic Area | Key Discussion Points |
|---|---|
| Management approach | ▪ Explain concept of multidisciplinary team (MDT)<br>▪ Outline who are the members of the MDT<br>▪ Explain how the MDT operates to coordinate care and make decisions regarding treatment options (i.e., surgery, radiotherapy, chemotherapy, or combined modality)<br>▪ Explain types of tests/investigations patients may be required to have as part of pretreatment planning |
| Role of key professionals | ▪ Discuss the key medical staff involved in management of patients with H&N cancer, including the: otolaryngologist, plastic and reconstructive surgeon, maxillofacial surgeon, radiation oncologist, radiologist<br>▪ Discuss who is taking the lead role for treatment (i.e., lead role will be dependent upon whether patient is having surgery or radiotherapy as initial treatment)<br>▪ Detail the role of key allied health staff involved in management of patients with H&N cancer, including: SLP, dietitian, social worker, physiotherapist<br>▪ Discuss the role of the nurse coordinator or clinical nurse specialist<br>▪ Outline the role of other professionals as appropriate (e.g., prosthodontist, facial prosthetics, psychologist, psychiatrist) |
| Timeline for recovery | ▪ Provide a realistic anticipated length of time in hospital postoperatively<br>▪ Outline the length of time required for completion of radiation and/or chemotherapy treatment and the expected recovery from both short-term and long-term side effects |
| Communication postsurgery | ▪ Discuss the implications of tracheostomy on speech and swallowing (where appropriate) during immediate postoperative/acute phase<br>▪ Discuss use of speaking valves during tracheostomy weaning (where appropriate)<br>▪ Investigate patient's ability to read/write for written communication option<br>▪ Discuss impairment to speech intelligibility and reinforce that SLP will provide exercises and strategies to maximize communication<br>▪ Discuss communication options available postlaryngectomy where appropriate, explaining the use of nonverbal communication systems, e.g., whiteboard, picture/word sheets, electrolarynx<br>▪ Discuss long-term communication needs if permanent tracheostomy expected |
| Swallowing postsurgery | ▪ Outline need for nil by mouth status postoperatively<br>▪ Provide timeline for expected return to oral intake<br>▪ Outline potential for diet and/or fluid modification to assist swallowing function<br>▪ Discuss potential for long-term dysphagia and long-term need for enteral nutrition<br>▪ Discuss role of SLP and dietitian to manage swallowing difficulties<br>▪ Discuss importance of pretreatment nutrition |
| Social and emotional support | ▪ Reinforce role of social worker, psychologist, and counselors to assist patient during all phases of treatment but especially during pretreatment phase<br>▪ Identify any significant social issues (e.g., patient with H&N cancer is carer for another person, and therefore may need assistance to organize respite care for that person, or increased services from local agencies such as housecleaning, meal delivery)<br>▪ Investigate what supports are available (i.e., family, spouse, friends)<br>▪ Discuss usual coping style/strategies with patient<br>▪ Consider referral to social worker to organize government benefits during H&N cancer treatment |
| Vocational | ▪ Establish patient's current employment status and interests<br>▪ Consider early referral to occupational therapist if patient still employed |
| Lifestyle changes | ▪ Discuss permanent lifestyle changes such as stoma and respiration for laryngectomee patients, difficulty eating out if modified diets/fluids required |

**Table 14–2.** Key Topics for Discussion Post-Treatment

| Topic Area | Key Discussion Points |
|---|---|
| Timelines for recovery | • Discuss healing of tracheostomy site (if appropriate) <br> • Detail expected edema and swelling as a result of treatment (common for both surgical and radiotherapy patients) and outline expected resolution of swelling/edema <br> • Seek patient's perception of edema resolution <br> • Outline the process and timeline to wound healing (both neck and skin graft/muscle flap sites), provide details of recovery <br> • Discuss appearance and aesthetics and potential long-term improvements and/or surgical treatments available |
| Long-term outcomes | • Discuss current status with patient and outline realistic long-term goals and what long-term outcome is likely to be |
| Rehabilitation options | • Inform patient of rehabilitation options (i.e., rehabilitation provided at current facility, or through another service supported by the treatment facility) <br> • Consider if inpatient rehabilitation is required to assist patient to return to home and/or adjust to life after treatment. |
| Ongoing review | • Explain the need for ongoing medical reviews as essential for prevention and monitoring of cancer recurrence <br> • Explain nature of medical reviews (i.e., frequent initially, then become less frequent and usually considered cured at 5 years post-treatment) <br> • Discuss ongoing relationship with SLP for laryngectomees <br> • Discuss ongoing review by dietitian and/or SLP for dysphagic patients |
| Support and equipment needs | • Outline the equipment patient will require post-treatment completion (e.g., laryngectomy equipment, humidifiers, suction equipment) <br> • Inform patient of appropriate support groups <br> • Inform patient of support services available in the community and within the hospital |

tion of family members who are unable to be present for the counseling sessions.

The preparation and skill of the clinician are also central to a positive counseling experience. In a study by Wiggers, Donovan, and Redman (1990), cancer patients rated the physicians' technical competence, as well as their interpersonal and communication skills, as being extremely important in achieving satisfaction with the care provided to them. It is critical that clinicians have all the relevant and up–to-date information, test results, and treatment options readily available while talking to the clients and their families. In a study of the counseling experiences of laryngectomy patients (Ward et al., 2003) the level of experi-

ence of the clinician and the familiarity with all aspects of H&N management was highlighted. When asked for suggestions regarding "optimal" patient counseling, a recurring theme from a number of patients was the need to ensure that all professionals involved in counseling and support be experienced and capable of discussing the issues of importance with the patient (Ward et al., 2003). Parker et al. (2001) examined cancer patients' and their families' preferences for the provision of information about their condition, and found that physician expertise, in terms of provision of information on their condition and treatment options, were of greatest importance to the patients they studied. The patients requested information be provided in clear and simple language and in an appropriate environment. They also suggested that they be given enough time to ask the physician all the questions that they have.

## Multidisciplinary Management of Special Populations

The final sections of this chapter are dedicated to detailed discussion of the multidisciplinary support needs of three special populations: patients who undergo total laryngectomy, pediatric patients with H&N cancer, and patients requiring palliative care. Although all patients with H&N cancer undergo considerable life readjustments, these populations in particular face significant issues that require sensitive, coordinated multidisciplinary care in order to optimize patient well-being. These populations are discussed with particular references to the role of the SLP.

## Total Laryngectomy

Surgical removal of the larynx is a devastating prospect for any individual. Although cure rates following laryngectomy are high the by-products of this surgery remain significant rehabilitation challenges. It is well known that total rehabilitation of the laryngectomee requires the expertise of numerous specialists and should begin at the multidisciplinary treatment planning meeting.

### Preoperative Counseling and Support

Preoperative education is essential and ideally should commence following diagnosis and treatment planning. This education and counseling session should be completed prior to the patient's admission to hospital to allow the patient time to process the large volume of information that he or she will receive. This session should be completed in the SLP's office where possible or a similar quiet area. Naturally there are occasions where time or logistics do not permit a preoperative education and counseling session and in these situations it is recommended that education be provided at a point when the patient has recovered enough to be able to participate and process the information provided (i.e., not within first 48 hours postoperatively).

The preoperative education and counseling session usually has two main components, which will be discussed in more detail in the following sections. These include:

1. Discussion of anatomical, physiological, and lifestyle changes postlaryngectomy, typically supplemented with the viewing of a patient education video outlining laryngectomy, recovery, communication, and return to life outside hospital
2. Arranged meeting with a laryngectomy support visitor

**Anatomical, Physiological, and Lifestyle Changes Postlaryngectomy.** The preoperative session is designed to give the patient sound insight into laryngectomy surgery and its impact on communication, swallowing, and other significant lifestyle issues. When asked about the types of information that they would have wanted to be included in preoperative counseling, three quarters of laryngectomy patients reported the surgery itself, difficulties eating and drinking, difficulties tasting and smelling, communication options and being unable to blow your nose, loss of voice, difficulty with some recreational activities, having a shower, being unable to laugh or cry, and breathing through a stoma as the most important things to be discussed (Ward et al., 2003). Table 14–3 outlines these key changes. Although it is recognized that there are a number of negative consequences associated with laryngectomy, with rehabilitation and good support services, many patients adjust well to life following laryngectomy (see CD: Chapter 14: Video: "Life since Laryngectomy").

**The Laryngectomy Support Visitor.** The laryngectomy support visitor (LSV) is a laryngectomee who, with basic training in patient counseling, is asked to visit patients who are about to undergo surgery. The LSV shares his or her experiences with someone who is about to undergo total laryngectomy. This discussion

**Table 14–3.** Anatomical, Physiological, and Lifestyle Changes Postlaryngectomy

**Anatomical**

| | |
|---|---|
| Stoma | • Explain role of stoma—air inhaled/exhaled via stoma; permanent opening in neck<br>• Inform patient of the need to wear a stoma cover<br>• Discuss potential change in employment/activities due to dusty/strong chemical environments<br>• Discuss altered body image<br>• Inform patient he or she will learn how to care for stoma; it will become part of daily routine like brushing hair and cleaning teeth |
| Flap sites | • Discuss use of muscle flaps and/or skin grafts and cosmetic/esthetic impairment afterwards |
| Scars and aesthetics | • Discuss the presence of suture lines along the neck and around stoma as well as any suture lines around areas of muscle flaps and skin grafts<br>• Discuss aesthetics associated with suture lines and altered symmetry of neck due to neck dissection<br>• Discuss potential strategies to manage altered body image, i.e., scarves around neck until suture lines heal well |
| Resuscitation | • Explain need to place oxygen mask on neck over stoma, mouth to stoma<br>• Provide patient with resuscitation card that may be carried in wallet to alert strangers to neck breathing status in case of emergency |

**Physiological**

| | |
|---|---|
| Breathing and humidification | • Outline air inhalation/exhalation via stoma with no involvement of nose/mouth for breathing purposes<br>• Explain loss of nose for filtering and warming of air and therefore need to provide extra humidification and filtering<br>• Outline process of humidification as part of daily routine (i.e., use of HME steam in shower, using vaporizers)<br>• Reinforce need to wear stoma covers to provide filter against dirt/dust/environment |
| Coughing | • Discuss inability to cough as previously and explain use of "huff" to clear secretions from airway<br>• Explain the need to cover the airway, not mouth, when "coughing"<br>• Discuss increased mucus production as consequence of surgery<br>• Explain importance of maintaining clear airway and removing mucus<br>• Discuss feelings about mucus and stoma maintenance, i.e., may be embarrassing in public<br>• Inform patient of need to carry tissues/handkerchief for removing mucus from stoma |
| Swallowing | • Explain altered anatomy removes risk of aspiration<br>• Discuss potential changes to saliva production post-radiotherapy treatment<br>• Discuss potential impairment secondary to fibrosis of the neck tissues<br>• Outline types of swallowing strategies that may be of assistance, e.g., modified diets (e.g., pureed or soft diets), cyclic ingestion (altering food and fluids so that fluids are used to "wash down" food), use of smaller but more frequent meals (especially for patients who have gastric pull-up) |
| Taste | • Outline potential change to flavor perception and taste secondary to the lack of air passing through the nasal passages and/or as a result of radiation damage<br>• Explain how to optimize flavor perception and taste (e.g., use of food additives to increase taste, increased chewing) |

**Table 14–3.** *continued*

**Physiological** *continued*

| Smell | • Discuss why smell is impaired (due to lack of air moving through nose)<br>• Outline the implications for emergency/danger warning (such as leaking gas), as well as the implications for personal hygiene and influence on appetite<br>• Explain why they may still be able to smell strong odors, and discuss treatment options for reestablishing olfaction |
|---|---|
| Speech and communication | • Explain why communication is altered and a new method of speech is required<br>• Present the communication options available postlaryngectomy (where possible use past laryngectomee to demonstrate speech technique)<br>• Outline the pros and cons of each communication option and reinforce it will be patient's choice, not clinician's; clinician will guide decision<br>• Discuss the grief associated with loss of natural voice; encourage patient to consider audio- or videotaping voice before surgery<br>• Discuss implication of new voice on occupation, interests, schooling/education, and social interactions<br>• Highlight impact on body image due to new method of speech production<br>• Explain temporary communication options available until preferred option available (i.e., use of electrolarynx before TE speech)<br>• Outline SLP support for communication therapy until patient achieves desired communication option |
| Blowing nose | • Explain reason why patient unable to blow nose in same manner as preoperatively (i.e., unable to direct air into nasal passage to clear nose secretions)<br>• Discuss ability of some patients to learn how to direct (shunt) air up into nasal cavity; reinforce this is difficult for many |

**Lifestyle**

| Showering | • Explain that airway is unable to be protected in same manner as preoperatively due to direct opening at neck<br>• Inform patient of need to wear a shower cover or use a handheld shower rose<br>• Explain how some patients are able to shower with normal shower but direct water away from neck/stoma (e.g., have water spray onto lower back) |
|---|---|
| Swimming and water sports | • Explain loss of ability to protect airway means patient unable to swim without laryngectomee swimming device<br>• Laryngectomee swimming device requires in-depth training and practice before patient is competent to use independently<br>• Advise patients on the risks of water sports such as fishing from a boat, sailing, water skiing due to the high risk of drowning even with a life jacket on |
| Lifting | • Explain that lifting will be difficult due to inability to develop pressure in the thorax secondary to inability to close the airway<br>• Discuss the need to consider changing some activities or employment if lots of lifting is required as patient is likely to be fatigued quickly or strain significantly<br>• Outline that some patients may be able to learn compensatory strategies but still usually tire more easily with strenuous exercise |
| Relationships and sexual activity | • Discuss the potential for relationships and sexual activities to be different postoperatively due to altered body image and the need to wear stoma covers; some patients also become conscious of stoma odors<br>• Inform patients that some people have difficulty talking during sexual activity<br>• Remind the patient that these issues can be discussed with the social worker, psychologist, or counselor |

*continues*

**Table 14–3.** *continued*

**Lifestyle** *continued*

| | |
|---|---|
| Airline travel | • Explain that the patient may require different oxygen masks in the event of an emergency<br>• Instruct the patient to contact the airline before travel<br>• Inform the patient that he or she may require use of metal instruments to assist removal of crusts and mucus during long flights. The patient will require a letter from the SLP to enable these items to be carry-on luggage |
| Laughing/crying/shouting | • Explain the altered ability to express the emotions of crying, laughter, and shouting due to altered communication methods<br>• Ensure the patient is aware that sometimes this can be misinterpreted by the listener, especially during the early recovery period |
| Occupation | • Encourage patients to return to work and activities where possible<br>• Inform patients that some people need to change employment due to communication difficulties or anatomical/structural reason (i.e., can't do heavy lifting or bend over) |

between the patient and the rehabilitated laryngectomee can provide invaluable support as the two share a common experience, and this is not the same as the support offered by the health professionals. The role of the LSV is to show the patient how to be able to communicate after surgery and that readaptation is a reality and return to a meaningful life is possible. The LSV provides emotional support, encouragement, and motivation for the planned surgery and recovery period ahead of the patient. LSVs are encouraged to be a friend to the patient, not another professional. The significance of the LSV is highlighted in the video clip contained on the CD (Chapter 14: Video: "Laryngectomy Support Visitor"), in which a patient describes how the LSV gave her hope and a goal to aim for in her rehabilitation.

The timing of the LSV visit is frequently determined by the timing of the initial referral to the SLP, but may also be determined by the patient's previous exposure to laryngectomees, the patient's readiness to meet a LSV, and the availability of a suitable LSV. The LSV usually meets with the patient prior to surgery but may also visit the patient after surgery to provide ongoing reassurance during the postoperative recovery period. If the LSV is unable to meet with the patient prior to surgery the session should be arranged as soon as the patient is able to participate in the session (i.e., not in the first 48 hours after surgery).

The LSV must be selected carefully, and in many hospitals the responsibility for selection and training of LSV is the SLP's. Some surgeons may have patients they refer to; however, in many settings the surgeon will still direct the referral through the SLP. Ideally, the LSV should be matched for gender and be as close as possible in age, interests, and culture to the patient.

There are a number of attributes for a good support visitor and the SLP should consider the following criteria when selecting a LSV. They should:

- be 6 months past their own surgery
- have functional to good communication skills
- be physically and emotionally well—have adjusted well and have a positive attitude about life postlaryngectomy
- be a good listener
- be warm and supportive
- have neat presentation (well groomed and dressed)

The LSV must be able to act under the supervision of the SLP at all times and remember that the purpose of the visit is to provide support to the patient and not to cast doubts or to confuse. LSVs must be prepared to discuss the physical changes that have occurred postoperatively and how they have coped emotionally after the surgery. The LSV can explain how to communicate after surgery but must remember that the patient may not use the exact same method of communication (depending upon availability of the LSV required). The LSV must understand that he or she does not have to know the answers to all questions and it is appropriate to be honest and say, "I don't know." They also need to remember that they are not there to provide clinical information, rather to provide insight based on their own experience.

The SLP must prepare the LSV adequately before the visit. They should undergo some form of training to ensure they are able to complete their role appropriately and successfully. Specifically training should include detailed discussion about the role and responsibilities of the LSV, including discussion about the potential questions they may be asked (i.e., Will I speak as well as you? Will the surgery cure my cancer? How long will it take me to speak again?) and the level of information that should be provided. Training should also explore what information the LSV believes would be beneficial information to provide to a new patient and information that may not be of benefit.

The SLP is encouraged to act as a facilitator and be present during the session to help guide questions and information exchange (this is less necessary with experienced LSVs). The SLP should help guide how much information is provided and how long the meeting should be. For some patients it is enough to meet with someone for just 5–10 minutes particularly considering the patient may be feeling overwhelmed at this initial stage. Sometimes the SLP may monitor this more accurately than the LSV. It is also crucial to be guided by the learning style of the individual patient. Some patients do not require a large amount of information but prefer to learn little bits as they progress. In a survey of the counseling and support services provided pre- and postsurgically to patients undergoing laryngectomy, the LSV was rated as the third main provider of presurgical information by the responding patients (Ward et al., 2003).

## Multidisciplinary Involvement Post-Treatment

Due largely to the intensive nature of the rehabilitation required to reestablish both speech and swallowing postlaryngectomy, the SLP is perceived by most patients as the primary health professional involved in

postoperative counseling and information dissemination (Ward et al., 2003). Chapters 8 to 13 of this textbook contain specific details of the support and rehabilitation process provided by speech pathology. As a result of such intensive involvement with the patient, the SLP is often the person that patients feel most comfortable with discussing issues and concerns. Because of this it is often the SLP who instigates unscheduled referrals to other team members as required postsurgery. Other team members who are commonly referred to in this phase are the dietitian, physiotherapist, and social worker.

**Laryngectomee Support Groups.** Organized laryngectomee support groups are common across many countries and states. They provide a variety of services for laryngectomees, their caregivers, and families, although all vary slightly in their programs. Many groups see their main role to provide information that can only come from the experience of living after laryngectomy. This support is provided to the patient, caregiver, and family before and/or after surgery. Laryngectomee support groups have numerous benefits that include information sharing, friendship, support, and understanding. They provide a safe environment for the new laryngectomees to hone their speech skills and interact with people who have been through the same challenges, obstacles, highs, and lows. The benefits patients experience from being involved in this supportive environment are exemplified by the comments on the video clip titled "Laryngectomy Support Group" on the CD (Chapter 14: Video: "Laryngectomy Support Group"). They also provide a venue for patients to discuss their problems and hear how others have found solutions (see CD: Chapter 14: Video: "Managing Dysphagia").

Many of the members of support groups are regular attendees over many years. However, it is equally important to acknowledge that the support group environment does not suit everyone. Some laryngectomees do not enjoy group activities and have no desire to attend a support group meeting, instead preferring to access information and support via other methods. It is crucial to recognize the individual choice and never force someone to attend against his or her wishes.

Support groups may be attached to large tertiary teaching hospitals that have specialized H&N units and highly experienced staff. These hospitals may coordinate regular meetings at the hospital for laryngectomees. The SLP is usually the leader in the organization of these meetings. The meetings may be delivered in a formal arrangement or may be held in the form of an informal social activity, such as a lunch or morning tea. There are also support groups that run independently of hospitals and clinicians and are based upon geographical location. These support groups are usually led by the laryngectomees themselves with input from SLPs sought out when required. Table 14–4 outlines general objectives of these groups.

Additionally there are groups at a national and international level, for example the International Association of Laryngectomees (IAL) and the National Association of Laryngectomee Clubs (NALC). The IAL is composed of approximately 250 member clubs and regional organizations across the globe. The IAL describes its purpose as to promote and support the total rehabilitation of laryngectomees by the exchange and dissemination of information to member clubs and to the public, to facilitate the formation of new clubs, to foster improvement in laryngectomee programs, and to improve the minimum standards for teachers of postlaryngectomy speech. At the IAL annual meeting a voice institute is run which trains laryngectomees and prospective SLPs. Further information about the IAL is available at: http://www.larynxlink.com/. Similarly, the NALC is comprised of nearly 100 member clubs across the United Kingdom and aims to unite all clubs across the British Isles whose objectives are to promote the welfare of laryngectomees and improve the treatments and availability of medical services for laryngectomees locally and nationally. Like the IAL the main focus is upon dissemination of information and support for laryngectomees. The NALC also produces a range of material including information brochures for patients and families and educational videos. Further information can be accessed via: http://www.nalc.ik.com/.

In addition to support groups there are many on-line services now available to laryngectomees. An Internet based newsletter called *WebWhispers* is a monthly on-line newsletter where laryngectomees can send in information and stories to share with others. This site can be accessed at: http://www.laryngectomees.inuk.com/whispers.html.

## Head and Neck Cancer in Childhood

When discussing pediatric H&N cancer in the current chapter, the term pediatric is used broadly to refer to both children and adolescents. Head and neck cancer due to squamous cell carcinoma is less common in the pediatric population with only 60 cases of juvenile laryngeal carcinoma reported since 1868 (Simon, Kahn, Schnider, & Pirsig, 1994). The gender distribution is also different. In the adult population, H&N cancer

**Table 14–4.** Key Objectives of Laryngectomy Clubs

**Objectives**

- Support and promote the rehabilitation of laryngectomees through laryngectomy support visitor programs

- Provide a support network for laryngectomees and their families through meetings and social gatherings of fellow laryngectomees and their partners

- Facilitate access to equipment and resources (e.g., stoma covers, electrolarynx)

- Collect, coordinate, and disseminate information relevant to laryngectomees through regular meetings and guest seminars

- Enhance community awareness and assist in the training and education of health professionals through lectures to community groups, students (schools, universities), and other professions (nursing, media, etc.)

- Provide a nonthreatening environment for people to practice their new modes of communication, gain confidence, and enjoy social interaction traditionally presents with a higher ratio of men to women, with a ratio of 10:1 (male:female) for laryngeal cancer. In comparison, pediatric H&N cancer appears more evenly distributed with a ratio of 6:4 (male:female) for laryngeal cancer. Although the incidence of H&N cancer in the pediatric population is lower than adults, the evidence suggests the disease is much more aggressive, with mortality rates for pediatric laryngeal cancer as high as 41% (Zalzal, Cotton, & Bove, 1987).

The themes of grief, loss, and trauma are at the forefront of our clinical experience with patients with H&N cancer. However, these themes appear magnified when working with young children/adolescents. For children and young adults, the negative consequences of cancer and its management seem heightened, and its impact even more devastating. Consequently, in addition to the support needs of the patient, there should also be consideration given to the support needs of the clinicians caring for these patients, assisting them to manage their own associated concerns and grief. Caring for pediatric patients with H&N cancer is emotionally demanding, and clinicians need to ensure they have close communication with their multidisciplinary team members and their colleagues to debrief.

## Physiological Differences

As detailed earlier in Chapter 1 of this textbook, laryngectomy is most common in the sixth and seventh decades of life and the factors most frequently associated with development of laryngeal cancer are cigarette and alcohol abuse. Therefore, adults usually present with lungs that have been exposed to many years of smoking which results in significant diseases of the airways (e.g., chronic obstructive pulmonary disease). This is in stark contrast to the pediatric laryngectomee who usually presents with healthy, clear lungs. This important physiological difference usually allows the child to adapt more easily to having a stoma and needing to remove secretions via the stoma. Similarly the sputum/mucus produced by the pediatric laryngectomee is usually thinner, clear, and more easily expectorated.

## Management Issues

While a child from a theoretical/medical perspective may manage the anatomical and physiological changes more easily, the impact of these changes psychologically is enormous, and perhaps greater for the child/adolescent. Having a stoma is far from ideal for an adolescent child who is increasingly conscious of appearance and body image. Similarly pediatric patients who undergo surgery and/or radiotherapy for removal of other types of H&N cancers may also need to deal with altered physiological characteristics, e.g., altered saliva production, skin reactions, and impaired oral movements. Managing temporary physiological changes associated with surgery such as tracheostomy, edema, pain, drain tubes, and feeding tubes in addition to being in the hospital and being unable to communicate verbally is an exceptionally confronting experience for the child or adolescent. Many children have minimal experience of hospitals and may never have been to a hospital before, therefore heightening their anxiety and the need for well coordinated support from the multidisciplinary team. The multidisciplinary team must ensure they explain procedures and physiological changes in lay terms the child/adolescent can understand.

Pediatric patients need to feel in control of what is happening at most points during the treatment and rehabilitation process. When working with adults who undergo cancer treatment, experience has shown that generally, but not always, adults will want directions from the clinician and want to see the clinician as the "expert." Adults more frequently are willing to follow the lead of the clinicians, though still remaining active in decision making. In contrast the child/adolescent definitely needs to be actively included in decision making, and not have decisions deferred to parents or caregivers. To be included and make some decisions is very important as it enables the child/adolescent to have a sense of being in control. The SLP must understand that, when working with patients beginning their adolescence, no matter how tight the plan was, you must demonstrate an ability to bend and flex with the adolescent to achieve the best outcome.

The pretreatment education session is crucial for the pediatric patient with H&N cancer. The information must be presented in a format appropriate to the age of the patient, which may mean usual visual aids and written material will need to be modified. It is important to encourage parents, grandparents, and siblings to try to be present so that the family and immediate others also understand what is happening and why. Experience has shown that even at the conclusion of pretreatment education sessions, children/

adolescents may have difficulty comprehending the magnitude of their H&N cancer and the treatment they will undergo. The clinician must be attuned to the questions children/adolescents are asking as this provides valuable information about how much information they have understood. Of equal importance is the need to explore silence. If no questions are being asked, they need to clarify if the child has understood or encourage him or her to discuss particular fears.

Another significant issue in the management of children with H&N cancer is the child's complete dependence on family. For example the child is often unable to attend any appointment independently but must rely on the adults to bring them. This becomes difficult when you have a family who does not communicate very well and where perhaps the parents are separated and theoretically share responsibility.

By the time most adults undergo treatment for H&N cancer they are well established as a person and know "who" they are. At this point, the benefit of staying alive often outweighs the embarrassment of the altered anatomy and physiology, new methods of communication, and the discomfort of changes even as significant as a stoma. However, adolescents who are still searching for their own identity do not necessarily see things this way, despite support and reassurance. Fear of an uncertain future and fear of recurrence are both at the forefront of the pediatric patient's mind for the duration of treatment and rehabilitation process. They require significant support to cope with the fact that their cancer and treatment have changed some aspects of their lives permanently and they are just beginning to experience many activities and events that now will not be "normal," i.e., going to parties, eating out, talking to the opposite sex, establishing intimate relationships.

There are significant and considerable adjustment issues for pediatric patients with H&N cancer. The child/adolescent will require close support from family and friends but would also be encouraged to call on the support of the multidisciplinary team members including the social worker, psychologist, nurse, and SLP. It is possible that the child may require long-term formal, professional support. Within Australian health settings, such assistance is often available from Child and Adolescent Mental Health departments. This support is highly encouraged; however, it is important to acknowledge that these services are usually only available up until age 17. Once the child/adolescent turns 18 he or she is no longer eligible for such services and must be referred on to appropriate adult services. This change is important as many of these adolescents will still benefit from ongoing psychological support as they continue to adjust to the new demands and challenges they face entering adulthood. The SLP and other professionals should be mindful of this and commence planning for treatment handover prior to the adolescent's turning 18; this will ensure there is a smooth transition of care and no "gap" in service provision.

It is also important to consider how adult and pediatric SLPs may work together to jointly manage a pediatric patient. Many pediatric clinicians have little experience with managing H&N cancer and therefore require the support and assistance of therapists who work with adult populations. It is a careful balance to ensure each clinician takes responsibility without getting in the other one's way or confusing the patient. It is important to realize that, as individual clinicians, neither adult or pediatric clinicians will have all of the specialist skills and knowledge required to manage a pediatric H&N patient on their own. Rather, working together enables the two clinicians to complement each other's expertise. To achieve this, both must recognize how to consult with each other to impart knowledge and skills to bridge the gaps, and be clear in each person's role so as not to confuse the child/adolescent.

There are also issues relating to equipment that need to be solved when working with the pediatric patient. Much of the equipment used with an adult laryngectomee is not appropriate for use with a child/adolescent because of size (e.g., tracheostoma tubes, oxygen masks, etc.). It is important that these issues have been considered and appropriate pediatric equipment sourced for the patient, particularly while admitted for surgery in an adult setting.

## Communication and Swallowing

For the pediatric laryngectomee, alaryngeal communication is extremely different from their "normal voice." Particularly for young female pediatric laryngectomees, tracheoesophageal (TE) speech is a radical departure from an adolescent girl's voice and they are understandably embarrassed by the deep quality of the new voice. Consequently the new form of communication may not be accepted. As a result, the pediatric laryngectomee may withdraw from communication. The SLP may find the new voice is used in clinic but not transferred to other settings. The child/adolescent may refuse to use new voice outside the clinical environment, therefore delaying any progress. In some cases the child/adolescent may use two forms of TE voice, a "soft" TE voice and true TE voice. The "soft" TE voice may be characterized by decreased volume and range and is used by the child/adolescent to avoid attracting attention and ensure only the immediate listener or communication partner can hear the voice. This voice often sounds more like a whisper. The child/adolescent may be able to produce the true TE voice just as easily, but is conscious of the deep quality of the voice and believes it draws unwanted attention because it sounds very different. Examples of a pediatric laryngectomee using her soft and loud voice is demonstrated on the CD segment titled "Two Voices" (Chapter 14: Video: "Two Voices").

Communication is integral to daily activities and there are many interactions people take for granted until communication is impaired. Verbal communication in the school classroom becomes very daunting for the patient who has undergone H&N surgery and may have mild to severely impaired speech. For the child/adolescent who has undergone oral surgery, intelligibility may be impaired while the child/adolescent laryngectomee has a completely different voice. It may take an enormous amount of encouragement and support for the child/adolescent to feel comfortable enough to speak verbally in front of classmates. Sometimes the SLP can tailor intervention to practice verbal tasks that might be required in the classroom to help facilitate the transfer of skills and confidence from the clinical setting into the everyday classroom setting. It may also be worth considering small group work with the child/adolescent and 2-4 friends first before attempting to speak with the entire class.

Similarly, the child/adolescent's parents and family must reinforce communication strategies and intervention techniques. The SLP only spends a limited amount of time with the child/adolescent and therefore must ensure the parent/family is well educated about the goals of rehabilitation and the strategies to successfully facilitate and enhance communication.

As earlier chapters have indicated patients undergoing laryngectomy are unable to eat/drink orally for a

period of 1-2 weeks postoperatively. This is often difficult for children/adolescents to accept even though they have been informed and understand that they are unable to. The child/adolescent will frequently ask if he or she can have small amounts of oral intake (i.e., "But I'll just have a couple of sips") or small candies/chocolates. In some cases surgeons are willing to be a little flexible and allow the child/adolescent to suck on candy (e.g., Soft Jubes) or commence clear fluids a little earlier than usual. The SLP may find it useful to complete swallowing assessments with the favorite food/drink of the child; this can be discussed in the days leading up to oral intake trials so that it becomes an anticipated reward. The SLP must be careful not to discuss oral intake plans without a clear picture from the surgeons regarding wound healing and likely oral intake commencement; otherwise the SLP may be presenting inaccurate information and setting the child/adolescent up for disappointment. See the video segment on the CD titled "Chocolate Thickshake" to hear this issue discussed.

Delayed or poor wound healing may result in longer periods of nil by mouth status. As we know death of muscle flaps used for reconstruction of the pharynx will result in long delays commencing oral intake. This is particularly distressing for the child/adolescent who has already endured a large operation and significant hospitalization without some of the comforts of favorite foods and drinks and now must endure a second large procedure that will result in further delayed oral intake commencement. Support and counseling from the SLP and other team members is crucial during this period.

As with adults the child/adolescent who has undergone reconstruction of the pharynx may have a significant motility disorder, which may result in difficulty swallowing food and/or fluids. The need for a child/adolescent to remain on a modified diet can be distressing and socially isolating, particularly in the long term. The child/adolescent often does not want to consider a modified diet, particularly not in front of friends and school mates.

## *Eesthetics*

Teenagers have to cope with many changes both physical and emotional. They are faced with growing independence, mood swings, and the development of sexual and emotional awareness. Self-image is extremely important and impacts upon their self-esteem. The teenage years are known to be the most bewildering and challenging of all years, so when you consider the impact of a stoma, the loss of the ability to communicate normally, and decreased autonomy, such changes can only intensify the changes the patient is experiencing as an adolescent. On the CD is a video segment "Adjusting to Changes" (Chapter 14: Video: "Adjusting to Changes") containing a young girl discussing some of these changes postsurgery.

The presence of a stoma for pediatric laryngectomee patients is devastating as it is a permanent reminder of the surgery and that the anatomy and physiology is different and will always look different to their friends and others around them. Some young girls enjoy wearing clothing that has low-cut necklines and shoestring straps, both of which are unable to disguise the presence of the stoma. Thus the child or adolescent girl must consider changing her choices of clothing and/or find suitable items to cover the stoma, which is not an easy or desired task. Adults who undergo laryngectomy do not face this difficulty as men are usually content to wear standard stoma protectors and women either hand make more attractive stoma covers or find a piece of jewelry that will be worn on a necklace to cover the stoma. Female pediatric laryngectomees are often unable to find suitable pieces of jewelry that will match the rest of their appearance, i.e., school uniform. Jewelry is often too ornate and considered "too old" for the child or adolescent. It may also be unacceptable from a school uniform regulation perspective (i.e., no jewelry allowed to be worn) therefore drawing attention to the pediatric laryngectomee if she is given an exception and allowed to wear the jewelry.

The impact of other radical surgical procedures will often leave patients with asymmetrical structures that are visible to others due to the location of the surgery. For example radical neck dissections will result in a loss of tissue bulk on the operated side, thus resulting in a significant asymmetry of the neck. The suture lines along the neck from surgery are another cosmetic defect that the child/adolescent must adjust to, in a world that is heavily focused upon body image. The use of reconstructive flaps for wound closure and restoration of function and cosmesis can result in different color skin tissue in visible places of the face,

neck, and/or throat. Depending upon the location of the donor site for the muscle flap the patient may have additional scar(s) along the arm, leg, or stomach. While the scar on the arm (for radial forearm free flaps) is on the underside of the forearm it is still significantly noticeable when wearing short sleeves. The use of jejunum flaps or gastric pull-ups will result in scars across the abdomen which may be upsetting to the female patient as this area of the body is frequently exposed these days with fashion focused on wearing midriff tops and two-piece swimsuits.

## Return to School/Friends/Social Life

Involvement of the school is essential for management of the pediatric H&N cancer patient to assist the patient to return to "normal life." It is important to include teachers in the group of people who should be educated to understand the cancer treatment and expected outcomes. It is recommended that education/counseling sessions be available for some or all of the teachers involved with the child/adolescent receiving treatment. It is usually most practical to visit the school and provide a short in-service to a larger group of teachers and then spend more time with one or two of the main teachers. It is also important to recognize the importance of friends for children and adolescents and to include them in education or treatment sessions where appropriate and agreed to by the patient. Sometimes the positive reinforcement from a friend can significantly influence the performance of the patient.

Integration aid assistance is available in many schools in Australia and can be a tremendous help and would be encouraged for any pediatric patient being treated for H&N cancer. This assistance is often a huge boost to the child's confidence and social development as well as facilitating a successful return to school often after several months away from school having treatment. Sessions with integration staff can also be used to encourage use of new methods of communication (e.g., TES speech). It is essential that the SLP ensures the integration staff is up to date with current goals and stages of recovery from treatment. These sessions can facilitate new learning and transfer of skills from within the formal clinical setting to the "real world."

For pediatric laryngectomees the inability to swim and restricted physical activity is a significant issue while at school where there are compulsory physical education classes and activities such as swimming. The pediatric laryngectomee will require particular support, understanding, and empathy during these times.

Returning to a normal life after treatment for H&N cancer will also include returning to socializing and going out with friends. This time can be particularly confronting for adolescents who are beginning to establish closer relationships with the opposite sex, starting to go to parties that are more focused on meeting the opposite sex ,and even beginning sexual relationships. These social functions can be challenging to the adolescent who has residual communication and/or swallowing difficulties post-treatment. It is even more confronting for the adolescent laryngectomee who is grappling with the use of TES speech. These social functions are often accompanied by loud music, which makes verbal communication difficult for anyone, let alone someone who is trying to use TES speech that does not have the volume range required to speak over loud background music. While there are no easy solutions to these difficulties, it is important to be aware of them and acknowledge them with the adolescent and attempt to find creative ways to adapt/manage these social functions.

# Palliative Care

Palliative care is care provided for a person with an active, progressive, advanced disease who has little or no prospect of cure, and for whom the primary treatment goal is quality of life (QOL) (Palliative Care Australia, 2003). The focus of palliative care is on the quality of the patient's life, with the aim of maintaining comfort and dignity, from diagnosis throughout the disease progression and into bereavement. Palliative care also refers to the care provided for the patient's partner, family, and caregivers.

Dying is an integral and inevitable part of life and quality palliative care helps to enable people to die in a way that is congruent with their life choices and personal wishes (Steinhauser, Clipp, McNeilly, Christakis, McIntyre, & Tulsky, 2000). As one can imagine, people's needs vary widely as death approaches, but commonly include the need to understand what is happening, resolve issues with family and friends, achieve a sense of completion emotionally and spiritually, and accept

significant life changes. Palliative care can support this process by relieving pain and other symptoms, addressing practical and financial problems, and providing appropriate psychological, social, and spiritual support.

*Palliative care* can be described as a concept of care that provides coordinated medical, nursing, and allied health services for people who are terminally ill and, where possible, is delivered in the environment of the patient's choice. Specialist palliative care is delivered by clinicians with specialist and accredited training in palliative care. *Palliative interventions* are treatments used to palliate symptoms (e.g., surgery, radiotherapy); they are not palliative care, but are offered simultaneously with palliative care.

## *Primary Aims of Palliative Care*

The primary aims of palliative care are to enable people facing death to:

- be as free as possible from suffering (physical, emotional, and spiritual)
- maintain their dignity and independence during the disease experience
- be cared for in the environment of their choice
- have their grief needs recognized and responded to
- neither to hasten or delay death
- be assured that their families' needs are also being met by offering a support system to help both patients and family/caregivers
- enhance QOL and potentially positively influence the course of illness (Palliative Care Australia, 2006)

Promotion of individuals' QOL is a central tenet in the context of palliative care. In cases when treatment has become noncurative, quality rather than quantity of life becomes important and is considered the primary outcome to assess. QOL is a broad concept that encompasses physical, social, psychological, and spiritual domains. While there are negative aspects about a patient's illness and impending end of life, many patients report positive outcomes that have come from their illness. This attribute of QOL often helps the health care professional to shift focus from the negative issues such as loss and distress, to focus instead on the strengths and positive capacities of the patient within the context of care. Many palliative care organizations (e.g., Palliative Care Australia) publish comprehensive documents that outline a framework for palliative care services (Palliative Care Australia, 2006). These documents aim to provide guidance for those working with patients with cancer and to cover all aspects of the patient care journey.

Some patients may initially view palliative care as another one of the many services burdening them and their family/caregiver. However, in reality the care from palliative care services is offered over time, with different teams or caregivers involved as appropriate. Palliative care moves with the patient and is available in a variety of settings including the patient's home, hospice, or inpatient hospital bed. There are numerous benefits for patients, including:

- pain control
- control of other symptoms such as nausea and vomiting, constipation, breathlessness
- improved sleep patterns
- reduced anxiety
- spiritual well-being
- connection with family
- improved patient and caregiver satisfaction

Similarly there are benefits for family and/or caregivers, including:

- grief resolution and bereavement adjustment
- reduced anxiety and depression, leading to improved health related quality of life
- adequate home support, reducing need for multiple hospital readmissions.

## Palliative Care Service Team Members

The palliative care team must consist of specialized staff who are accredited and experienced in delivering palliative care services. For patients with H&N cancer, a specialist medical oncologist and clinical nurse specialist typically lead the team. The multidisciplinary team is crucial to the success of palliative care services. They must work in an interdisciplinary model and be flexible to provide rapid response. Usually only a small percentage of patients with H&N cancer receiv-

ing palliative care have direct involvement with palliative care specialists. This may be due to a number of reasons, including availability of specialist palliative care services, medical staff preferences, and patients' wishes. Sometimes palliative care is provided by H&N health care professionals such as surgeons, oncologists, radiation oncologists, allied health, and nursing in the normal delivery of care. However, it is crucial to understand the benefits of the specialist palliative care teams, and when they are available, patients should be referred. The treating medical staff and allied health staff have often developed close relationships with their patients due to the ongoing monitoring and intervention over many years. Some may not want to lose the opportunity to support the patient through this final stage of life. However, often the care can be provided in a collaborative way, with ongoing input from all staff familiar to the patient.

## Palliative Care in Head and Neck Cancer Population

Most H&N cancers if caught early are curable and can be treated successfully with single or multimodality treatments (e.g., surgery, radiotherapy, combined chemotherapy and radiotherapy). However, it is still not uncommon for patients to present to the multidisciplinary clinic with advanced malignancies, preventing the possibility of curative treatment. Similarly, there is the population of patients who present with unchecked or recurrent disease following failed treatment attempts, who are not for curative management. In both scenarios, palliative care becomes appropriate and should be immediately instigated, as opposed to waiting until later stages of disease when death is imminent.

Many of the problems faced by the H&N patient are not peculiar to the disease and are faced by many patients with terminal illness. The problems that are specific to the patient with H&N cancer include management of airway obstruction, dysphagia, and speech/communication problems.

## When to Refer to Palliative Care?

It is important to note that referral to a palliative care service is appropriate at any time of the disease trajectory. Referral may be initiated when the patient or family/caregiver has identified needs that are not being addressed adequately. These needs may be based on physical, emotional, psychological, or spiritual issues. Palliative care referrals should be instigated early in the illness. Late referrals to palliative care are often "crisis" referrals with high levels of distress and frustration. In some cases patients are not referred at all, which may be detrimental to the patient's last wishes.

There are a number of referral indicators that can help identify the need for palliative care services for patients with H&N cancer. These can include:

- *Physical symptoms.* Fatigue, weakness, and drowsiness are prevalent problems in patients with H&N cancer. These symptoms may be related to poor oral intake (and dysphagia), which is a common characteristic of patients with H&N cancer. Poor appetite and loss of weight would also highlight the need for palliative care referrals. Physical problems of the family members as well as those of the patient can have a negative effect on the psychological health of the family, including reduced mental health and cognitive functioning during and after the patient's illness.

- *Psychological symptoms.* Younger patients are at higher risk of developing depression. A diagnosis of depression may be complicated by the presence of physical symptoms and may be missed in situations in which depression is presumed to be a normal response to the situation. Patients who believe they are a burden, perceive they have lost their dignity, are depressed, and/or with poor symptom control present with higher risk of wishing to hasten their end of life. Patients with cognitive impairments may benefit from palliative services as cognitive dysfunction can sometimes be the result of a biomedical condition such as the effects of drugs, sepsis, or brain metastases. If recognized and treated, significant improvements can be made.

- *Cultural and social issues.* The level of palliative care received by the patient and his/her family can have implications for the functioning of the family during bereavement. Female patients with cancer report greater unmet support needs than male patients;

and younger patients and their families have greater unmet social needs than older patients, indicating that cancer has greater psychosocial effects on younger patients and their families. The need for support from nonfamilial sources such as health professionals was expressed by 77% of the patients with women reporting greater need for support from health professionals than men (McIllmurray, Thomas, Francis, Morris, Soothill, & Al-Hamad, 2001).

- *Caregiver issues.* Females and younger caregivers, especially wives, may be at increased risk of psychological morbidity. Similarly caregivers with small social networks, high levels of anxiety and anger, and long histories of caring for patients with unrelieved physical and/or psychological symptoms are also at greater risk developing psychological disorders and benefit from referral to palliative care services. It is also worth noting it is difficult for caregivers to express their own needs unless asked specifically away from the hearing of the patient, and so health care professionals should be encouraged to invite caregivers for discussions away from the bedside so that the caregivers are able to honestly express how they are feeling.

- *Other patient or health professional issues.* It is evident that given the high financial burden associated with having or caring for a person with a terminal illness, health professionals need to be aware of the financial situation of their patients with advanced cancer. Patients also need to be aware of the financial implications when making ongoing care decisions. It is also imperative that patients and their families are informed of services and programs that may assist with meeting financial needs. Developing and implementing advance care planning and creating advance directives are increasingly becoming an important quality of care issue. An advance directive is sometimes called a "living will." It is a document that describes one's future preferences for medical treatment in anticipation of a time when one is unable to express these preferences due to illness or injury. Advance directives can result in increased patient satisfaction, patients believing that their doctors had a better understanding of their wishes, and greater comfort making end-of-life decisions.

## Conclusion

Patients who present with H&N cancer have complex care needs and require input from multiple specialist clinicians across all areas of treatment. This multidisciplinary team consists of medical, nursing, and allied health staff. The multidisciplinary team framework enhances patient care by improving coordination, reducing duplication, and facilitating evidence based practice. It is essential that clinicians working in H&N cancer care have a sound understanding of the role of each multidisciplinary team member and when each should be involved. Knowledge and awareness of the multidisciplinary team will ensure that the most appropriate clinicians are referred to in a timely manner.

## References

Association of Oncology Social Work. Retrieved May 11, 2006 from http://www.aosw.org/

Clarke, L. (1998). Rehabilitation for the head and neck cancer patient. *Oncology, 12*(1), 81-89.

Edwards, D. (1998). Head and neck cancer services: Views of patients, their families and professional. *British Journal of Oral and Maxillofacial Surgery, 36*(2), 99-102.

Fallowfield, L. (1993). Giving sad and bad news. *Lancet, 341*(8843), 476-478.

Gates, G. A., Ryan, W., & Lauder, E. (1982). Current status of laryngectomee rehabilitation, IV. Attitudes about laryngectomee rehabilitation should change. *American Journal of Otolaryngology, 3*(2), 970-1003.

Gourdji, I., McVey, L. & Loiselle, C. (2003). Patient satisfaction and importance ratings of quality in outpatient oncology center. *Journal of Nursing Care Quality, 18*(1), 43-55.

Hutton J., & Williams, M. (2001). An investigation of psychological distress in patients who have been treated for head and neck cancer. *The British Journal of Oral & Maxillofacial Surgery, 39*(5), 333-339.

Leydon, G., Boulton, M., Moynihan, C., Jones, A., Mossman, J., Boudioni, M., & McPherson, K. (2000). Cancer patients' information needs and information seeking behaviour: In depth interview study. *British Medical Journal, 320*, 909-913.

Mathog, R. (1991). Rehabilitation of head and neck cancer patients: Consensus on recommendations from the international conference on rehabilitation of the head and neck cancer patient. *Head & Neck, 13*(1), 1-14.

McIllmurray, M., Thomas, C., Francis, B., Morris, S., Soothill, K., & Al-Hamad, A. (2001). The psychosocial needs of cancer patients: Findings from an observational study. *European Journal of Cancer Care, 10*(4), 261-269.

National Institute for Health & Clinical Excellence. (2004). *Improving outcomes in head and neck cancers—The manual.* Retrieved June 1, 2006, from http://www.nice.org.uk/page.aspx?o=csghn guidance

Newell, R., Ziegler, L., Stafford, N., & Lewin, R. (2004). The information needs of head and neck cancer patients prior to surgery. *Annals of Royal College of Surgeons of England, 86*(6), 407-410.

Palliative Care Australia. (n.d.). Retrieved May 10, 2006, from http://www.pallcare.org.au/Default.aspx?tabid=301

Palliative Care Australia. (2003). Palliative care service provision in Australia: A planning guide 2003 (2nd ed.). Retrieved May 10, 2006, from: http://www.pallcare.org.au/Portals/9/docs/publications/Planning%20guide2003.pdf

Palliative Care Australia. (n.d.). Standards for providing quality palliative care services for all Australians. Retrieved May 10 2006, from http://www.pallcare.org.au/Portals/9/docs/Standards%20Palliative%20Care.pdf

Parker, A., Baile, W., Moor, C., Lenzi, R., Kudelka, A., & Cohen, L. (2001). Breaking bad news about cancer: Patient's preferences for communication. *Journal of Clinical Oncology, 19*(7), 2049-2056.

Ptacek, J. T., & Ptacek, J. J. (2001). Patient's perceptions of receiving bad news about cancer. *Journal of Clinical Oncology, 19*(21), 4160-4164.

Renner, M. J. (1995). Counselling laryngectomees and their families. *Seminars in Speech and Language, 16*(5), 215-219.

Rutten, L., Arora, N., Bakos, A., Aziz, N., & Rowland, J. (2005). Information needs and sources of information among cancer patients: A systematic review of research (1980-2003). *Patient Education and Counselling,* 57(3), 250-261.

Simon, M., Kahn, T., Schnider, A., & Pirsig, W. (1994). Laryngeal carcinoma in a 12-year-old child—Association with human papillomavirus 18 and 33. *Archives of Otolaryngology-Head and Neck Surgery, 120,* 277-282.

South Western Sydney Area Health Service Liverpool Hospital Cancer Therapy Centre. (n.d.). *Counselling & support services.* Retrieved May 10, 2006, from http://www.swsahs.nsw.gov.au/cancer/counslng&supprt.asp

Steinhauser, K. E., Clipp, E. C., McNeilly, M., Christakis, N. A., McIntyre, L., & Tulsky, J. A. (2000). In search of a good death: Observation of patients, families and providers. *Annals of Internal Medicine, 132*(10), 825-832.

Ward, E. C., Hobson, T. K., & Conroy, A. (2003). Pre- and post-operative counselling and information dissemination: Perceptions of patients undergoing laryngeal surgery and their spouses. *Asia Pacific Journal of Speech, Language and Hearing, 8,* 44-68.

Wiggers, J. H., Donovan, K. O., & Redman, S. (1990). Cancer patient's satisfaction with care. *Cancer, 66,* 610-616.

Zalzal, G., Cotton, R., & Bove, K. (1987) Carcinoma of the larynx in a child. *International Journal of Paediatric Otorhinolaryngology, 13,* 219-225.

# Chapter 15

# MANAGEMENT OF HEAD AND NECK CANCER: AN INTERNATIONAL PERSPECTIVE

Elizabeth C. Ward, Robyn A. Burnett, Ann-Louise Morton, Julie A. G. Stierwalt, Kimberly R. Wilson, Edwin M. Yiu, and Corina J. van As-Brooks

## Introduction

Head and neck cancer is a global concern. Internationally, clinicians working with this population strive to achieve optimal outcomes for their patients through establishing the best practice models of care. Yet it must be acknowledged that even when the goal is to embrace evidence-based health care, clinicians face a number of hurdles that can impact on the ability to adopt "new" or "best practice" within their clinical settings, including: national health priorities, health care service differences, costs and economic constraints, differing clinical roles and scope of care, cultural diversity, and even medical and personal bias. As a consequence, national patterns of health care evolve which have elements that are both similar and unique on the international stage.

The current chapter has been designed to provide the reader with some insight into international differences, and the nature of the challenges facing different countries as they seek to provide optimal health care and support services for their population of patients with head and neck cancer. To achieve this goal, the authors of the current chapter have identified some of the key service issues that face clinicians and patients with head and neck cancer in Australia, the United Kingdom (UK), the United States of America (USA), China, and parts of Europe. Across each of these settings, different terminology is used to describe professionals involved in speech pathology practice, including speech pathologists (Australia), speech language therapists (UK), speech-language pathologists (USA), and speech therapists (China). In each international section the relevant professional terminology will be used, while the term speech-language pathologist will be used in the European section as various different terms are used in different European settings.

## Australia

Cancer surveillance in Australia is governed under state and territory legislation and routine collection of cancer statistics has been universal in all states and territories since 1982. The cancer incidence data collected through this national process indicates that Australia has a high incidence of squamous cell carcinoma of the head and neck mucosa, with approximately 853 new cases identified in 2001 representing 3.8% of all cancers in men and 1.9% of all cancers in women (Australian Institute of Health and Welfare [AIHW] report: Cancer in Australia, 2001). The incidence rate for most head and neck cancers in Australia, in comparison to world incidence data, is represented in Table 15–1.

As cancer incidence data within Australia are collected within each state and territory, this allows both state and national data analysis. Figures in the 2001 national cancer report reveal that incidence rates for smoking related cancers vary between Australia's states and territories, with the Northern Territory currently having the highest smoking related cancer incidence rates for both males and females, and also the highest death rates from cancers attributed to smoking (AIHW report, 2001). This pattern is expected to shift in future years in alignment with the changes in smoking related behaviors reported between the states and territories documented in the 2001 National Health Survey (Australian Bureau of Statistics [ABS], 2002). The national interest and investment in cancer management and research continues to grow in Australia. In 2000–2001, $215 million dollars was spent on cancer research, representing 18% of all health research expenditure in Australia (AIHW report, 2001).

## The Australian Health Care System

Within Australia, spending on health care is not overly high in comparison to similar advanced countries, with approximately 9.7% ($78.6 billion) of gross domestic product (GDP) being spent on health care in 2003–2004 (Health Expenditure Australia 2003-4, 2005). Yet although this annual expenditure may not be as high as other countries, such as the United States (in excess of 14% GDP expenditure), currently Australians experience life expectancies and years of good health which fall among the highest in the world. However, it is noted that current demands facing the Australian health system, including rising costs, growing workforce shortages, maldistribution of the available workforce, the aging population, and job dissatisfaction, are placing increased pressures on the current

**Table 15–1.** Cancer incidence data expressed as per 100,000 per population and age standardized (AS) to both the Australian 2001 standard population and the WHO 2000 World Standard Population (AIHW Report, 2001).

| Cancer Subtype | Males | | Females | | Sex Ratio M:F |
|---|---|---|---|---|---|
| | Australian AS Rate | World AS Rate | Australian AS Rate | World AS Rate | |
| Lip | 7.7 | 6.0 | 2.5 | 1.8 | 3.1 |
| Tongue | 3.2 | 2.5 | 1.5 | 1.1 | 2.1 |
| Mouth | 2.9 | 2.2 | 1.7 | 1.3 | 1.7 |
| Salivary gland | 1.7 | 1.2 | 0.8 | 0.6 | 2.1 |
| Tonsil | 1.6 | 1.3 | 0.4 | 0.3 | 3.7 |
| Other oropharynx | 0.6 | 0.5 | 0.1 | 0.1 | 4.3 |
| Nasopharynx | 0.8 | 0.6 | 0.3 | 0.2 | 2.7 |
| Hypopharynx | 1.3 | 1.0 | 0.2 | 0.2 | 5.8 |
| Pharynx unspecified | 0.6 | 0.5 | 0.2 | 0.1 | 2.9 |
| Larynx | 5.8 | 4.3 | 0.5 | 0.4 | 11.2 |

workforce and health service (Health Systems Review Final Report, 2005).

Particular issues with demonstrated impact on the management of the head and neck population include the current shortage of health care workers, including speech pathologists, and the issue of distribution of health care services in rural and remote areas of Australia. It is currently recognized that speech pathology services throughout Australia are inadequate, with speech pathology identified as one of the 14 non-information technology professions on the National Skills Shortage list (Department of Employment and Workforce Relations, 2006). In addition to national shortages, distribution of speech pathologists across urban and rural settings shows imbalance, with the supply of health workers decreasing dramatically with increasing remoteness (Australia's Health Workforce, 2005). This data is significant, considering that approximately 30% of Australia's population of 19.5 million people live in the more rural and remote areas of the continent. Consequently, it is widely accepted that this proportion of the population have limited choice in available health care providers, and are often expected to travel long distances to access health services provided in the larger urban centers.

Within Australia, patients can be managed through either the public or private health care systems, though the majority of patients utilize the public health care system for all or part of their ongoing cancer care. Funding for public health is managed largely at the state government level, resulting in differences in health services between the states and territories. Consequently, pathways to care for patients across Australia can differ slightly between each state. For the most part, however, each follows a relatively similar service model, with one or two key large urban public hospitals within the state serving as specialist centers for patients with head and neck cancer. These centers operate multidisciplinary head and neck clinics that consider the patient's presenting issues and determine as a team the treatment approach (nonsurgical +/– surgical), intent (palliative, curative), and the management plan. In most cases, all necessary services (medical, surgical, oncology, and allied health) are located either within the hospital complex or within close proximity, facilitating cohesive and integrated care.

## Speech Pathology Management of Head and Neck Cancer in Australia

Within the multidisciplinary service model, the speech pathologist has input into management decisions and commences interaction with the patient from the point of initial access to the hospital system. This provides improved continuity of care and ensures optimal counseling, education, and patient support. The multidisciplinary model of care is then maintained throughout the clinical management of the patient.

In 2001, Burnett examined patterns of clinical care for patients following laryngectomy in Australia. Detailed questionnaires were sent to 38 acute hospital speech pathology departments across all states and territories with responses returned by 27 units. Information was gathered regarding the acute care of the laryngectomy inpatient, examining preferred alternative feeding routes, time frames for commencing oral intake, and the regimes used for upgrading diets. Voice rehabilitation options and the decision-making process were explored, as were management practices. In general, management of the acute inpatient and voice rehabilitation options for laryngectomy patients was found to be very similar across settings in Australia, though some slight variations in the timelines for various aspects were noted.

In relation to patterns of vocal rehabilitation, research has demonstrated that within Australian settings tracheoesophageal speech (TES) is the predominant method of voice restoration for patients following total laryngectomy. Approximately two thirds of patients use TES compared to only one third of patients using an artificial larynx (Ward, Koh, Frisby, & Hodge, 2003). In contrast, in current practice very few laryngectomy patients are trained in esophageal speech. Within Australia, the majority of equipment/devices necessary for alaryngeal vocal rehabilitation are provided free of charge through the public health system allowing patient suitability and personal preference to be the key determining factors influencing rehabilitation method. National patterns (Burnett, 2001) have revealed a predominant use of Blom-Singer products, with a less extensive use of the Provox or Bivona prosthesis to address individual needs. These patterns have largely evolved due to funding issues and cost containment at the speech pathology department level. Similarly Servox is the primary brand of artificial larynx used by patients within Australia, due to the distribution of this particular electrolarynx device to public patients through the national Medical Aids Subsidy Scheme.

## Ongoing Services and Clinical Support

Although the Australian health system is currently facing many service challenges, postoperative patient support services for patients following both surgical and nonsurgical management of head and neck cancer are generally perceived as good. A survey of laryngectomy patients in Queensland revealed a high level of satisfaction with the postoperative counseling and support services provided (Ward, Hobson, & Conroy, 2003). Typically, in the early postdischarge phase, patients have access to free therapy services through the public hospital system. Outpatient care is then ongoing and intensity varies depending on the needs of the patient.

In addition to ongoing clinical support services, most states have organized laryngectomy support groups, which are nonfunded organizations run by laryngectomy patients and serve to provide a network of information and support for patients and their families both prior to and following surgery. These state groups often have an alliance with the Cancer Council of Australia, which provides some assistance with the running of the organization. Many of the large specialist hospitals within Australia also have smaller hospital based support groups for their patients, which are typically organized by the staff of the speech pathology departments.

Providing optimal and ongoing postdischarge patient support can, however, be particularly challenging within Australia in light of the large rural/remote population. Because only a few key specialist centers exist within each state, many patients need to travel out of town to receive services. Indeed, recent data on the pre and postoperative counseling and support services provided to laryngectomy patients in Queensland (Ward, Hobson et al., 2003) revealed that almost one third of respondents lived greater than 100 km from the hospital that conducted their surgery. Hence, long-term, postdischarge care necessitates either lengthy travel or seeking the support services of clinicians less familiar with specialist head and neck services. In relation to the levels of satisfaction with services received, the study found that a number of participants who lived in rural or remote communities reported dissatisfaction with postoperative support, contrary to the high levels of satisfaction reported by the urban respondents. The difficulty associated with accessing professional services due to distance was identified as a significant issue by a proportion of respondents. Respondents noted that rural health professionals are often inexperienced in the specialty area of laryngectomy rehabilitation and, therefore, they had experienced difficulty receiving adequate services and appropriate advice.

The use of telecommunication and the new information technology currently available have the potential to solve or assist many of the health care delivery issues facing rural and remote communities in Australia (Yellowlees, 2000). Indeed, telemedicine can be viewed as a practical tool that can assist health care professionals to close the gap between medical resources and the health care needs of the rural and remote patient. Remote consultation with specialists (i.e., "telerehabilitation" services) that can be offered locally or even to the home offers an opportunity to provide more timely access to health services and reduce unnecessary referrals and travel to urban centers, as well as help minimize the expense, social isolation, and carer burden associated with accessing services in distant urban centers. Currently the lead author of this chapter and colleagues (Ward, White, Russell, & Theodoros) from the Telerehabilitation Research Group at the University of Queensland, Australia, are evaluating the ability to conduct laryngectomy patient review assessments via telehealth services. In the next decade it is anticipated that services delivered by systems such as eREHAB may emerge as a viable supplement to traditional postsurgical care, particularly for patients returning to rural settings, where distance prevents timely and cost-effective service, or where specialized service is unavailable.

## The United Kingdom

Head and neck cancer is not common and represents less than 5% of all cancers in the United Kingdom (UK) (Yorkshire Cancer Network, 2003). Mouth, lip, and oral cavity cancer (oral cancer) has the highest incidence,

with cancers of the larynx and pharynx second and third respectively. The incidence of cancers of the mouth and pharynx has risen by over 20% over the last 30 years particularly among people under the age of 65. This increase is counterbalanced somewhat by a recent decrease in the numbers of laryngeal cancer (Quinn, Babb, Brock, Kirby, & Jones, 2001 cited in the National Institute for Clinical Excellence [NICE] Guidelines, 2004). As with many other countries, the incidence of and mortality from head and neck cancers are higher among disadvantaged populations and there are marked regional variations of incidence throughout the UK (Thorne, Etherington, & Birchall, 1997). Survival rates for each of the common head and neck cancer sites vary depending on the site and stage of the cancer; however, research has demonstrated that there have been minimal improvements in the survival rates of patients with head and neck cancer over recent decades (Soutar & Robertson, 2001).

## Overview of the Health Care System in the United Kingdom

Within the UK, the National Health Service (NHS) is the organizational body that delivers health care services throughout England, Wales, Scotland, and Northern Ireland. The system is financed mainly through general taxation with the additional element of National Insurance contributions. Though approximately 10% of the population in the UK take out private health insurance, the Health Service Act of 1977 and subsequent legislation provide that anyone in the UK is eligible for free health care. This system has, however, been subject to rationing on the basis of scarce resources. Over the past decade, the NHS has experienced significant budget increases in its monetary investment from £33 billion in 1996/1997 to £67.4 billion in 2004/05. This means an increase in the average spending per head of population from £680 to £1,345 (Department of Health, 2004).

In recent times, there has also been a stronger focus in the NHS on the importance of clinical governance and the development and implementation of National Service Frameworks. These changes in the last decade have resulted in an improvement in the quality of patient care by placing emphasis on evidence based interventions which demonstrate better health outcomes. Progress has been made within the NHS in tackling the country's largest killer diseases with premature deaths from diseases, such as cancers for instance, falling at the fastest rate of any European country (Department of Health, 2004).

## Services for Patients with Head and Neck Cancer in the United Kingdom

The lack of coordination of specialized services for patients with head and neck cancer has been identified as an issue in the UK. In a recent national study, slightly less than half of the hospitals had multidisciplinary teams for managing head and neck cancer compared to the treatment of more common forms of cancer such as breast cancer (Commission for Health Improvement/Audit Commission, 2001). Furthermore, in a major audit carried out in 1999/2000, it was revealed that the majority of patients in the south and west of the UK were treated by consultants who carried out 10 or fewer procedures for head and neck cancer each year (South West Cancer Intelligence Service, 2001). Processes are now firmly in place to rectify these problems to improve service delivery to head and neck cancer patients.

In 1995, the Calman Hine Report set out the direction of changes for cancer services throughout the UK (The Expert Advisory Group on Cancer to the Chief Medical Officers of England & Wales, 1995) and recognized the need for the establishment of national standards for cancer care. Following from this, in 2004 NICE formulated guidelines titled "Improving Outcomes in Head and Neck Cancers" (NICE, 2004). These guidelines heralded the move towards the centralization of cancer services to identified specialized centers, with ongoing high level support provided to local hospitals and primary and community care centers throughout the patient journey. Some of the key recommendations from the NICE guidelines (2004) have endorsed that over the next few years, services for patients in the UK with head and neck cancers should:

- be commissioned at the cancer network level
- have multidisciplinary teams with a wide range of specialists each managing at least 100 new cases of head and neck cancer per year
- have referral arrangements streamlined at each stage of treatment
- have a wide range of support services such as speech language therapists, clinical nurse specialists, dietitians, restorative dentists, and other health professionals as required both pre- and postoperatively until rehabilitation is complete
- have coordinated local support teams to provide long-term support and rehabilitation for patients in the community
- have accurate and complete information collection and audit procedures
- carry out research into the effectiveness of management that incorporates not only clinical trials but quality of life and patient satisfaction

A number of consensus documents in the UK have also been developed in the last 5 years that have focused on treatment guidelines for the management of head and neck cancer. These documents can be accessed on http://www.cancerbacup.org.uk. Primary treatment for most head and neck cancers in the UK is generally with surgery or radiotherapy or a combination of both. UK practice has also followed the shift observed in many other countries for the use of combined chemoradiotherapy for some patients as a primary mode of treatment of head and neck cancers (Pignon, Bourhis, Domenge, & Designe, 2000). Like many health services around the world, there can be delays in the NHS for patients to access certain investigations, procedures, and interventions, and in turn such delays may impact on the mode of treatment provided. The recent NHS Cancer Services Collaborative "Improving Partnership" target is to reduce the time from initial referral for suspected cancer to first definitive treatment to 62 days (Department of Health: Cancer Services Collaborative, 2006).

The British Association of Head and Neck Oncologists (BAHNO) has also begun a process of nationwide audit, supported by the National Clinical Audit Support Program (NCASP). The project known as DAHNO (Data for Head and Neck Oncology) will be mandatory for the multidisciplinary team to complete for every patient and will significantly improve the data available on outcomes of treatment in the NHS. For the first time, this should help to provide a more equitable service. The Department of Health grant to establish this information management system also included the remit to establish a data set for laryngectomy and surgical voice restoration in order to collect "real" figures in British practice. A speech language therapist chairs the steering committee for this project.

## Challenges Facing Speech-Language Therapy Services in the United Kingdom

The role of the speech language therapist in the management of patients with head and neck cancer is well established throughout the UK. In most specialist centers, the speech language therapist plays an important role in contributing to multidisciplinary team discussions on treatment planning and in the ongoing assessment and management of communication and swallowing function. There is however considerable regional variability in the provision of coordinated multidisciplinary services. Some patients feel they have very little support in some centers, while others praise the wide-ranging services, and report a high level of satisfaction in particular with speech therapy services (Edwards, 1997). In an audit carried out in 2001 by the Southwest Cancer Intelligence Service, it was revealed that 80%, 72%, and 32% of patients who had surgery to the larynx, hypopharynx, and posterior third of tongue, respectively, saw a speech language therapist. Overall, just 64% of patients saw a speech language therapist during their treatment, despite an agreed standard throughout the region covered by the audit that this was best practice.

While improvements are being made throughout the NHS in terms of funding and overall patient outcomes, a number of issues impact on the provision of speech and language therapy services to the head and neck cancer population. The main factor is a national shortage of skilled professionals. It is documented that there are currently only approximately 10,000 speech language therapists registered within the UK (Royal College of Speech and Language Therapists, 2005). As a result, speech therapy services have been identified

as one of the professions in the Tier 1 National Skills Shortage List (United Kingdom Immigration Work Permit and Visa Services, 2005) with the workforce strongly supported by locum or temporary contract staff largely from Australia, New Zealand, and South Africa.

This locum workforce has considerable budget implications for the NHS, with temporary contract staff often earning more per hour than permanent staff members with similar expertise. In addition, locum staff by nature are more transient, which raises issues in relation to consistency of services across the patient care episode. Funding for continuing professional development of locum staff is also not routinely provided by the NHS, and consequently, this has an impact on maintaining competencies of staff and standards of services provided. Speech language therapists who are trained in the UK receive basic dysphagia training at the undergraduate level to meet the minimum competencies established by the Royal College of Speech and Language Therapists (RCSLT). Once in the workforce, specialized dysphagia training must be undertaken by individual therapists and there are well-established courses that deliver this training.

In 1998, funding was obtained through Macmillan Cancer Relief for the appointment of a national consultant in surgical voice restoration. The primary responsibility of this position is in promoting and providing an equitable service to all surgical voice restoration patients nationally. A large proportion of this role is in the development and provision of training on surgical voice restoration to UK speech language therapists as this is mandatory prior to commencing work in this area. This process is well established with 534 professionals receiving basic level training throughout the UK and 900 professionals having attended the courses from 1998 to date (Edels, personal communication, November 16, 2005). An accredited university module is also currently being proposed. To the best of our knowledge, this module will be a world first as no post-graduate university accredited courses in surgical voice restoration currently exist. The appointee to this position has also established "The Advice Line" which is manned daily and has taken over 800 individual calls from speech language therapists around the UK and abroad. Each call is documented and categorized and the data have been audited several times in order to identify trends in areas of difficulty and lack of knowledge.

Ongoing professional development and peer support is also provided through the Head and Neck Special Interest Groups with two groups operating in England and one in each of Scotland and Wales. These groups have a high profile among the profession and are well attended by speech language therapists working within the realm of head and neck cancer. It is recognized that speech language therapists working in this field should have specialist expertise or have the close support of a specialist therapist. The NHS is currently undergoing a major review of the job descriptions and pay scales for all NHS staff known as "Agenda for Change" and this may have an impact on the level of services provided to speciality areas such as head and neck cancer.

## United Kingdom Speech-Language Therapy Practices

Speech language therapy services to patients with oral and pharyngeal cancers in the UK are primarily focused on the management of dysphagia with less time devoted to communication assessment and rehabilitation. This pattern is predominantly related to resource pressures and reflects what is happening in other patient groups throughout the UK. Videofluoroscopy and fiberoptic endoscopic evaluation of swallowing (FEES) are commonly used in the UK in the assessment and rehabilitation of dysphagia in head and neck cancer patients. Speech language therapists independently scope once they have achieved the competencies documented in the Royal College of Speech and Language Therapist Fiberoptic Endoscopic Evaluation of Swallowing policy (Kelly, Hydes, McLaughlin, & Wallace, 2005). Multidisciplinary videofluoroscopy and FEES clinics are common in most centers treating head and neck cancer and an increasing number of centers are using this instrumentation as a biofeedback approach for managing the swallowing and speech problems that arise from the treatment of head and neck cancers.

In relation to vocal rehabilitation, Ryan, Yong, Pracy, and Simo (2004) examined the current trends in voice restoration following laryngectomy in the UK via a national questionnaire. A total of 166 questionnaires were sent out to otolaryngologists throughout the UK and data was obtained from 77. Of these, it was revealed that 92% of the surgeons listed tracheoesoph-

ageal valve as their first choice of voice rehabilitation. Similarly, the large majority of surgeons performed primary punctures and most routinely performed myotomy. In the 1980s, when surgical voice restoration was in its infancy, the majority of surgeons commonly performed secondary punctures. However, as this data revealed, in the UK as with many other countries, the trend has changed with the recognition of surgical voice restoration as an excellent choice for many patients postlaryngectomy. Now, in the large centers, surgeons tend to exclusively perform primary punctures with the exception of extensive surgical reconstruction (e.g., jejunal interposition) when the anastomosis lies very close to the tracheoesophageal puncture. Regarding postsurgical management, there are some centers in the UK where the surgeon plays an integral role in surgical voice restoration particularly in relation to the placement and day-to-day troubleshooting. In larger centers with specialist speech language therapists on staff, this role is managed by the speech therapists with active consultation with the surgeon and the wider multidisciplinary team as required. In their survey, Ryan et al. (2004) noted that all responding surgeons (100%) involved speech language therapists in their rehabilitation teams.

In terms of voice prosthesis selection, Blom-Singer and Provox products are commonly used in the UK with certain regions tending to use one product brand over another. These decisions traditionally have been based more on product familiarity and what is most commonly used in the local region. This pattern of product use, however, is changing with therapists and surgeons now tending to choose the prosthesis according to its properties rather than according to its brand name. Regarding other forms of voice restoration, most laryngectomy patients within the UK are offered a Servox electrolarynx at some stage in their rehabilitation; however, an electrolarynx is primarily offered as a secondary method of communication for patients who continue to use surgical voice restoration as their primary means of communication. Very few patients are taught esophageal speech in centers in the UK primarily due to the success rate of surgical voice restoration. Some of the patients who use tracheoesophageal speech develop esophageal speech in the long term but in general adopt it only as a supplemental mode of communication, choosing to retain tracheoesophageal speech as their primary mode.

## Ongoing Services

Prior to leaving the hospital, patients are supplied with the relevant equipment for discharge home. In the case of oral and pharyngeal cancer patients, this may include supplies such as a fluid thickening agent and modified feeding devices. For laryngectomy patients, equipment such as the heat moisture exchange system and laryngectomy tubes is provided at no charge to the patient. In the UK, all ongoing equipment needs can be sourced through the NHS by prescription from the patient's general practitioner on recommendation by the speech language therapist or clinical nurse specialist. Surgical voice restoration equipment is supplied by the treating hospital and is funded from the speech therapy or otolaryngologist budget depending on the individual health care organization.

The importance of support groups in the UK for head and neck cancer is well recognized. In a British study of head and neck cancer care, patients who were members of support groups reported that their attendance at these groups provided them with a lifeline and described the relief they felt of meeting other people that had been though similar experiences (Edwards, 1998). Many of the patients reported a desire to have been informed of the groups earlier in their head and neck cancer management (NICE, 2004). There are well-established support groups in the UK for laryngectomees, patients with facial disfigurement, and those with dental problems. Specific details for these can be found on the NHS Direct Web site (www.nhsdirect.nhs.uk). Information on the National Association of Laryngectomee Clubs can be accessed on www.nalc.ik.com. Many of the larger head and neck cancer centers in the UK have hospital based support groups which tend to be patient led and involvement of the speech language therapist as part of these groups is common.

## The United States of America

As in many countries worldwide, cancer is a major health concern in the USA. Following heart disease, cancer is the second leading cause of death (Benninger & Grywalski, 1998). National incidence figures for the USA predict that there will be 1,372,910 new cases of cancer in 2005 (American Cancer Society, 2005). Additional estimates suggest that around 40,000 will involve cancers of the head and neck (National Cancer Institute, 2005), with 20% of those cases involving laryngeal cancer (Anderson & Sataloff, 2005). Examination of the national incidence figures for cancer in the USA point to geographic and cultural influences, with urban areas of dense population representing much higher incidence figures than less populated regions. For example, the primarily urban state of New Jersey has an anticipated incidence of around 43,000 new cases of cancer in 2005. In contrast, the state of Montana, which is a much larger state geographically, is primarily rural and thus the incidence for 2005 is anticipated to be much lower at 4,910 new cases. While contributors to general cancer types are not well known, cancers of the head and neck are primarily linked to tobacco use (Anderson & Sataloff, 2005; Boone & McFarlane, 2000).

The National Cancer Institute estimates that the prevalence of those living with cancer either cured or in treatment is around a million (American Cancer Society, 2005). While these estimates are staggering in terms of cost to individuals and institutions, there is hope on the horizon. Advances in treatment and early detection methods have led to increased 5-year survival rates from approximately 50% in the mid-1970s to 64% in the late 1990s. While this trend is promising, access to cutting edge advances and early detection methods is not universal. That unfortunately is a reflection of the health care system in the USA, which contains highly complex, multifaceted delivery systems.

## Delivery of Health Care in the United States of America

In the USA, the delivery of health care services has undergone dramatic change in the past 10–15 years. The impetus for that change was health care costs that in 1960 accounted for approximately 5% of the country's gross national product but by the mid-1990s had spiraled to 16%. Without reform, at that rate of growth, health care costs alone would have consumed the country's total annual resources by the year 2050 (Banja, 1994). As a consequence, the provision of health care moved from a model that operated primarily on a "fee for service" model to one of "managed care" (Pietranton, 1998). The fee for service model was one in which individual patients were provided with the services covered in their health plan as long as was deemed clinically necessary. The speech-language pathologist submitted charges, reported patient progress on the required documentation, and payment for the service was rendered.

Attempts at cost containment resulted in the model shift for the delivery of services. The model of managed care consisted of contractual agreements with capitation of costs (typically determined by diagnosis). With capitation, predetermined allotments of resources were allocated, regardless of the procedures and/or treatments administered. Obviously then it was in the best interest of facilities to maximize the efficiency of their services delivered. The benefit of that efficiency was realized when the cost of an individual's total care was under the allotment defined by capitation resulting in a profit for the facility. On the other hand, when health care services for a specific individual exceeded the allotment, the facility was responsible for the deficit.

Given today's framework of managed care, health care in the USA is multifaceted, driven largely by reimbursement systems that vary both in cost as well as in the extent of services that are covered. Primary methods to cover health care expense in the USA include: commercial health insurance, Veterans Affairs benefits, government benefits, and finally, other systems that fall outside the purview of these categories. The following discussion will describe these services and what they offer to individuals in the USA.

## Health Insurance

Many individuals in the United States receive health care services that are reimbursed through commercial health insurance. Typically, individuals receive at least a portion of their health care benefit through employment (Golper & Brown, 2004). Services offered through commercial health care insurance vary across individuals and plans. Since insurance companies adopt methods to contain the costs of health care, most plans do not offer unlimited access to services. Instead there are restrictions and coverage limits. For example, when a new plan is initiated, any condition that was preexisting may not be covered in the plan. Another example that has been discussed previously is capitation or the

act of limiting coverage based on an average payment typically determined by diagnosis. The limit for services is determined based on a review of data from a large number of patients, across an array of facilities. For the average patient, this method of reimbursement is adequate. However, for those patients who present with extraordinary circumstances or with a particularly difficult case, the funding limit may be restrictive.

## Veterans Health Care Benefits

Veterans Affairs benefits are offered to individuals and their families who have served in any branch of the military (e.g., USA Army, Air Force, Marines, National Guard, and Reserves). Like other health care systems in the USA, benefits are not universally applied. Instead, individuals who qualify and apply for these benefits are assigned to a priority group in an attempt to adequately allocate resources to those in greatest need (Department of Veterans Affairs, 2005). Assignment to one of eight priority groups is based on the percent of disability and employment status. For example, the highest level of care would be offered to individuals in Priority Group 1 that includes veterans with at least a 50% or more service-related disability and are unemployed due to their condition. At the other end of the continuum are individuals enrolled in Priority Group 8, who are nonservice veterans with zero disability who are willing to offer a co-payment for a portion of the health care service.

## Government Benefits

Medicare is the government health care benefit offered to individuals who are of retirement age and older (also eligible are younger individuals who are disabled or have end-stage renal disease). Individuals who are employed in the United States support Medicare. Such individuals pay Medicare taxes across the span of their employment. At the typical retirement age of 65, individuals are eligible to apply for this health care benefit (Medicare Web site, 2005). Medicare is comprised of several component pieces.

Medicare Part A is the primary component that covers the following:

- inpatient hospitalization
- stay in a skilled nursing facility

▓ some home health care (for those who qualify)

▓ hospice (care for end-stage, terminally ill)

Medicare Part B is an optional component that offers supplemental insurance to cover expenses not covered by Part A. There is a monthly premium ($88.50/month in 2006) for this option as well as a 20% co-payment for any services incurred. Additional services provided by Part B include:

▓ physician services not covered by Part A

▓ outpatient services (including outpatient therapy)

▓ home health visits without a hospitalization or nursing home stay

▓ medical equipment

Another alternative is sometimes called Part C or Medicare Advantage. In order to obtain this plan you must be eligible for Medicare A and B and depending on the plan you may pay an additional monthly premium. Medicare Part C acts as one comprehensive plan, without the need for several separate pieces. Finally, the advent of 2006 brought with it Medicare Part D which includes a number of prescription drug plans. Members enrolled in Medicare plans are to examine the many prescription drug options available in Medicare Part D and enroll in the benefit that is best suited to their needs. Because Part D is a new development, there are currently many educational tools to assist in the decision-making process. For a comprehensive outline of all Medicare benefits visit www.medicare.gov.

Individuals who do not qualify for any of the health plans listed (i.e., commercial insurance, Veterans benefits, and Medicare) may be eligible for Medicaid. Medicaid is the other primary government health care benefit for low-income adults and children who qualify. While Medicare is a government benefit, regulations are imposed by state government, resulting in a good deal of variability across the country (Centers for Medicare and Medicaid Services, 2005). Eligibility for Medicaid is based on a number of factors including age, income, and resources just to name a few. Although Medicaid is available for children and adults, it is the primary means for low-income, medically fragile, or developmentally delayed children to receive health care and early intervention services.

While the health care systems just described cover the vast majority of individuals in the USA, there are other delivery systems. For individuals injured on the job or as a result of job related exposure, workman's compensation goes into affect. Workman's compensation is provided by the employer of the injured/disabled party and is one of the most comprehensive of systems. In order to treat and rehabilitate injured workers so that they recover to the fullest extent possible, workman's compensation covers any and all procedures and treatments necessary.

Perhaps the most familiar health care concept of all, regardless of benefit, is "out of pocket" expense. No matter how comprehensive the health care plan, there will be some element of expense that is not covered. The expense may be in the form of a co-payment for physician visits and pharmaceuticals, or it may be a service that is not covered by the plan. There are even some outpatient offices that due to their small size and staffing constraints do not process insurance claims; thus they only accept cash payment (Golper & Brown, 2004).

At a glance, an overview of health care options in the USA may seem overwhelming. Fortunately for individuals, their own plans become very familiar and manageable. Where does the patient with head and neck cancer fall in this puzzle? Well, they are puzzle pieces that fall within every service delivery option available. Like all patients, they do the best they can with the health care coverage that is available to them.

## Role of the Speech-Language Pathologist in the United States of America

A team-based approach has become the standard in the USA for treatment of individuals with head and neck cancer (Johnson & Jacobson, 1998). As reviewed earlier in this text, the team includes professionals from a variety of health care professions including speech-language pathologists (SLPs). Such a team provides a collective body of expertise that can assist patients in the decision-making process regarding their cancer treatment. In the USA, it is typically the otolaryngologist who acts as the primary physician leading the team in educating the patient and guiding the course of action for treatment. In many settings, a clinical nurse specialist may also be utilized as a coordinator to ensure that all scheduled evaluations and treatments are coordinated with the patient and family for optimum continual care (Benninger & Grywalski, 1998). Services by the speech-language pathologist can only be provided through physician referral (Golper & Brown, 2004); therefore, the importance of a close working relationship among team members cannot be emphasized strongly enough. Team cohesion results in the best possible care for patients.

# Asia

In comparison to other regions of the world, some specific types of cancers are more prevalent in the Asian population. The incidence of oral cancer is high in Asia (Moore, Johnson, Pierce, & Wilson, 2000). This is probably due to poor oral hygiene, smoking, and alcohol consumption. Similarly, the incidence of nasopharyngeal carcinoma is particularly high in the Chinese populations in the South China region. In Hong Kong, the incidence is between 20–30 per 100,000 population (Parkin, Whelan, Ferlay, Raymond, & Young, 1997). In comparison, nasopharyngeal carcinoma is relatively uncommon in most other non-Asian countries, with an incidence of less than one per 100,000 population (Parkin et al., 1997). Dietary, genetic, and viral infection factors are believed to be contributing to this high incidence particularly in the South China region. Figure 15-1 shows the world map representing the incidence of nasopharyngeal cancer in males for all countries.

Health care practices and services in Asia vary between countries. Consequently, it is not possible to review how all the different health care systems across the Asian countries manage head and neck cancer patients. Rather, the following content will attempt to highlight just some of this diversity by reviewing two very different systems that exist within the one Asian country: (a) the region of mainland China, which covers the largest population in the world, and (b) Hong Kong, a special administrative area of China. The following sections will also outline some of the factors influencing the management of patients with head and neck cancer specific to Asia and the Chinese population in particular.

## The Mainland China Health Care System

The reform of China's health care services has turned the public health service in mainland China into basically a self-paying system. This means that patients in the public health system have to pay for all the costs associated with their medical expenses. With the per capital annual disposable income of urban households reported to be around US $1059 and the net income of rural households only around US $328 (National Bureau of Statistics of China, 2004), many individuals in mainland China cannot easily afford medical expenses.

In light of such cost issues, it is not uncommon to find that many patients delay in seeking medical advice until the symptoms and signs of cancer have developed into the late stage. This often prevents early detection and makes the management of head and neck cancers more difficult. For individuals diagnosed at relatively late stages of cancer, or for those patients who live in distant, rural areas of China, the use of radical treatment is a common approach in order to reduce the chance of recurrence (Wei, 2002). This approach unavoidably causes more loss of function.

The concept of rehabilitation is also relatively new in mainland China. The roles of speech therapy, physiotherapy, or occupational therapy are not clearly defined in the rehabilitation framework. These different types of therapies are often provided by medical practitioners who work as rehabilitation physicians. The extent of training of these rehabilitation physicians, however, varies greatly from center to center. Therefore, the availability of allied health rehabilitation after surgery may not be a standard service for many individuals with head and neck cancers.

## The Hong Kong Health Care System

Contrary to this self-paying public health system, the health care system in Hong Kong, which is a special administrative area of China, inherited the public-funded health care system of the former British government. Consequently, it offers both public-funded and private health schemes. This has a significant impact on the management of individuals with head and neck cancer in Hong Kong. In the public health

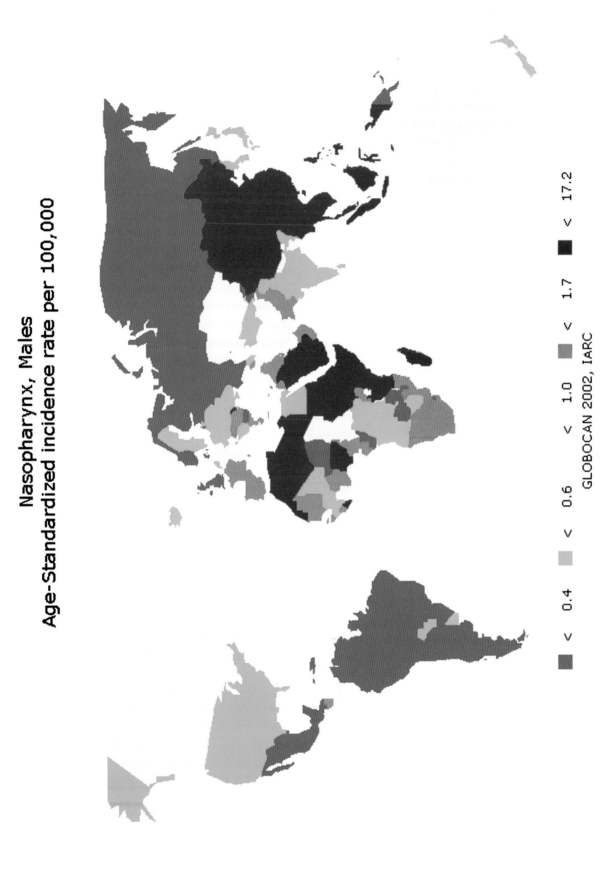

**Figure 15–1.** Incidence of nasopharyngeal cancer in males for all countries. (Note. From *GLOBOCAN 2002 Database*, via Cancer Mondial Web site, www_dep.iarc.fr) (Printed with permission.)

system, Hong Kong residents are only required to pay a daily nominal fee of approximately US $15 to cover all medical costs. This daily charge includes all laboratory tests, surgery, medications, and all related expenses. In comparison, non-Hong Kong residents or individuals who choose the private system have to meet all costs associated with their medical care.

As the costs for major surgeries for head and neck cancers are substantial, most surgical procedures and rehabilitations are taken care of by the public-funded health system. Within Hong Kong, the allied health systems (which include speech pathology, physiotherapy, and occupational therapy) and the medical social welfare system are relatively well established, although the availability of these services is still inadequate to meet the demand.

## Management of Head and Neck Cancer in China

As mentioned previously, due to the costs associated with medical care, many patients present with late stage cancers, necessitating radical management. Radiotherapy is generally the choice of treatment for nasopharyngeal cancer (Wei & Sham, 2005). There are, however, a number of undesirable side effects following radiotherapy. Most of these are the result of the radiation effects to the head and neck areas (Wei & Sham, 2005). Such effects include cranial nerve palsies, sensorineural hearing loss, otitis media, dysphagia, cognitive dysfunction, and memory loss (Wei & Sham, 2005). For oral and laryngeal cancers, surgery is typically the treatment of choice. This is often followed by postoperative radiotherapy to ensure that cancer cells at primary and secondary sites are eradicated completely. Chemotherapy is occasionally used instead of or in addition to radiotherapy as well. These treatment regimes often delay the rehabilitation process as the side effects of radiotherapy or chemotherapy may prevent patients from attending the rehabilitation sessions.

## Specific Issues Related to Speech Rehabilitation in China

Speech rehabilitation for Chinese alaryngeal speakers poses specific challenges for clinicians. Although all available forms of alaryngeal speech methods are employed in China (i.e., electrolaryngeal, pneumatic, esophageal, and tracheoesophageal speech), the availability and affordability of alaryngeal speech options restrict the choice available to many patients. Tracheoesophageal voice restoration is primarily offered to patients as a primary procedure if the surgeons decide that the patient will have a good chance of developing and using tracheoesophageal speech (Wong, Yuen, Cheung, Wei, & Lam, 1997). The cost associated with tracheoesophageal voice restoration is often not an issue for residents of Hong Kong, as these will be either covered by patients who can afford this option or by the social security system. However, in mainland China the cost and ongoing support associated with this form of alaryngeal rehabilitation can be a limitation for some patients.

Similarly, speech rehabilitation using electronic devices is cost prohibitive for the majority of patients. Many alaryngeal speakers cannot afford the more expensive models of electrolarynx. As a result, relatively cheaper alaryngeal speaking devices, such as the Taiwan-made pneumatic device (see Figure 15–2), costing around US$20, are a popular alternative. In rural China, however, for many patients, writing (or gestures only if they are illiterate) may be the only option for postsurgical communication.

Another key challenge in speech rehabilitation specific to the Chinese population is the nature of the language. Chinese is a lexical tone language. This means that a lexical word can have different tones that represent different meanings. For example the word "ma" with a falling tone means "mother" but with a rising

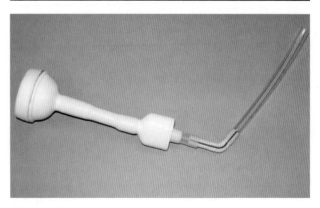

**Figure 15–2.** Taiwanese pneumatic device. (Note. From Hong Kong New Voice Club.)

tone it means "a horse." Speech rehabilitation involving production of correct lexical tone in alaryngeal speech is a difficult issue and poses a challenge to alaryngeal speech rehabilitation. It has been shown that speech produced using an electrolarynx is unable to produce intelligible words with different lexical tones (Yiu, van Hasselt, Williams, & Woo, 1994; Ng, Lerman, & Gilbert, 1998). In comparison, tracheoesophageal speech, pneumatic devices (Yiu et al., 1994), and esophageal speech (Ng et al., 1998) have been suggested to be more useful in conveying lexical tones in alaryngeal speech. Of these options, a Taiwan-made pneumatic device (Chalstrey, Bleach, Cheung, & van Hasselt, 1994; Yiu et al., 1994) (see Figure 15-2) has gained much popularity because of its relatively low cost and its capability of producing intelligible lexical tone words.

## Europe

Europe consists of a large number of different countries. All of these countries have their own cultural and historical background, leading to differences in for example health care systems and the incidence of various types of cancer. It is beyond the scope of this chapter to discuss each of these countries individually; therefore, the current section will provide a general explanation of the European health care systems, discuss European cancer incidence figures for oral cavity, pharyngeal, nasopharyngeal, and laryngeal cancers, and then focus on the country of the Netherlands as an example.

## Health Care Systems in Europe

Basically, Europe has two different types of health care financing systems (Belien, 2006), the *single payer* system and the *social insurance* or *sickness fund* system. In the single payer system, health care is paid for and organized by the government with money from income taxes. The countries using this type of system are the Scandinavian countries, the United Kingdom, Ireland, Italy, Spain, and Portugal. In the social insurance or sickness fund system, health care is financed through mandatory premiums calculated as a percentage of wages. The countries using this type of system

are Austria, Belgium, France, Germany, Luxembourg, and the Netherlands. Both Germany and the Netherlands have a sickness fund system, but part of the population is also privately insured. Switzerland is the only country in Europe that has a health care system totally based on private insurance.

In the Netherlands, there are both catastrophic health insurance, which is handled according to the single payer system, and routine health care, which is handled according to the sickness fund system. About 35% of the population is privately insured for routine health care. This is defined by the person's level of income, as once their income reaches a certain level, they need to take out private insurance.

## Incidence of Head and Neck Cancer in Europe

The International Agency for Research on Cancer (IARC) Web site (www-dep.iarc.fr) provides access to the GLOBOCAN 2002 database. This database provides the most recent *estimates* of the cancer incidence, mortality, and prevalence by sex and cancer site for all countries in the world. Dividing Europe into four regions (Northern, Southern, Western, and Central/Eastern), data can be found on the following cancers of the head and neck: oral cavity, nasopharynx, other pharynx, and larynx.

The estimated incidence of *laryngeal cancer* is considerably higher in males compared to females in all European regions. In general, the Southern European region has the highest estimated average incidence (age-standardized [world] rate, per 100,000) of laryngeal cancer in males of 10.9, followed by Central and Eastern Europe (9.2), Western Europe (7.2), and Northern Europe (4.3). In females, the highest estimated average incidence of laryngeal cancer is found in Western Europe (0.8), followed by Northern and Southern Europe (0.7), and Central and Eastern Europe (0.4). The estimated incidence varies largely from country to country; for example, the estimated incidence of laryngeal cancer in males in the Netherlands is 5.3, while for France it is 10.8, and for Sweden it is 2.0. For females, the estimated incidences of laryngeal cancers for these countries are 0.9, 0.7, and 0.4 respectively. Figure 15-3 shows the world map representing the incidence of laryngeal cancer in males for all countries.

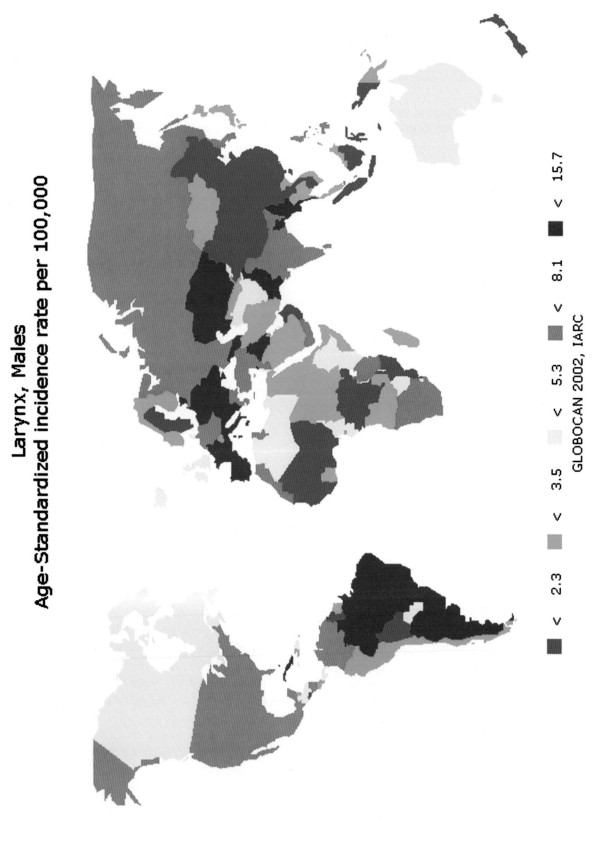

**Figure 15–3.** International pattern of laryngeal cancer incidence for males. (Note. From *GLOBOCAN 2002 Database*, via Cancer Mondial Web site, www_dep.iarc.fr) (Printed with permission.)

As can be seen, the incidence of laryngeal cancer varies within Europe and across the world, and is for example high in Southern and Eastern Europe and South America.

The estimated incidence of *pharyngeal cancer* in males is highest in Western Europe (9.7), followed by Central and Eastern Europe (5.4), and Southern and Northern Europe (5.3). For females, these numbers are 1.7 for Western Europe, 0.7 for Northern Europe, and 0.5 for Southern Europe and Central and Eastern Europe. For the *oral cavity cancers*, the estimated incidence in males is highest for Western Europe (11.3), followed by Southern Europe (9.2), Central and Eastern Europe (8.6), and Northern Europe (5.3). As for the other head and neck cancers, the estimated incidence is again much lower for females (i.e., Western: 2.7; Northern: 2.6; Southern: 2.0; Central and Eastern: 1.6).

In contrast to Asian countries, the incidence of *nasopharyngeal cancer* is very low in Europe. For males it is 1.1 in Southern Europe, 0.8 in Western Europe, 0.6 in Central and Eastern Europe, and 0.4 in Northern Europe. For females, the incidence is even lower with 0.5 in Southern Europe and 0.2 in the other parts of Europe.

In the Netherlands (population roughly 16 million), the estimated number of patients with laryngeal cancer per year is 738 (629 males, 109 females), the estimated number of patients with pharyngeal cancer is 427 (321 males, 106 females), the estimated number of patients with oral cavity cancer is 1083 (645 males, 438 females), and the estimated number of patients with nasopharyngeal cancer is 66 (54 males, 12 females).

## The Netherlands: Health Care and Laryngectomee Rehabilitation

The Netherlands is a relatively small country, with a total area of only 41,526 square kilometers. This figure not only includes land, but also rivers, canals, and lakes. The population however is approximately 16 million; therefore, each square kilometer accommodates on average 449 people, making the Netherlands one of the most densely populated countries in the world. This dense population has its implications for health care: a doctor, hospital, or major university hospital or dedicated cancer center is usually in close proximity for most patients.

Historically, the Netherlands has a large academic interest in laryngectomee rehabilitation. The first Ph.D. thesis on this topic was written in 1937, and so far a total number of 25 Ph.D. theses have appeared in this small country, 15 in the last 10 years alone. Four different types of indwelling voice prostheses have also been developed by academic institutions in the Netherlands: the Provox, Groningen, Nijdam, and Voicemaster. Especially the first two have found more widespread (international) use.

## Services for Patients with Head and Neck Cancer in the Netherlands

The Netherlands has eight major centers that treat the majority of the head and neck cancer patients. Those eight centers all participate in the Dutch Cooperative Group for Head and Neck Tumors. The members of this group consist of physicians and allied health professionals and their common goal is to improve the quality of care of patients with head and neck cancer in the Netherlands. They organize for example symposia and scientific meetings, carry out internal evaluations, and develop guidelines. The group has developed national guidelines for the treatment of laryngeal cancer (Kaanders & Hordijk, 2002) and oral cavity and oropharyngeal cancer (in Dutch, can be downloaded from www.nwhht.nl). The group is currently working on guidelines for cancer of the hypopharynx. These guidelines are based on available evidence from international literature and when no evidence is available it is based on the consensus of the cooperative group.

## Role of the Speech-Language Pathologist

The role of the speech-language pathologist in the multidisciplinary team treating the patient with head and neck cancer is well described in the national guidelines. The National Guideline for Oral Cavity/ Oropharyngeal Cancers (in Dutch, can be downloaded from www.nwhht.nl) states that the SLP should be part of the multidisciplinary team treating these patients. The tasks of the SLP are to provide pretreatment information about expectations and treatment regarding speech and swallowing; to provide more specific post-treatment information when the impact of the treatment is clearer; to evaluate and diagnose speech and swallowing problems; to rehabilitate speech and swallowing, and to provide the patient with exercises to prevent speech and swallowing problems (for example range of motion exercises before and during chemoradiotherapy).

The National Guideline for Cancer of the Larynx states that the SLP should play a role in providing voice therapy to patients that have voice complaints after treatment (radiotherapy/laser resection) for smaller laryngeal tumors. In laryngectomy patients, the SLP should provide preoperative counseling and postoperative voice and speech rehabilitation. It is stated that each patient should receive the option to achieve tracheoesophageal speech, and that esophageal speech training and artificial larynx training should be offered to the patient as well.

In the Netherlands, the vast majority of patients receive a primary puncture and primary placement of an indwelling voice prosthesis. Replacement of the voice prosthesis is generally carried out by the otolaryngologist. The SLP focuses on optimal rehabilitation of voice and speech. It is also stated in the guideline that pulmonary rehabilitation should be an essential part of postoperative rehabilitation and that the use of heat and moisture exchangers (HMEs) (see Chapters 11 and 12 for further discussion of HMEs) should be stimulated.

## Conclusion

Across the international area there are differences in the management of patients with head and neck cancer. In the current sample of countries, financial and cost issues, linguistic differences, and health service issues were revealed, and their contribution to the unique patterns of patient management in each setting discussed. The current chapter highlights that there are many challenges facing clinicians managing patients with head and neck cancer. It is up to these clinicians to remain aware of international practices and address local obstacles preventing the implementation of best practice, in order to continue to improve patient outcomes.

## References

American Cancer Society. (2005). *Cancer facts & figures 2005*. Atlanta, GA: American Cancer Society.

Anderson, T. A., & Sataloff, R. T. (2005). Laryngeal cancer. In R. T. Sataloff (Ed.), *Treatment of voice disorders* (pp. 307–324). San Diego, CA: Plural.

Australian Bureau of Statistics (ABS) (2002). *National Health Survey, summary of results*. (Cat. No. 4364.0). Canberra, Australia: Australian Bureau of Statistics.

Australian Institute of Health and Welfare (AIHW). (2001). Report: Cancer in Australia. Retrieved March 15, 2006, from www.aihw.gov.au/publications/index.cfm/title/10083

Australian Institute of Health and Welfare. (2005). *Health expenditure Australia 2003–4*. Retrieved October 20, from www.aihw.gov.au/publications/index.cfm/title/10204

Australia's Health Workforce. (2005). Productivity commission position paper. Retrieved October 20, 2005, from www.pc.gov.au/study/healthworkforce

Banja, J. D. (1994). Ethics, outcomes, and reimbursement. *REHAB Management, 7*(1), 61–65.

Belien, P. (2006). Best buy: Privatised healthcare systems in Europe. Retrieved May 12, 2006, from www.brusselsjournal.com/node/665

Benninger, M. S., & Grywalski, C. (1998). Rehabilitation of the head and neck cancer patient. In A. F. Johnson & B. H. Jacobson (Eds.), *Medical speech-language pathology: A practitioner's guide* (pp. 669–684). New York: Thieme.

Boone, D. R., & McFarlane, S. C. (2000). *The voice and voice therapy* (6th ed.). Boston: Allyn and Bacon.

Burnett, R. (2001). *Unpublished speech pathology departmental survey*. Contact Robyn Burnett, Royal Adelaide Hospital, Adelaide, South Australia.

Centers for Medicare and Medicaid Services. (2005). *Medicaid program, general information*. Retrieved October 25, 2005, from http://www.cms.hhs.gov/MedicaidGenInfo/

Chalstrey, S. E., Bleach, N. R., Cheung, D., & van Hasselt, C. A. (1994). A pneumatic artificial larynx popularized in Hong Kong. *Journal of Laryngology and Otology, 108*(10), 852–854.

Commission for Health Improvement/Audit Commission. (2001). *NHS cancer care in England and Wales*. London: Department of Health.

Department of Employment and Workforce Relations. (n.d.) Retrieved May 24, 2006, from www.health.nsw.gov.au/amwac/pdf/4_relations.pdf

Department of Health, NHS. (2004, June). *The NHS improvement plan: Putting people at the heart of public services.* Presented to parliament by the Secretary of State for Health by Command of Her Majesty, London, England.

Department of Health, NHS. (n.d.). *Cancer services collaborative improvement partnership.* Retrieved February 13, 2006, from www.cancerimprovement. nhs.uk

Department of Veterans Affairs (n.d.). *Veterans benefits and services.* Retrieved December 9, 2005, from www.1.va.gov/health_benefits

Edwards, D. (1997). *Face to face: Patient, family and professional perspectives of head and neck cancer care.* London: Kings Fund.

Edwards, D. (1998). Head and neck cancer services: Views of patients, their families and professionals. *British Journal of Oral and Maxillofacial Surgery, 36,* 99–102.

Golper, L. A., & Brown, J. E. (2004). *Business matters: A guide for speech-language pathologists.* Rockville, MD: American Speech-Language-Hearing Association.

Health Systems Review Final Report—September 2005. (2005). Queensland Health Systems Review. Retrieved November 22, 2005 from www.health. qld.gov.au/health_sys_review/final/default.asp

Johnson, A. F., & Jacobson, B. H. (1998). *Medical speech-language pathology: A practitioner's guide.* New York: Thieme.

Kaanders, J. H., & Hordijk, G. J. (2002). Carcinoma of the larynx: The Dutch national guideline for diagnostics, treatment, supportive care and rehabilitation. *Radiotherapy and Oncology, 63,* 299–307.

Kelly, A. M., Hydes, K., McLaughlin, C., & Wallace, S. (2005). Fiberoptic endoscopic evaluation of swallowing (FEES): The role of speech language therapy. *RCSLT Policy Statement.* Royal College of Speech Language Therapists, www.rcslt.org

Medicare Web site. (n.d.). Retrieved October 25, 2005, from www.medicare.gov

Moore, S. R., Johnson, N. W., Pierce, A. M., & Wilson, D. F. (2000). The epidemiology of mouth cancer: A review of global incidence. *Oral Diseases, 6,* 65–74.

National Bureau of Statistics of China. (2004). *2004 China statistical yearbook.* Beijing: China Statistics Press.

National Cancer Institute/U.S. National Institutes of Health. (n.d.) *National Cancer Institute fact sheet: Head and neck cancer.* Retrieved October 24, 2005, from http://www.cancer.gov/cancertopics/factsheet/ Sites-Types/head-and-neck/print?page&k

National Institute for Clinical Excellence (NICE). (2004). *Improving outcomes in head and neck cancers.* Retrieved November 9, 2005 from www. nice.org.uk

Ng, M. L., Lerman, J. W., & Gilbert, H. R. (1998). Perceptions of tonal changes in normal laryngeal, esophageal, and artificial laryngeal male Cantonese speakers. *Folia Phoniatrica et Logopaedica, 50,* 64–70.

Parkin, D. M., Whelan, S. L., Ferlay, J., Raymond, L., & Young, J. (Eds.). (1997). *Cancer incidence in five continents* (Vol VII). IARC Scientific Publications, Oxford University Press.

Pietranton, A. (1998). Clinical service reform. In A. F. Johnson & B. H. Jacobson (Eds.), *Medical speech-language pathology: A practitioner's guide* (pp. 669–684). New York: Thieme.

Pignon, J. P, Bourhis, J., Domenge, C., & Designe, L. (2000). Chemotherapy added to locoregional treatment for head and neck squamous-cell carcinoma: Three meta-analyses of updated individual data. MACH-NC Collaborative Group. Meta-analysis of chemotherapy on head and neck cancer. *Lancet, 355,* 9208.

Royal College of Speech and Language Therapists. (2005). Retreived 16 November, RCSLT Website www.rcslt.org

Ryan, C., Yong, L., Pracy, P., & Simo, R. (2004). Current trends in voice rehabilitation following laryngectomy in Britain. *Australian Journal of Oto-laryngology, 7*(1), 26–30.

Soutar, D., & Robertson, G. (2001). Head and neck cancers. *Cancer scenarios: An aid to planning cancer services in Scotland in the next decade.* Edinburgh: The Scottish Executive.

South West Cancer Intelligence Service. (2001). *Second head and neck audit report (SWAHNII).* Referenced in National Institute for Clinical Excellence (NICE). (2004). *Improving outcomes in head and neck cancers.* Retrieved November 9, 2005 from www.nice.org.uk

The Expert Advisory Group on Cancer to the Chief Medical Officers of England & Wales (1995). *The Calman Hine report: A policy framework for commissioning cancer services.* Retrieved April, 1995, from www.dh.gov.uk

Thorne, P., Etherington, D., & Birchall, M. A. (1997). Head and neck cancer in South West England: Influence of socio-economic status on incidence and secondary primary tumours. *European Journal of Surgical Oncology, 23,* 503–508.

United Kingdom Immigration Work Permit and Visa Services. (2005). *UK skills shortage occupations.* Retrieved February 13, 2006, from www.skillclear.co.uk/skilllist.asp

Ward, E. C., Hobson T. K., & Conroy, A. (2003). Pre- and post-operative counselling and information dissemination: Perceptions of patients undergoing laryngeal surgery and their spouses. *Asia Pacific Journal of Speech, Language and Hearing, 8,* 44–68.

Ward, E. C., Koh, S. K., Frisby, J., & Hodge, R. (2003). Differential modes of alaryngeal communication and long-term voice outcomes following pharyngolaryngectomy and laryngectomy. *Folia Phoniatrica et Logopaedica, 55,* 39–49.

Wei, W. I. (2002). Commentary: Head and neck carcinomas in the developing world. *British Medical Journal, 325,* 827.

Wei, W. I., & Sham, J. S. T. (2005). Nasopharyngeal carcinoma. *The Lancet, 365,* 2041–2054.

Wong, S. H., Yuen, A. P., Cheung, C., Wei, W. I., & Lam, L. K. (1997). Long-term results of voice rehabilitation after total laryngectomy using primary tracheoesophageal puncture in Chinese patients. *American Journal of Otolaryngology, 18*(2), 94–98.

Yellowlees, P. M. (2000). Intelligent health systems and third millennium medicine in Australia. *Telemedicine Journal, 6,* 197–200.

Yiu, E. M., van Hasselt, C. A., Williams, S. R., & Woo, J. K. (1994). Speech intelligibility in tone language (Chinese) laryngectomy speeches. *European Journal of Disorders of Communication, 29*(4), 339–347.

Yorkshire Cancer Network. (2003). *Head and neck cancer treatment guidelines.* Retrieved November 24, 2005, from www.yorkshire-cancer-net.org.uk/

# INDEX